Ear, Nose and Throat Histopathology

Springer

London
Berlin
Heidelberg
New York
Barcelona
Hong Kong
Milan
Paris
Singapore
Tokyo

Leslie Michaels and Henrik B. Hellquist

Ear, Nose and Throat Histopathology

Second Edition

With 436 Figures
Including 172 Colour Plates

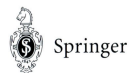 Springer

Leslie Michaels, MD, FRCPath, FRCP(C), D Path, FCAP
Professor Emeritus, University of London, Royal Free and UCL Medical School
  and
Honorary Consultant Pathologist, Royal National Throat, Nose and Ear Hospital,
London
Department of Histopathology, UCL Medical School, Rockefeller Building,
University Street, London WC1E 6JJ, UK

Henrik B. Hellquist, MD, PhD, SAPath(Stockh), FCAP
Professor of Pathology, Haukeland University Hospital, Bergen, Norway
  and
Chairman, Department of Laboratory Medicine and Pathology,
Hamad Medical Corporation, Doha, Qatar

Cover illustrations: Front cover (top to bottom): Figure 36.7, supraglottic verrucous squamous carcinoma; Figure 42.18, salivary duct carcinoma; Figure 10.4a, otosclerosis. Back cover: Figure 13.5d, allergic fungal sinusitis – branching fungal hyphae in inspissated mucus.

British Library Cataloguing in Publication Data
Michaels, L. (Leslie), 1925–
    Ear, nose and throat histopathology. – 2nd ed.
    1. Otolaryngology – Histopathology
    I. Title II. Hellquist, Henrik B.
    617.5'1'07583
ISBN 354076142X

Library of Congress Cataloguing-in-Publication Data
Michaels, L. (Leslie)
    Ear, nose, and throat histopathology/Leslie Michaels and Henrik B. Hellquist. – 2nd ed.
        p. ; cm.
    Includes bibliographical references and index.
    ISBN 354076142X (alk. paper)
    1. Ear – Diseases. 2. Nose – Diseases. 3. Throat – Diseases. 4. Histology, Pathological. I. Hellquist, Henrik B.
II. Title.
    [DNLM: 1. Otorhinolaryngologic Diseases–pathology. 2. Otorhinolaryngologic Neoplasms–pathology.
WV 140 M621e 2000]
RF47.5.M53 2000
617.5'107–dc21   00-044031

ISBN 3-540-76142-X 2nd edition Springer-Verlag Berlin Heidelberg New York
ISBN 3-540-17130-4 1st edition Springer-Verlag Berlin Heidelberg New York
ISBN 0-387-17130-4 1st edition Springer-Verlag New York Berlin Heidelberg
a member of BertelsmannSpringer Science+Business Media GmbH
http://www.springer.co.uk

Typeset by EXPO Holdings, Malaysia
Printed and bound by Kyodo Printing Co. (S'pore) Pte. Ltd., Singapore
28/3830-54321   Printed on acid-free paper   SPIN 10881791

Preface

I wrote the first edition of this work in 1987 with the object of providing a review of the aetiology, pathogenesis and morphological basis of diseases of the ear, nose and throat. Since that time important changes have taken place in the disciplines of both histopathology and otorhinolaryngology. Pathology has shifted its research orientation towards a molecular one; notable successes with new medical and surgical treatments in ENT have resulted in a striking expansion of that field. To provide a précis of the scientific principles of a subject lying between two such mobile territories was a daunting prospect. Help was indeed necessary and I welcome Henrik Hellquist as the co-author of this second edition. He has had a longstanding interest in both head and neck and molecular pathology and has not only produced scholarly publications, but has also played an important role in enhancing international cooperation in this combined field.

We have striven in this edition to introduce where possible the modern molecular viewpoint of our discipline, without, however, losing sight of the important purpose of helping the pathologist in his diagnostic work. Although the material is considerably revised, the pattern of chapters in this book is similar to that of the first edition, but we have added completely new parts on salivary gland diseases and on the neck, these areas now also usually being under the clinical aegis of the ENT specialist. We hope that this book will be of interest and of value to clinicians as well as histopathologists.

Acknowledgements

We wish to thank the very large number of our associates who have helped us directly or indirectly in the production of this work. On the professional side the list is so large that to name particular individuals would be invidious in regard to those who might be inadvertently excluded. On the publishing side, however, we are delighted to name staff at Springer-Verlag, London, Nick Mowat, Medical Editor and Roger Dobbing, Production Manager. We appreciate their encouragement, support and expertise. At the same time, we must also express our indebtedness to the late Michael Jackson, an earlier Medical Editor at Springer, without whose patient efforts the first edition would not have seen the light of day.

The following photographs have been published in other works and permission to reproduce them is gratefully acknowledged. Source details are as follows:

Michaels L. Chapter 14. The ear. In: Sternberg SS (ed) Histology for pathologists, 2nd edn. Lippincott-Raven, Philadelphia, 1997, pp 337–366
Fig. 1.15, Fig. 1.18, Fig. 1.21, Fig. 1.28, Fig. 1.33, Fig. 1.34

Michaels L. Chapter 80. The ear. In: Damjanov I, Linder J (eds) Anderson's pathology, 10th edn. Mosby Year Book Inc., St. Louis, Missouri, 1996, pp. 2876–2900
Fig. 1.36, Fig. 2.9, Fig. 2.10, Fig. 4.2, Fig. 4.3, Fig. 4.7, Fig. 4.8, Fig. 8.8

Michaels L. Examination of specimens of larynx. J Clin Pathol, ACP Broadsheet 1990; 1–4
Fig. 28.4

Slack RWT, Wright A, Michaels L *et al.* Inner hair cell loss and intracochlear clot in the preterm infant. Clin Otolaryngol 1986; 11:443–446
Fig. 7.2

Gill H, Michaels L, Phelps PD *et al.* Histopathological findings suggest the diagnosis in an atypical case of Pendred syndrome. Clin Otolaryngol 1999; 24:523–526
Fig. 6.2

Slootweg PJ, De Groot JAM. Surgical pathological anatomy of head and neck specimens. Springer-Verlag, London, 1999, p. 96, Fig. 5.1a
Fig. 12.6

Leslie Michaels
London, 2000

Contents

Part A The Ear

Part B The Nose and Paranasal Sinuses

Part C **The Nasopharynx**

Part D **The Palatine Tonsil**

Part E **The Larynx and Hypopharynx**

Part F **Major Salivary Glands**

Part G **The Neck**

A

The Ear

1 The Normal Ear

Development

The ear is not a single organ, but two, being the peripheral receptor site both for stimuli derived from sound waves and for changes of posture. The structures subserving both of those functions are developed from an invagination of ectoderm early in embryonic life – the otocyst – to produce the epithelia of the membranous labyrinth of the inner ear. Superimposed upon, and developing slightly later, the first and second branchial arch systems provide structures which augment the hearing function. The endodermal component of the first branchial system, the branchial pouch, gives rise to the Eustachian tube and middle ear epithelia and the corresponding ectodermal outgrowth, the first branchial cleft, to the external ear epithelia. The connective tissue part of the local branchial system, the first and second branchial arches, produces the ossicles. The eighth cranial nerve outflow from the central nervous system grows to link up with the sensory epithelia lining the otocyst-derived cochlear and vestibular labyrinths and the cartilaginous, bony and muscular conformations of the ear are developed from the mesenchyme surrounding these early epithelia.

External Ear

The pinna is developed from the fusion of six small protuberances arising at the outer end of the first and second branchial arches, which fuse to form the auricular structures including the helix, antihelix and tragus. The external auditory meatus is derived from the first branchial cleft, a depression of the ectoderm between the first (mandibular) arch and the second (hyoid) arch. The deep extremity of this groove meets the outer epithelium of the corresponding first pharyngeal pouch, separated from it by a thin layer of connective tissue only. The point of meeting produces the tympanic membrane. In the course of this development a complex series of changes take place, which have been shown to be related to the function of auditory epithelial migration.[1,2,3]

Auditory Epithelial Migration

The stratified squamous epithelium of the tympanic membrane, like all epithelia of this type, matures continuously to produce keratin squames at its surface. In moist mucosal areas this material is carried away by fluid. The surface of the tympanic membrane is, of necessity, dry, in order to facilitate its delicate vibrations. A mechanism for removal of the keratin must exist, otherwise it would accumulate on the surface, resulting in defective sound transmission. This mechanism has been termed auditory epithelial migration. It has been studied by observation of the movement of ink daubs placed on the eardrum. In the process the whole epithelium with its keratin had been observed by earlier workers to move radially from the region of the centre of the eardrum across the pars tensa and then away from the tympanic membrane on to the deep external canal. The final part of its course was then laterally as far as the cartilaginous canal.[4] The development of the meatal plate, a ribbon of epithelium growing from the fundus of the first branchial cleft from which the pars tensa and deep external canal-covering epithelium arise, has been found to be in a similar direction. It may be hypothesized from this observation that auditory epithelial migration is the persistence of developmental growth in the mature ear.[1]

Two pieces of evidence support this hypothesis:

1. Development of the pars flaccida and handle of malleus-covering epithelia takes place from the fundal extension plate, a primordial evagination (Fig. 1.1) that grows posterosuperiorly (Fig. 1.2) in contrast to the meatal plate, which grows radially (Fig. 1.3). It would be expected, therefore, if auditory epithelial migration is the persistence of developmental growth, that there would be two separate pathways of migration, one for the pars flaccida/handle-covering epithelium, and the other for the pars tensa epithelium. When serial photography of the tympanic membrane is carried out after dots of ink are daubed on its surface, two separate and discrete pathways of migration can indeed be identified.[5] The first is upward over the handle of the malleus and then posterosuperiorly

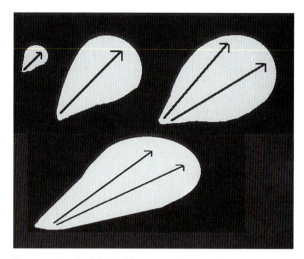

Figure 1.2 Growth of the fundal extension plate in the fetus to produce the pars flaccida and handle of the malleus-covering epithelium, as shown in an en face view. Growth takes place in a posterior-superior direction

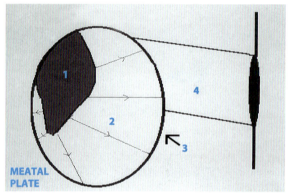

Figure 1.3 Growth of the meatal plate in the fetus to produce the pars tensa-covering epithelium. Growth of the ribbon of epithelium takes place in a radial direction away from the pars flaccida and handle of the malleus-covering epithelium

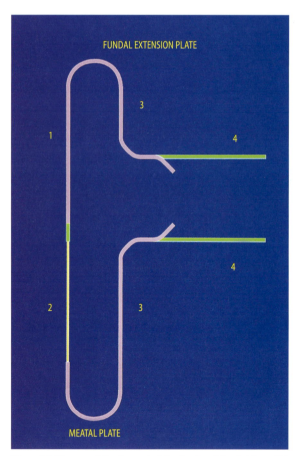

Figure 1.1 Diagram of development of the fundus of the first branchial groove. The numbers represent the growth areas of the epithelium and deep external canal: *1*, over pars flaccida and adjacent deep external canal; *2*, over pars tensa; *3*, over most of deep external canal

across the pars flaccida, from which epithelium passes laterally over the deep canal (Fig. 1.4). This is also the pathway of developmental growth of this epithelium. The second pathway is radially away from the handle of the malleus and pars flaccida-lower edge to the periphery of the eardrum and then to the deep canal, as mentioned above (Fig. 1.5). Again, this is precisely the pathway of growth of this epithelium, which is derived from the meatal plate (Fig. 1.3).

2. The movement of ink particles along the external canal has been observed to terminate beyond the junction of the deep, non-adnexal-bearing skin with superficial, adnexal-bearing skin.[4] The mechanism of shedding of the spent migratory epithelium has been stated to be by desquamation, and a flattening of the hair

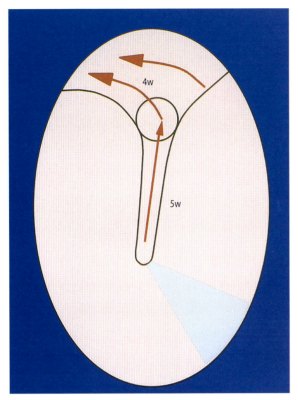

Figure 1.4 Pathway of ink dot migration over the pars flaccida and handle of malleus. The numerals repesent the time in weeks for a dot to completely traverse the region

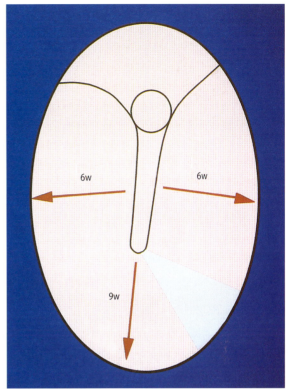

Figure 1.5 Pathway of ink dot migration over the pars tensa. The numerals represent the time in weeks for a dot to completely traverse the region

follicles, which has been observed at the superficial/deep epidermal junction, has been regarded as a bridge for the shedding of keratin.[6] Histological observation of this junction shows no convincing excess of keratinization. It is more likely that the epithelium is lost by a process of apoptosis (organised cell death), the standard way in which cells are routinely eliminated. Such an activity has been identified by us in the deep external canal, manifested as a ballooning of cells with condensed semilune nuclei (unpublished observations). The apoptotic activity in this region is absent during active growth of the ear tissues (up to 30 weeks gestation), very marked during the phase of reconstruction (30 weeks gestation to 2 years post-partum) (Fig. 1.6) and moderate in amount in the mature ear (after 2 years post-partum). These findings are further evidence for the hypothesis that auditory epithelial migration is the persistence of developmental growth.

Middle Ear

The malleus and incus are developed from Meckel's cartilage, itself a product of the first branchial arch. The stapes is formed from Reichert's cartilage, derived from the second branchial arch. The auditory ossicles develop from cartilage with a single centre of ossification for each and no epiphyseal ossification. The persistence of cartilage in each of the ossicles and the bifurcation of the stapes to form the crura with the obturator foramen between them (see below) distinguishes the auditory ossicles from other long bones. The vestibular wall of the stapes footplate is derived from tissue adjacent to the otocyst. The tympanic cavity and mastoid air cells arise from the growing end of the Eustachian tube (first pharyngeal pouch). The fetal middle ear is filled with loose primitive mesenchyme, which is interposed between the epithelium and the bone (Fig. 1.7), but this has largely disappeared by 9 months gestation. The basis for the disappearance of primitive mesenchyme at about 9 months gestation has been obscure. A strong case has been put forward, based on image analysis of the volume of primitive mesenchyme and that of the middle ear cavity as a whole at different stages of development,

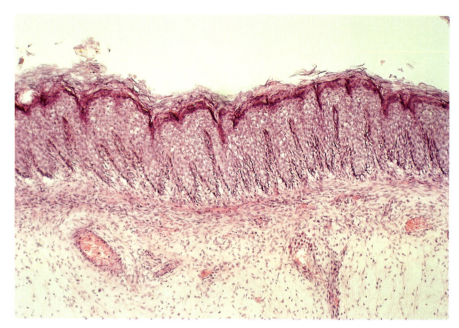

Figure 1.6 Deep external canal epidermis in a 32-week fetus showing marked ballooning of squamous cells with condensed semilune nuclei. These changes are interpreted as active apoptosis

that primitive mesenchyme does not disappear, but simply fails to grow, so that it becomes relatively insignificant in the mature ear.[7] The presence of a pathologically low volume of amniotic fluid surrounding the fetus (oligohydramnios) has been correlated with an increased amount of mesenchyme in the middle ear.[8]

The Epidermoid Formation

A stratified squamous cell rest is frequently found in the middle ear of fetuses and young infants, always in the same position.[9,10] This epidermoid formation is prominent during early development when it may act as an organiser at the head of the upwardly migrating tubotympanic recess.[11] It lies usually in the epithelium at the junction of the Eustachian tube with the middle ear, in the region of the anterior-superior quadrant of the tympanic membrane and about 0.3 mm anterior to it, adjacent to the bony annulus (Fig. 1.8). Recent studies have shown that this structure may sometimes be sited over the anterior-superior part of the eardrum, posterior to its anterior edge and even suspended into the tympanic cavity from the eardrum by a short stalk.[12] The epidermoid formation may appear as an elongated structure sometimes with a superficial cap of keratin (Fig. 1.9). It may be spherical, often with central keratinization, sometimes featuring a space

among the epidermoid cells. It may be flat and superficial or even sited in a fold of epithelium, which is frequently seen in relation to the epidermoid formation (Fig. 1.10). The epidermoid formation may be present as late as 2 years 7 months after birth,[13] but is not seen in older children or adults.

It is almost certain that continued growth of the epidermoid formation beyond fetal life gives rise to the lesion of congenital cholesteatoma, which has been described recently with increasing frequency in young children. This is frequently situated in the anterior-superior part of the tympanic cavity in many cases, the same position as the epidermoid formation[14,15] (see Chapter 3).

Inner Ear

The otocyst, after its initiation by invagination of ectoderm, becomes separated from the surface ectoderm and, by branching and coiling, gives rise to the whole endolymphatic system (Fig. 1.11). The sensory epithelia of the cochlear duct, vestibular endolymphatic adjuncts and endolymphatic duct and sac are differentiated from the inner lining surface cells of this otocyst. The bony labyrinth (otic capsule) is formed from the surrounding mesoderm, with the prior development of a cartilaginous framework, as in the long bones.

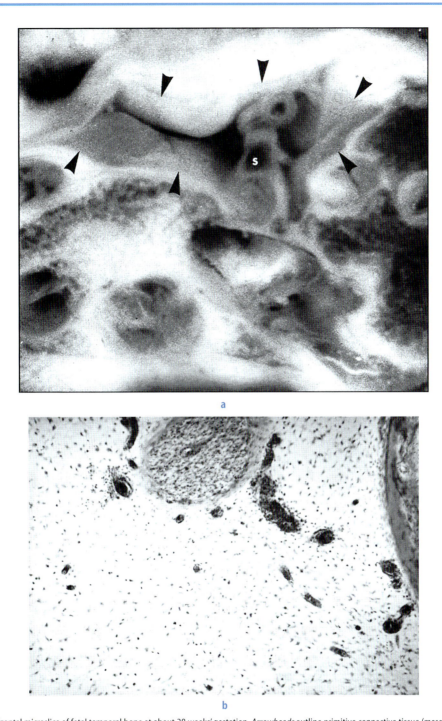

a

b

Figure 1.7 a Horizontal microslice of fetal temporal bone at about 28 weeks' gestation. *Arrowheads* outline primitive connective tissue (mesenchyme); *S,* stapes. **b** Section of middle ear from 28-week-old fetus in region of chorda tympani nerve (*above*) and handle of malleus (*right*) to show primitive mesenchyme

Anatomy and Functions

The anatomy of the ear (Fig. 1.12) may be considered by reference to its functions in hearing and balance.

The pinna and external canal conduct sound waves in air to the tympanic membrane, which transmits them by very delicate vibrations. The middle ear enhances this sound energy transmission by conveying vibrations from the larger area of the

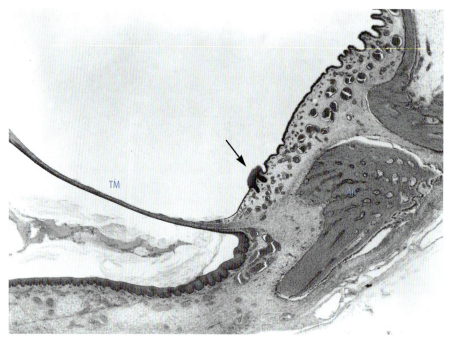

Figure 1.8 Epidermoid formation (*arrow*), situated in its characteristic position at the junction of the middle ear with the Eustachian tube epithelium, just anterior to the tympanic membrane (*TM*) and adjacent to the bony anterior limb of the annulus (*An*)

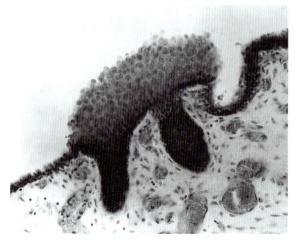

Figure 1.9 Higher power of part of Fig. 1.8 showing epidermoid formation with two rete ridges and superficial keratinised cells. Note cuboidal middle ear epithelium on left and columnar Eustachian tube epithelium on right of epidermoid formation

tympanic membrane through the ossicular chain (malleus, incus and stapes) to the much smaller area of the footplate of the stapes, which lies in the oval window of the vestibule in contact with perilymph. In this way vibrations representing sound are conducted to the fluids of the inner ear. The air space of the middle ear cavity is magnified by the mastoid air cells, which are complex expansions into the mastoid bone. There is a connection of the middle ear space with the nasopharynx and so with the external air through the Eustachian tube, by which air pressure can be adjusted.

From the vestibular perilymph, vibrations derived from sound waves pass directly via the scala vestibuli into the spirally coiled perilymphatic spaces of the cochlea, where an upper compartment, the scala vestibuli, ascending from the vestibule and oval window and a lower compartment, the scala tympani, may be recognised. The latter descends to the round window membrane, a connective tissue disc separating the perilymph compartment from the middle ear. Between the scalae vestibuli and tympani there is an endolymph-containing coiled middle compartment, the cochlear duct (scala media), which houses the sensory organ of sound reception, the organ of Corti. Waves of vibration are conveyed from the perilymph to the walls of the scala media, from which, through the endolymph, they affect the sensory cells of the organ of Corti.

The cochlear duct communicates with the vestibular endolymph-containing sacs through two fine canals so that the endolymphatic system of cochlea and vestibule is continuous, like the perilymphatic one. Gravitational acceleration of the head is detected in a sensory organ arranged within endolymph-containing sacs in the vestibule (the utricle and saccule), and angular acceleration is detected within tubes emanating in three dimensions from the utricle (lateral, posterior and superior semicircular canals). The sensory cells are located as a thickened portion of epithelium, the

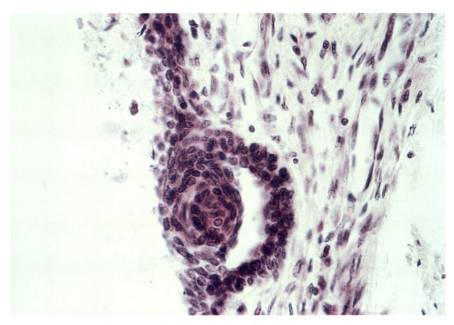

Figure 1.10 Epidermoid formation situated in a fold of Eustachian tube

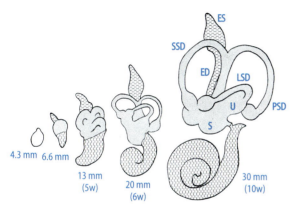

Figure 1.11 Diagram of the development of the labyrinthine system from the otocyst (*far left*), based on literature sources. *Horizontal hatches*, endolymphatic duct (*ED*) and sac (*ES*); *vertical hatches*, cochlear duct; *dotted*, vestibular system; *SSD*, semicircular duct; *S*, saccule; *U*, utricle; *LSD*, lateral semicircular duct; *PSD*, posterior semicircular duct. Embryo and fetal stages are given in mm crown-rump length and weeks gestation

macula, in the saccule and utricle and a raised prominence of epithelium, the crista, in expansions of each semicircular canal, the ampullae. The vestibular aqueduct contains the endolymphatic duct and sac, which are a blind offshoot of the endolymphatic system, probably functioning in absorption of endolymph. The cochlear aqueduct is a communication between the cerebrospinal fluid in the subarachnoid space to the perilymph of the scala tympani near the round window. Cochlea, vestibule and semicircular canals are surrounded by very dense bone, the otic capsule.

The cochlear and vestibular sensory structures are supplied by a double nerve, the audiovestibular nerve or eighth cranial nerve, which enters the temporal bone through the internal auditory meatus. The facial nerve or seventh cranial nerve enters the temporal bone through the same canal, and after a right-angled bend in the genu, where the geniculate ganglion is located, reaches the posterior wall of the middle ear, from which it passes down through the mastoid to emerge in the region of the parotid salivary gland, after which it provides motor nerve supply for the muscles of the face.

Gross Features

Microslice preparation of the temporal bone (see below) yields a series of specimens in which the gross and radiographic features of external, middle and inner ears and their neighboring tissues can be delineated (Fig. 1.13). The deeper osseous portion of the external auditory meatus terminating in the tympanic membrane, with its attached handle of the malleus, is identified. The ossicles themselves and the joints between the malleus and the incus and between the incus and the stapes can be seen. The Eustachian tube is observed, opening onto the anterior wall of the middle ear and passing medially toward the nasopharynx. The tensor tympani muscle lies in a canal lateral to and above the Eustachian tube. The facial nerve is present in the posterior wall of the middle ear. Mastoid air cells are abundant also in the posterior wall of the external

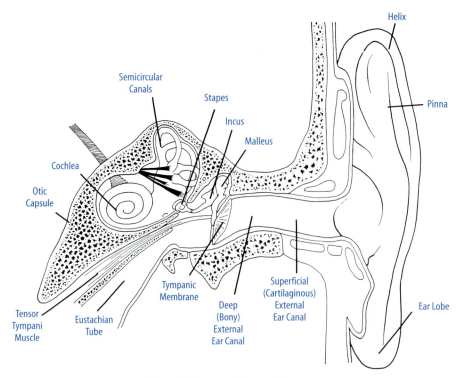

Figure 1.12 Anatomical diagram of the ear

canal. In the inner ear the vestibule and the cochlea are easily made out. Although not notable in the two photographs, the three semicircular canals – superior, lateral and posterior – are easily seen in slices at different levels.

External Ear

Gross Features

Diagonal Earlobe Crease

A crease in the earlobe has been reliably associated with coronary heart disease (Frank's sign)[16] and so may be of interest to pathologists when performing an autopsy. Earlobes may be free or attached, the "soldered" form being an extreme version of the latter.[17] Diagonal creases occur in all three forms of earlobe. The crease runs diagonally backward and downward across the lateral surface of the earlobe from the external meatus. The crease may be classified as Grade 2 if it is superficial and runs across the whole earlobe; or if it is deep, but runs across more than 50%, but less than 100%, of the earlobe. Grade 1 is a crease less than Grade 2. It is Grade 3 if it is deep and runs across 100% of the earlobe (Fig. 1.14). Bilateral Grades 2 and Grades 3

are associated with a significantly higher risk of death from atherosclerosis and myocardial infarction.[18] Not only is there an increased cardiac mortality associated with diagonal creases,[19] but also an increased cardiac morbidity.[20]

Light Microscopy

Pinna

The pinna consists of elastic cartilage with a covering of skin containing appendages: hair with sebaceous glands, eccrine sweat glands, and a few ceruminous glands. There is hardly any subcutaneous connective tissue in the pinna except in the ear lobe, where the elastic cartilage is absent and is replaced by a pad of adipose tissue. The perichondrium is composed of loose vascular connective tissue, and is important as the tissue from which the avascular cartilage is nourished by diffusion from a network of capillary blood vessels derived from small arteries and arterioles running in a plane parallel to the surface of the cartilage. Extensive collections of blood or pus following trauma or infection, respectively, may develop over the perichondrium and by compression of vessels there, may lead to cartilage necrosis.

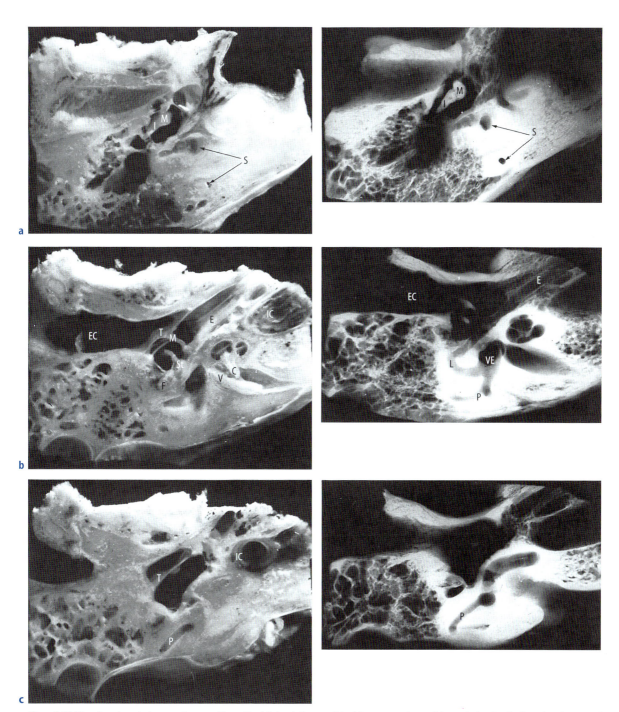

Figure 1.13 Microslices through the normal temporal bone. The *left-hand photograph* is of the gross specimen of the particular slice. On the *right* is the X-ray of that slice. **a** Microslice passing through the attic region of the middle ear and showing incudomalleal joint. **b** Microslice to include mid-modiolar region of cochlea and showing stapes. The tendon of the stapedius muscle may be seen on the gross photograph, attached to the posterior crus of the stapes. **c** Microslice taken through the basal coil of the cochlea and hypotympanum. *C*, cochlear branch of eighth nerve; *E*, Eustachian tube; *EC*, ear canal; *F*, facial nerve; *I*, incus; *IC*, internal carotid artery; *L*, lateral semicircular canal; *M*, malleus; *P*, posterior semicircular canal; *S*, superior semicircular canal; *St*, stapes; *T*, tympanic membrane; *V*, vestibular branch of eighth nerve; *VE*, vestibule

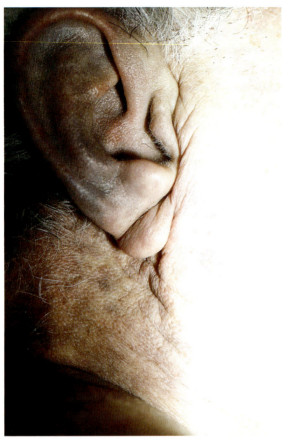

Figure 1.14 Diagonal ear-lobe crease. This crease is deep and runs across 100% of the earlobe so that it should be classified as Grade 3

External Auditory Meatus

The skin over the cartilaginous portion of the external auditory meatus contains hair follicles with sebaceous glands and apocrine (ceruminous) glands, but no eccrine glands. The ceruminous glands, of which there are between 1000 and 2000 in the average ear,[21] closely resemble the apocrine glands of the axillary and pubic skin. They are found in the dermis deep to the level of the sebaceous glands and just superficial to the perichondrium. The inner secretory cells of the ceruminous glands display an apocrine-type secretion, which appears as buds of cytoplasm that bulge from the surface of the cell into the lumen. There are yellow-brown pigment granules near the nucleus that are acid fast and show reddish fluorescence in ultraviolet light. Peripheral to the secretory cells are flattened myoepithelial cells (Fig. 1.15). The ducts of the ceruminous glands do not show apocrine or myoepithelial cells and terminate in a hair follicle or on the skin surface. The rare benign tumour of ceruminous glands, the ceruminal adenoma, usually displays both apocrine and myoepithelial cells (see Chapter 2).

In the deep bony portion of the external canal there are no adnexal structures, and the subcutaneous tissue and periosteum form a single thin layer. The distance between the epidermal surface and underlying bone is consequently small, which explains the tendency for exostoses of the tympanic bone to develop in this region in cold-water swimmers. The water dribbles into the deep canal and

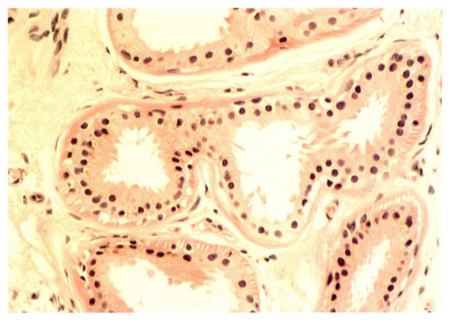

Figure 1.15 Apocrine glands of external auditory meatus. Note buds of cytoplasm, some of which are lying loosely, projecting into the lumen. An outer myoepithelial layer may be identified in the glands[50]

cools the nearby periosteum, stimulating it to produce new bone (see Chapter 2).

Tympanic Membrane

The pars tensa consists of an externally-placed epidermis of stratified squamous epithelium, a central bilaminated zone (lateral radially arranged, and medial circularly arranged, collagenous fibres), and an internal mucosal middle ear layer. It is a mark of previous inflammatory damage if this architecture is absent. The middle ear surface is a single layer of cubical epithelium, which rests on a thin lamina propria (Fig. 1.16).

Middle Ear

Light Microscopy

Epithelium

The epithelial covering of the middle ear is a single layer of flattened or cubical cells. In newborns several layers of cubical epithelium may be seen in a few areas in response to inflammation and true

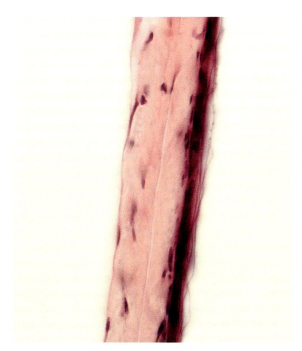

Figure 1.16 Section of pars tensa of tympanic membrane. The following layers may be distinguished from right to left: stratified squamous epithelium, lamina propria, radial arrangement of collagenous fibres, circular arrangement of collagenous fibres (i.e. *at right angles to former layer*), lamina propria, middle ear epithelium

stratified squamous epithelium is found as the epidermoid formation in fetal life (see above) and in cholesteatoma, but claims that stratified squamous epithelium is frequent in the middle ear as a result of squamous metaplasia[22] have not been confirmed (see Chapter 3).

Ciliated pseudostratified columnar epithelium can be seen in small patches among the cubical epithelial cells of the middle ear, particularly following inflammatory changes associated with perforation of the tympanic membrane. Inflammatory aural polyps, which grow from the medial surface of the middle ear (see Chapter 3), often show a partial covering of true ciliated epithelium.

Periodic acid–Schiff-positive (neutral mucopolysaccharide-containing) and alcian blue stains (acid mucopolysaccharide-containing) cells have been found in the middle ear, mostly adjacent to the Eustachian tube in adults and children.

Glandular Metaplasia

The epithelium of most of the respiratory tract, including that of the cartilaginous portion of the Eustachian tube, contains tubuloalveolar glands, often with mucous and serous elements (see below). The middle ear, however, does not normally display these structures. Under pathological conditions, however, the middle ear epithelium comes to resemble other parts of the respiratory tract by the formation of glands, but the middle ear glands consist only of a simple tubule of mucus-producing cells. Glandular metaplasia of the middle ear has been described as the main lesion of children with secretory otitis media[23] and is also a prominent feature of the middle ear of patients with AIDS[24] (see Chapter 3).

Mastoid Air Cells

The mastoid air cells are a network of intercommunicating spaces that emanate from the tympanic cavity. Each air cell has a thin frame of lamellar bone, covered by a periosteum on which the middle ear epithelium rests. In acute otitis media, the mastoid air cells become filled with pus.

Middle Ear Corpuscles

Middle ear corpuscles are smooth, translucent, pear-shaped or oval swelling usually found growing on fibrous septa, which appear in the mastoid air cells with advancing age[25] (Fig. 1.17). Microscopically

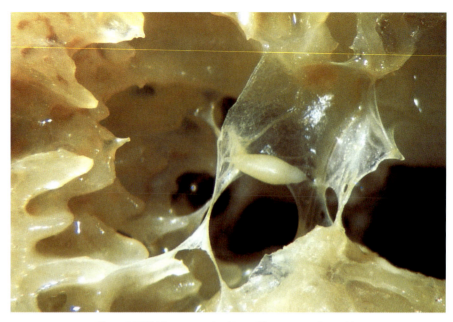

Figure 1.17 Middle ear corpuscle arising on fibrous septum of mastoid

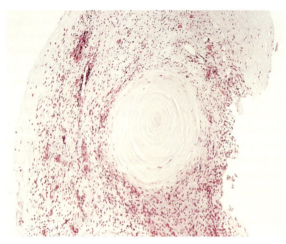

Figure 1.18 Middle ear corpuscle within inflammatory tissue of mastoid[50]

they are concentrically laminated masses of collagen, resembling corpora amylacea of the lung or prostate (Fig. 1.18). In frozen sections carried out on the middle ear, usually during operations for squamous cell carcinoma, they may be mistaken for pearls of keratinising neoplasm. They have also been confused with pacinian corpuscles, but they lack the fine innervation and the nucleated concentric layers of the latter.

Eustachian Tube

The Eustachian tube is covered by ciliated pseudostratified columnar (respiratory) epithelium (Fig. 1.19), about a fifth of which is composed of goblet cells; the proportion of the latter increases in middle ear infection.[26] Beneath the epithelium are groups of lymphocytes, "Gerlach's tubal tonsil", probably the result of inflammation.[27] Seromucinous glands are seen in the submucosa of the cartilaginous portion of the tube, but not near the tympanic end of the tube (Fig. 1.20). They are also increased in chronic otitis media.[28,29] The cartilage at the nasopharyngeal end of the Eustachian tube is of hyaline type. The mucosa of the osseous portion of the Eustachian tube is separated from the carotid canal by a plate of bone, which is less than 1 mm in

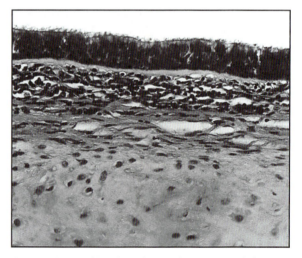

Figure 1.19 Mucosa of Eustachian tube in cartilaginous region. The lining is of ciliated columnar epithelium. In the lamina propria beneath there are numerous lymphocytes, which are probably the result of inflammation. Cartilage fills the *lower part of the illustration*

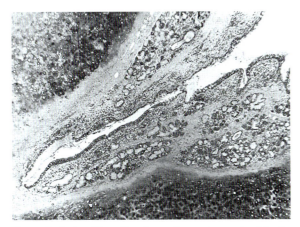

Figure 1.20 Section of Eustachian tube near its nasopharyngeal end showing abundant seromucinous glands and outer cartilaginous layer.

thickness and frequently shows dehiscence[30] (Fig. 1.21). This can easily be penetrated by squamous carcinoma of the middle ear and Eustachian tube to reach the carotid canal, where it tends to spread widely[31] (see Chapter 5). Thin bone also separates the tube from the tensor tympani muscle superiorly and air cells inferiorly and laterally.

Auditory Ossicles

Stapes

Cartilage is retained as a thin horizontal lamina on the vestibular aspect of the footplate of the stapes and also covers the articular surfaces of the stapediovestibular joints (annulus fibrosus) (Fig. 1.22). The vestibular surface of the stapes is lined by a single flattened layer of cells characteristic of the perilymphatic space. A thin layer of bone is exterior to the cartilage on the middle ear surface of the footplate. Occasionally it contains areas of cartilage, which extend from the vestibular to the tympanic surface.

The crura are formed of periosteal bone only. Endochondral bone, which covered the inner part of the crura earlier in development, is completely eliminated during later development of the obturator foramen. The head of the stapes is composed of endochondral bone capped by a cartilaginous layer at the incudostapedial joint.

In a small proportion of temporal bone sections, an artery, the persistent stapedial artery, is present, which arises from the internal carotid artery, passes into the middle ear and then runs through the obturator foramen of the stapes, eventually entering the middle cranial fossa through the Fallopian canal of the facial nerve.

Specimen after Stapedectomy

Stapedectomy is performed to remove the fixation caused by otosclerosis. The fixed stapes is then replaced by a mobile prosthesis. The surgical pathology specimen of stapes is composed either of the superstructure (the head and crura) alone without

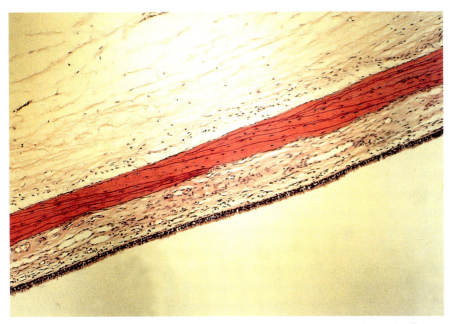

Figure 1.21 Thin layer of bone between Eustachian tube below and canal of internal carotid artery above[50]

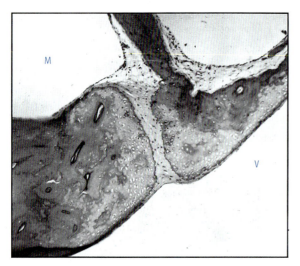

Figure 1.22 Stapediovestibular joint (*centre*), part of footplate of stapes (*upper right*), adjacent bony labyrinthine wall (*left*) and crus of stapes (*upper right*). The footplate shows a lamina of cartilage on its vestibular surface, which is continuous with the cartilage of the articular surface of the stapediovestibular joint. *M*, middle ear cavity; *V*, cavity of vestibule

the footplate or of the whole ossicle including the footplate. Otosclerosis is seen within the stapes only in the footplate because the fixation causing deafness is often the result of extension of the otosclerotic process from the adjacent temporal bone across the annulus fibrosus (stapediovestibular joint) (see Chapter 10). In many cases not even the footplate will show otosclerosis because fixation has been caused only by pressure onto the footplate as a result of the swelling of the otosclerotic process in the adjacent temporal bone.

Malleus and Incus

The structure of malleus and incus is more like that of a typical long bone than is that of the stapes. There is an outer covering of periosteal bone and an inner core of endochondral bone, both showing well-formed Haversian systems (Fig. 1.23). Both layers are subject to removal and replacement by new bone. Bone removal may give rise to pits on the surface of the ossicles, which should not necessarily be interpreted as the erosive effects of inflammation. The sites of fresh bony deposition are indicated by the presence of cement lines. Islands of endochondral bone with cartilage similar to the globuli ossei of the otic capsule (see below) are sometimes found in the incus and malleus.

Most of the malleus handle does not have a shell of periosteal bone; instead, there is a layer of retained cartilage. The handle merges with the middle collagenous layer of the tympanic membrane.

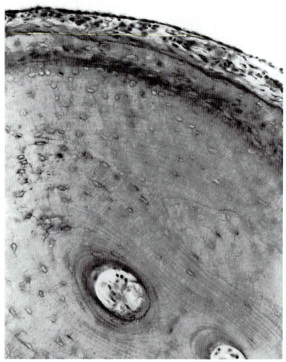

Figure 1.23 Long process of incus. There is an outer covering of periosteal bone and an inner core of endochondral bone. Note flat middle ear epithelium on surface

Superiorly the malleus handle is separated from the eardrum by a ligament covered by middle ear epithelium. Lower down, the malleus handle is invested by the middle fibrous layer of the tympanic membrane. The inner core of the whole of the malleus handle is composed of endochondral bone like that of the rest of the malleus. The articular process of the malleus is covered by cartilage. The anterior process of the malleus is, unlike the rest of the malleus, formed in membrane early in fetal life and merges with the malleus soon after its formation.

The short process of the incus shows a tip of unossified cartilage. Cartilage also covers the articular surfaces of the incus at its two joints.

Middle Ear Joints

The incudomalleal and incudostapedial joints are diarthrodial. The space between the articular ends is occupied largely by fibrocartilage – the articular disc. The joint capsule is lined on its outer surface by middle ear epithelium and on its inner surface by synovial membrane. The capsule is of fibrous tissue with a very high elastic fibre content (Fig. 1.24).

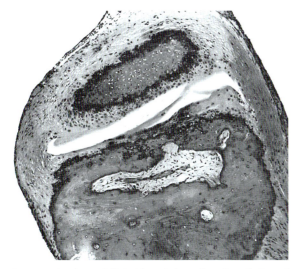

Figure 1.24 Incudostapedial joint. The articular cartilage shows fraying and small areas of calcification. These are manifestations of advancing age

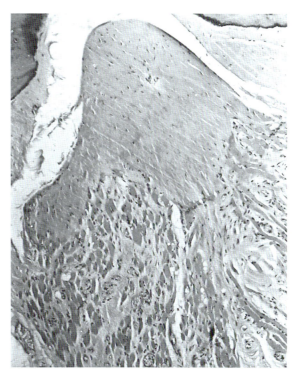

Figure 1.25 Stapedius muscle and tendon. The skeletal muscle fibres and fibrous bands between them radiate to a tendon

The cartilaginous edge of the footplate of the stapes, the stapediovestibular joint, is bound to the cartilaginous rim of the vestibular window by a fibrous connection, the annular ligament. A small cavity is present in most adult annular ligaments.[32] Elastic fibres are prominent near the surfaces of the ligaments.

In the bone just anterior to the joint, a canal is often seen linking the middle ear with vestibule, the fissula ante fenestram. We have found that it develops as a slit filled with fibrous tissue, often with associated cartilage. Its presence has been thought to be related to otosclerosis because both are seen in a similar position, but this is not yet confirmed.

Middle Ear Muscles

The tensor tympani and stapedius muscles are composed of fibres with a penniform (i.e., feather-shaped) arrangement, showing a central tendon formed by elastic tissue with muscle fibres radiating from it (Fig. 1.25). The tensor tympani often has a prominent content of adipose tissue (Fig. 1.26), which may serve to insulate the nearby cochlea from the electric effects of its contraction.

Ageing Changes

Changes have been described in the incudomalleal and incudostapedial joints in the elderly, which are thought to cause a mild conductive deafness.[33] The joint capsule and articular disc show hyalinisation and later calcification. The articular cartilage frequently shows fraying, vacuolation, fibrillation and even calcification. The joint becomes narrowed and eventually obliterated.[34]

Inner Ear

Light Microscopy

Otic Capsule

The otic capsule surrounds and replicates the outline of the membranous labyrinth contained within it. Its extreme denseness is probably necessary to insulate and safeguard the extremely delicate vibrations of the fluids that it encloses, which subserve the functions of hearing and balance. Three layers may be recognised: an outer periosteal layer, which corresponds to the circumferential lamella of long bones; an inner layer, next to the membranous labyrinth, which is another periosteal layer (although usually referred to as the "endosteal" layer of the otic capsule, suggesting, wrongly, correspondence to the osseous layer next to the bone marrow of long bones); and a middle layer in which there are foci of bluish-staining ground substance, the "globuli interossei" or "globuli ossei" (Figs 1.27, 1.28). The latter have been shown to be the empty

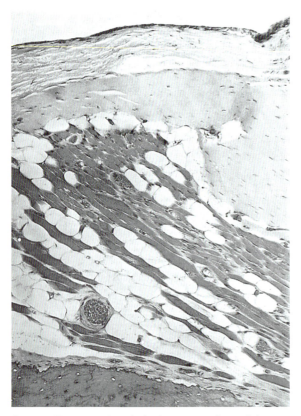

Figure 1.26 Tensor tympani muscle showing numerous adipose cells between the skeletal muscle fibres

lacunae of the cartilage remnants, which are infiltrated by osteoblasts.[35] The bony architecture of the adult otic capsule is neither lamellated nor woven bone, but somewhere in between. Thus, the otic capsule bone differs from other areas of adult bone formed in cartilage by incomplete removal and replacement of calcified cartilaginous matrix and of primitive bone. The interweaving of these persisting structures form a unique tissue that is of extremely hard consistency.

Cochlea

The modiolus is an axial core of spongy bone centrally placed in the cochlea. It is penetrated by blood vessels and the nerve bundles of the cochlear branch of the eighth nerve. At the origin of the three cochlear coils and forming nests within the modiolus lie the nerve cells of the spiral ganglion, to which the axons derived from the sensory hair cells, carrying impulses of hearing, arrive and from which axons pass to the cochlear nucleus in the brain stem. The spiral ganglion cells are each surrounded by Schwann cells.

The spaces of the cochlear coils are divided into two compartments, the scala vestibuli and the scala tympani, by a partially bony membrane, the spiral lamina, which emanates from the modiolus in a spiral manner. Each scala contains perilymph. The scala vestibuli winds towards the apex of the cochlea at the helicotrema, where it becomes the scala

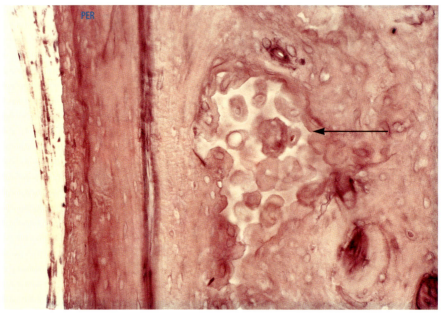

Figure 1.27 Otic capsule bone showing globuli ossei (*arrow*) and periosteal layer (*PER*)

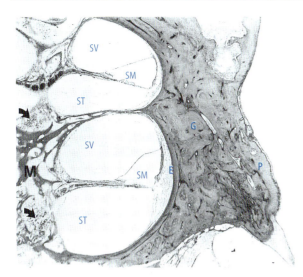

Figure 1.28 Half of two coils of cochlea bony cochlea and modiolus. *E,* endosteal layer; *G,* endochondral layer containing globuli interossei; *M,* modiolus; *P,* periosteal layer; *SM,* scala media; *ST,* scala tympani; *SV,* scala vestibuli; *arrows,* spiral ganglion cells[50]

tympani, which coils back towards the round window (Fig. 1.28).

The inner zone of the spiral lamina is the osseous spiral lamina, which is composed of thin trabeculae of bone, the habenulae perforata. These surround nerve fibres that are composed of both afferent fibres, which run from the organ of Corti to the acoustic nerve, and efferent fibres supplying the outer hair cells. The efferent fibres are derived from the olivocochlear system of Rasmussen and follow the course of the cochlear branch of the eighth cranial nerve through the modiolus to enter the osseous spiral lamina and basilar membrane, eventually to supply the outer hair cells for arcane functions related to hearing. The outer zone of this lamina is known as the basilar membrane. At the attachment of the latter to the cochlear wall, the periosteal connective tissue is thickened to form the spiral ligament. This appears in section as a crescentic collagenous structure with a protruding peak on its concave surface to which the basilar membrane is anchored.

Sections of the scala tympani in the region of the basal coil and round window membrane usually show the cochlear aqueduct near its scala tympani opening (Fig. 1.29); this canal passes from the latter to the subarachnoid space near the jugular foramen. Thus, there is a connection between the labyrinth and the cerebrospinal fluid. The lumen of the aqueduct at its cochlear end is often filled by a meshwork of fibrous reticular tissue, but it still remains patent. Contaminated cerebrospinal fluid from the subarachnoid space in meningitis and red cells from subarachnoid haemorrhage can be conveyed to the perilymphatic space of the labyrinth along this channel.[36]

The cochlear canal is further subdivided by a thin membrane, Reissner's membrane, that extends from the osseous spiral lamina to the outer wall of the bony cochlea, so producing an additional scala, the scala media or cochlear duct, which is inserted

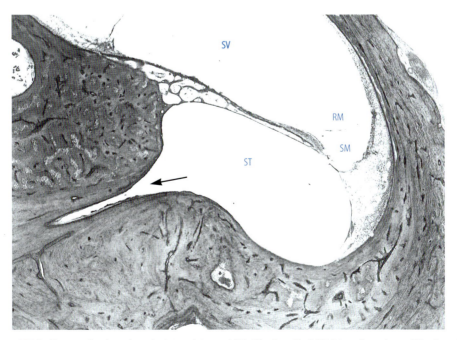

Figure 1.29 Cochlear aqueduct (*arrow*) opening into scala tympani (*ST*). *SV,* scala vestibuli; *RM,* Reissner's membrane; *SM,* scala media

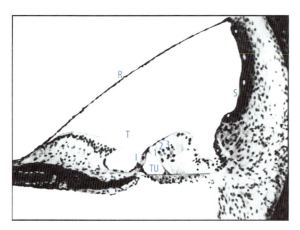

Figure 1.30 Scala media from cochlea of rhesus monkey. *I*, inner hair cell; *R*, Reissner's membrane; *S*, stria vascularis; *T*, tectorial membrane; *Tu*, tunnel of Corti; *1*, *2* and *3* = first, second and third rows of outer hair cells

between the other two (Figs 1.28–1.30). Reissner's membrane consists of two thin layers of cells: an inner is ectodermal in origin and often contains epithelial-appearing clusters; an outer layer is mesodermal in origin and shows large, flat, and elongated cells. Reissner's membrane bulges upward into the scala vestibuli in conditions producing hydrops, notably Ménière's disease.

The outer vertical wall of the cochlear duct is the stria vascularis. Under the light microscope lightly staining basal cells and darkly staining epithelial-like marginal cells can be recognised. The stria vascularis is frequently altered in ototoxic conditions such as those produced by the diuretic drugs frusemide and ethacrynic acid, and by the cytotoxic agent cisplatin (see Chapter 7).

The spiral prominence is a bulge of connective tissue covered by epithelial cells, which lies at the outer end of the basilar membrane over the spiral ligament. The outer hair cells are present in rows, which, in the mammalian organ of Corti, vary from three to five. They are separated from the single row of inner hair cells by the pillar cells that enclose the tunnel of Corti. In many sectioned preparations of human organ of Corti, the cochlear hair cells are not seen because of autolysis; stereocilia are, moreover, observed with great difficulty only in sections. On the other hand, not only stereocilia and hair cells but also supporting cells, pillar cells and nerves can be well shown by the surface preparation method using ordinary staining and light microscopy (see below). Supporting cells separate outer hair cells. The spiral limbus is a bulge of periosteal connective tissue in the upper surface of the osseous spiral lamina. The fibres of this structure show a vertical arrangement to produce the "auditory teeth of Huschke". Epithelial cells on the upper margin of the spiral limbus, the interdental cells, secrete the tectorial

membrane, a linear bundle of amorphous protein in which hairs of the outer hair cells lie (Fig. 1.30).

Vestibular Structures

The end of each semicircular duct is expanded to form the ampulla. The epithelium of the floor of the three ampullae is formed into a transverse ridge, the crista, and is their sensory epithelium. A viscous protein polysaccharide formation, known as the cupula, rests above each crista. The remainder of the ampullary and semicircular duct lining is formed by flattened cells (Fig. 1.31).

The two main membranous structures of the vestibule, the utricle and saccule, are in part lined by a sensory epithelium, the macule (Fig. 1.32). The sensory cells of the maculae and the cristae are of two types when examined by transmission electron microscopy. The type 1 cell is flask-shaped with a swollen basal portion. The type 2 cell is cylindrical. Type 1 cells are attached to the fibres of the sensory nerves by a wide chalice-like terminal. The terminal of type 2 cells is by button-like attachments of the nerve (Fig. 1.33).

Overlying the hairs of the sensory cells of the maculae are large numbers of crystalline bodies, known as otoliths, which are composed of a mixture of calcium carbonate and a protein, suspended in a jelly-like polysaccharide.

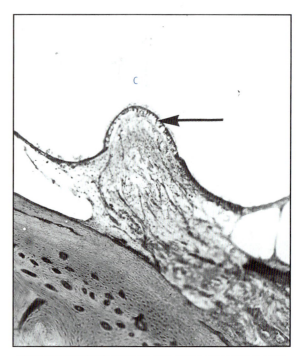

Figure 1.31 Ampulla of semicircular canal. *Arrow* points to crista; *C*, cupula

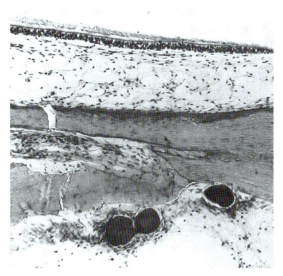

Figure 1.32 Macule of the saccule. Note dark concentrically laminated structures (calcified arachnoid villi) in internal auditory meatus below

Cochleovestibular Nerve

The eighth cranial (cochleovestibular) nerve lies in the internal auditory meatus in its passage to the peripheral end organs in the cochlea and vestibule. The afferent ganglion for the vestibular structures – the vestibular ganglion – is seen at the termination of the main part of the vestibular division of the nerve in the internal auditory meatus. The afferent ganglion for the cochlear division, the spiral ganglion, lies in the modiolus (see above). Near the entrance to the internal auditory meatus, where the cochlear and vestibular divisions are fused, the nerve changes from pale-staining proximally to dark-staining distally. This appearance is produced by the abrupt transition of the coverings of the nerve fibres from the pale-staining oligodendroglia to the darker Schwann cells. It has been suggested that vestibular schwannomas (acoustic neuromas) are formed in the nerve at this junction, which could represent a region of Schwann cell instability.

Facial Nerve

The facial nerve enters the temporal bone through the internal auditory meatus, where it lies above the eighth cranial nerve. It then passes Bill's bar, a pointed projection of bone that separates it from the superior division of the vestibular nerve. The facial nerve then enters the fallopian canal, making a right-angled bend at the genu. A bulge in the facial nerve below Bill's bar in the internal auditory meatus has mistakenly been regarded as a pathological feature of Bell's palsy. It is, in fact, a normal finding present in all temporal bones. The facial nerve then lies in a bony canal in the posterior wall of the middle ear. It is surrounded here by a sheath of blood vessels. The bony covering separating the facial nerve from middle ear is often lacking. Such a "dehiscence" makes the nerve particularly vulnerable to damage by pathological change, especially inflammation, originating in the middle ear.

Paraganglia

Small paraganglia with a structure similar to the carotid body have been described in the ear.[37] More than 50% of these structures are situated in relation to the jugular bulb; a minority are found under the mucosa of the middle ear in the region of the medial promontory wall (Fig. 1.34). The tumours arising from the paraganglia in these situations form the more frequent jugular paraganglioma (glomus jugulare) and the less frequent tympanic paraganglioma (glomus tympanicum), respectively.

Vestibular Aqueduct and Endolymphatic Duct and Sac

The endolymphatic duct is linked by short canals to the utricle and saccule and passes posteriorly across the petrous bone to terminate in the blind endolymphatic sac, which projects into the dura in the poste-

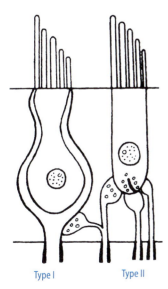

Type I   Type II

Figure 1.33 Diagram of structure and mode of attachment to afferent nerve of sensory hair cells types I and II of macules and cristae[50]

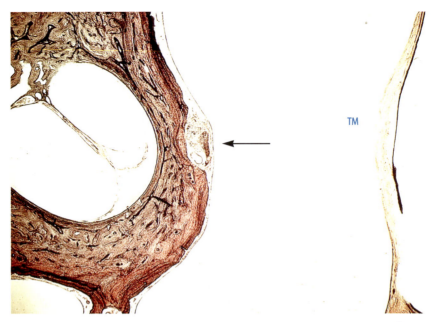

TM

Figure 1.34 Tympanic paraganglion on promontory of cochlea (*arrow*). *TM*, tympanic membrane[50]

rior cranial fossa. In its course through the bone, the endolymphatic duct is housed within the vestibular aqueduct. The latter is identified easily in microsliced temporal bones and particularly in their radiographs. The lining epithelium of the upper endolymphatic duct is low cubical, that of the lower suct and endolymphatic sac taller and papillary (Fig. 1.35).

Examination in the Histopathology Laboratory

Removal of Temporal Bone at Autopsy

Piecemeal removal of individual parts of the ear for post-mortem examination is not satisfactory

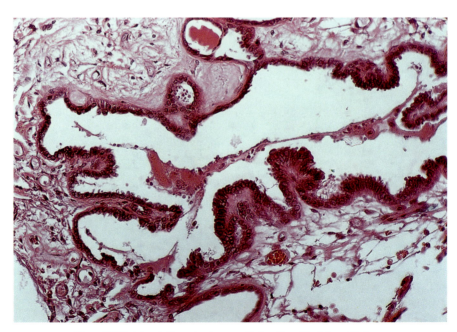

Figure 1.35 Endolymphatic sac showing normal tall papillae of the lining epithelium

because the relationship of changes in adjacent structures is always important in ear disease and this is destroyed by such a means of examination. To examine the ear adequately the whole temporal bone should be removed as one block.

Autopsy and removal of the temporal bone should be carried out as soon after death as possible. Useful information may, however, still be obtained even 20 hours after death and longer. Autolysis of labyrinthine structures is prevented to some degree if 20% formalin is injected into the middle ear through the tympanic membrane soon after death. Such an injection will, of course, damage the tympanic membrane and some middle ear structures. For examination of the membranous labyrinth, perfusion of the perilymphatic space with fixative soon after death is preferable (see below). The cadaver should be refrigerated as soon as possible after death.

The standard method of approaching the temporal bone at post-mortem involves prior removal of the skull cap and brain. In doing so the dura should be treated carefully and left adherent to the temporal bone in order not to damage the endolymphatic sac (see below). The seventh and eighth cranial nerves should be cut at the orifice of the internal auditory meatus so as to leave portions of the nerve trunks within the temporal bone specimen. A vibrating electric saw is satisfactory for removing the petrous temporal bone. A blade of triangular shape, measuring at least 5 cm (2 inches) from attachment to vibrating saw to edge is required. The more commonly employed circular blade is unsatisfactory for this purpose. Three vertical cuts and one horizontal cut are made with the saw (Fig. 1.36).

1. The first cut is set medial to the internal auditory meatus and extends vertically through the petrous temporal bone at right angles to the superior and posteromedial surfaces to a depth of approximately 2.5 cm.

2. The second cut is made parallel with the first and at least 2.5–3 cm posterolateral to it at the lateral end of the temporal bone. It also passes vertically to a depth of 2.5 cm. This cut leaves out most of the mastoid air cell system. A more extensive procedure by which these cells may be removed involves extending cut **3** laterally to the lateral surface of the squamous temporal bone anterior to the bony orifice of the external auditory meatus, after dissecting the pinna, scalp, and cartilaginous canal away from the latter. Cut **4** is also extended laterally posterior to the mastoid process and the two cuts are joined together below the bony ear canal. With care this extended temporal bone resection does not result in an unsightly external disfigurement

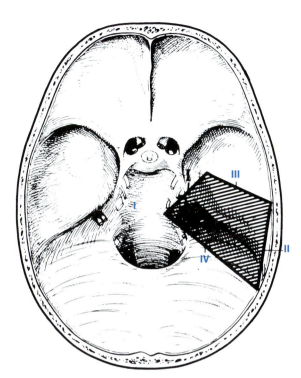

Figure 1.36 Base of skull showing position of four saw cuts (*Roman numerals*), which are required in removal of temporal bone[51]

produced by skull base collapse as long as cut **1** on each side is placed just medial to the internal auditory meatus and not further medially.

3. The third vertical cut is made connecting the forward ends of the two previous cuts, approximately parallel with the free (posterior) end of the petrous temporal bone at the anterior extent of the middle cranial fossa.

4. A horizontal cut is made beneath the petrous temporal bone at about 2.5 cm below the upper surface and parallel with it. The block can now be removed by gently "rocking" and cutting the ligamentous structures on its inferior surface. So removed it will include the deeper part of the external ear canal, the tympanic membrane, the middle ear, the labyrinthine structures and the petrous portion of the seventh and eighth cranial nerves.

A method has been devised of removing and processing the temporal bone so as to include the whole length of the Eustachian tube.[38]

Handling of Temporal Bone Site and Specimen

After removing the specimen, plaster of Paris may be inserted in the space previously occupied by the temporal bone. To assist the subsequent embalming process, the internal carotid arteries may be clamped in the neck before removal of the temporal bones and then ligated after removal has been completed.

The specimen is then placed in fixative in a large screw-top plastic jar. For most purposes the fixative may be buffered 4% formaldehyde solution. In some centres another fixative is preferred, e.g. Heidenhain Susa solution, but this is unsatisfactory if modern immunochemical procedures are to be applied to sections.

Preparation of Autopsy Temporal Bones for Histological Examination and Molecular Techniques

The standard technique available for histological examination of the temporal bone as a whole has been to decalcify it and then embed it in celloidin and then to cut it into serial sections for histological staining. Hair cells in particular are not well displayed, since their most characteristic feature, the stereocilia, are hardly visible in such sections. A more satisfactory method for examining the hair cells of the cochlea is by means of surface preparations of the basilar membrane. This has previously called for skilled drilling in exposing the inner ear.[39] A method is available whereby slices of the undecalcified bone are first inspected and chosen parts are then subjected to histological section. With suitably perfused material, surface preparations can, as an alternative, be obtained from the samples sliced by this method (see below).

Technique of Serial Sectioning after Celloidin Embedding

Fixation is required for approximately 4 weeks. The bone should be roughly sawn to size before fixation. To decalcify the whole temporal bone, it is placed in 10% formic acid for a period of 4–8 weeks, taking X-rays every week to check the progress of decalcification. On its completion the final trimming of the specimen can be done by using a strong-bladed knife. It is important to keep the size of the bone to a minimum to allow adequate diffusion of impregnating substances during the processing of the bone; the trimmed block should measure not more than 4.0 cm long by 2.5 cm wide by 5.5 cm high. Dehydration of the whole specimen is carried out by placing it for 1 day in ascending grades of alcohol and alcohol–ether as follows: 30%, 50%, 95%, 100%, 100%, equal parts alcohol and ether.

Impregnation in a celloidin base dissolved in a mixture of equal parts of alcohol and ether is then required. For microtomy a long heavy stellite-tipped knife is preferable. This should be sharpened to a final cutting edge bevel of about 28°. Sections are cut at 20 μm thickness and it is necessary only to stain every tenth section, keeping the intermediate sections interleaved in vellum tissue, which may be stored indefinitely with the uncut blocks in 70% alcohol. Staining of sections may be carried out by the hematoxylin and eosin method (preferably using Ehrlich's hematoxylin) as well as by a variety of other routine histological stains, but immunohistochemical methods are difficult to apply to celloidin-embedded material, although a technique for this purpose has been described (see below).

Disadvantages of the Serial Sectioning Method

Gross examination, an important prerequisite of the histological analysis of all other organs, cannot be carried by the serial sectioning method after celloidin.

Prolonged decalcification must precede embedding and marked alterations in the histological appearances of some of the tissues takes place as a result of this. Some of the microscopic alterations ascribed to post-mortem autolysis in serially sectioned temporal bones are likely to be the result of damage by acid. Decalcification by ethylenediamine tetracetate (EDTA) rather than acid is less damaging and is carried out in some laboratories. Decalcification by EDTA is, however, very slow, a much longer time being required than with the use of acids.

The serial sectioning method after celloidin embedding makes special microscopic studies including histochemistry, immunohistochemistry, electron microscopy and molecular biological investigations particularly difficult.

Processing of the whole temporal bone in toto is extremely slow, since not only decalcification but also dehydration and embedding each require a long exposure. It takes at least 9 months from the autopsy to produce serial sections. This is discouraging in maintaining a sustained interest for research and teaching.

Serial sectioning of the embedded whole temporal bone is technically difficult and demands a high degree of skill on the part of the histologist in cutting sections through the whole of this structure, which is both tough and fragile.

Large numbers of serial sections are produced from a single temporal bone. A limited number only are mounted and stained; the rest have to be stored in jars of alcohol. Sometimes the serial examination of a specific portion of the temporal bone is important, but most of the sections are, as a rule, not required.

Slicing Method

A method has been devised to obviate these disadvantages and to facilitate the examination of the temporal bone in the general histopathology laboratory.[40] The temporal bone is removed at postmortem as described above. Fixation should take place for a minimum of 4 days. The bone is trimmed so that it is no larger than about 2.5 × 2.5 × 2.5 cm. The undecalcified bone is next cut into a series of slices of about 4 mm thickness using a machine specially designed for the purpose. We use a Microslice 2 Precision Annular Saw, but several similar machines are now available. Each slice may now be X-rayed with a laboratory X-ray machine (such as the Faxitron system made by Hewlett Packard).

After careful examination of the slices with a hand lens or dissecting microscope, the whole series, a single slice, or selected areas may be subjected to celloidin embedding or paraffin embedding for light microscopy, special histological or histochemical methods, or even for electron microscopy (in the case of structures that have been sufficiently well preserved).

Surface Preparation Method

The surface preparation method has been applied mainly to the analysis of the hair cells of the organ of Corti and can be used in temporal bones in which the perilymphatic space has been perfused by fixative within 24 hours after death; the autolysis that takes place in the hair cells beyond that time renders them unsuitable for this type of examination. Electron microscopy, particularly by the scanning method, is also frequently used to study specimens that have been perfused within 3 hours after death. This is often before permission for the autopsy has been granted and local legal restrictions have to be taken into account before this technique can be applied. A satisfactory method for perilymphatic perfusion has been described and has been well tested in a large number of cases.[41] The procedure may be carried out directly on the cadaver in the autopsy room or in the histopathology laboratory on a temporal bone that has been removed by the method described above. By using an ear speculum, the upper posterior part of the tympanic membrane may be folded forward. With a curette any bony overhang is removed to expose the oval and round windows. The incudostapedial joint is divided

and the stapes is luxated from the oval window. It can be left in the middle ear hanging from the stapedial muscle tendon or removed for further study. The round window membrane is perforated with a small hook directed forward (towards the Eustachian tube).

A glass pipette of tip diameter 0.5–1 mm or a syringe with an unsharpened needle of the same diameter is filled by aspiration with 1–2 ml of fixative solution at room temperature. The tip is directed toward the oval window and the fixative injected. This causes a slight increase in pressure in the vestibule and some fixative will enter the scala vestibuli (see below) and perfuse the cochlea. The perilymphatic spaces are perfused in this way for 15 min or at least ten times. The fixative preferred if electron microscopy is to be carried out is the "reduced Karnovsky" solution.[42] If surface preparation and staining by a light microscopic method is to be carried out (see below), fixation by buffered formaldehyde solution is preferred.

Technique of Sampling the Membranous Labyrinth

The method of drilling away the bony labyrinth to sample the membranous labyrinth is described by Johnsson and Hawkins.[39] The method is difficult, requiring special training and a detailed knowledge of temporal bone anatomy. Because of its difficulty, damage to the membranous labyrinth is likely until the operator has acquired a high degree of skill in the procedure. Even then the drilling method requires hours of work on a single specimen. A further disadvantage is that in order to expose the membranous labyrinth in this way, it is necessary to destroy other parts of the middle and inner ear, which cannot thereafter be subjected to routine microscopic methods.

By contrast, the microsliced temporal bone prepared by the method described above may be used to sample the membranous labyrinth without drilling and with but slight damage to inner ear structures. By this method the whole inner ear may be exposed within minutes. Moreover there is no destruction of the rest of the ear. Thus, after portions of the inner ear have been selected and removed for the surface specimen technique, the rest of the temporal bone may be put through for routine histological study.

Staining the Surface Preparation

The standard method for examination of the surface preparation, in both human and experimental investigations, has been to post-fix the sample of the membranous labyrinth in osmic acid solution and then to mount and view it microscopically by the phase-contrast or Nomarski method. The following method of staining allows the microscopical examination of the specimen by ordinary light. After a short period of post-fixation in dilute osmic acid solution, the sample is stained by an Alcian blue solution followed by phloxine-eosin counterstain. Hairs (stereocilia), hair cells, supporting cells, pillar cells and nerves are well shown by this method using ordinary light microscopy.

Surgical Specimens

The great majority of surgical biopsy specimens from the ear are small. Many contain some bone and brief decalcification is required. After decalcification, resection specimens of stapes superstructure or of the whole stapes should be oriented for embedding so that the outline of the whole ossicle is revealed in the section; transverse sectioning is unsatisfactory. Care should be taken in orienting any skin or mucosal surface correctly in small biopsies during paraffin embedding so that sections will be cut at right angles to the epithelial surface. This can be carried out by observation with a hand lens or dissecting microscope at the time of embedding. Frozen sections from the ear region require no special handling procedures.

Occasionally larger resection specimens are submitted, usually derived from the surgical treatment of squamous carcinoma of the external and/or middle ear. These include resection of the pinna and deep external canal and "petrosectomy". The latter is far from being a resection of the whole petrous temporal bone, but consists usually of the external canal, tympanic membrane and middle ear contents. The surviving normal anatomical structures should be identified in these specimens and resection margins should be carefully sampled for evidence of tumour extension.

Molecular Techniques

Although soft tissue specimens removed from the ear are fully amenable to modern methods of immunohistochemistry and molecular biology, a start has only just been made on the exploration of the bone-encapsulated tissues of the hearing and balance organ by these methods. There are large numbers of archival temporal bone sections available in many centres; if molecular methods could be adapted to their particular milieu they might

enhance understanding of pathologic processes in this region. The biggest hurdles to be overcome are the prolonged exposure to acid decalcifying agents and the widespread use of celloidin as an embedding medium.

The prolonged acid decalcification which the majority of archival temporal bone sections have undergone may destroy antigens that are tested for by immunohistochemistry.

In one study in which temporal bones were embedded in paraffin wax after decalcification in 10% formic acid, sections showing cells with cytomegalovirus inclusions on haematoxylin and eosin staining did not display the virus antigen on immunohistochemistry.[24] This failure was ascribed to the acid decalcification process. A technique for antigen retrieval in celloidin-embedded human temporal bone sections has recently been described, in which the sections are immersed in a saturated solution of sodium hydroxide in methanol before performing immunohistochemistry. Using this method on sections of temporal bone that had been decalcified in 5% trichloracetic acid, antigens of keratin, vimentin, neurofilament, glial fibrillary acidic protein and desmin intermediate filament proteins[43] and antigen of S-100 protein[44] were successfully demonstrated. The sodium hydroxide method has also been successfully carried out in another centre on acid decalcified celloidin sections of temporal bones for retrieval of the following antigens: CD3, CD43 (T lymphocytes), CD20 (B lymphocytes), CD45 (leucocyte common antigen) and CD68 (macrophages);[45] OPD4 (helper-inducer T cells), CD8 (cytotoxic and suppressor T cells), CD57 (natural killer T cells), CD30 (activated T and B cells), CD15 (granulocytes and monocytes);[46] intercellular adhesion molecule.[47]

Studies have also been carried out in which the effects of celloidin embedding and decalcification on molecular biological methods have been examined. The polymerase chain reaction (PCR) is an extremely sensitive method for augmenting small amounts of DNA and by its use specific DNA fragments have been isolated in decalcified celloidin sections.[48] Using PCR for the detection of *p53* gene DNA in temporal bone sections, we have found that after the use of a variety of decalcifying agents, temporal bone celloidin-embedded sections yield ample amounts of the shorter fragments (gene exon 7: 38 base pairs), but longer fragments (gene exon 8 + 6: 38 base pairs, and gene exon 7–9) were not amplified. EDTA-decalcified temporal bones also provide amplification of longer fragments (gene exon 8 + 6: 320 base pairs), but not gene exon 7–9: 780 base pairs. Although there has been a reduced yield of *p53* gene DNA from acid-decalcified specimens, herpes virus type 1 DNA has been successfully amplified from the geniculate ganglion of an acid-decalcified paraffin-embedded temporal bone of a patient with Bell's palsy.[49]

Although the use of the PCR reaction in particular on archival sections of temporal bone is hopeful for future studies, it seems likely that prospectively planned investigations using optimally processed material from temporal bones may allow more significant results. The temporal bone material in inner ear investigations, for instance, would best be perfused with fixative into the perilymphatic space soon after death (see above) and temporal bone would be subjected to microslicing (see above). Decalcification may be carried out with EDTA solution followed by paraffin embedding. This technique will allow the immunohistochemical identification of many antigens subsequently. To avoid the necessity for decalcification samples of the soft tissues of basilar membrane, stria vascularis, spiral ganglion and eighth nerve, for instance, could be sampled by dissection from the microslices and embedded in paraffin wax. The techniques of immunohistochemistry, in situ hybridization and PCR could then all be applied to the paraffin sections.

References

1. Michaels L, Soucek S. Development of the stratified squamous epithelium of the human tympanic membrane and external canal: the origin of auditory epithelial migration. Am J Anat 1989;184:334–344
2. Michaels L, Soucek S. Stratified squamous epithelium in relation to the tympanic membrane: its development and kinetics. Int J Ped Otolaryngol 1991;22:135–149
3. Michaels L, Soucek S. Auditory epithelial migration: III. Development of the stratified squamous epithelium of the tympanic membrane and external canal in the mouse. Am J Anat 1991;191:280–292
4. Alberti, PW. Epithelial migration on the tympanic membrane. J Laryngol Otol 1964;74:808–830
5. Michaels L, Soucek S. Auditory epithelial migration. II. The existence of two discrete pathways and their embryologic significance. Am J Anat 1990;189:189–200
6. Johnson A, Hawke M, Berger G. Surface wrinkles, cell ridges, and desquamation in the external canal. J Otolaryngol 1984;13:345–354
7. Piza JE, Northrop CC, Eavey RD. Neonatal mesenchyme temporal bone study: typical receding pattern vs increase in Potter's sequence. Laryngoscope 1996;106:856–864
8. Eavey RD. Abnormalities of the neonatal ear: otoscopic observations, histologic observations, and a model for contamination of the middle ear by cellular contents of amniotic fluid. Laryngoscope 1993;103(suppl 58):1–31
9. Michaels L. An epidermoid formation in the developing middle ear; possible source of cholesteatoma. J Otolaryngol 1986;15:169–174
10. Wang R-G, Hawke M, Kwok P. The epidermoid formation (Michaels' structure) in the developing middle ear. J Otolaryngol 1987;16:327–330
11. Michaels L. Evolution of the epidermoid formation and its role in the development of the middle ear and tympanic membrane during the first trimester. J Otolaryngol 1987;17:22–27
12. Lee T-S, Liang J, Michaels L et al. A reinvestigation of the epidermoid formation and its affinity to congenital cholesteatoma. Clin Otolaryngol 1998;23:449–454
13. Levine JL, Wright CG, Pawlowski KS et al. Postnatal persistence of epidermoid rests in the human middle ear. Laryngoscope 1998;108:70–73
14. Michaels L. Origin of congenital cholesteatoma from a normally occurring epidermoid rest in the developing middle ear. Int J Pediatr Otolaryngol 1988;15:51–65
15. McGill TJ, Merchant S, Healy GB et al. Congenital cholesteatoma of the middle ear in children: a clinical and histopathological report. Laryngoscope 1991;101:606–613
16. Frank ST. Aural sign of coronary heart disease. N Engl J Med 1973;289:327–328
17. Overfield T, Call EB. Earlobe type, race and age: effects on earlobe creasing. Am J Geriatr Soc 1983;31:479–481
18. Patel V, Champ C, Andrews PS et al. Diagonal earlobe creases and atheromatous disease: a postmortem study. J R Coll Physicians Lond 1992;26:274–277
19. Tranchesi Jr B, Barbosa V, de Albuquerque CP et al. Diagonal earlobe crease as a marker of the presence and extent of coronary atherosclerosis. Am J Cardiol 1992;70:1417–1420
20. Elliott WJ, Harrison T. Increased all-cause and cardiac morbidity and mortality associated with the diagonal earlobe crease: a prospective cohort study. Am J Med 1991;91:247–254
21. Perry ET. The human ear canal. Charles C Thomas, Springfield, IL, 1957
22. Sade J. The biopathology of secretory otitis media. Ann Otol Rhinol Laryngol 1974;11(suppl):59–70
23. Tos M. Pathogenesis and pathology of chronic secretory otitis media. Ann Otol Laryngol 1980;89(suppl 68):91–97
24. Michaels L, Soucek S, Liang J. The ear in the acquired immunodeficiency syndrome: I. Temporal bone histopathologic study. Amer J Otol 1994;15:515–522
25. Michaels L, Liang J. Structure and origin of middle ear corpuscles. Clin Otolaryngol 1993;18:257–262
26. Bak-Pedersen K. Goblet cell population in the pathological middle ear and Eustachian tube of children and adults. Ann Otol Rhinol Laryngol 1977;86:209–218
27. Aschan G. The Eustachian tube. Histologic findings under normal conditions and in otosalpingitis. Acta Otolaryngol (Stockh) 1954;4:295–311
28. Berger G. Eustachian tube submucosal glands in normal and pathological temporal bones. J Laryngol Otol 1993;107:1099–1105
29. Matsune S, Sando I. Distributions of Eustachian tube goblet cells and glands in children with and without otitis media. Ann Otol Rhinol Laryngol 1992;101:750–754
30. Moreano EH, Paparella MM, Zelterman D et al. Prevalence of carotid canal dehiscence in the human middle ear: a report of 1000 temporal bones. Laryngoscope 1994;104:612–618
31. Michaels L, Wells M. Squamous cell carcinoma of the middle ear. Clin Otolaryngol 1980;5:235–248
32. Bolz EA, Lim DL. Morphology of the stapediovestibular joint. Acta Otolaryngol (Stockh) 1972;73:10–17
33. Glorig A, Davis H. Age, noise and hearing loss. Ann Otol Rhinol Laryngol 1961;70:556–571
34. Etholm B, Belal A. Senile changes in the middle ear joints. Ann Otol Rhinol Laryngol 1974;83:49–54
35. Rauchfuss A. On the endochondral ossification of the otic capsule: formation of the globuli ossei and the interglobular spaces. (In German). Arch Otorhinolaryngol 1981;233:237–250
36. Walsted A, Garbarsch C, Michaels L. Effect of craniotomy and cerebrospinal fluid loss on the inner ear. An experimental study. Acta Otolaryngol (Stockh) 1994;114:626–631

37. Guild SR. The glomus jugulare, a nonchromaffin paraganglion, in man. Ann Otol Rhinol Laryngol 1953;62:1045–1071

38. Sando I, Doyle W, Takahara T et al. How to remove, process, and study the temporal bone with the entire Eustachian tube and its accessory structures: a method for histopathological study. Auris Nasus Larynx 1985;12(suppl 1):21–25

39. Johnsson LG, Hawkins JE. A direct approach to cochlear anatomy and pathology in man. Arch Otolaryngol 1967;85:599–613

40. Michaels L, Wells M, Frohlich A. A new technique for the study of temporal bone pathology. Clin Otolaryngol 1983;8:77–85

41. Iurato S, Bredberg G, Bock G. Functional histopathology of the human audio-vestibular organ. Eurodata hearing project. Commission of the European Communities, 1982

42. Karnovsky MJ. A formaldehyde-glutaraldehyde fixative of high osmolality for use in electron microscopy. J Cell Biol 1965;27:137A–138A

43. Shi S, Tandon AK, Haussmann RR et al. Immunohistochemical study of intermediate filament proteins on routinely processed, celloidin-embedded human temporal bone sections using a new technique for antigen retrieval. Acta Otolaryngol (Stockh) 1993;113:48–54

44. Shi S, Tandon AK, Cot C et al. S-100 protein in human inner ear: use of a novel immunohistochemical technique on routinely processed, celloidin-embedded human temporal bone sections. Laryngoscope 1992;102:734–738

45. Ganbo T, Sando I, Balaban C et al. Immunohistochemistry of lymphocytes and macrophages in human celloidin-embedded temporal bone sections with acute otitis media. Ann Otol Rhinol Laryngol 1997;106:662–668

46. Kamimura M, Balaban CD, Sando I et al. Cellular distribution of mucosa-associated lymphoid tissue with otitis media in children. Ann Otol Rhinol Laryngol 2000;109:467–472

47. Ganbo T, Sando I, Balaban CD et al. Inflammatory response to chronic otitis media in DiGeorge syndrome: a case study using immunohistochemistry on archival temporal bone sections. Ann Otol Rhinol Laryngol 1999;108:756–761

48. Wackym PA, Simpson TA, Gantz BJ et al. Polymerase chain reaction amplification of DNA from archival celloidin-embedded human temporal bone sections. Laryngoscope 1993;103:583–588

49. Burgess RC, Michaels L, Bale JF et al. Polymerase chain reaction amplification of herpes viral DNA from the geniculate ganglion of a patient with Bell's palsy. Ann Otol Rhinol Laryngol 1994;103:775–779

50. Michaels L. Chapter 14. The ear. In: Sternberg SS (ed) Histology for pathologists, 2nd edn. Lippincott–Raven, Philadelphia, 1997, pp 337–366

51. Michaels L. Chapter 80. The ear. In: Damjanov I, Linder J. Anderson's pathology, 10th edn. Mosby Year Book Inc., St. Louis, Missouri, 1996, pp 2876–2900

2 Non-neoplastic Lesions of the External Ear

In this chapter a variety of non-neoplastic conditions will be considered. Inflammation of the middle ear is dealt with separately (see Chapter 3).

Malformations

Malformations of the external ear include:

1. Partial or complete absence of the auricle.
2. Accessory auricles.
3. Preauricular sinus. This usually shows a stratified squamous epithelial lining, but occasionally it may be of respiratory epithelium, deep to which the connective tissue is chronically inflamed (Fig. 2.1). There is often elastic cartilage in the deep wall of the sinus.
4. Atresia of the external auditory meatus, which may present as a blind sac or may be completely absent. Abnormalities of chromosome 18 have been demonstrated in some cases of atresia of the deep external auditory meatus[1,2] and it seems possible that a gene on this chromosome may help to provide the DNA blueprint for the normal maturation of this region. A few cases of atresia of the external canal fall into the category of the oto-branchial renal syndrome (see Chapter 6).
5. Abnormalities of the shape and size of the auricle.

Inflammatory Lesions

The external ear is subject to a wide variety of inflammatory lesions. Some of these are identical with those occurring elsewhere on the skin. Others are specific to or most common in the region of the external ear and only these will be considered here.

Infections

Diffuse External Otitis

Diffuse external otitis is a common condition which affects the external auditory meatus. A variety of organisms, but most commonly *Pseudomonas aeruginosa*, have been recovered from the inflammatory exudate in diffuse external otitis. It is likely that bacterial infection is only one of the causative factors contributing to the lesion. Probably equally significant are a hot, humid environment and local trauma to the ear canal.

The skin of the ear canal is erythematous and oedematous and gives off a greenish discharge. In the severe form of the condition histological examination of the epidermis reveals marked acanthosis, hyperkeratosis and an acute inflammatory exudate in the dermis, particularly around apocrine glands.

Perichondritis

Perichondritis most commonly affects the pinna, where it may follow surgical trauma. As in the diffuse acute inflammation of the ear canal, *Ps. aeruginosa* is the most common infecting organism. Pus accumulates between the perichondrium and cartilage of the pinna. This may interfere with the blood supply of the cartilage and so lead to its necrosis.

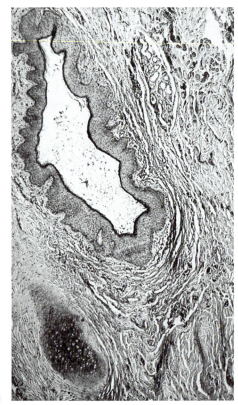

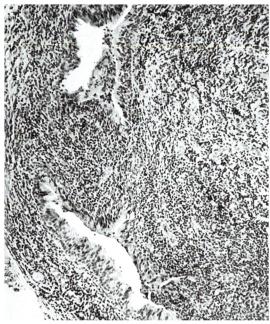

Figure 2.1 Preauricular sinus. **a** In this case the sinus is lined by squamous epithelium and shows sweat glands and elastic cartilage in the underlying connective tissue. **b** Another case in which the sinus is lined by ciliated respiratory epithelium and shows marked chronic inflammation

Malignant Otitis Externa

Malignant otitis externa was first described as a severe infection of the external auditory canal.[3] It usually (but not always[4]) affects elderly diabetics, resulting in unremitting pain, purulent discharge and invasion of cartilage, nerve, bone and adjacent soft tissue. The causative agent in all cases is said to be *Ps. aeruginosa*. The condition frequently goes on to ninth, tenth, eleventh and twelfth cranial nerve palsies, and meningitis and death may result.

Microscopic Appearances

Histopathological changes in the temporal bones of two patients who had been diagnosed clinically as having "malignant otitis externa" and were thought to have died of this condition[5] were those of severe otitis media and osteomyelitis of the jugular foramen secondary to it. In another case in which the temporal bone was examined histologically, evidence of spread of infection was present by way of the submucosal vasculature of the air spaces rather than through the air spaces themselves.[6]

Tissues removed from the deep external canal are often received for pathological examination during surgical attempts to drain the inflammatory process. Necrotic changes of external canal bone, accompanied by osteomyelitis with osteolytic and osteogenic reaction, are observed.

It seems likely that the manifestations of "malignant otitis media" are due to the spread of inflammation from the tympanic cavity and mastoid air spaces to the petrous apex through bone marrow spaces by a process of osteomyelitis[7] (see Chapter 8). The frequency of this condition in elderly patients with diabetes mellitus is probably due to the tendency of diabetics and old people to suffer serious degrees of otitis media. Otitis externa is a common complication of otitis media with perforation of the tympanic membrane, and the inflammation of the external ear may obscure that of the middle ear. The role of *Ps. aeruginosa* is poorly understood. It is a frequent cause of infection in diabetics and commonly infects the external ear (see above). Infection by anaerobic organisms in malignant otitis externa has been discovered in some cases.

Acquired Immunodeficiency Syndrome

In recent years several patients with the acquired immunodeficiency syndrome (AIDS) have been reported to have malignant otitis externa, and in one of them the presence of acute osteomyelitis of the skull base in addition, supported the concept of osteomyelitis as the pathologic basis for malignant otitis externa put forward above.[8]

Non-infectious Inflammatory Lesions

Starch Granuloma

Granulomatous inflammatory lesions due to contamination by corn starch glove powder were often encountered in the peritoneum and pleura after surgery when starch granules were used to powder gloves. Granulomatous inflammatory lesions in reaction to starch granules have also been seen in the ear canal and middle ear.[9] The starch in the latter cases has been derived not from surgical glove powder but from insufflations of antibiotic, in which it is used as a vehicle in the treatment of external or middle ear otitis. Microscopically there is an exudate of histiocytes and lymphocytes. Granules of starch are easily recognised as spherical or polyhedral basophilic bodies, 10–20 μm in diameter, often within histiocytes. The granules show a Maltese cross birefringence and a brilliant red colouration after staining with periodic acid–Schiff reagent.[10]

Hair Granuloma

Biopsy sections taken from inflammatory lesions of the ear canal in surgical or post-mortem temporal bone specimens show quite commonly in the subcutaneous tissue a granulomatous reaction of foreign body type. Within the granuloma foreign body type, giant cells are seen surrounding and engulfing hair shafts (Fig. 2.2). There is usually no middle ear inflammation and the tympanic membrane is intact. The hairs in hair granulomas of the ear canal are derived from the patient's own hair, possibly by ingrowth from those near the orifice of the canal, in the same fashion as occurs in cases of pilonidal sinus of the sacro-iliac skin. In some instances the hair may enter the ear canal after hair-cutting.

Inflammatory Lesions of Unknown Origin

Relapsing Polychondritis

Relapsing polychondritis is a disease characterised by recurring bouts of inflammation affecting cartilaginous structures and the eye. Although the cartilage of the external ear is most frequently involved and that of the nose next in frequency, it is the inflammation with destruction of the cartilages of the respiratory tract, particularly those of the

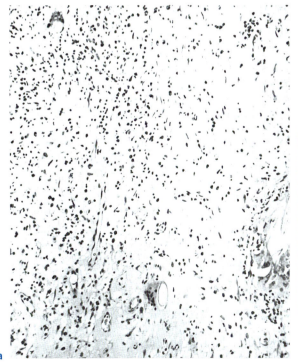

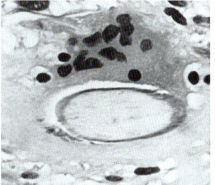

Figure 2.2 Hair shaft granuloma of ear canal. **a** Three hair shafts are present within the chronic inflammatory reaction. **b** Higher power of hair shaft from **a**. Note foreign body type giant cell, which has engulfed the shaft

larynx, which threatens life, and in most cases where death has resulted from the condition it is from respiratory obstruction due to such cartilage damage.

Age and Sex Incidence

Relapsing polychondritis may commence at any age, but 80% of patients have first symptoms between the ages of 20 and 60 years. The incidence is equal between the sexes.

Clinical Features

Presenting symptoms are related to inflammation of a wide variety of cartilages, the various tissues of the eye, and the aortic valve.

The commonest site of the disease is the cartilage of the pinna, which becomes recurrently acutely inflamed (Fig. 2.3). An unexplained conductive or, more rarely, sensorineural deafness and attacks of vertigo may be present. Examination of histologic sections of the temporal bone of a patient with

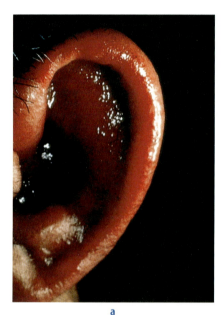

a

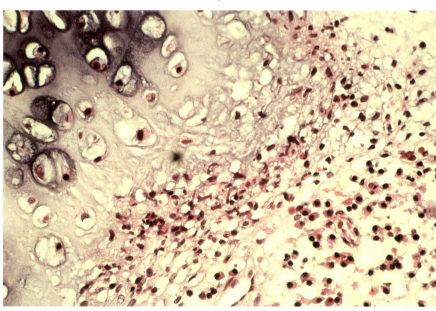

b

Figure 2.3 Relapsing polychondritis. **a** Pinna showing red, swollen ear, produced by inflammation of cartilage. **b** Erosion of cricoid cartilage by inflammatory tissue

relapsing polychondritis and sensorineural hearing loss showed, however, no histologic abnormality of the inner ear (unpublished personal observations). After numerous attacks of inflammation, the pinna shrinks and falls forwards. Inflammation of the joints is usually manifested as transient arthralgia, mainly involving the large joints of the extremities. The nasal cartilages are often affected, and the inflammation of the nasal septum leads to a sinking of this structure, producing a "saddle nose" appearance. Involvement of laryngeal and tracheal cartilages is associated with tenderness over the larynx. Inflammation of the eye usually takes the form of episcleritis or scleritis, but iritis, conjunctivitis or keratitis may also be found in relapsing polychondritis. The affection of the rib cartilages is manifested as tenderness over the ribs anteriorly and the xiphoid process. Heart lesions are characteristically aortic, showing signs of regurgitation. Mitral and tricuspid dilatations are also encountered occasionally in some patients. Features of rheumatoid arthritis, systemic lupus erythematosus, ankylosing spondylitis and Reiter's disease have sometimes been seen coexisting with relapsing polychondritis.[11]

Gross Appearances

The lobule is usually normal. In the acute stage the auricle is erythematous (Fig. 2.3). The anterior surface may have a cobblestone appearance and the auricle may eventually become atrophic.

In the larynx the epiglottic, thyroid and cricoid cartilages show loss of cartilage substance and fibrosis. The result may be a loss of normal cartilaginous support, particularly in the cricoid region, which may lead to laryngeal obstruction.

Microscopic Appearances

The histological appearances suggest a primary affection of cartilage prior to invasion by inflammatory tissue. The ground substance of the cartilage becomes acidophilic (except for basophilia around some surviving lacunae), and shows deeper staining by the periodic acid–Schiff method. In cartilage near the interface with inflammatory tissue there is compression of lacunae, which often appear linear. Focal calcification and dystrophic ossification of the degenerated cartilage have been described.[12] The early inflammatory exudate is composed of neutrophils. Later it is formed mainly by plasma cells and lymphocytes, with some areas of histiocytes. These cells invade the cartilage from the perichondrium. Fibroblasts multiply, and eventually a dense,

poorly cellular scar results. A late stage of the disease is cystic spaces containing gelatinous fluid in the degenerated cartilage.[11]

Immunological Findings

Autoantibodies to type II, IX and XI collagen have been found in cases of relapsing polychondritis.[13,14,15] It is of interest, in view of the frequent occurrence of ocular inflammation in relapsing polychondritis, that type II collagen is a constituent of both eye and cartilage.

Direct tissue studies suggest that relapsing polychondritis may be associated with deposition of immune complexes in the vicinity of chondrocytes,[16] and it has been suggested that direct immunofluorescence may allow a diagnosis of relapsing polychondritis before clinical criteria or routine histologic evaluation suggest a definite diagnosis.[17] Anti-neutrophil cytoplasmic antibodies, usually associated with Wegener's granuloma, have also been found by standard indirect immunofluorescence in occasional cases of relapsing polychondritis.[18]

Keratosis Obturans; Keratosis of the Tympanic Membrane; Keratin Implantation Granuloma

In keratosis obturans the keratin produced by exfoliation from the skin of the tympanic membrane and external canal is retained on the epithelial surface and forms a solid plug. This enlarges and may cause erosion of the bony canal. Cholesterol deposition and secondary infection with *Pseudomonas* sp., *Proteus* sp. or *Staphylococcus aureus* may occur within the keratinous mass.

The conditions labelled keratosis obturans and cholesteatoma of the external auditory meatus have usually been considered to be the same process. It has been suggested, however, that the term keratosis obturans should be preferred for the condition described above, which is usually associated with a thickened tympanic membrane and frequently with chronic sinusitis or bronchiectasis. Cholesteatoma of the external canal, on the other hand, is stated to be a process of localised erosion of the inferior and posterior ear canal wall by a squamous epithelial-lined sac derived from the epidermis of the canal.[19] It seems unlikely, however, that there is any fundamental difference between the two named conditions.

The aetiologic basis of keratosis obturans has been considered to be a defect of the migratory properties of the squamous epithelium of tympanic membrane and adjacent ear canal which causes the accumulation of keratinous debris.

Recent studies of the pattern of auditory epithelial migration in two cases of keratosis obturans showed that this was, indeed, abnormal in each case.[20] A condition of keratosis of the tympanic membrane in which deposits of keratin grow on the eardrum and cause tinnitus has also been found to be associated with absent or defective auditory epithelial migration.[21]

A granulomatous process may result in the external ear canal when keratin squames become implanted into the deeper tissues following traumatic laceration.[22] The granuloma contains foreign body type giant cells, histiocytes, lymphocytes, plasma cells and flakes of keratin. The latter are strongly eosinophilic and birefringent in polarised light. Aural polyps frequently contain such granulomas, but the keratin is then more likely to be derived from a middle ear cholesteatoma (see Chapter 3).

Petrified Auricle

Petrified auricle is an uncommon condition in which the elastic cartilage of the auricle becomes calcified. This may be the result of ectopic calcification caused by local trauma or systemic diseases such as Addison's disease, hypopituitarism, thyroid or parathyroid disorders or radiation therapy. The other form of petrified auricle is ectopic ossification, in which the elastic cartilage is replaced by bone.[23] The latter condition is usually preceded by severe acute hypothermia (frostbite). In neither form of petrified auricle is the cartilage of the superficial external canal affected.

Grossly in both forms the auricle is stony hard and moves as a rigid unit. Microscopically in ectopic ossification the cartilage is replaced by bony trabeculae, which may have haversian canals and marrow spaces.

Metabolic Conditions

Several metabolic conditions may become manifest in the tissues of the ear.

Gout

Gout is manifested both as an acute arthritis which is related to deposits of urates in the joint capsule, most frequently in the big toe joint, and as tophi in non-articular tissues. The external ear is one of the most frequent places for the latter and deposits may occur in the helix and anti-helix. They may ulcerate, discharging a creamy white material, within which needle-like crystals of sodium urate may be detected on microscopy.

Histologically the gouty tophus is composed of basophilic masses of amorphous material surrounded by foreign body giant cells and histiocytes. The sodium urate crystals are soluble in water and so are dissolved in the formaldehyde solution usually used for fixation (Fig. 2.4). For this reason

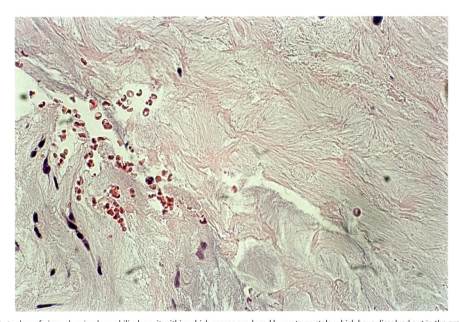

Figure 2.4 Gouty tophus of pinna showing basophilic deposit within which spaces produced by urate crystals, which have dissolved out in the processing, may be observed (Courtesy of Dr. B.Z. Pilch)

fixation in alcohol is preferred when a gouty tophus is suspected. A few crystals may then remain in the basophilic material as brownish, closely packed, needle-like structures which are birefringent.

Ochronosis

Ochronosis (alkaptonuria) is an inherited disease of metabolism in which a step in tyrosine metabolism is disturbed, resulting in accumulation of homogentisic acid in a variety of places, but especially cartilages. The substance is colourless in the urine when first passed, but darkens to a black or brown polymer on standing. The disease is inherited as an autosomal recessive.

In the external ear there may be one or both of two manifestations: (a) dark colour of the wax; when seen in a child this may be the first manifestation of ochronosis; (b) dark colour of the aural cartilage due to the binding of the homogentisic acid to the cartilage ground substance.

Xanthoma Associated with Hyperlipoproteinaemia

Hyperlipoproteinaemia is classified into types I–IV, depending upon which fraction of lipoprotein is prominent on electrophoretic fractionation of the plasma. All of the hyperlipoproteinaemic conditions are transmitted by inheritance on a dominant or recessive basis. Some are associated with cutaneous and tendinous xanthomas and severe atherosclerotic coronary artery disease. In rare cases, deposits of lipid with an associated histiocytic reaction may be found infiltrating bone trabeculae and marrow spaces of the mastoid.[24]

The appearances are similar to those of cholesterol granuloma (see Chapter 3), except that there is no trace of haemorrhage or hemosiderin, foam cells are more numerous than usual in cholesterol granuloma and the lipid deposits and their cellular reaction mainly involve the bone itself and not the mucosa of the mastoid air cells[25] (Fig. 2.5).

Lesions Simulating Neoplasms

A variety of lesions may be found in the external and middle ears that may show some similarity to neoplasms.

Malakoplakia

Malakoplakia is a chronic inflammatory condition characterised by accumulation of macrophages and

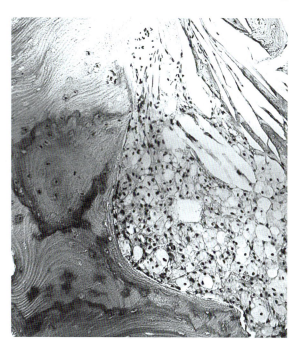

Figure 2.5 Xanthomatous deposit in mastoid associated with type V hyperlipoproteinaemia. Marrow spaces and bone trabeculae are infiltrated by foam cells and cholesterol clefts, the latter accompanied by a foreign body type giant cell reaction

the presence of characteristic microscopic lamellated structures (see below). The lesion may be confused with neoplasm. This lesion may affect the external canal with involvement also of the tympanic cavity and mastoid.[26,27] Microscopic examination shows macrophages with abundant cytoplasm containing diastase-resistant, PAS-positive granules (von Hansemann cells). Lamellated, calcified (Michaelis-Gutmann) bodies, often within macrophages, are also frequently present (Fig. 2.6).

Malakoplakia is usually associated with a coliform infection and a defective response to phagocytised *Escherichia coli* has been identified in that condition. It is possible that malakoplakia may be commoner in the middle and external ears than would appear by the few case reports that have been published, since otologists frequently do not submit material for histological examination from chronic inflammatory conditions of the ear.

Chondrodermatitis Nodularis Chronica Helicis

In chondrodermatitis nodularis chronica helicis, sometimes known as Winkler's disease,[28] a small nodule forms on the auricle, usually in the superior portion of the helix. About 70% of the patients are males.[29] The lesion is found in middle-aged or older patients. Pain is often a prominent feature.

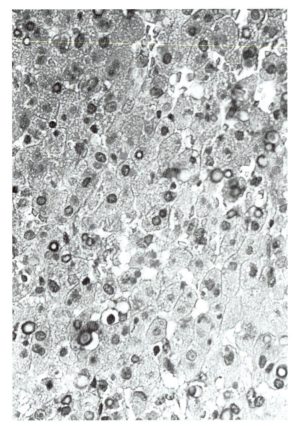

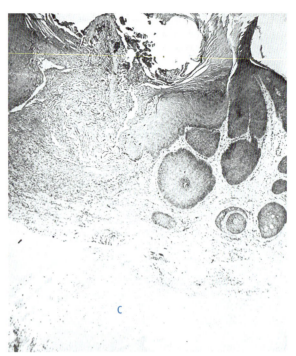

Figure 2.7 Chondrodermatitis nodularis chronica helicis. There is an irregular acanthosis at the margins of an ulcer, the crater of which is occupied by necrotic eosinophilic material. Inflammation extends down into the cartilage of the pinna

Figure 2.6 Malakoplakia of the middle ear. The tissue is composed of macrophages with abundant granular cytoplasm. Note also numerous calcified Michaelis-Gutmann bodies, often within macrophages

Histologically the nodule usually shows ulceration with marked irregular acanthosis at its margins. The collagen in the centre shows increased eosinophilia, is often degenerated, and is surrounded by chronic inflammatory granulation tissue. The perichondrium adjacent to the lesion is usually involved by the inflammatory tissue and the elastic cartilage of the auricle is also often degenerated (Fig. 2.7). There is evidence that the lesion may evolve from inflammation of the infundibular portion of local hair follicles.[30] It seems most likely that chondrodermatitis nodularis is related to poor blood supply at the periphery of the auricle and in the opinion of Winkler[28] there was an association with frostbite; this opinion is still commonly held by many, although some published reports do not support it.[29] An association with the limited form of systemic sclerosis has been described.[31]

Spectacle Frame Acanthoma (Granuloma Fissuratum)

Spectacle frame acanthoma occurs behind the ear in the region of the postauricular groove, where it is commonly mistaken for basal cell carcinoma at clinical examination. A similar reaction may occur on the bridge of the nose or above the malar area. The cause is irritation by the frame of spectacles. Grossly there is a raised pink nodule with a linear depression running through its centre. The spectacle frame usually fits exactly into the depression when in its usual position.[32,33] Histologically there is acanthosis and chronic inflammation of the dermis. A shallow sulcus may be seen at the centre of the specimen containing keratin and parakeratotic material (Fig. 2.8).

The acanthoma is readily treated by making appropriate alterations in the shape of the spectacle frame so that it no longer presses into the skin.

Epithelioid Haemangioma and Kimura's Disease

Synonyms for epithelioid haemangioma are benign angiomatous nodules of face and scalp, atypical pyogenic granuloma, angiolymphoid hyperplasia with eosinophilia and several other terms. Although this entity was first described by Kimura, "Kimura's disease" is now believed to be a different condition.

Benign angiomatous nodules may occur anywhere in the skin, especially on the scalp and face, but there is a particular predilection for the external

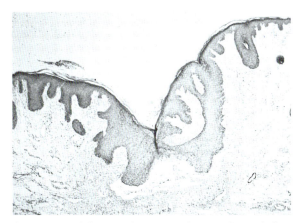

Figure 2.8 Spectacle frame acanthoma. Note moderate acanthosis and inflammation of dermis. There is a sulcus in the epidermis produced by the spectacle frame

auricle and external auditory meatus. It is a lesion of young and middle-aged of both sexes and all races.

Grossly there are sessile or plaque-like red or reddish-blue lesions from 2 to 10 mm in diameter, which may coalesce to form large plaques that obstruct the ear canal. On transection the lesion is seen to be present in the dermis and subcutaneous tissue. Microscopically there is a mixture of two proliferated elements in the dermis: blood vessels and lymphoid tissue. The blood vessels are mainly capillaries lined by plump, often protruding (hobnailed), sometimes multilayered, endothelial cells (Fig. 2.9). Occasionally an artery or vein showing intimal fibrous thickening is part of the vascular component. Solid clusters of cells, which are often vacuolated and show features intermediate between endothelial cells and histiocytes, are also observed.[34] The lymphoid tissue may possess germinal centres. Eosinophils (often extremely numerous), mast cells and macrophages may also be prominent.

Kimura's disease is more common in Orientals, mainly affecting young males. It involves the subcutaneous and deep soft tissues; lymph nodes are frequently affected.

Microscopically in Kimura's disease the main lesion is the lymphoid hyperplasia. Vascular proliferation is not marked, comprising mainly high endothelial venules in the lymphoid tissue.[35] A comparison of epithelioid haemangioma with Kimura's disease using lymphocyte markers showed T-cell lymphoid aggregates with well-formed B-cell germinal centres in Kimura's, and nodular and diffuse T-cell infiltration with small B-cell clusters in epithelioid haemangioma.[36]

Both epithelioid haemangioma and Kimura's disease are benign entities. Recurrence is rare in the former if it is completely excised. It is more frequent in the latter, but eventually becomes stationary. A nephrotic syndrome may rarely occur in Kimura's disease.

Idiopathic Cystic Chondromalacia (Pseudocysts)

Idiopathic cystic chondromalacia (pseudocysts) is an unusual lesion of the cartilage of the auricle.[37,38] It occurs mainly in young and middle-aged adults. The gross appearance is one of a localised swelling of the auricular cartilage. Cut surface shows a well-

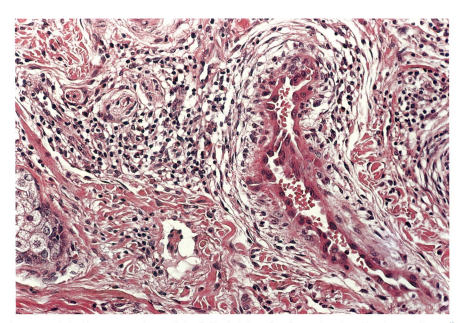

Figure 2.9 Epithelioid haemangioma showing "hobnailed" endothelium of capillary on the right and lymphocytic infiltration[41]

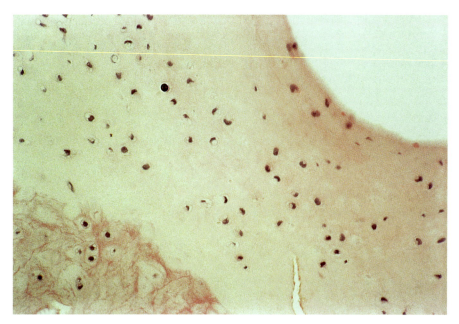

Figure 2.10 Idiopathic cystic chondromalacia of cartilage of auricle. Note the cystic cavity in the cartilage lined by normal cartilage[41]

defined cystic cavity in the cartilage, which is distended with yellowish watery fluid. Microscopically the cyst is a simple space with a lining of normal cartilage[39] (Fig. 2.10). Its association with severe atopic eczema in four children[40] suggested that minor trauma from repeated rubbing of the auricle may play a part. Simple curettage will eliminate the lesion.

Keloid

Keloid, a common benign skin lesion, follows injury to the skin of the ear, often after piercing the earlobes for wearing an ear-ring, particularly in black people. Grossly there is a lobulated swelling covered by normal skin. Microscopically the dermis is enlarged by deposits of eosinophilic, poorly cellular collagen.

References

1. Chrobok V, Simakova E. Temporal bone findings in trisomy 18 and 21 syndromes. Eur Arch Otorhinolaryngol 1997;254:15–18
2. Schinzel A, Hayashi K, Schmid W. Structural aberrations of chromosome 18. II. The 18q-syndrome. Report of three cases. Humangenetik 1975;26:123–132
3. Chandler JR . Malignant external otitis. Laryngoscope 1968;78:1257–1294
4. Shpitzer T, Stern Y, Cohen O et al. Malignant external otitis in nondiabetic patients. Ann Otol Rhinol Laryngol 1993;102:870–872
5. Wells M, Michaels L. "Malignant otitis externa": a manifestation of chronic otitis media with complications? Clin Otolaryngol 1984:9:131(abstract)
6. Kohut RI, Lindsay JR. Necrotizing ("malignant") external otitis histopathologic processes. Ann Otol Rhinol Laryngol 1979;88:714–720
7. Ostfeld E, Segal M, Czernobilsky B. External otitis: early histopathologic changes and pathogenic mechanism. Laryngoscope 1982;91:965–970
8. Weinroth SE, Schessel D, Tuazon CU. Malignant otitis externa in AIDS patients: case report and review of the literature. Ear, Nose & Throat J 1992;73:772–774
9. Rock EH. Surgeon's glove powder (starch) middle ear granuloma. Arch Otolaryngol 1967;86:8–17
10. Michaels L, Shah N. Dangers of corn starch powder (letter). Br Med J 1973;2:714
11. Hughes RA, Berry CL, Seifert M et al. Relapsing polychondritis. Three cases with a clinicopathological study and literature review. Q J Med 1972;41:363–380
12. Verity MA, Larson WM, Madden SC. Relapsing polychondritis. Report of two necropsied cases with histochemical investigation of the cartilage lesion. Am J Pathol 1963;42:251–269
13. Anstey A, Mayou S, Morgan K et al. Relapsing polychondritis: autoimmunity to type II collagen and treatment with cyclosporin A. Br J Dermatol 1991;125:588–591
14. Joliat T, Seyer J, Bernstein J et al. Antibodies against a 30 kilodalton cochlear protein and type II and IX collagens in the serum of patients with inner ear diseases. Ann Otol Rhinol Laryngol 1992;101:1000–1006
15. Yang CL, Brinckmann J, Rui HF et al. Autoantibodies to cartilage collagens in relapsing polychondritis. Arch Dermatol Res 1993;285:245–249
16. Valenzuela R, Cooperrider PA, Gogate P et al. Immunomicroscopic findings in cartilage of ear biopsy specimens. Hum Pathol 1980;11:19–22
17. Helm TN, Valenzuela R, Glanz S et al. Relapsing polychondritis: a case diagnosed by direct immunofluorescence and coexisting with pseudocyst of the auricle. J Am Acad Dermatol 1992;26:315–318

18. Geffriaud-Ricouard C, Noel LH, Chauveau D et al. Clinical spectrum associated with ANCA of defined antigen specificities in 98 selected patients. Clin Nephrol 1993;39:125–136

19. Piepergerdes JC, Kramer BM, Behnke EE. Keratosis obturans and external auditory canal cholesteatoma. Laryngoscope 1980;90:383–390

20. Corbridge RJ, Michaels L, Wright A. Epithelial migration in keratosis obturans. Am J Otolaryngol 1996;17:411–414

21. Soucek S, Michaels L. Keratosis of the tympanic membrane and deep external canal: a defect of auditory epithelial migration. Eur Arch Oto-rhino-laryngol 1993;250:140–142

22. Hawke M, Jahn AF. Keratin implantation granuloma in external ear canal. Arch Otolaryngol 1974;100:317–318

23. DiBartolomeo JR. The petrified auricle: comments on ossification, calcification and exostoses of the external ear. Laryngoscope 1985;95:566–576

24. Koch HJ, Lewis JJ. Hyperlipemic xanthomatosis with associated osseous granulomas. A clinical report. N Engl J Med 1956;255:387–393

25. Emery PS, Gore M. An extensive solitary xanthoma of the temporal bone associated with hyperlipoproteinaemia. J Laryngol Otol 1982;96:451–457

26. Azadeh B, Ardehali S. Malakoplakia of middle ear: a case report. Histopathology 1983;7:129–134

27. Azadeh B, Dabiri S, Mosfegh M. Malacoplakia of the middle-ear. Histopathology 1991;19:276–278

28. Winkler M. Knotchenformige Erkrankung am Helix (Chondermatitis Nodularis Chronica Helicis). Arch Dermatol Syph 1915;12:278–285

29. Metzger SA, Goodman ML. Chondermatitis helicis. A clinical re-evaluation and pathological review. Laryngoscope 1976;86:1402–1412

30. Hurwitz RM. Painful papule of the ear: a follicular disorder. J Dermatol Surg Oncol 1987;13:270–274

31. Bottomley WW, Goodfield MD. Chondrodermatitis nodularis helicis occurring with systemic sclerosis – an under-reported association? Clin Exp Dermatol 1994;19:219–220

32. Barnes HM, Calman CD, Sarkany I. Spectacle frame acanthoma (granuloma fissuratum). Trans St. John's Hosp Dermatol Soc 1974;60:99–102

33. Tennstedt D, Lachapelle JM. Acanthome fissure. Revue de la litterature et diagnostic histopathologique differentiel avec le nodulc douloureux de l'oreille. Ann Dermatol Venereol 1979;106:219–225

34. Barnes L, Koss W, Nieland ML. Angiolymphoid hyperplasia: a disease that may be confused with malignancy. Head & Neck Surg 1980;2:425–434

35. Chan Jk, Hui Pk, Ng CS et al. Epithelioid haemangioma (angiolymphoid hyperplasia with eosinophilia) and Kimura's disease in Chinese. Histopathol 1989;15:557–574

36. Helander SD, Peters MS, Kuo TT et al. Kimura's disease and angiolymphoid hyperplasia with eosinophilia – new observations from immunohistochemical studies of lymphocyte markers, endothelial antigens, and granulocyte proteins. J Cutaneous Pathol 1995;22:319–326

37. Hansen JE. Pseudocysts of the auricle in Caucasians. Arch Otolaryngol 1967;l85:1314

38. Santos VB, Pilisar IA, Ruffy ML. Bilateral pseudocysts in a female. Ann Otol Rhinol Laryngol 1974;83:911

39. Heffner DK, Hyams VJ. Cystic chondromalacia (enchondral pseudocysts of the auricle). Arch Pathol Lab Med 1986;110:740–743

40. Devlin J, Harrison CJ, Whitby DJ et al. Cartilaginous pseudocyst of the external auricle in children with atopic eczema. Br J Dermatol 1990;122:699–704

41. Michaels L. Chapter 80. The ear. In: Damjanov I, Linder J. Anderson's pathology, 10th edn. Mosby Year Book Inc., St. Louis, Missouri, 1996, pp 2876–2900

3 Otitis Media

Infection of the middle ear causes not only generally known inflammatory changes but also others peculiar to the site. Otitis media is one of the most common of all diseases, particularly in young children. The clinical forms of the acute and chronic conditions correspond to the pathological changes, but intermediate or mixed states are frequent. Perforation of the tympanic membrane may occur at any phase of otitis media, but an effusion is often present behind an intact tympanic membrane. It is important that an advanced degree of otitis media may exist, but may remain undetected clinically and even be undetectable.[1]

Microbiology

In the acute phase, *Streptococcus pneumoniae* and *Haemophilus influenzae* are the most common causative organisms. *Staphylococcus aureus* and *Streptococcus pyogenes* are also causative in a lesser number.[2] Anerobic organisms, notably *Propionibacterium acnes* and *Peptococcus* have been seen in significant numbers.[3] Epidemiological studies have indicated that the respiratory viruses, influenza viruses A and B, enterovirus, rhinovirus, parainfluenza virus, adenovirus, and respiratory syncytial virus, may be agents in the early phases of the illness.[4,5,6] In the chronic phase, Gram-negative organisms, particularly *Proteus* and *Pseudomonas* are found, although *Staphylococcus pyogenes* and beta-haemolytic streptococci are sometimes isolated from the discharging pus of chronically inflamed ears. Anaerobes may sometimes be isolated, including anaerobic Gram-positive cocci, *Bacteroides* sp. and *Clostridium* sp.[1]

Although much less frequent than the above organisms, *Mycobacterium tuberculosis* may be the causative agent of chronic inflammation of the middle ear. In such cases the inflammatory reaction is quite distinct (see below).

General Pathological Changes
(Table 3.1)

Not only is the acute phase of otitis media characterised by severe congestion of the mucosa of the middle ear and the tympanic membrane, but a similar change is also present in chronic otitis media. The exudation of blood products may leave a

Table 3.1. Pathological processes in otitis media

Process	Cell or tissue	Pathological change
Congestion Exudation	Plasma	Serous otitis media
	Histiocytes, lymphocytes, plasma cells	Chronic inflammation
	Red cells	Haemorrhage Cholesterol granuloma
Proliferation	Columnar epithelium	Glandular change
	Squamous cell epithelium	Cholesteatome
	Blood vessels, fibroblasts, mononuclear cells	Granulation tissue
	Fibroblasts, collagen	Adhesive otitis Tympanosclerosis
	Bone	Woven and lamellar bone formation
Necrosis	Tympanic membrane	Perforation
	Bone	Rarefying osteitis

deposit of fibrin in the tissues or in the tympanic and mastoid air cell cavities. A fluid or gelatinous exudate in the middle ear cavity is frequently a prominent component of the inflammatory reaction, giving rise to a specific form of the disease known as otitis media with effusion (serous otitis media or glue ear). In these cases mucus may be secreted by newly formed glands in the middle ear mucosa and contribute to the fluid "exudate".

In acute inflammation neutrophils are prevalent. It is likely that the immigration of these cells is mediated by the local production of cytokines, such as interleukin-1, interleukin-2 or tumour necrosis factor.[7] In chronic inflammation, histiocytes, lymphocytes and plasma cells are the characteristic infiltrate. There is evidence that cytokine production is also present in the chronic phase of otitis media. The amount of interleukin-1 has been correlated with the early stages of chronic otitis media, while that of tumour necrosis factor has been correlated with persistence of disease.[8]

Organisms are rarely seen in routinely stained histological sections of acute or chronic inflammation of the middle ear. In newborn infants an inflammatory reaction may be the result of the contamination of the middle ear by inhaled amniotic squames (see below and Chapter 6). In these cases the histiocytes reacting to the foreign material fuse to form giant cells.

Haemorrhage is a common result of the congestion of otitis media. It may lead to cholesterol granuloma (see below).

Local tissue cells frequently react to the inflammatory process by dissolution or proliferation. Necrosis may occur, as is characteristic of perforation of the tympanic membrane or rarefying osteitis of the ossicles. Several factors may produce the necrosis. It is likely that rupture of the tympanic membrane takes place as a result of ischaemic necrosis caused by pressure at a focal point. Ossicular loss may, on the other hand, be caused by cytokine substances such as tumour necrosis factor-alpha.[8,9]

At the same time as the process of necrosis, proliferative activity of middle ear tissue occurs and may represent an important part of the pathological picture. The columnar epithelium of the middle ear has, in the presence of inflammation, the remarkable property of invaginating itself to produce glands, which often develop luminal secretion. The glandular transformation of the middle ear mucosa may be seen in any part of the cleft, including the mastoid ear cells. The secretion of the glands contributes to the exudate in otitis media with effusion. Fibrous tissue proliferation may also occur in combination with glandular transformation – a process which, in the advanced state, has been called "fibrocystic scler-osis". Squamous cell epithelium may likewise proliferate in the middle ear – a process known as cholesteatoma. A specific form of reparative reaction following inflammation is the development of granulation tissue. In this process the endothelium of blood vessels and fibroblasts are the newly formed cells. Mononuclear inflammatory cells usually accompany the latter. Fibroblasts and collagen are abundant in the terminal phase of the reparative stage. A normal degree of cellularity in the fibrous reaction is seen in adhesive otitis. A peculiar form of scar tissue production occurs in the middle ear, in which the collagen is poorly cellular and hyalinised. This condition, known as tympanosclerosis, is characterised also by deposition of calcium salts in the hyaline fibrous tissue. The bony walls of the middle ear frequently react to the inflammatory process by a new formation of bone. This is woven in the early stages and lamellar later.

Acute Otitis Media

Incidence and Clinical Features

The incidence of acute otitis media as seen in hospital practice in developed countries has declined over the past 25 years because of the ready availability of antibiotics and improved socio-economic conditions. Children are more often affected than adults.

The clinical features are general signs of infection, pain, particularly in the mastoid area, tenderness and swelling in the post-auricular region and oedema of the posterosuperior wall of the external auditory meatus. The tympanic membrane is initially hyperaemic and then bulges as more pus collects in the middle ear, until eventually it may burst.

Pathological Appearances

The appearances of the middle ear mucosa as seen in the bone chips removed at mastoidectomy indicate congestion and oedema of the mucosa of the mastoid air cells. Haemorrhage may be severe and the mucosa and air cells are filled with neutrophils. Pus destroys bone, the actual dissolution being carried out by osteoclasts. At the same time new bone formation takes place, commencing as osteoid, later becoming woven and finally lamellar. Fibrosis may also be active even in the acute stage.

Acute inflammatory changes are also prominent in other parts of the middle ear. The tympanic membrane shows marked congestion, the dilated vessels distending the connective tissue layer. Pus cells fill the middle ear cavity. The acute inflammation may spread deep into the temporal bone as osteomyelitis.

Chronic Otitis Media

Clinical Features

The inflammation, while often indolent, may at times give rise to serious complications and even cause death. The hearing loss that is a constant concomitant also contributes to the immense socioeconomic problem. Chronic otitis media sometimes, but not always, follows an attack of the acute disease.

The major feature is discharge from the middle ear. Sometimes polyps may occlude the external auditory meatus. The tympanic membrane is usually perforated in the pars tensa.

Gross Appearances

There has been little study of the gross appearances of chronic otitis media, except at surgery when the examination of the middle ear cleft is limited to the operative field. With the use of the microslicing method (see Chapter 1) a more complete gross examination of the whole middle ear may be carried out at post-mortem. An important feature of chronic otitis media is the variation in the degree and extent of the inflammation. The tubotympanic region is the most frequently involved and mastoid air cells are also often affected. Mucopurulent material often fills the middle ear space in the tubotympanic region and may also be seen within mastoid air cells. In the inflamed regions the mucosa is thickened and congestion may be severe. Granulation tissue formation may be extensive, showing as red thickened areas particularly on the promontory, in the epitympanum, in the round and oval window niches and in the mastoid. The granulation tissue on the promontory mucosa may be of sufficient thickness to protrude through the perforation in the tympanic membrane. Such a lesion is the common aural polyp presenting clinically in the ear canal.

A variable degree of loss of ossicular bone may be observed. The most frequently affected ossicle is the incus, particularly in the region of its long process, but dissolution of other ossicles may also occur.

In post-mortem temporal bones with chronic otitis media, large cavities are sometimes visible in the mastoid region. These are the results of operations to remove infected parts of the mastoid to drain the middle ear cleft.

Yellow localised areas seen anywhere in the middle ear cleft are regions of cholesterol granu-

loma and pearly white patches particularly in the attic are likely to be cholesteatomas, which are frequently present in association with chronic otitis media (see below).

Microscopic Appearances

The most characteristic feature of the pathology of chronic otitis media is the presence of inflammatory granulation tissue. This cellular reaction has two components. On the one hand there is the presence of lymphocytes, plasma cells and macrophages. On the other hand there is granulation tissue, constituted by newly formed capillaries and by fibroblasts. Granulation tissue formation takes place in the early stages of healing after the inflammatory destruction of tissue. Chronic inflammatory leucocytes and granulation tissue may be found in the middle ear in chronic otitis media independently of each other. The two forms of cellular reaction are seen together in aural polyps. This lesion is frequently subjected to biopsy in the investigation of cases of chronic otitis media. The polyp is usually covered by columnar epithelium, which is often ciliated (Fig. 3.1). Sometimes the epithelium is squamous. This may be produced by metaplasia in the middle ear or by irritation of the polyp when it reaches the ear canal. The core of the polyp is made up of chronic inflammatory granulation tissue.

Using a whole mount method, in which the entire middle ear mucosa is removed and stained with PAS-Alcian blue, in chronic otitis the numbers of goblet cells were found to be greatly increased to a level similar to those in other parts of the respiratory tract.[10,11]

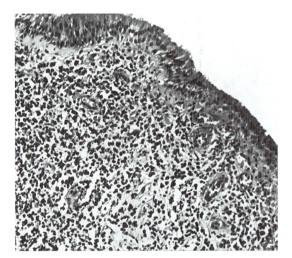

Figure 3.1 Aural polyp composed of chronic inflammatory granulation tissue and lined by columnar epithelium, which is partially ciliated

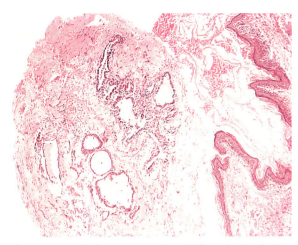

Figure 3.2 Biopsy of inflammatory tissue from middle ear showing glandular transformation. Note strand of cholesteatoma on right

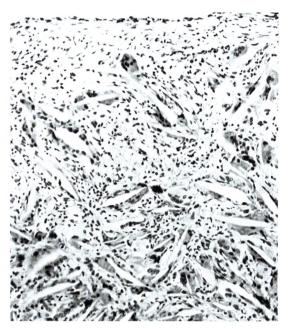

Figure 3.3 Cholesterol granuloma of middle ear. The lesion is composed of cholesterol clefts surrounded by foreign body type giant cells and other chronic inflammatory cells

Under conditions of chronic inflammation, however, the middle ear epithelium comes to resemble the rest of the respiratory tract by the formation of glands. They consist usually of simple tubules of mucus-producing cells (Fig. 3.2). Gland formation is particularly active in children with secretory otitis media. Glandular transformation may take place in the mastoid air cells as well as the main middle ear cavity. The secretion derived from the glands is an important component of the aural discharge in chronic otitis media.

The mastoid air cells show fibrosis and their bony walls are markedly thickened. Cement lines in the lamellar bone are numerous and irregular, often forming a mosaic pattern. This indicates the recent active deposition and resorption of bone as a result of the inflammatory process. The product of these reparative processes in the mastoid is a patchy sclerosis with some cystic cavities representing distended air cells. The obliteration of mastoid air cells as a result of chronic otitis is referred to as secondary sclerosis.

In some ears the mastoid air cells lack pneumatisation from an early age. This has been ascribed to inflammatory change, but such an interpretation has been doubted by others who have regarded the sclerosis as primary, perhaps due to genetic factors.[12] The appearance of the mastoid in primary arrest of pneumatisation is said to be unlike that following otitis media, in that in the former the mastoid air cell system is small and the bone is diffusely sclerotic.

Cholesterol Granuloma

Yellow nodules are found in the tympanic cavity and mastoid in many cases of chronic otitis media. These are composed microscopically of cholesterol crystals (dissolved away to leave empty clefts in paraffin-embedded histological sections) surrounded by foreign body type giant cells and other chronic inflammatory cells (Fig. 3.3). Such cholesterol granulomas are almost always found in the midst of haemorrhage in the middle ear mucosa. Hemosiderin is often present among the cells surrounding the cholesterol granuloma. Cholesterol granuloma in the mastoid air cells must be distinguished from lipid deposits of hypercholesterolaemic xanthomatosis (see Chapter 2).

Pathogenesis

The lipid in cholesterol granulomas of the middle ear has been found to be mainly cholesterol with only very small amounts of cholesterol esters. In serum the reverse is the case: a high proportion of cholesterol ester is present, but little cholesterol.[13] These findings are compatible with an origin of the lipid material in cholesterol granuloma from red cell membranes, in which cholesterol exists mainly in the free, not esterified state.

Tympanosclerosis

Tympanosclerosis is a special form of fibrosis, which is often encountered in chronic otitis media.

Deposits of dense white tissue are laid down in the middle ear mucosa, not only on the tympanic side of the tympanic membrane, which is particularly likely to occur in otitis media with effusion, but also, following chronic suppurative otitis media, on the crura of the stapes, within the tympanic cavity and sometimes in the mastoid. On dissection, the tympanosclerotic deposit may show a lamellated onion-skin-like structure.

Microscopically the material is composed of hyaline collagen deposited in the mucosa. The collagen stains with acid aniline dyes and is birefringent. Deposits of calcium salts, appearing as basophilic dust-like areas, are irregularly distributed through the collagen. A multilayered structure corresponding to the gross appearance of lamellation is frequently observed. Bone is also often present in tympanosclerotic plaques (Fig. 3.4).

Ultrastructurally the tympanosclerotic plaque shows degeneration of collagen and reticulin fibrils with calcified deposits of electron-dense material of spindle or spherical shape in the areas of degeneration. The calcium salts appear as crystalline formations. Tympanosclerosis, although the result of otitis media, is not an ordinary form of fibrous tissue reaction, but resembles the type of collagen deposition seen in the silicotic nodules of the lung and leiomyomas of the uterus. There may be an autoimmune factor in its development, which leads to degeneration of collagen. This is possibly enhanced by trauma, as in the use of ventilating tubes, which have been observed to lead to the development of tympanosclerosis of the tympanic membrane in 11% of the patients in which they are used.[14]

Cholesteatoma

Cholesteatoma is an important concomitant of many cases of chronic otitis media. It is a mass of keratin produced by a layer of stratified squamous epithelium within the middle ear cavity. The term cholesteatoma is an unfortunate one, because the entity it designates bears no relation to either cholesterol granuloma or to a neoplasm. Since the term is so well established and the pathology and natural history of the disease are now well understood, it would present much difficulty (and is probably unnecessary) to change it.

It has now become apparent that there exists a congenital or primary form of cholesteatoma, which is present behind an intact tympanic membrane, that is quite distinct from an acquired form, in which there is a perforation of the tympanic membrane. The term congenital cholesteatoma is also applied to a squamous epithelial cyst arising at the petrous apex of the temporal bone, which causes damage by erosion of the skull (see Chapter 11). This is quite a different entity from the middle ear cholesteatoma. In the following account only the form in the tympanic cavity behind an intact tympanic membrane will be considered.

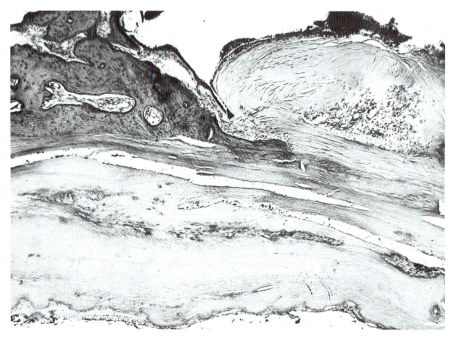

Figure 3.4 Tympanosclerotic plaque of middle ear mucosa. Layers of hyaline poorly cellular collagen thicken the mucosa. *Darker areas* (basophilic in the original) represent zones of calcification. An area of ossification is seen in the *top left*

Both aquired and congenital cholesteatoma may take one or other of the two classical forms presented in the older literature: (1) a closed, keratinous cyst or (2) an open lesion comprising multiple layers of keratinous squames, which is carpeted by cholesteatoma matrix that covers part of the middle ear surface.[15,16] In most cases of acquired cholesteatoma the lesion is open. Most cases of congenital cholesteatoma, on the other hand, are described as being in the first category, presenting as a simple closed cyst.

Acquired Cholesteatoma

Clinical Features

A small cholesteatoma may be present with normal hearing and no discharge. Typically, however, there is a foul-smelling discharge and conductive hearing loss. On examination of the tympanic membrane there is, in most cases, a perforation of the superior or posterosuperior margin.

Gross Appearances

The cholesteatoma appears as a pearly grey or pale-yellow cyst-like structure in the middle ear cavity (Fig. 3.5). The wall of the cyst may often be seen as a thin membrane.

The cholesteatoma is usually situated in the upper part of the middle ear cleft and discharges usually through a perforation of the pars flaccida of the tympanic membrane, sometimes through a perforation located at the edge of the tympanic membrane near the annulus. The cholesteatoma may extend

through the aditus into the mastoid antrum and mastoid air cells. Frequently the outline of the cholesteatomatous sac is adapted to that of normal structures such as ossicles. Chronic inflammatory changes are always present. In most cases at least one ossicle is seriously damaged, so interrupting the continuity of the ossicular chain. The scutum, the upper part of the bony ring of the tympanic opening, is eroded in most cholesteatomas.

Microscopic Appearances

Under the microscope the pearly material of the cholesteatoma consists of dead, fully differentiated anucleate keratin squames. This is the corneal layer of the squamous cell epithelium. Sometimes biopsy material shows only squames when the so-called capsule has not been excised. This capsule, often called the matrix, is composed of fully differentiated squamous epithelium similar to the epidermis of skin, and resting on connective tissue. As in any normal stratified epithelium there are one to three basal layers of cells above which is a prickle (malpighian or spinous) layer composed of five or six rows of cells with intercellular bridges (Fig. 3.6). The deeper layers of the epithelium of the cholesteatoma matrix frequently show evidence of activity in the form of downgrowths into the underlying connective tissue (Fig. 3.7). These often separate the cholesteatoma into lobules. A thin granular layer lies between the malpighian layer and the extensive corneal layer.

The eroded ossicles may be invested by the squamous epithelial wall of the sac. There is always, even in these circumstances, a layer of granulation tissue in contact with the bone and it seems likely that it is the chronic inflammatory covering, not the squamous epithelium, that produces the erosion.

Pathogenesis

Four concepts of the pathogenesis of acquired cholesteatoma have been put forward. It has been suggested that it may arise:

1. From invasion of canal and tympanic membrane epithelium into the middle ear.
2. From invagination of tympanic membrane in the form of a retraction pocket.
3. From metaplasia of the epithelia of the middle ear.
4. From trauma such as blast injury or insertion of ventilation tubes into the eardrum.

There is evidence to favour (1), (2) and (4) and it is likely that cholesteatoma may arise as a

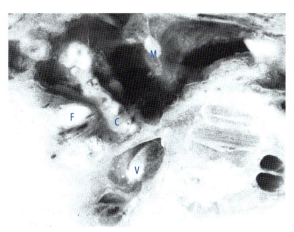

Figure 3.5 Microsliced temporal bone showing cholesteatoma sac (*C*), which is situated in posterior wall of the middle ear. *F*, facial nerve; *M*, handle of malleus; *V*, vestibule

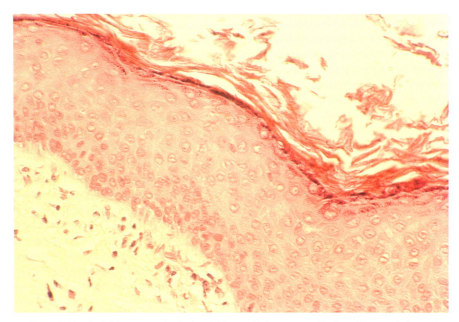

Figure 3.6 Acquired cholesteatoma showing keratinising stratified squamous epithelium with a granular layer

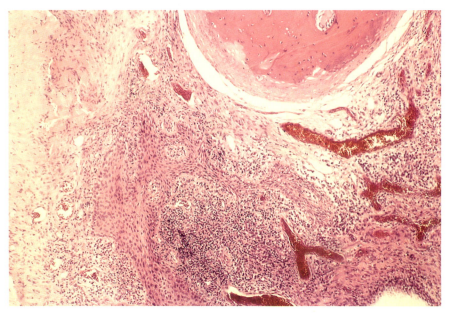

Figure 3.7 Acquired cholesteatoma showing downgrowths from deeper layer of cholesteatoma epithelium. Note marked inflammatory exudate and erosion of surface of long process of incus at top

result of different mechanisms under different circumstances.

Medial Growth of Epithelium

Squamous epithelium may grow in from the tympanic membrane or ear canal through a perforation to line parts of the middle ear, sometimes exten-

sively. Such a growth does frequently occur, but is not usually accompanied by true cholesteatoma,[17] even though there may be progressive invasion of skin from the ear canal to line most of the middle ear and its attic.

Light or ultrastructural examination of cholesteatoma epithelium reveals the presence of Langerhans (dendritic) cells, as does ear canal skin. When counts are carried out using S-100 protein, immunohistochemical staining for these cells, cholesteatoma shows a higher number of dendritic cells than does normal canal wall skin.[18] This observation has been taken as evidence in favour of the migratory origin of cholesteatoma. The prominence of these cells in cholesteatomatous squamous epithelium may be explained, however, on the basis of the marked exposure of the epithelium to foreign antigens rather than on the basis of its mode of origin.

Cytokeratin Markers and External Canal Origin. The intermediate filaments of the cytokeratins expressed by epithelia comprise 19 polypeptides classified into two families: (1) basic polypeptides with large molecules known by cytokeratin numbers 1–8 and (2) acidic polypeptides with small molecules known by cytokeratin numbers 9–19. There is copolymerisation of acidic and basic polypeptides together, the pairs of which when expressed are characteristic of particular epithelia. The cytokeratin expression of simple (cuboidal) middle ear epithelium on the one hand and that of stratified squamous epithelium of the external canal and tympanic membrane on the other, has been compared with the cytokeratin expression of cholesteatomatous epithelium, to seek evidence for the source of the cholesteatoma. In several studies[19,20,21] external ear and cholesteatoma epithelium both expressed cytokeratin 10 and other cytokeratins characteristic of mature stratified squamous epithelium, but middle ear epithelium was not expressed. Middle ear epithelium, in contrast, expressed cytokeratins 4, 8, 18 and 19, a pattern characteristic of simple epithelia, but these cytokeratins were not expressed by cholesteatoma or external ear epithelium. It could be inferred from these researches that cholesteatoma is derived from external ear epithelium; however, an origin from simple middle ear epithelium metaplastic to stratified squamous epithelium could not be excluded, nor could an origin from a rest of stratified squamous epithelium in the middle ear. Indeed, in one of the investigations[21] material from cases of congenital cholesteatoma, a lesion known to be derived from an ectodermal cell rest in the middle ear (see Chapter 1) was examined and found to express a similar pattern of cytokeratins to those of stratified squamous epithelium of the external canal and tympanic membrane and of acquired cholesteatoma.

Hyperproliferation Markers and Differentiation Factors. The strong expression of cytokeratin 16 by cholesteatoma, but its absence in middle ear and external ear epithelium, except in the annulus region of the external tympanic membrane epithelium, has also been emphasised.[21] CK16 is a marker for hyperproliferative keratinocytes and this finding gives

molecular support for the frequent clinical observations of the active nature of cholesteatomatous growth in the middle ear and the appearance of downgrowths on histological observation of cholesteatoma (see above). They also support the previous suggestions of great activity of the annulus region epithelium; this region has even been invoked as the generation centre for auditory epithelial migration.[22] The strong expression of the hyperproliferation marker cytokeratin 16 by cholesteatoma has been confirmed and extended using antibodies against the antigen Ki-67, which is a marker of proliferative activity throughout most of the growth cycle.[23] Such findings have been found to be valid not only in the frozen sections used for the earlier work, but also in paraffin sections of cholesteatoma using MIB-1, an antigen related to Ki-67.[24] The site of the most concentrated expression of increased proliferative activity was in the epithelial downgrowths (see above).

In a study of acquired cholesteatoma, using counts of silver-stained argyrophil nucleolar organiser regions, a technique which likewise displays proliferative activity, significant differences between cholesteatoma and deep meatal skin could be identified.[25]

In Chapter 1 the biological zones of stratified squamous epithelium of the meatal skin and tympanic membrane based on developmental studies were outlined. It was shown in fetal material that the zone of epithelium over the pars flaccida and handle of the malleus, and also the epithelium of the deep external canal, especially over the annulus, had a higher proliferative activity using Ki-67 than others and it was inferred from morphological observations that this relative activity is present throughout life. In only a single study of either the cytokeratin or the expression of hyperproliferative antigen was an attempt made to examine differentially these biologically disparate areas of the meatal epithelium.[21] Further use of such a differential approach might provide clues as to the exact source of meatal epithelium from which cholesteatoma is derived. One investigation in which such a consideration was addressed was focussed on the spatial organisation of the keratinocytes.[26] A highly ordered vertical architecture, with cell stacking, is found in the stratum corneum of cholesteatoma as well as in the normal pars flaccida and deep external canal. The corneocytes of the pars tensa, on the other hand, appear randomly arranged. Thus pars flaccida and deep external canal epidermis are more akin to cholesteatoma, further evidence that cholesteatoma may be derived from these epithelia.

In company with the hyperproliferative activity of cholesteatoma, there is evidence of overexpression of a variety of peptides that are known to provide a regulatory function in differentiation.[27] Thus, together with the surrounding inflammatory cells, but not the middle ear epithelium, cholesteatomatous epithelium showed a high concentration of IL-1, TGF-alpha, EGF-R and 4F2, all being growth factors.[28] It would thus seem that cholesteatoma manifests molecular evidence of greater growth and differentiating activity than does normal epidermis. Acquired cholesteatoma, however, exists usually in an ambience of severe infection and inflammation. The question has not yet been addressed as to whether the greater activity of cholesteatoma is a primary, innate quality, perhaps endowed by the deep external ear epithelium from which it is derived, or rather a secondary one stimulated by the background in which it exists.

Tissue Culture. Explant cultures of cholesteatoma grow in vitro,[29,30] but have a lower colony-forming efficiency than those from normal skin.[31] A phenomenon observed in the course of the first 2 weeks of the explant in some cultures is the rapid en masse movement of a portion of the explanted cells across the culture dish. It is tempting to explain this as an in vitro correlate of auditory epithelial migration, but the same change may also occasionally be seen in cultures of normal external skin (Dr. I.M. Cheshire, Birmingham, UK, personal communication). The cultured cholesteatoma cells express a similar pattern of cytokeratin, as do uncultured cholesteatoma cells in frozen section.[20] Parathyroid hormone-related protein is found in the conditioned medium of primary and secondary cell cultures of cholesteatoma, which may explain the increased incidence of bone resorption in the disease.[31]

Experimental Cholesteatoma from Penetration of Squamous Epithelial Cells through the Tympanic Membrane. Manipulations of the middle ear in animals have successfully induced penetration of stratified squamous epithelium through the intact tympanic membrane to enter the middle ear and produce cholesteatoma. The placement of irritants[32,33] or bacteria[34] into the middle ear cavity of animals provoked an otitis media, which was associated with epidermal invasion through the tympanic membrane with the subsequent development of cholesteatoma. The early stages of this process were studied after the instillation of propylene glycol solution into the middle ears of chinchillas.[35,36] Destruction of the epithelium of both middle ear and lateral tympanic membrane surfaces in the days after the application of the propylene glycol was followed by re-epithelialisation with hyperplastic epidermal cells and, in 2–3 weeks, penetration of the thickened fibrous layer of the tympanic membrane by the epidermal cells to reach the middle ear cavity. The cells then reproduced to form keratinous masses typical of cholesteatoma. The findings also suggested that the stratified squamous epithelium of the invasive process may undergo necrosis and lead to a perforation of the tympanic membrane with viable epidermal cells at its margins.

These experimental findings seem to clarify somewhat the pathogenesis of human acquired cholesteatoma. Histological findings in the human of similar penetration of stratified squamous epithelium through the tympanic membrane, however, have been rare. In a case of chronic otitis media, thin strands of epidermoid cells were found to extend from the outer tympanic membrane surface into the middle ear.[37] Similar thin bands of squamous epithelium were seen extending from retraction pockets into the middle ear[38] (see below).

It thus seems possible that with a severe disturbance of the tissues of the tympanic membrane as a result of otitis media, the epithelium on the lateral surface of the eardrum may still possess a fetal-like growth potential, but, lacking the local control mechanisms of the normal eardrum, it may enter the fibrous layer of the tympanic membrane to reach the middle ear, growing to cholesteatoma there.

Cholesteatoma from Retraction Pocket

A retraction pocket is an invagination of part of the tympanic membrane into the middle ear cavity as a result of chronic otitis media. It is usually the pars flaccida that is so indented. It frequently becomes adherent to the posterior wall of the middle ear in the region of the facial nerve or stapes or to the promontory. Histological sections of the wall of the retraction pocket show an absence of the normal, tympanic membrane connective tissue, which may have been destroyed by inflammation.[39] The retraction pocket may show a moderate amount of keratin in the lumen of the sac, but inflammatory cells are not usually seen.

Histological examination of 12 retraction pockets in post-mortem temporal bones[38] showed no evidence of development of cholesteatoma or of obstruction of the mouth of a retraction pocket, which could lead to the eventual development of cholesteatoma. In two of the retraction pockets, however, small keratinising epidermoid foci, connected to the squamous epithelium of the retraction pocket by a band of non-keratinising squamous epithelium, were seen on the malleus and incus within the middle ear (Fig. 3.8). Similar active downgrowths of pars flaccida epithelium have been described in eardrums not affected by retraction pocket.[17,40] If retraction pocket gives rise to

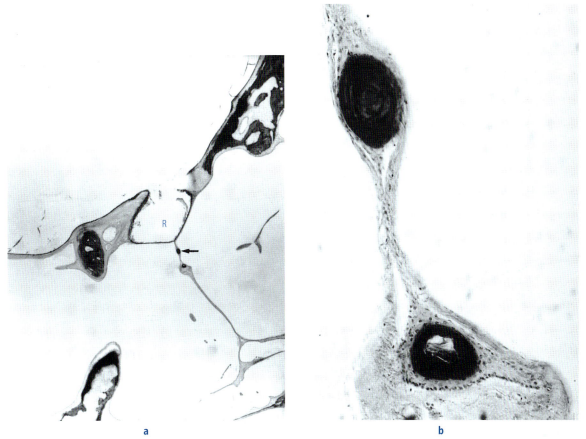

Figure 3.8 a Retraction pocket from the fundus of which a fibrous band extends into the middle ear. Two keratinous microcysts, the upper one marked with an arrow, are present in the fibrous band. **b** Higher power of keratinous cysts in **a** showing that they are connected by a band of non-keratinising stratified squamous epithelium, which, in fact, extends in the fibrous band from the fundus of the retraction pocket

cholesteatoma, it may do so through such an invasive activity rather than by any failure of its drainage.

Experimental Retraction Pocket Cholesteatoma. A form of cholesteatoma has been produced in Mongolian gerbils by cauterising the Eustachian opening in the nasopharynx.[41] An acute otitis media results and by 16 weeks some of the animals have retraction pockets filling the middle ear. These have evidently arisen in a similar fashion to the spontaneous "cholesteatoma" found in nearly one-half of older animals of this species.[42] In the latter condition the deep ear canal is filled with keratinous material, which causes an inward bulging and distension of the pars flaccida. The distended sac of eardrum eventually comes into contact with the cochlear and other bony walls of the middle ear and leads to their erosion.

Personal observation of the early stages of this process in experimental material of Dr. A. Cecire (New Zealand) has shown us that in the first weeks after the nasopharynx has been cauterised, the epithelium of the pars flaccida and deep ear canal becomes thickened. Later the thickened epithelium shows acute inflammation and this process gives rise to purulent exudate mixed with keratin squames, which fills the lumen of the deep external canal and eventually distends the eardrum to produce the retraction-pocket-like inversion of this membrane.

The gerbil seems to possess an unusual propensity for such "retraction pocket formation"; a similar distension results from ligation of the external canal in this species but not in a variety of other small mammals.[43]

Experimental "retraction pocket cholesteatoma" of the gerbil in these experiments is thus not necessarily the direct result of the middle ear inflammation caused by the Eustachian tube cauterisation, but, in view of the fact that spontaneous retraction-pocket-like formations are so common in the gerbil,[42] it is possible that the experimentally induced form may instead be associated with the deterioration of the animal's general condition that undoubtedly follows the surgical trauma.

In human retraction pocket cholesteatoma the external canal skin is normal and retraction pockets do not form as a result of the pressure of debris against the tympanic membrane. It would thus seem that the gerbil "retraction pocket" is not an appropriate model for human cholesteatoma.

Cholesteatoma from Metaplasia

Islands of metaplastic squamous cell epithelium in the middle ear from which acquired cholesteatoma could originate have been reported,[44] but not confirmed. The concept of metaplasia as a source of cholesteatoma must thus at present be considered unproven.

Experimental Vitamin A Deficiency. In rats with diet-induced vitamin A deficiency, squamous metaplasia of large areas of normally columnar, ciliated epithelium of the middle ear was observed without frank cholesteatoma formation. In most of the animals acute otitis media with effusion was also found.[45] This extreme experimental situation, while representing a process of squamous metaplasia in the rat middle ear, would seem to be irrelevant to squamous metaplasia or cholesteatoma of the middle ear in the human.

Trauma (Blast Injury or Ventilation Tubes)

Cholesteatoma is found at tympanoplasty up to 18 months after blast injury in 7.6% of ears that have suffered perforation of the tympanic membrane at the time of the injury. The incidence of cholesteatoma increases with the severity of the perforation so produced.[46]

Congenital Cholesteatoma

In contrast to acquired cholesteatoma, which has been established as a clinicopathologic entity for more than a century, congenital cholesteatoma has been recognised only recently. Although not common, it is seen now with some regularity in parts of North America, although still described as rare in other parts of the world. The mean age of presentation is 4.6 years. Many patients present with a lesion in the anterosuperior part of the middle ear (Fig. 3.9). In one-quarter of patients the cholesteatoma occupies much of the tympanic cavity. In 3% of patients the congenital cholesteatoma is bilateral.[47] Possible reasons for the much greater recent frequency of this entity, which

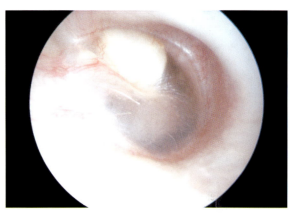

Figure 3.9 Congenital cholesteatoma seen as a small cyst in the anterosuperior part of the middle ear (Courtesy of Dr. Mark Levenson, New York City)

was formerly considered extremely rare, are: (1) the use of the operating microscope in diagnosis, (2) the improved lighting of otoscopes by the use of the halogen bulb, (3) the screening of tympanic membranes of normal young children by paediatricians and (4) the possibility that many cases of congenital cholesteatoma which formerly underwent "spontaneous abortion" following acute otitis media may now survive with the cure of the otitis with antibiotics.[47]

Gross Appearances and Appearances at Surgery

Congenital cholesteatoma has until recently been seen in most cases as a spherical whitish object in the anterosuperior part of the tympanic cavity behind an intact tympanic membrane (Fig. 3.9). More recently the proportion of cases of this lesion seen in the posterosuperior part of the middle ear has increased (Dr. Simon Parisier, New York, personal communication). In some cases the lesion may fill most of the tympanic cavity.

At operation the cholesteatoma is reported usually to be a cyst measuring 3 mm or more in diameter, which is situated in close relation to the tympanic membrane, tensor tympani tendon, neck of the malleus and mouth of the Eustachian tube. The cyst may have no firm attachments to the wall of the tympanic cavity[48] or there may be only a thin tenuous connection to the wall.[47] Bone erosion is not present when the cholesteatoma is small. In larger lesions some degree of this change is present[49] and eventually may enlarge to involve the mastoid and even grow into the middle cranial fossa.[50]

In approximately 10% of cases the cholesteatoma is open and shows layers of squames and a matrix which is plastered to the wall of the tympanic cavity.[51] In one study the open type of congenital cholesteatoma was reported to be more frequent and it was suggested that super-added middle ear inflammation may be the factor contributing to the change from the open to the closed variety.[52]

Microscopic Appearances

The microscopic appearances of the matrix of congenital cholesteatoma are those of skin epidermis, comprising a single row of basal cells, several rows of malpighian cells and a thin granular layer. The surface of dead, keratinous squames merges with the keratinous contents of the cyst, or lamellae in the case of the open type. When the histological appearances of these cases are compared with those of acquired cholesteatoma, little difference can be seen and it seems likely that there is a similar degree of activity to that described above in acquired cholesteatoma. The epithelium of congenital cholesteatoma has not been subjected to a similar study for growth activity to that of acquired cholesteatoma (see above).

In opportune cases, a double layer of epithelium may be seen surrounding the keratin squames forming the main bulk of the lesion. On the outside a single layer of middle ear epithelium may be present, which is continuous with the epithelium covering the stalk of the cholesteatoma. Separated from the middle ear epithelium only by a thin and often markedly inflamed lamina propria is the basal layer of the stratified squamous epithelium of the congenital cholesteatoma.[47]

Small epidermoid cysts attached to the middle ear side of the tympanic membrane, labelled intratympanic cholesteatomas, were found in five temporal bones of adults in three patients.[53] In two of the patients the cysts were identified in the same position of the bone on each side, in the anterosuperior part of the eardrum in one and in the posterosuperior pars tensa in the other. In the third patient the cyst was behind the umbo region. The significance of these lesions is not clear. Chronic otitis media was present in all, but the specimens were selected only from temporal bones that had this change. It is tempting to relate the lesion to an alteration in a pre-existing epidermoid formation; although most of these structures are found near the anterosuperior part of the tympanic membrane, some are found more posteriorly (see Chapter 1).

Pathogenesis

Two suggestions have been put forward regarding the pathogenesis of congenital cholesteatoma. They may arise:

1. From an epidermoid cell rest which has arisen during development in the middle ear epithelium.
2. From amniotic squames, which reach the middle ear during parturition.

Epidermoid Cell Rests

Cell rests of epidermoid tissue have been suggested from time to time as the origin of the primary form of cholesteatoma. The discovery of a cell rest in the anterosuperior part of the middle ear in 1936[54] was forgotten, but rediscovered in 1985 – the epidermoid formation (EF)[55]; and confirmed in 1987.[56] The features of this cell rest are described in Chapter 1.

Although the cell rest is now generally accepted as the source of congenital cholesteatoma by most workers, a few arguments have been put forward to suggest difficulties in the acceptance of this concept. One such argument is that when the congenital cholesteatoma is small, there is often a distinct margin between it and the tympanic annulus anteriorly.[39] This argument can be countered by the observations that the EF is normally very close to the edge of the eardrum, sometimes even over it. Moreover, the epitympanum is angled relative to the anterior edge of the eardrum. A small congenital cholesteatoma arising from the EF would thus be easily visible to the otoscopist and may appear to have normal tissue anterior to it.

A further argument is that no intermediate stage lesion in the temporal bone between the EF and congenital cholesteatoma has yet been discovered.[49] Such lesions have indeed been seen: large EFs (> 1 mm in diameter) have been observed and indeed the histology of a very extensive anterosuperior open cholesteatoma has been displayed.[57]

Amniotic Squames

Mechanisms other than by a preceding cell rest have been suggested as an origin for congenital cholesteatoma. Amniotic fluid cellular content is frequently observed in the fetal and neonatal middle ear[58] and an origin of cholesteatoma from growth of some of these cells has been suggested. In favour of this concept, it has been adduced, is that the cells desquamated into amniotic fluid have the property of powerful growth in tissue culture when removed by amniocentesis. Against this argument, however, is that these cells grow in vitro as fibroblasts, not as epithelial cells. The numbers of apparently viable nucleated squames in the material are, moreover, small, and it is difficult to see how they could embed themselves in the mucosa to set up a cholesteatoma. Other columnar epithelia, e.g. those of bronchus and nose, are exposed to even greater numbers of amniotic squames during fetal life, but cholesteatoma-like processes are not a feature of these areas. The propensity of this lesion to occur in the anterosuperior part of the middle ear would not, moreover, be explained on this basis.

Chemical Factors in Bone Resorption by Cholesteatoma

A number of chemical factors have been incriminated in the bone resorption of cholesteatoma. All of these are derived from the accompanying chronic otitis media or the infection associated with it. Specimens of cholesteatoma, which include the underlying matrix, have been found to show strong collagenase activity.[59] It is likely that this collagenase plays a part in resorption of bone. Endotoxins may also play a part and this is particularly likely because they are derived from Gram-negative bacilli, which are prominent in infection associated with cholesteatoma.[60]

Otitis Media with Effusion (OME)

Synonyms commonly in use for OME are: secretory otitis media, serous otitis media, catarrhal otitis media, tubotympanitis and glue ear. It is a very common cause of hearing loss in children, characterised by an effusion behind a non-perforated eardrum in the absence of frank symptoms of acute infection. Few biopsy or temporal bone pathologic studies have been described. All the features of chronic otitis may be present, including cholesterol granuloma, chronic inflammatory granulation tissue, ossicular destruction and tympanosclerosis. The most prominent feature of the histopathology in childhood OME seems to be new formation of glands in the middle ear mucosa.

OME also occurs in adults, often in association with neoplasms of the nasopharynx, probably as a result of occlusion of the distal orifice of the Eustachian tube. Histopathologic examination of the middle ear mucosa in adult OME at autopsy in one study also showed such glandular metaplasia accompanying the secretion, but with more inflammatory infiltrate than in the childhood cases of OME.[61]

In a post-mortem study of patients with AIDS, OME was found in 60% of 49 temporal bones, characterised by the extensive exudation of fibrin into the middle ear spaces, as well as the features of OME mentioned above. In one case, cytomegalovirus infection was present in the middle ear mucosa. Changes of a more active otitis media with suppuration in the middle ear cleft were identified in 23%, a much higher number than was found in a large clinical study carried out concomitantly, suggesting that severe otitis media may occur frequently in terminally sick patients with AIDS, perhaps on the site of a middle ear mucosa already weakened by OME.[62]

Complications of Otitis Media

The inflammatory process may extend from the middle ear to involve adjacent structures. Inflammation of the labyrinth may occur as a result of extension of the infection through the round or oval windows. The petrous bone may become involved by spread of the inflammation through the bone marrow or air cells (see Chapter 8). Adjacent intracranial and cranial nerve structures may become inflamed by spread of the infection outside the temporal bone. Meningitis, sinus thrombophlebitis, extradural abscess or brain abscess are important possible sequelae of otitis media.

Tuberculous Otitis Media

Tuberculous otitis media is an unusual form of chronic otitis media, which is generally associated with active pulmonary tuberculosis.

In the initial stages, multiple perforations of the tympanic membrane develop. Granulations in the middle ear are pale and profuse and complications, especially involvement of the facial nerve, are more frequent than in the commoner form of chronic otitis media.

Culture of the middle ear tissue may produce tubercle bacilli. Histological examination shows tuberculoid granulation tissue composed of epithelioid cells, Langhans giant cells and areas of caseation situated in the middle ear mucosa (Fig. 3.10). There is much bone destruction. Acid-fast bacilli are found with difficulty in the granulomatous material.

In two cases of tuberculous otitis media, in otherwise healthy adult males with no evidence of tuberculosis of lung or other internal organ, there were vast numbers of acid-fast bacilli present in the granulomas. They were confirmed as *Mycobacterium tuberculosis hominis* by culture.[63]

Sarcoidosis

Sarcoidosis is very rare in the middle ear, but has been identified as producing granulomatous

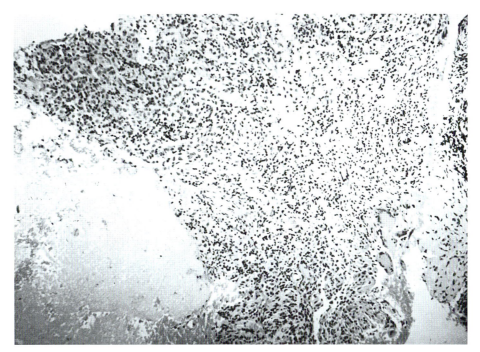

Figure 3.10 Tuberculosis of middle ear. Note caseation on *left*. To the *right* of this there are epithelioid cells, lymphocytes and some Langhans giant cells

changes in the middle ear in patients in whom typical manifestations of the disorder were present in the lungs.[64]

Actinomycosis

Actinomycosis of the middle ear, an uncommon infection caused by the anaerobic organism *Actinomycosis israeli*, cannot usually be identified without open operation on the middle ear in order to obtain samples of tissue containing the organism (see Chapter 45).

Wegener's Granulomatosis

Wegener's granulomatosis is a systemic inflammatory condition affecting the kidneys, lungs and often the nose and many other organs (see Chapter 14). Unfortunately, cases of otitis media without renal or pulmonary manifestations, or even histological evidence of Wegener's granulomatosis, such as angiitis, have been given the label of Wegener's granulomatosis on the basis only of a positive C-ANCA test and apparent success in treating the condition with cyclophosphamide.[65] Pathologists should be cautious in interpreting such cases as a "locoregional" form of Wegener's granulomatosis.

References

1. Paparella MM, Kimberley BP, Alleva M. The concept of silent otitis media. Its importance and implications. Otolaryngol Clin N Amer 1991;24:763–773
2. Sugita R, Fujimaki Y, Deguchi K. Bacteriological features and chemotherapy of adult acute purulent otitis media. J Laryngol Otol 1985;99:629–35
3. Brook I, Anthony BF, Finegold SM. Aerobic and anaerobic bacteriology of acute otitis media in children. J Ped 1978;92:13–16
4. Henderson FW, Collier AM, Sanyal MA et al. A longitudinal study of respiratory viruses and bacteria in the etiology of acute otitis media with effusion. N Engl J Med 1982;306:1377–1383
5. Chonmaitree T, Howie VM, Truant AL. Presence of respiratory viruses in middle ear fluids and nasal wash specimens from children with acute otitis media. Pediatrics 1986;77:698–702
6. Buchman CA, Doyle WJ, Skoner DP et al. Influenza A virus-induced acute otitis media. J Infect Dis 1995;172:1348–1351
7. Catanzaro A, Ryan A, Batcher S et al. The response to human RIL-1, RIL-2, and RTNF in the middle-ear of guinea-pigs. Laryngoscope 1991;101:271–275
8. Yellon RF, Leonard G, Marucha PT et al. Characterization of cytokines present in middle-ear effusions. Laryngoscope 1991;101:165–169
9. Amar MS, Wishahi HF, Zakhary MM. Clinical and biochemical studies of bone destruction in cholesteatoma. J Laryngol Otol 1996;110:534–539
10. Tos M, Bak-Pedersen K. Goblet cell population in the normal middle ear and Eustachian tube of children and adults. Ann Otol Rhinol Laryngol 1976;85(suppl 25):44–50
11. Tos M, Bak-Pedersen K. Goblet cell population in the pathological middle ear and Eustachian tube of children and adults. Ann Otol Rhinol Laryngol 1977;86:209–218

12. Albrecht W. Pneumatisation und Konstitution. Z Hals-Nasen-und Ohrenheilkunde 1924;10:51–55

13. Sadé J, Teitz A. Cholesterol in cholesteatoma and in the otitis media syndrome. In: Sadé J (ed) Cholesteatoma and mastoid surgery. Proceedings of the second international conference. Kugler, Amsterdam, 1982, pp 125–132

14. Goldstein NA, Roland JT, Sculerati NN. Complications of tympanostomy tubes in an inner-city clinic population. Int J Pediatr Otorhinolaryngol 1996;34:87–99

15. Politzer A. Das Cholesteatom des Gehörgans vom anatomischen und klinischen Standpunkte, Wiener Medizinische Wochenschrift 1891;8:329–333

16. McKenzie D. The pathogeny of aural cholesteatoma. Proc Roy Soc Med 1931;24:332–362

17. Palva T, Karma P, Makinen J. The invasion theory. In: Sadé J (ed) Cholesteatoma and mastoid surgery. Proceedings of the second international conference. Kugler, Amsterdam, 1982, pp 249–264

18. Frankel S, Berson S, Godwin T et al. Differences in dendritic cells in congenital and acquired cholesteatomas. Laryngoscope 1993;103:1214–1217

19. Van Blitterswijk CA, Grote JJ, Lutgert RW et al. Cytokeratin patterns of tissues related to cholesteatoma pathogenesis. Ann Otol Rhinol Laryngol 1989;98:635–640

20. Lee RL, Sidey C, Narula AA et al. The nature of the epithelium in acquired cholesteatoma: part 3 – cytokeratin patterns in aural epithelial and cholesteatoma cells grown in cell culture. Clin Otolaryngol 1994;19:516–520

21. Broekaert D, Couke P, Leperque S. Immunohistochemical analysis of the cytokeratin expression in middle ear cholesteatoma and related epithelial tissues. Ann Otol Rhinol Laryngol 1992;101:931–938

22. Litton WB. Epithelial migration in the ear: the location and characteristics of the generation centre revealed by utilizing a radioactive desoxyribose nucleic acid precursor. Acta Otolaryngol (Stockh) 1968;240(suppl):1–39

23. Bajia J, Schilling V, Holly A et al. Hyperproliferation-associated expression in human middle ear cholesteatoma. Acta Otolaryngol 1993;113:364–368

24. Sudhoff H, Bujia J, Fisselereckhoff A et al. Expression of a cell-cycle-associated nuclear antigen (MIB1) in cholesteatoma and auditory meatal skin. Laryngoscope 1995;105:1227–1231

25. Sudhoff H, Fisseler-Eckhoff A, Stark T et al. Argyrophilic nucleolar organizer regions in auditory meatal skin and middle ear cholesteatoma. Clin Otolaryngol 1997; 22:545–548

26. Youngs R, Rowles P. The spatial organisation of keratinocytes in acquired middle ear cholesteatoma resembles that of external canal skin and pars flaccida. Acta Otolaryngol (Stockh) 1990;110:115–119

27. Stammberger M, Bujia J, Kastenbauer E. Alteration in epidermal differentiation in cholesteatoma. Am J Otol 1995;4:527–531

28. Sudhoff H, Bujia J, Holly A et al. Functional characterization of middle ear mucosa residues in cholesteatomatous samples. Am J Otol 1994;15:217–221

29. Proops DW, Hawke WM, Parkinson EK. Tissue-culture of migratory skin of the external ear and cholesteatoma – a new research tool. J Otolaryngol 1984;13:63–69

30. Boxall JD, Proops DW, Michaels L. The specific locomotive activity of tympanic membrane and cholesteatoma epithelium in tissue culture. J Otolaryngol 1988;17:140–144

31. Cheshire IM, Blight A, Proops DW. An in-vitro growth study on cholesteatoma and normal skin. Clin Otolaryngol 1995;20:453–456

32. Ruedi L. Cholesteatoma formation in the middle ear in animal experiments. Acta Otolaryngol (Stockh) 1959; 50:233–242

33. Fernandez C, Lindsay JR. Aural cholesteatoma: experimental observations. Laryngoscope 1960;70:1119–1141

34. Friedmann I. The comparative pathology of otitis media. Experimental otitis and human. 11. The histopathology of experimental otitis of the guinea pig with particular reference to experimental cholesteatoma. J Laryngol Otol 1955;69:588–601

35. Wright CG, Meyerhoff WL, Burns DK. Middle ear cholesteatoma: an animal model. Am J Otolaryngol 1985; 6:327–341

36. Masaki M, Wright CG, Lee DH et al. Experimental cholesteatoma. Epidermal ingrowth through tympanic membrane following middle ear application of propylene glycol. Acta Otolaryngol (Stockh) 1989;108:113–121

37. Palva T, Johnsson L. Findings in a pair of temporal bones from a patient with secretory otitis media and chronic middle ear infection. Acta Otolaryngol 1984;98:208–220

38. Wells MD, Michaels L. Role of retraction pockets in cholesteatoma formation. Clin Otolaryngol 1983;8:39–45

39. Schuknecht HF. Pathology of the ear, 2nd edn. Lea & Febiger, Philadelphia, 1993

40. Ruedi L. Pathogenesis and treatment of cholesteatoma in chronic suppuration of the temporal bone. Ann Otol Rhinol Laryngol 1957;66:283–304

41. Chole RA. Experimental retraction pocket cholesteatoma. Ann Otol Rhinol Laryngol 1986;95:639–641

42. Chole RA, Henry KR, McGinn D. Cholesteatoma: spontaneous occurrence in the Mongolian gerbil, *Meriones unguiculatis*. Am J Otol 1981;2:204–210

43. McGinn MD, Chole RA, Henry KR. Cholesteatoma induction. Consequences of external auditory canal ligations in gerbils, cats, hamsters, guinea-pigs, mice and rats. Acta Otolaryngol Stockh 1984;97:297–304

44. Sadé J. The biopathology of secretory otitis media. Ann Otol Rhinol Laryngol 1974;11(suppl):59–70

45. Chole RA. Squamous metaplasia of the middle ear mucosa during vitamin A deprivation. Otolaryngol Head Neck Surg 1979;87:837–844

46. Kronenburg J, Ben-Shoshan J, Modam M et al. Blast injury and cholesteatoma. Am J Otol 1988;9:127–130

47. Friedberg J. Congenital cholesteatoma. Laryngoscope 1994;104(suppl):1–24

48. Derlacki EL. Congenital cholesteatoma of the middle ear and mastoid: a third report. Arch Otolaryngol. 1973;97:177–182

49. McGill TJ, Merchant S, Healy GB et al. Congenital cholesteatoma of the middle ear in children: a clinical and histopathological report. Laryngoscope 1991;101:606–613

50. Grundfast KM, Ahuja GS, Parisier SC et al. Delayed diagnosis and fate of congenital cholesteatoma (keratoma). Arch Otolaryngol Head Neck Surg 1995;121:903–907

51. Cohen D. Locations of primary cholesteatoma. Am J Otol 1987;8:61–65

52. Iino Y, Imamura Y, Hiraishi M et al. Mastoid pneumatization in children with congenital cholesteatoma: an aspect of the formation of open-type and closed-type cholesteatoma. Laryngoscope 1998;108:1071–1076

53. Jaisinghani VJ, Paparella MM, Schachern PA. Silent intratympanic membrane cholesteatoma. Laryngoscope 1998;108:1185–1189.

54. Teed RW. Cholesteatoma verum tympani: its relationship to the first epibranchial placode. Arch Otolaryngol 1936;24:455–474

55. Michaels L. An epidermoid formation in the developing middle ear; possible source of cholesteatoma. J Otolaryngol 1986;15:169–174

56. Wang R-G, Hawke M, Kwok P. The epidermoid formation (Michaels' structure) in the developing middle ear. J Otolaryngol 1987;16:327–330

57. Eggston A, Wolff D. Histopathology of the ear, nose and throat. Williams and Wilkins Co., Baltimore, 1947, p 432

58. Northrop C, Piza J, Eavey RD. Histological observations of amniotic fluid cellular content in the ear of neonates and infants. Int J Pediatr Otorhinolaryngol 1986;11:113–127

59. Abramson M, Huang C. Cholesteatoma and bone resorption. In: McCabe BF et al. (eds) Cholesteatoma. First international conference. Aesculapius, Birmingham Ala, 1977, pp 162–166

60. Yin ET. Endotoxin, thrombin and the limulus amebocyte lysate test. J Lab Clin Med 1975;86:430–434

61. Ishii T, Toriyama M, Suzuki J-I. Histopathological study of otitis media with effusion. Ann Otol Rhinol Laryngol 1980;89(suppl 68):83–86

62. Michaels L, Soucek S, Liang J. The ear in the acquired immunodeficiency syndrome: I. Temporal bone histopathologic study. AmeJ Otol 1994;15:515–522

63. Buchanan G, Rainer EH. Tuberculous mastoiditis. J Laryngol Otol 1988;102:440–446

64. Tyndel FJ, Davidson GS, Birman H et al. Sarcoidosis of the middle ear. Chest 1994;105:1582–1583

65. Macias JD, Wackym PA, McCabe BF. Early diagnosis of otologic Wegener's granulomatosis using the serologic marker C-ANCA. Ann Otol Rhinol Laryngol 1993;102:337–341

4 Neoplasms of the External Ear

The external ear is a specialised appendage of the skin, so that its neoplasms are most frequently those derived from skin. Bony neoplasms also occur, as would be expected from the presence of bone nearby, but the cartilage of the ear seems to have no neoplastic propensity. The following account will deal only with those tumours that have a predilection for that region and those that pose special diagnostic histological and clinical problems.

Epithelial Neoplasms

Solar Keratosis

Solar keratosis usually occurs in Caucasians as multiple lesions in areas of the body, such as the face and the dorsa of the hands, that are particularly exposed to sunlight over many years with inadequate protection. The pinna of the ear is occasionally involved and, rarely, the commencement of the external auditory meatus. The lesion takes the form of a small erythematous flat plaque. Histologically there is hyperkeratosis, epidermal hyperplasia and dysplasia of the epidermis. The upper dermis shows elastic tissue degeneration and a chronic inflammatory exudate. There is a decided tendency to malignant change, but squamous carcinomas arising in solar keratosis rarely metastasise.

Basal Cell Papilloma (Seborrhoeic Keratosis)

Basal cell papilloma is a very common lesion of the trunk and face. It is sometimes present on the pinna or in the ear canal. It is a well-demarcated pigmented elevation, which looks as if it has been stuck on to the skin surface. Histologically it is elevated above the surrounding skin so that the lower border with dermis forms a straight line. The proliferated tissue is composed of basal cells with numbers of keratin cysts embedded within them. In the cysts keratinisation occurs by sudden transformation from the basal cells without interposition of a stratum granulosum. Melanocytes are frequently present. The condition is benign.

Pilomatricoma (Pilomatrixoma, Calcifying Epithelioma of Malherbe)

Pilomatricoma is a tumour of the skin of children or young adults, with a decided preference for the skin of the external ear, although it is also seen elsewhere on the face, neck and arms. It often assumes the form of a cyst with a lumen of cheesy material, but may show a solid pinkish cut surface. Pilomatricoma is usually situated under the skin.

The peripheral part contains islets of basophilic cells, which have little cytoplasm and prominent nucleoli. These cells blend with or are sharply demarcated from "ghost" cells, which are groups of degenerated epidermal cells staining only in a faintly eosinophilic fashion. The central part of the lesion contains amorphous debris, keratin and often calcified and even ossified areas.

The neoplasm is almost always benign, although an invasive variant has recently been described.[1]

Squamous Papilloma

Squamous papillomas are common tumours of the external auditory meatus and do not differ significantly from similar tumours growing from the mucous surface of the nasal septum (see Chapter 15) or vocal cord (see Chapter 33). They show cylinders of squamous epithelium growing outwards on central cores of fibrous tissue. Sometimes the fibrous component is more prominent in an ear canal tumour, meriting the term "fibro-epithelial polyp". Neither of these lesions are malignant.

Keratoacanthoma

Keratoacanthomas may occur on the external ear as well as the skin of the face. Their special features are: (1) a resemblance to low-grade squamous carcinoma of the skin and (2) a tendency to disappear spontaneously after 6–8 weeks of growth.

Microscopically the centre of the lesion is composed of a crater of keratin. This is surrounded by trabeculae of squamous cell epithelium, which are well differentiated. The outer edge of the lesion is clear-cut with no extension of tongues of growth. In surgical pathology practice, keratoacanthoma is frequently difficult to distinguish from low-grade squamous carcinoma and when in doubt it is probably safer to diagnose squamous carcinoma.

Sebaceous Adenoma

Sharply defined tumours of sebaceous gland origin may be found in the external auditory meatus. The neoplasm is made up of small lobules comprising two types of cell. Situated around the periphery of the lobules the cells are undifferentiated germinative. More centrally they can be recognised as sebaceous.

Sebaceous Epithelioma

Sebaceous epithelioma – a malignant variant of sebaceous adenoma – is sometimes seen in the ear canal. It is locally infiltrative, but does not metastasise and may be a form of basal cell carcinoma.

Basal Cell Carcinoma

The great majority of malignant epithelial neoplasms of the pinna are basal cell carcinomas,[2] a small number only being squamous cell carcinomas. The few basal cell carcinomas that occur in the ear canal arise near the external opening. Their preference for the exposed part of the external ear is in keeping with the accepted view that sunlight is in most cases the causal factor in skin insufficiently protected by melanin pigment.

Gross Appearances

The appearance of basal cell carcinoma is usually one of a pearly wax-like nodule, which eventually ulcerates. Twenty-five per cent of basal cell carcinomas of the pinna are of the morphea type (see below). The importance of this variety is that although the edge of the tumour tends to infiltrate subcutaneously, this cannot be recognised clinically or on gross pathological examination.

Microscopic Appearances

The classical and most frequent form of basal cell carcinoma is composed of solid masses of cells, which are seen to be arising from the basal layers of the epidermis or the outer layers of the hair follicles. The cells are uniform with basophilic nuclei and little cytoplasm. At the periphery of the neoplastic lobules the cells tend to be palisaded. Mitoses are frequent. Alveolar or cystic spaces are frequent. Squamous cell differentiation is also common. The splitting up of cell groups by much hyaline fibrous tissue, so that the carcinoma appears compressed into thin strands, is referred to as the morphea type of basal cell carcinoma (Fig. 4.1). The suggestion that tumours with this histology have a worse outlook is probably related to their tendency of insidious infiltration (see above). There is otherwise no convincing evidence of the relationship of a particular histological appearance to prognosis in basal cell carcinoma.

Natural History

This is not an aggressive neoplasm and in at least 90% of cases a 3-year cure can be easily achieved by surgical excision. In a few cases repeated recurrences with deep extension to the middle ear, mastoid and even cranial cavity may, however, take place. Metastasis is rare.

Squamous Cell Carcinoma

Incidence

Squamous carcinomas of the pinna occur predominantly in males; those of the ear canal mainly in

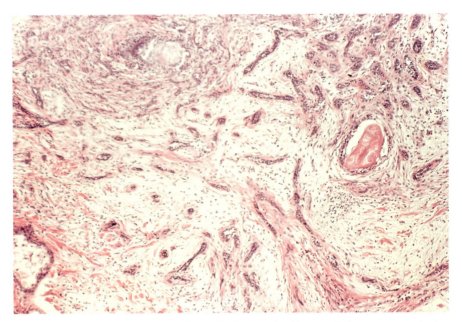

Figure 4.1 Morphea type of basal cell carcinoma showing thin downgrowths with stroma of inflammatory connective tissue

females. Ear canal cancers grow at a markedly younger age than those of the pinna. Metastatic spread derived from squamous carcinoma of the pinna and external auditory meatus takes place in but a small minority of cases. Tumours confined to the external ear usually have a good outlook after surgical therapy.

Gross Appearances

The gross appearances of the lesion are similar to those of the same tumour elsewhere in the skin and range from a papular nodule to an ulcerating mass. The appearances of this lesion in the ear canal are not diagnostic because of the narrowness of the structure.

Microscopic Appearances

This form of epidermoid carcinoma usually shows significant degrees of keratinisation. Evidence of origin from local epidermis is usually present. In cases arising deeply within the ear canal there is usually a concomitant origin from middle ear epithelium and dissolution of the tympanic membrane (see Chapter 5).

Natural History

Metastatic spread of squamous carcinoma of the pinna and external auditory meatus takes place in 8–25% of cases. The presence of such spread is, of course, important in the prognostic evaluation. Tumours confined to the external ear usually have a good outlook after surgical therapy.

Verrucous Squamous Cell Carcinoma

The verrucous form of squamous cell carcinoma has been seen in the external ear.[3] As is the case at other sites where this neoplasm occurs, the diagnosis may be delayed until several biopsies have been performed because of initial confusion with benign squamous papilloma (see Chapter 36). Image analysis may help in making this distinction.[4]

Neoplasms of Ceruminous Glands

External ear neoplasms derived from ceruminous glands are very uncommon. They can be benign or malignant entities. Only the adenoma can usually be categorised with certainty as being derived specifically from ceruminous glands since its component acini display an apocrine secretory struc-

Table 4.1. Classification of glandular neoplasms of the external canal

Benign
Adenoma (ceruminous adenoma)
Syringocystadenoma papilliferans
Chondroid syringoma – mixed tumour
Cylindroma

Malignant
Mucoepidermoid carcinoma
Adenocarcinoma
Adenoid cystic carcinoma

ture. Sometimes syringocystadenoma papilliferum shows areas of apocrine change. Adenoid cystic carcinoma of the external canal can sometimes be seen arising from ceruminous glands. Table 4.1 gives a classification of glandular neoplasms of the external auditory canal.

Adenoma (Ceruminous Adenoma)

Adenomas usually present with a blockage of the lateral part of the external auditory meatus, often associated with deafness and discharge. An important part of the clinical investigation of all glandular neoplasms of the ear canal is exclusion of origin in the parotid gland.

Gross appearances are those of a superficial grey mass up to 4 cm in diameter, which is covered by skin.

Microscopically this neoplasm lacks a definite capsule. It is composed of regular glands often with

intraluminal projections (Fig. 4.2). The glandular epithelium is distinctly bilayered, the outer layer being myoepithelial, but this may not be obvious in all parts of the neoplasm. The glands are often arranged in groups surrounded by fibrous tissue. In some ceruminomas, acid-fast fluorescent pigment may be found in the tumour cells, which is similar to that found in normal ceruminous glands[5,6] (see Chapter 1). Adenoma of ceruminous glands is a benign neoplasm. Recurrence should not be expected if it is carefully excised.

Syringocystadenoma Papilliferum

Syringocystadenoma papilliferum, a benign lesion, is seen in children or young adults and is usually found on the scalp or face. Occasionally it occurs in the ear canal. The histological appearance of the neoplasm is that of an invagination from the surface epithelium forming a cyst-like structure. Projecting into the lumen are papillae lined by bilayered glandular epithelium showing decapitation secretion. Apocrine (ceruminous) glands may be present in the wall of the cyst.

Cylindroma

Cylindroma is a benign tumour arising from the epidermal appendages, whether apocrine- or eccrine-

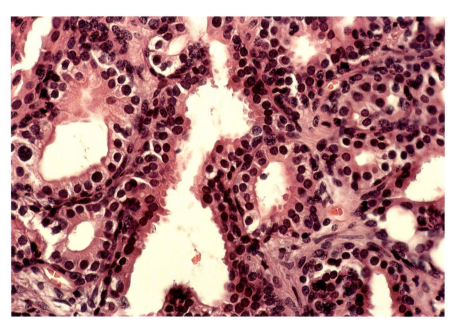

Figure 4.2 Ceruminoma of external canal. Note peg-like protrusions into the lumina, indicating apocrine secretion[19]

derived is not conclusively known. In the external ear the lesion may be present on the pinna or in the external canal. In these situations it may be part of a multiple "turban tumour" presentation of this neoplasm on the scalp. It forms a projecting smooth swelling beneath the skin and is composed histologically of rounded masses of small, darkly staining cells, which seem to fit together in a jigsaw-like pattern and are surrounded by pink-staining hyaline material. Hyaline globules are often present in the cellular masses and also larger cells with vesicular nuclei[7] (Fig. 4.3). Cylindroma in the external canal may be confused with primary adenoid cystic carcinoma of this location (see below). It differs from the latter in the absence of a cribriform structure, as well as in the presence of the larger cells with vesicular nuclei.

Chondroid Syringoma (Mixed Tumour)

A benign neoplasm of the skin with a structure similar to that of pleomorphic adenoma of salivary glands is also occasionally seen in the external auditory meatus. Cartilage, myoepithelial and adenomatous structures are features of this neoplasm. In some cases cartilage may be absent (Fig. 4.4).

Malignant Salivary Gland Type Neoplasms

Malignant glandular tumours of salivary gland type are sometimes seen in the ear canal, and an origin from ceruminous glands may then be reasonably postulated. It should again be stressed that exclusion of a primary site in the parotid gland is crucial. The most frequent of such tumours is adenoid cystic carcinoma. This malignant neoplasm has the gross and microscopic features of the corresponding major or minor salivary gland neoplasm (Fig. 4.5), including its tendency to invade along nerve sheaths. Relentless, although often delayed recurrence and eventual bloodstream metastasis, particularly to the lungs, is likewise a feature of this cancer.

Mucoepidermoid carcinoma arising as a primary neoplasm of the ear canal has been described. A malignant glandular neoplasm without adenoid cystic or mucoepidermoid structure may also arise in the ear canal. Its histology bears some similarity to adenoma of ceruminous glands, but the presence of nuclear atypia and mitotic figures enjoins a diagnosis of a malignant glandular neoplasm. A myoepithelial layer and decapitation secretion are not usually recognised in the malignant tumours.

Melanotic Neoplasms

Melanotic neoplasms are unusual in the external ear. Nevi arise mainly in the ear canal, but are rare on the auricle. Malignant melanomas, on the other hand, usually arise on the auricle; a single case only has been recorded in the canal.[8] Malignant melanoma of the external ear is a highly malignant disease. In a review of 16 patients with this condition, as many as nine showed invasion to Clark level IV or more.[9] It is likely that the parotid gland and cervical lymph nodes will be involved when malignant melanoma of the external ear is first diagnosed in a patient and early surgical excision of these two regions has been advised.[10]

Neoplasms of Bone and Cartilage

Benign Fibro-osseous Lesion (Fibrous Dysplasia)

In the section on osseous neoplasia of the nose and paranasal sinuses (see Chapter 21) it is suggested that, because of the difficulty of classifying a solitary benign neoplasm composed of woven bone and fibrous tissue into one or other of the classical groups – monostotic fibrous dysplasia or ossifying fibroma – the designation "benign fibro-osseous lesion" could be used in most circumstances without loss of accuracy. Lesions of a similar histological type are found in the temporal bone.

Nager et al.[11] have provided a detailed description of fibrous dysplasia and its involvement of the temporal bone. Sixty-nine patients were reviewed, of whom 38% had the monostotic form of fibrous dysplasia. More recently Megerian et al. reviewed 43 cases of fibrous dysplasia from the literature and added ten cases of their own. Seventy per cent of their 53 cases were monostotic.[12]

Extraskeletal Manifestations

Abnormal cutaneous and mucosal melanin pigmentation, usually in the midline of the body, is the commonest extraskeletal manifestation of fibrous dysplasia. It occurs in over 50% of polyostotic cases. The McCune-Albright syndrome is the association of precocious sexual development with polyostotic fibrous dysplasia. Goitre, hyperthyroidism, acromegaly, Cushing's disease, extrainsular hypothalamic diabetes mellitus and hyperparathyroidism are other endocrine lesions that may be associated with polyostotic fibrous dysplasia.

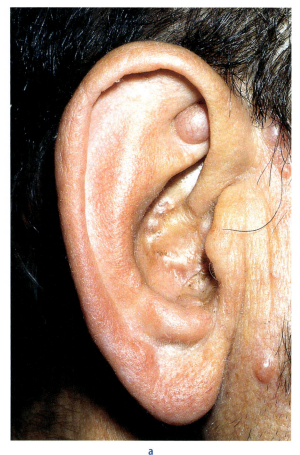

a

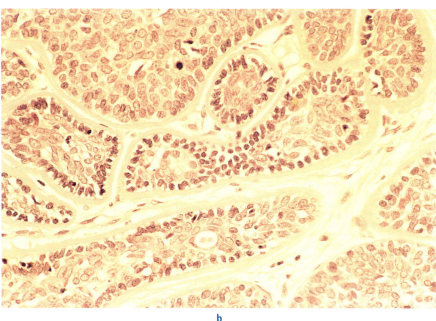

b

Figure 4.3 Cylindroma of pinna. **a** Multiple spherical tumours on pinna, face and temporal region. **b** Jigsaw-like pattern of cell groups surrounded by hyaline and enclosing some larger cells[19]

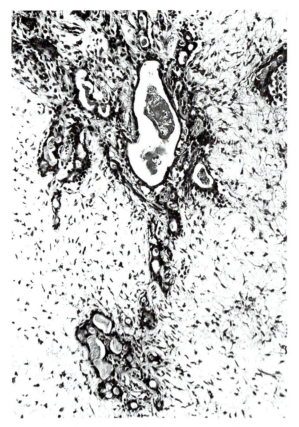

Figure 4.4 Mixed tumour of external auditory meatus. Note glandular epithelial elements and loosely lying myoepithelial cells

Clinical Features

The main clinical features are:

1. Progressive loss of hearing, conductive in most, sensorineural, which can be profound, in some.
2. Enlargement of the temporal bone with progressive bony occlusion of the external auditory meatus.
3. Facial nerve palsy is present in some patients due to involvement of the facial nerve by the pathological process.

Imaging Studies

Imaging studies show the sites of the disease to be in the tympanic, mastoid, squamous or petrous temporal bone. The internal auditory canal, the lateral semicircular canal and the ossicles may sometimes also be affected. Three radiographic patterns have been described:

1. Pagetoid, or "ground-glass", a mixture of dense and radiolucent areas of fibrosis; this is the most frequent radiological appearance.

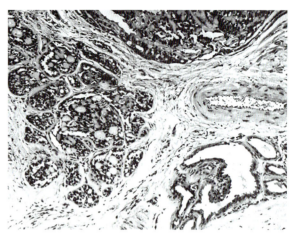

Figure 4.5 Adenoid cystic carcinoma of external auditory meatus. Lobules of neoplasm showing a cribriform pattern. Note normal ceruminous glands at *bottom right*

2. Sclerotic, homogeneously dense.
3. Cystic, a spherical or ovoid lucency surrounded by a dense boundary.

Pathological Appearances

The gross appearance of fibrous dysplasia is one of yellowish-white resilient tissue, which occasionally includes small cysts filled with an amber-coloured fluid. The transition to normal bone is sharp. Microscopically irregular trabeculae of woven bone are embedded in a connective tissue stroma (Fig. 4.6). The bony trabeculae are said to lack osteoblasts around their periphery, but this is by no means invariable. The constriction of the ear canal may cause an epidermoid cyst lateral to the tympanic membrane, referred to as "cholesteatoma" by Megerian et al.[12]

Malignant Transformation

Although fibrous dysplasia has been on rare occasions associated with malignant disease such as osteogenic sarcoma, fibrosarcoma, chondrosarcoma and giant cell tumour, the temporal bone is not one of the sites where this change has been described.

Osteoma and Exostosis

Two types of benign bony enlargement of the deeper bony portion of the external auditory meatus are recognised: osteoma and exostosis.

Osteoma is a spherical mass arising from the region of the tympanosquamous or tympanomas-

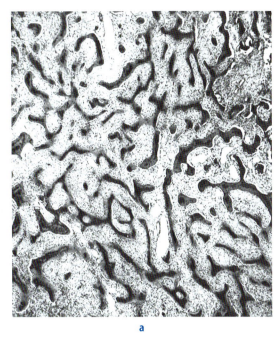

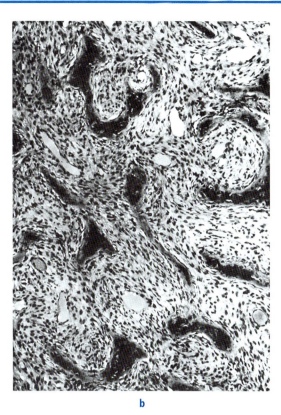

a										b

Figure 4.6 a Benign fibro-osseous lesion (fibrous dysplasia) of temporal bone. Irregular trabeculae of woven bone forming a "Chinese letter" pattern. Between the bony trabeculae is a stroma of cellular connective tissue. **b** Higher power of part of **a**, showing bony trabeculae partly lined by osteoblasts and cellular fibrous stroma

toid suture line by a distinct bony pedicle. Symptoms are usually those of ear canal obstruction (Fig. 4.7). Microscopically the osteoma is composed of lamellar bone and may show outer cortical and inner cancellous trabeculated areas, the latter with marrow spaces. There may be a thin layer of woven bone on the surfaces of the lamellar bone. The osteoma is covered by the normal squamous epithelium of the ear canal.

Exostosis is a broad-based lesion, which is often bilateral and symmetrical. It is usually situated deeper in the ear canal than osteomas. In the bony portion of the normal external auditory meatus there are no adnexal structures, and the subcutaneous tissue and periosteum merge to form a thin layer. The distance between the epidermal surface and underlying bone is consequently small. This explains the propensity for exostoses of the tympanic bone to develop in this region in those who swim frequently in cold water. It seems likely that the water, after dribbling into the deep external auditory canal, exerts a cooling effect on the bone surface and stimulates it to produce new bone. Unlike osteoma, the bone formations of exostosis

are said not to possess any marrow spaces (Fig. 4.8).

Osteoma and exostosis are often associated with infection of the external canal on their tympanic membrane side and surgical removal may be

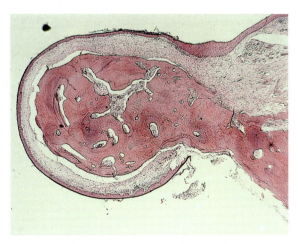

Figure 4.7 Osteoma of deep external canal[19]

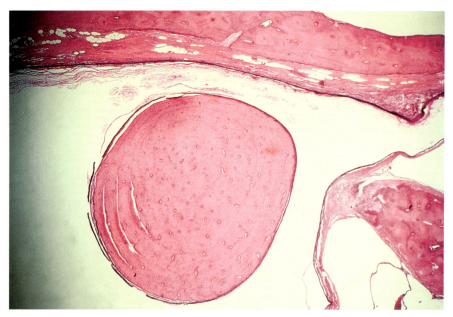

Figure 4.8 Exostosis of deep external canal. Note thin epidermal layer on the exostosis and canal skin and their proximity to the bone[19]

required to enhance drainage as well as to relieve the conductive hearing loss.

Fibro-osseous Lesion of the Superficial External Canal

Five cases of a benign circumscribed bony lesion of the external auditory canal distinct from exostosis and osteoma have recently been described.[13] They all showed a hard, round, unilateral, skin-covered mass occluding the superficial external auditory canal with no relationship to the cartilaginous tissue or to the bony structure surrounding that canal. Histologically the lesion displayed an osteoma-like bone formation with sparse osteoblastic areas; mature lamellar bone was observed in some cases, and also bone marrow containing adipose tissue and haematopoietic remnants. The bone showed irregular trabeculae, bordered by osteoid osteoblasts.

Neural Neoplasms

The only common neural neoplasm of the temporal bone is the schwannoma of the eighth cranial nerve (see Chapter 11). A schwannoma of the facial nerve is occasionally seen. Clinically the patient may present with facial palsy. Histologically the features are those of a typical neurilemmoma.

Neoplasms of Muscle

Rhabdomyosarcoma

Rhabdomyosarcoma is seen occasionally in the temporal bone. The usual age incidence is from 1 to 12 years, with an average of 4.4 years.[14] In most cases both the external canal and middle ear are involved by the neoplasm, so that the exact site of origin is difficult to determine. The child usually has a bloody discharge from the ear, when a tumour may be observed in the external auditory meatus. It is highly malignant and with widespread local invasion and lymph node and bloodstream metastases.

Grossly the tumour is lobulated and dark red with a hemorrhagic cut surface. Almost all temporal bone rhabdomyosarcomas are of the embryonal type (see Chapter 25).

Rhabdomyosarcoma of the temporal bone is highly malignant and spreads extensively into the cranial cavity, externally or to the pharyngeal region. Lymph node and bloodstream metastases frequently develop in these patients.

Kaposi's Sarcoma and Other Manifestations of AIDS

Kaposi's sarcoma is a neoplasm with histological features comprising a mixture of spindle cells and branching vascular channels. Multiple deposits of this tumour are seen in some patients with AIDS and have been seen in the tympanic cavity and external and internal ear in cases of HIV infection with AIDS.

Another manifestation of AIDS in the ear that has been found by direct pathologic examination of diseased tissue is that of infection with *Pneumocystis carinii*, including the skin of the external ear and the middle ear cavity.[15,16]

Reticuloendothelial Neoplasms

Langerhans' Cell Histiocytosis

Langerhans' cell histiocytosis (histiocytosis X, eosinophil granuloma, Hand-Schuller-Christian disease) sometimes affects the temporal bone as a bony lesion of the medial part of the external auditory meatus in children. It is characterised by multifocal proliferation of histiocyte-like cells with many foam cells. Eosinophils are often prominent. Polymorphonuclear leucocytes and plasma cells may also be abundant. A distinct feature on electron microscopy is the presence of a rod-shaped inclusion in the cytoplasm of the histiocytes. This is known as the Birbeck granule and is identical with the structures seen in the cytoplasm of the Langerhans cell of the epidermis (see also Chapter 22).

In the temporal bone the disease is usually manifested as a bony lesion of the medial part of the external auditory meatus in children, often with ear discharge.[17] In patients younger than 3 years of age, the disease process is more likely to be multifocal in the skull, i.e. to be of the Hand-Schuller-Christian disease variety and to have a worse outlook.

Malignant Lymphoma

Malignant lymphoma may appear in the external ear as part of a generalised process. Occasionally it may be primary in this situation, presenting as a B- or T-cell lymphoma of the skin of the pinna. Some cases may present a striking symmetry in deposition of the lymphoid neoplasia, each earlobe or both ear-lobes and helices on each side being similarly affected.[18]

References

1. Bremnes RM, Kvamme JM, Stalsberg H et al. Pilomatrix carcinoma with multiple metastases: report of a case and review of the literature. Eur J Cancer 1999;35:433–437
2. Bailin PH, Levine HL, Wood BG et al. Cutaneous carcinoma of the auricular and preauricular region. Arch Otolaryngol 1980;106:692–696
3. Stafford ND, Frootko NJ. Verrucous carcinoma in the external auditory canal. Am J Otol 1986;7:443–445
4. Cooper JR, Hellquist HB, Michaels L. Image analysis in the discrimination of verrucous carcinoma and squamous papilloma. J Pathol 1992;166:383–387.
5. Wetli CV, Pardo V, Millard M et al. Tumours of ceruminous glands. Cancer 1972;29:1169–1178
6. Cankar V, Crowley H. Tumours of ceruminous glands: a clinicopathological study of seven cases. Cancer 1964;17:67–75
7. Wolf BA, Gluckman JL, Wirman JA. Benign dermal cylindroma of the external auditory canal: a clinicopathological report. Am J Otolaryngol 1985;6:35–38
8. Milbrath MM, Campbell BH, Madiedo G et al. Malignant melanoma of the external auditory canal. Am J Clin Oncol 1998;21:28–30
9. Davidsson A, Hellquist HB, Villman K et al. Malignant melanoma of the ear. J Laryngol Otol 1993;107:798–802
10. Shah JP, Kraus DH, Dubner S et al. Patterns of regional lymph node metastases from cutaneous melanomas of the head and neck. Am J Surg 1991;162:320–323
11. Nager GT, Kennedy DW, Kopstein E. Fibrous dysplasia: a review of the disease and its manifestations in the temporal bone. Ann Otol Rhinol Laryngol 1982;91(suppl 92)
12. Megerian CA, Sofferman RA, McKenna MJ et al. Fibrous dysplasia of the temporal bone: ten new cases demonstrating the spectrum of otologic sequelae. Am J Otol 1995;16:408–419
13. Ramirez-Camacho R, Vicente J, Garcia Berrocal JR et al. Fibro-osseous lesions of the external auditory canal. Laryngoscope 1999;109:488–491
14. Wiatrak BJ, Pensak ML. Rhabdomyosarcoma of the ear and temporal bone. Laryngoscope 1989;99:1188–1192
15. Gherman CR, Ward RR, Bassis ML. *Pneumocystis carinii* otitis media and mastoiditis as the initial manifestation of the acquired immunodeficiency syndrome. Am J Med 1988;85:250–252
16. Smith MA, Hirschfield LS, Zahtz G et al. *Pneumocystis carinii* otitis media. Am J Med 1988;85:745–756.
17. Quesada P, Navarrete ML, Perrello E. Eosinophilic granuloma of the temporal bone. Eur Arch Otorhinolaryngol 1990;247:194–195
18. Goudie RB, Soukop M, Dagg JH et al. Hypothesis: symmetrical cutaneous lymphoma. Lancet 1990;1:316–318
19. Michaels L. Chapter 80. The ear. In: Damjanov I, Linder J. Anderson's pathology, 10th edn. Mosby Year Book Inc., St. Louis, Missouri, 1996, pp 2876–2900

5 Neoplasms and Similar Lesions of the Middle Ear

The middle ear is only occasionally the site of a new growth. Because of its deep-seated position, primary malignant tumours of the middle ear do not usually manifest themselves until they are well advanced. Table 5.1 lists the developmental tumour-like anomalies and neoplasms that have been located there.

Developmental Tumour-like Anomalies

A hamartoma is a focal overgrowth in improper proportions, of tissues normally present in that part of the body. A choristoma is similar to hamartoma, except that the tissues of which it is composed are not normally present in the part of the body where it is found. Choristomas are occasionally seen in the middle ear. They are composed of one or other of three types of tissue: salivary gland, glial or sebaceous glandular tissue.

Table 5.1. Neoplasms and similar lesions of the middle ear

Developmental tumour-like anomalies
Salivary choristoma
Glial deposit
Sebaceous choristoma

Primary neoplasms
Adenoma
Papillary adenocarcinoma
Meningioma
Paraganglioma
Squamous cell carcinoma

Secondary neoplasms
Metastatic neoplasms

Salivary gland choristomas consist as a rule of mixed mucous and serous elements like the normal submandibular or sublingual gland, but unlike the parotid gland (Fig. 5.1). The lesion typically consists of a lobulated mass of histologically normal salivary gland tissue in the middle ear attached posteriorly in the region of the oval window. Frequently the mass is intimately associated with the facial nerve. There are usually absent or malformed ossicles.[1] Glial masses are composed largely of astrocytic cells (Fig. 5.2), the identity of which may be confirmed by immunohistochemical staining for glial acidic fibrillary protein. When such masses are identified in biopsy material from the middle ear, a bony deficit with consequent herniation of brain tissue into the middle ear should be ruled out.[2] Three cases of heterotopic brain tissue in the middle ear associated with cholesteatoma have been reported.[3] It is possible that in all three, brain herniation occurred as a result of inflammatory damage to the tegmen tympani. Spontaneous herniations of brain (encephaloceles) may occur into the middle ear through a deficiency of the tegmen or other sites.[4]

A case of sebaceous choristoma of the middle ear has been described.[5] At middle ear exploration a mass was found in the hypotympanum, which showed at microscopy stratified squamous epithelium covering a large area of sebaceous gland tissue. The appearances in this case, although presenting sebaceous glands in the hypotympanum and skin, not hairy skin in the pharynx, bring to mind the recent interpretation by Heffner et al. of pharyngeal hairy polyps (see Chapter 23) as choristomatous developmental anomalies arising from the first branchial cleft area and representing accessory auricles.[6] An ectodermal cell rest, the epidermoid formation, is present in the tubotympanic recess (precursor of Eustachian tube and middle ear)

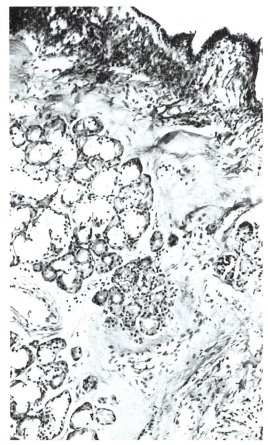

Figure 5.1 Salivary gland choristoma of middle ear. Lobules of salivary gland tissue are present in the mucosa. The acini are composed of both mucous and serous glandular elements

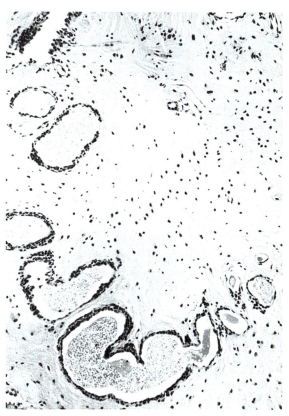

Figure 5.2 "Glioma" of middle ear. The deposit is composed of fibrillary astrocytes. Glands formed by irritated middle ear mucosa are also present

throughout development (see Chapter 1) and it seems possible that both the hairy polyp of the nasopharynx and the sebaceous choristoma of the middle ear may arise from full differentiation of the epidermoid formation to a skin-like condition.

Neoplasms

Adenoma

The epithelium of the middle ear has a propensity for gland formation in otitis media (see Chapters 1 and 3) and adenoma would seem to represent a benign neoplastic transformation of the epithelium along the same lines.

Clinical Features

Most patients complain of hearing loss, which is of conductive type. Pain, facial palsy and ear discharge are usually absent. The tympanic membrane is almost always intact and the neoplasm confined to the middle ear, sometimes extending to the mastoid spaces; in a few cases the tumour does extend externally through a perforation into the ear canal, or even may occasionally penetrate through an intact tympanic membrane.

Gross Appearances

The neoplasm has been described as being white, yellow, grey or reddish-brown at operation and unlike paraganglioma is usually not vascular. It seems to peel away from the walls of the surrounding middle ear with ease, although ossicles may sometimes be entrapped in the tumour mass and may even show destruction.

Microscopic Appearances

Adenoma is formed by closely apposed small glands with a "back-to-back" appearance (Fig. 5.3). In some places a solid or trabecular arrangement is present. Sheet-like, disorganised areas are seen in which the

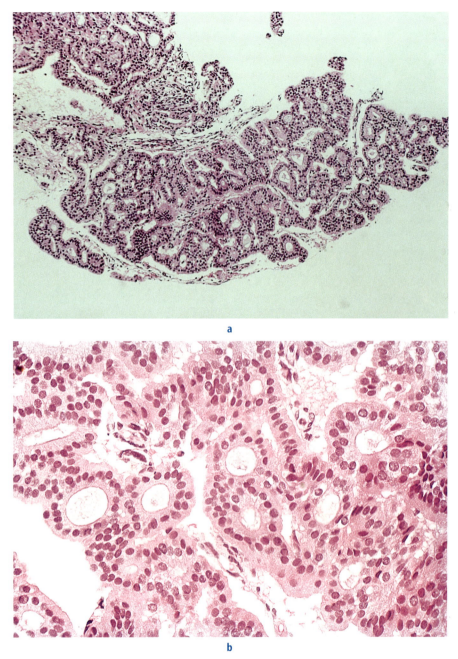

Figure 5.3 Adenoma of the middle ear. **a** Low-power view. **b** High-power view

glandular pattern appears to be lost. This may be artefactual and related to the effects of trauma used in taking the biopsy specimen on the delicate structure of the cells, but the appearance may erroneously lead one to suspect malignancy. The cells are regular, cuboidal or columnar and may enclose luminal secretion. A distinct and predominant "plasmacytoid" appearance of the epithelial cells of the neoplasm may be displayed.[7] No myoepithelial layer is seen. Periodic acid–Schiff and Alcian blue stains may be positive for mucoprotein secretion in the gland lumina and in the cytoplasm of the tumour cells.

Neuroendocrine Change and the Concept of "Carcinoid"

Historical Review

Benign glandular tumours of the middle ear were not described until 1976.[8,9] In 1975 Fayemi and

Toker had reported glandular tumours of the middle ear with a bland histological structure, but believed that they were adenocarcinomas.[10] Murphy et al. in 1980[11] were the first to report that a glandular tumour of the middle ear, otherwise identical to an adenoma, was Grimelius positive and on electron microscopy, showed numerous membrane-bound granules. These neuroendocrine features were held to indicate a neoplasm distinct from adenoma, which was termed "carcinoid", suggesting a similarity to carcinoid tumours of the small intestine and bronchus. Friedmann et al. in 1983 described membrane-bound granules on electron microscopy in the cytoplasm of the tumour cells of a glandular middle ear neoplasm, thereby categorising it as a potentially malignant "carcinoid".[12] In support of this assertion, they cited the supposed carcinoid-like morphology of the adenocarcinomas diagnosed by Fazemi and Toker in 1975,[10] but did not mention the possibility of any relationship to the benign glandular middle ear neoplasms described in 1976.[8,9]

From the time of the case report of Friedmann et al. until 1983 there has been a series of at least 16 further papers in which cases of "carcinoid tumours" were described, either ignoring the entity of adenoma altogether or claiming that carcinoid was a lesion distinct from it with the potential for more aggressive behaviour. The neuroendocrine aspect of these tumours could now, by the use of immunohistochemistry from 1987, be further confirmed[13] and a broad range of polypeptides was identified in the cytoplasm of the tumours in the process. We have inspected the illustrations of the histology of these neoplasms in the majority of these articles and find the morphological structure to be similar to that of adenoma of the middle ear. All of them, moreover, had findings at surgery and a benign clinical course identical to those of adenoma of the middle ear.

There can be no objection to the separation of a glandular tumour of the middle ear without neuroendocrine features from a glandular tumour with those features. The use of the term "carcinoid" for the latter, however, implies a potentially malignant activity that was not displayed in any of the cases. Thus the "carcinoids" described by Krouse et al. in 1990[14] were identified as "low-grade malignant neoplasms" only, because of their neuroendocrine features, although the authors believed that "recurrence (was) unlikely with adequate local excision".

The wrong choice of a diagnostic category can, unfortunately, lead to unnecessary treatment, which may be deleterious to the patients involved. It can also lead to further misinterpretations that can cloud over the illogicality of the original concept. After nearly 20 years of separation of a glandular neuroendocrine neoplasm of the middle ear as a "carcinoid" it was, perhaps, to be expected that a non-glandular neuroendocrine neoplasm of the middle ear would be labelled as "carcinoid tumour" and, with its manifestation of metastases, be hailed as the first carcinoid of the middle ear to metastasise. The patient described by Mooney et al. in 1999 had a "glomus jugulare" tumour (see below) of the right temporal bone, which was treated by surgery and radiotherapy.[15] The neoplasm recurred in the middle ear and 9 years later displayed metastases in cervical lymph nodes. The diagnosis was changed to "carcinoid" of the middle ear because it showed positivity for cytokeratin in both the original middle ear and in the cervical metastases, but despite the following features:

1. The origin of the neoplasm from the jugular region of the temporal bone that was implicit in the original diagnosis of "glomus jugulare", a paraganglioma spreading to the middle ear from the jugular region, as opposed to "glomus tympanicum", an entirely middle ear paraganglioma (see below).
2. The absence of an acinar or glandular morphology of the neoplasm in illustrations of biopsy sections either from the middle ear primary or from its lymph node metastases.

It would seem that there is insufficient evidence in this case at present to warrant its diagnosis as a glandular neuroendocrine neoplasm ("carcinoid") of the middle ear.

Neuroendocrine Features of Adenomas

A deeper understanding of the significance of the neuroendocrine changes in the benign glandular tumour of the middle ear was provided by the important study of Wassef et al. in 1989.[16] In a meticulous investigation of five cases of this neoplasm by normal light microscopic methods, immunohistochemistry and transmission electron microscopy, the glandular areas of the tumour in each patient showed a bidirectional mucinous and neuroendocrine differentiation. This was demonstrated by the presence of two cell types. Apically situated dark cells contained mucous granules; these cells were negative for neuroendocrine markers. Basally situated cells contained neuroendocrine granules; these cells were positive for neuroendocrine markers – vasoactive intestinal polypeptides or neuron-specific enolase. In the solid areas the tumour cells were composed mainly or exclusively of cells of neuroendocrine differentiation.

Wassef et al. indicated that the tendency to neuroendocrine as well as mucinous differentiation shown by these middle ear tumours is one that is widespread in neoplasms in general and particularly in neoplasms of endodermal origin.[17]

Conclusions

We would suggest that there is but a single benign glandular neoplasm of the middle ear. It is safer to give it the designation of adenoma. Neuroendocrine as well as mucinous differentiation is frequent, perhaps universal, in these neoplasms. The presence of neuroendocrine differentiation does not reflect a more aggressive potential.

Papillary Adenocarcinoma

Many glandular neoplasms in which a diagnosis of primary adenocarcinoma of the middle ear is at first suspected show features that allow their eventual classification as adenomas of the middle ear. Some, however, show too many atypical cellular features for a benign tumour and adenocarcinoma must be considered. In such cases every effort must be made to exclude the possibility of a secondary metastatic deposit. Tumours with a papillary adenocarcinomatous pattern with a close resemblance to papillary adenocarcinoma of the thyroid have been identified in the middle ear (Fig. 5.4). Their behaviour is that of a slowly growing but invasive neoplasm. In many cases the tumour has permeated widely into the temporal bone at presentation, producing a lytic lesion, seen by radiological examination and showing significant extension into the posterior cranial fossa.[18] Some, at least, of these cases would seem to fall into the category of low-grade adenocarcinoma of the endolymphatic sac (see Chapter 11).

Meningioma

Meningiomas are usually intracranial neoplasms. Extracranial meningiomas, however, may be found (see Chapter 18). Like the intracranial variety, they are thought to arise from arachnoid villi. These structures may be formed at a number of sites in the temporal bone, including the internal auditory meatus, the jugular foramen, the geniculate ganglion region and the roof of the Eustachian tube. Thus meningiomas may arise from a wide area within the temporal bone itself.[19] The commonest temporal bone site for primary meningioma is in the middle ear cleft. Symptoms are usually those of otitis media; involvement of the chorda tympani and the facial nerve may also occur.

Gross appearances are those of a granular or even gritty mass. Microscopically the neoplasm takes the same forms as any of the well-described intracranial types of meningioma. The commonest variety seen in the middle ear is the meningothelial type, in which the tumour cells form masses of epithelioid, regular cells often disposed into whorls. Fibroblastic and psammatous varieties are also sometimes seen in the middle ear.

Histological diagnosis of meningioma may be difficult because the above features are indistinct. Under these circumstances immunocytochemistry may be of some diagnostic value. Most of the markers are negative, including those for cytokeratins. Vimentin and epithelial membrane antigen are, however, positive in the majority of meningiomas.[20] Nager's review of temporal bone menin-

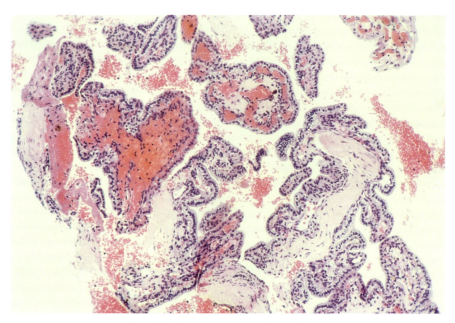

Figure 5.4 Papillary adenocarcinoma of the middle ear

giomas indicated that only two out of 30 patients survived a 5-year period.[19] More recent experience of middle ear meningiomas signals a better outlook after careful local excision. Nevertheless, meningiomas presenting in the middle ear and considered at surgery to be primary in that situation, will often be found on imaging studies to be arising from outside the petrous bone, probably on its external surface, and therefore actually to be invading the middle ear. Such tumours do not necessarily present with the symptoms of a space-occupying intracranial lesion.

Jugulotympanic Paraganglioma

Synonyms of this neoplasm are glomus tumour and chemodectoma. This tumour, which presents mostly in the middle ear, is slightly less frequent than squamous cell carcinoma in this situation.

Site of Origin

Most jugulotympanic paragangliomas arise from the paraganglion situated in the wall of the jugular bulb. These tumours have been referred to as jugular paragangliomas or glomus jugulare tumours. A minority of the tumours arise from the paraganglion situated near the middle ear surface of the promontory (see Chapter 1). These tumours have been referred to as tympanic parangliomas or glomus tympanicum tumours. The distinction between jugular and tympanic paragangliomas can easily be made by modern imaging methods. The jugular neoplasm is identified as arising from the jugular bulb region and shows evidence of invasion of the petrous bone. The tympanic neoplasm is confined to the middle ear. The gross and histological appearances of the two types of neoplasm in the middle ear are, however, identical.

Sex and Age Incidence

Solitary jugulotympanic paragangliomas arise predominantly in females. The neoplasm has been seen at ages between 13 and 85 years with a mean age of about 50 years.

Clinical Features

Most patients present with conductive hearing loss. Pain in the ear, facial palsy, haemorrhage, and tinnitus are also described as symptoms of this lesion. On examination a red vascular mass is seen either behind the intact tympanic membrane or sprouting through the latter into the external canal. Surgical approach to the mass at biopsy often results in severe bleeding.

Genetic Aspects

Jugulotympanic paragangliomas may be multicentric or coexist with tumours of other types. They may be bilateral in the same patient and coexist with carotid body paragangliomas, which may be bilateral.[21] They may also coexist with adrenal gland pheochromocytomas, which can produce hypertension. A familial tendency to grow paragangliomas has been noted, particularly in cases with multiple tumours of this type. In such family groups of patients with head and neck, including jugulotympanic, paragangliomas there is, unlike the solitary jugulotympanic paraganglioma (see above) a preponderance for the male sex and inheritance is autosomal dominant, with an increased penetrance with age.[22] There is evidence from molecular genetic studies that the gene underlying familial paragangliomas is located on chromosome 11q proximal to the tyrosinase gene locus.[23]

Gross Appearances

The neoplasm is a reddish sprouting mass at its external canal surface. In the jugular variety the petrous temporal bone is largely replaced by red, firm material and the middle ear space is occupied by soft neoplasm as far as the tympanic membrane. The bony labyrinth is rarely invaded by paraganglioma. Investigation of a paraganglioma in an autopsy temporal bone by the microslicing method showed the shape of the jugular bulb to be retained, but the lumen to be completely replaced by neoplasm (Fig. 5.5).

Microscopic Appearances

The neoplasm in a typical section shows some resemblance to the carotid body tumour. Epithelioid, uniform cells are separated by numerous blood vessels. The tumour cells often form clusters or "Zellballen" with peripheral flattened cells (Fig. 5.6). Nuclei are usually uniform and small, but diagnosis is sometimes made difficult by the presence of bizarre or multinucleate cells. These appearances do not denote a malignant origin. A fibrous stroma is sometimes encountered in these tumours.

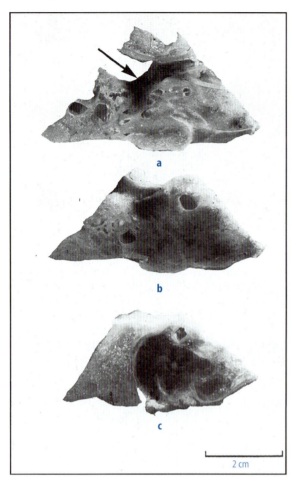

Figure 5.5 Microslices of temporal bone in a case of jugular paraganglioma. The tumour appears as dark areas, bright red in the original. In **c** it has expanded to the shape and position of the jugular bulb, where it has arisen. In **b** tumour is extending through the temporal bone and has reached the middle ear. In **a** tumour is entirely in the middle ear, but has not penetrated the tympanic membrane, which is marked by an *arrow*

Reticulin stain usually shows groups of tumour cells surrounded by reticulin, without reticulin fibres between the cells.

Immunohistochemistry and Electron Microscopy

Jugulotympanic paragangliomas express neuron-specific enolase and chromogranin A on immunocytochemical investigation, but cytokeratins are consistently negative.[24]

Normal paraganglionic tissue contains two types of cell: chief or type I cells, which are neuroendocrine cells, and sustentacular or type II cells, which are not neuroendocrine, but contain S-100 protein. The observation that the S-100 protein-containing sustentacular cells are diminished in hyper-

plasia and neoplasia of the adrenal medulla[25] has led to investigations of the status of the sustentacular cells in benign as opposed to malignant neoplasms of paraganglionic tissue at other sites.[26] Sustentacular cells were identified by their positivity to S-100 protein and glial fibrillary acidic protein (GFAP). Low-grade tumours, i.e. those that were not recurrent, locally aggressive or metastatic, contained sustentacular cells (Fig. 5.6). The majority of intermediate-grade paragangliomas, i.e. those that were recurrent or locally aggressive, had diminished or absent reactivity to S-100 protein and GFAP. All malignant paragangliomas were devoid of sustentacular cells except in one case, which showed only rare S-100 protein-positive cells. Jugulotympanic paragangliomas usually have sparse, but not absent, S-100 protein-staining sustentacular cells, implying a rather aggressive, but not fully malignant, activity.

Electron-microscopic examination of paragangliomas shows membrane-bound, electron-dense neurosecretory granules in the cytoplasm of the tumour cells, indicating a significant catecholamine

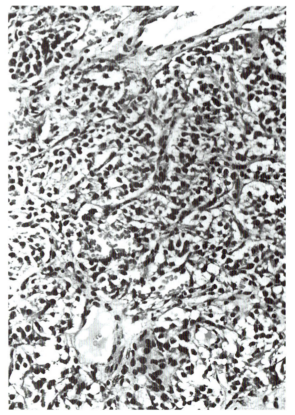

Figure 5.6 Jugular paraganglioma. The cells form small clusters, each surrounded by a row of flattened cells, probably sustentacular cells, and separated by blood vessels

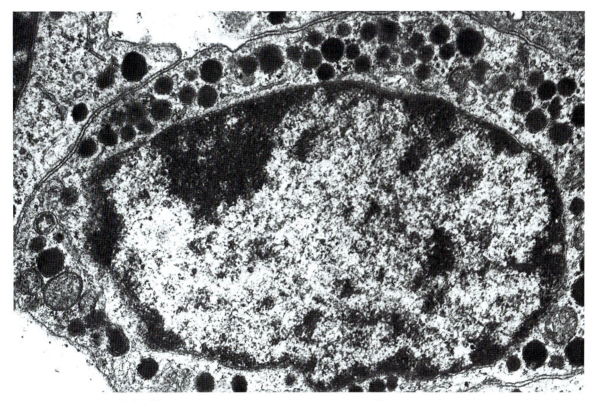

Figure 5.7 Electron micrograph of a cell from a jugular paraganglioma. Membrane-bound granules of between 170 and 260 nm are present in the cytoplasm of the tumour. Original magnification × 30 000

(epinephrine and norepinephrine) content[27] (Fig. 5.7), but the incidence of clinically functioning paraganglioma is only 1–3%. Symptoms and signs are those of norepinephrine excess, particularly hypertension. Neurone-specific enolase as demonstrated by the immunoperoxidase method is present in the cells of this neoplasm.

Spread and Natural History

Jugulotympanic paraganglioma is a neoplasm of slow growth. The jugular variety infiltrates the petrous bone, but distant metastasis is rare. Radiation therapy, and in some cases surgery, offers a high rate of cure for these neoplasms and the number of patients who do badly after such therapy is very small.

Squamous Carcinoma

Squamous carcinoma of the middle ear is very uncommon.

Age and Sex Incidence

There is an equal incidence between the sexes. The age range is 34–85 years, with an average of 60 years.[28]

Clinical Features

Aural discharge and conductive hearing loss are present in all patients. Pain in the ear, bleeding and facial palsy are common.

Site of Origin and Microscopic Appearances

In microscopic sections the tumour may be seen arising from the surface squamous epithelium, itself metaplastic from the normal cubical epithelium. In certain areas an origin from the basal layers of cubical or columnar epithelium may be seen. This feature is present also in some cases of squamous carcinoma of the larynx (see Chapter 34). In some the tumour arises from the external as well as the middle ear, and the squamous epithelium of the ear canal (identified by its sebaceous and apocrine adnexa) is confirmed histologically as the source of part of the tumour. There is no doubt that such cases arise concomitantly from both external and middle ear epithelia, rather than by subepithelial spread of tumour from one to the other. Such widespread field change is a frequent feature of squamous carcinoma of the head and neck (see Chapters 16, 27, 35 and 39).

There is no evidence at present that the epidermoid formation, a cell rest which occurs normally in the middle ear during development (see Chapter 1) may be a source of squamous carcinoma in some cases.

The neoplasm is an epidermoid carcinoma, similar in its range of keratinisation and epithelial differentiation to neoplasms of the same histological type elsewhere in the upper respiratory tract. Carcinoma in situ may be seen in some parts of the middle ear epithelium adjacent to the growth.

Spread

The mode of spread of the neoplasm from the middle ear epithelium was ascertained in temporal bone autopsy sections by Michaels and Wells[28] and has been confirmed radiologically in living patients. The carcinoma tends to grow into and erode the thin bony plate which separates the medial wall of the middle ear, at its junction with the Eustachian tube, from the carotid canal. This bony wall is normally up to 1 mm in thickness and may be recognised radiologically. Having reached the carotid canal, the growth will extend rapidly along the sympathetic nerves and the tumour is then impossible to eradicate surgically (Fig. 5.8). Another important method of spread is through the bony walls of the posterior mastoid air cells to the dura of the posterior surface of the temporal bone. From there it spreads medially, enters the internal auditory meatus and may then invade the cochlea and vestibule. Spread into the lamellar bone in both of these situations is along vascular channels between bone trabeculae. A similar type of bone invasion may also occur from other parts of the middle ear surface such as in the region of the facial nerve. The special bone of the bony labyrinth is, on the other hand, peculiarly resistant to direct spread of growth from tumour within the

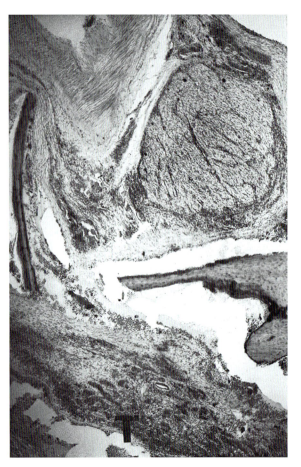

Figure 5.8 Squamous carcinoma of middle ear growing from the epithelium of the Eustachian tube (*T*) has penetrated the thin bar of bone separating it from the carotid canal and is growing in the nerve plexus around the internal carotid artery

middle ear; even the round window membrane is not invaded. When invasion does occur it takes place after entry of the tumour into the internal auditory meatus and penetration of the bone by way of the filaments of the vestibular and cochlear divisions of the eighth nerve. In the later stages tumour grows extensively in the middle cranial fossa and may invade the condyle of the mandible. Death is usually due to direct intracranial extension. Lymph node metastasis is unusual and spread by the bloodstream even more so.

Metastatic Neoplasms

Metastasis of malignant neoplasms to the temporal bone including the middle ear is not uncommon. Hill and Kohut[29] listed breast, lung, kidney, stomach and larynx as primary sources of metastatic

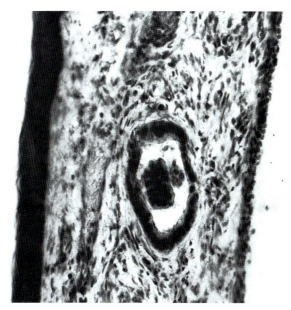

Figure 5.9 Metastastic adenocarcinoma of temporal bone. Section of tympanic membrane. Adenocarcinoma has grown from the bony tympanic ring into the connective tissue layer of the membrane

tumours, in that order of frequency. Jahn et al.[30] drew attention to malignant melanoma as a common source of metastasis and noted two distinct modes of spread of all metastatic neoplasms within the temporal bone. These correspond to the two modes of spread described in primary squamous carcinoma above: (1) along vascular channels in the petrous bone and (2) along nerves emanating from the internal auditory meatus into the labyrinthine structures and bone. A striking rarity that we have observed in a case of metastatic adenocarcinoma is one in which the neoplasm grew along the connective tissue of the tympanic membrane between the epidermis and middle ear epithelium (Fig. 5.9).

References

1. Hinni ML, Beatty CW. Salivary gland choristoma of the middle ear: report of a case and review of the literature. Ear Nose Throat J 1996;75:422–424
2. Kamerer DB, Caparosa RJ. Temporal bone encephalocele. Diagnosis and treatment. Laryngoscope 1982;92:878–881
3. McGregor DH, Cherian R, Kepes JJ et al. Case reports: heterotopic brain tissue of middle ear associated with cholesteatoma. Am J Med Sci 1994;308:180–183
4. Iurato S, Bux G, Colucci S et al. Histopathology of spontaneous brain herniations into the middle ear. Acta Otolaryngol (Stockh) 1992;112:328–333
5. Nelson EG, Kratz RC. Sebaceous choristoma of the middle ear. Otolaryngol Head Neck Surg 1993;108:372–373
6. Heffner DK, Thompson LD, Schall DG et al. Pharyngeal dermoids ("hairy polyps") as accessory auricles. Ann Otol Rhinol Laryngol 1996;105:819–824
7. Ribe A, Fernandez PL, Ostertarg H et al. Middle-ear adenoma (MEA): a report of two cases, one with predominant "plasmacytoid" features. Histopathology 1997;30:359–364
8. Hyams VJ, Michaels L. Benign adenomatous neoplasms (adenoma) of the middle ear. Clin Otolaryngol 1976;1:17–26
9. Derlacki EL, Barney PL. Adenomatous tumours of the middle ear and mastoid. Laryngoscope 1976;86:1123–1135
10. Fayemi AO, Toker C. Primary adenocarcinoma of the middle ear. Arch Otolaryngol 1975;101:449–452
11. Murphy GE, Pilch BZ, Dickersin GR et al. Carcinoid tumour of the middle ear. Am J Clin Pathol 1980;73:816–823
12. Friedmann I, Galey FR, House WF et al. A mixed carcinoid tumour of the middle ear. J Laryngol Otol 1983;97:465–470
13. Stanley MW, Horwitz CA, Levinson RM et al. Carcinoid tumours of the middle ear. Am J Clin Pathol 1987; 7:592–600
14. Krouse JH, Nadol JB Jr, Goodman ML. Carcinoid tumours of the middle ear. Ann Otol Rhinol Laryngol 1990;99:547–552
15. Mooney EE, Dodd LG, Oury TD et al. Middle ear carcinoid: an indolent tumour with metastatic potential. Head Neck 1999;21:72–77
16. Wassef M, Kanavaros P, Polivka M et al. Middle ear adenoma. A tumour displaying mucinous and neuroendocrine differentiation. Am J Surg Pathol 1989; 13:838–847
17. Sidhu GS. The endodermal origin of digestive and respiratory tract APUD cells: histopathologic evidence and a review of the literature. Am J Pathol 1979;96:5–20.
18. Mills ES, Fechner RE, Intemann SR et al. Aggressive papillary middle-ear tumours. A clinico-pathologic entity distinct from middle-ear adenoma. Am J Surg Pathol 1988;12:790–797
19. Nager GT. Meningiomas involving the temporal bone. Charles C Thomas, Springfield Ill, 1963
20. Shanmugaratnam K (ed) Histological typing of upper respiratory tract tumours, 2nd edn. Springer, Berlin, 1991
21. Ophir D. Familial multicentric paragangliomas in a child. J Laryngol Otol 1991;105:376–380
22. van Baars FM, Cremers CW, van den Broek P et al. Familiar non-chromaffinic paragangliomas (glomus tumours). Clinical and genetic aspects. Acta Otolaryngol Stockh 1981;91:589–593
23. Mariman EC, van Beersum SE, Cremers CW et al. Analysis of a second family with hereditary non-chromaffin paragangliomas locates the underlying gene at the proximal region of chromosome 11q. Hum Genet 1993;91:357–361
24. Martinez-Madrigal F, Bosq J, Micheau C et al. Paragangliomas of the head and neck. Immunohistochemical analysis of 16 cases in comparison with neuro-endocrine carcinomas. Pathol Res Pract 1991; 187:814–823
25. Lloyd RV, Blaivas M, Wilson BS. Distribution of chromogranin and S100 protein in normal and abnormal adrenal medullary tissues. Arch Pathol Lab Med 1985;109:633–635
26. Kliewer KE, Duan-Ren W, Pasquale A et al. Paragangliomas: assessment of prognosis by histologic, immunohistochemical and ultrastructural techniques. Hum Pathol 1989; 20:29–39
27. Schwaber MK, Glasscock ME, Jackson CG et al. Diagnosis and management of catecholamine secreting glomus tumours. Laryngoscope 1984;94:1008–1015

28. Michaels L, Wells M. Squamous cell carcinoma of the middle
     ear. Clin Otolaryngol 1980;5: 235–248
29. Hill BA, Kohut RI. Metastatic adenocarcinomas of the tem-
     poral bone. Arch Otolaryngol 1976;102:568–571

30. Jahn AF, Farkashidy J, Berman JM. Metastatic tumours in the
     temporal bone – a pathophysiologic study. J Otolaryngol
     1979;8:85–95

6 Malformations of the Middle and Inner Ear

Middle Ear

Most of the clinically important malformations affecting the ear involve the inner ear. For convenience a short section here describes the malformations of the middle ear.

The ossicles and skeletal structure of the middle ear are formed by a complex association of the first and second branchial arches with that of the skull bones (see Chapter 1). The malleus is more often malformed than the stapes and incus. It may be fused with the body of the incus, or fixed to the epitympanum by bone. The incus may also be fixed to the medial wall of the epitympanum. Its long process can be short and placed in an abnormal position in the middle ear cleft. The stapes may be congenitally fixed, or the crura distorted. The stapes may show a variety of other anomalies, including complete absence. In one lesion the anterior crus of the stapes is markedly bowed so that the whole of it appears to be curved forwards over the promontory. Congenital dehiscence of the bony facial canal in the region of the oval window occurs frequently. Persistence of the stapedial artery and total absence of the round window are rare conditions. The whole middle ear cavity may be incompletely developed, retaining primitive mesenchyme. Anomalies of the internal and external ear are usually present in conjunction with this lesion.

Syndromes Involving the Middle Ear

A number of congenital syndromes are seen in which middle ear lesions are combined with abnormalities elsewhere.[1]

Treacher Collins Syndrome (Mandibulofacial Dysostosis)

Treacher Collins syndrome is a hereditary malformation, predominantly due to abnormal development of the first branchial arch. The ossicles may be small, deformed or absent, producing mainly conductive deafness. Other anomalies of this syndrome include notching of the lower eyelids, diminished frontonasal angle, flatness of the cheeks, receding mandible, anomalies of the teeth and deformity of the auricle. The defect is usually bilateral but may be unilateral.

Crouzon's Syndrome (Craniofacial Dysostosis)

Crouzon's syndrome is characterised by hypertelorism, exophthalmus, optic atrophy, underdeveloped maxillae and craniosynostosis. Convulsions and dementia can also occur. Conductive deafness is due to fixation of the stapes footplate and deformed crura. The malleus and incus may also be fixed.

Hunter-Hurler Syndrome (Gargoylism, Mucopolysaccharidosis type II)

Hunter-Hurler syndrome, an X-linked disorder, is one of the mucopolysaccharidoses, characterised by a deficiency of the lysosomal enzyme iduronate sulphatase. It produces skeletal deformity, blindness, deafness, low-set ears, mental deficiency and hepatosplenomegaly. The changes are due to the deposition of glycosaminoglycans in many tissues, particularly of the head and neck. Deafness is conductive and sensorineural. The middle ear mucosa and vestibular and spiral ganglia of the inner ear may be filled with foamy histiocytes containing one of the abnormally metabolised mucopolysaccharides in their cytoplasm ("gargoyle cells"). This material stains positively by the periodic acid–Schiff reaction.[1] An association with childhood otosclerosis has been claimed.[2]

Klippel-Feil Syndrome

Klippel-Feil syndrome consists of congenital fusion of the cervical vertebrae, causing shortening of the neck, low hair-line posteriorly and deafness. The conductive component in the deafness is due to deformed and ankylosed ossicles, the sensorineural to a rudimentary cochlea and labyrinth.

Inner Ear

The development of the inner ear is described in Chapter 1. Malformations may relate to (a) deficiencies in the degree of branching and coiling of the otocyst-derived tubular structures, (b) absence or poor development ("dysplasia") of the sensory epithelia and (c) deficiencies in the cartilaginous and bony framework. (a) and (b) may arise separately or jointly, but if (c) is present, the underlying membranous structures are always defective or, more usually, absent. Neural elements of the inner ear are derived from the neuroectoderm and its coverings. Malformations of these structures will thus tend to be associated with other brain and skull deformities.

Classifications

Eponymous

A classification of inner ear malformations widely used until recently was that of Ormerod.[3] Although eponymous, the system was approximately based on the developmental processes outlined above. Four broad types of lesion were delineated:

1. Michel type: complete lack of development.
2. Mondini-Alexander, more usually known as the Mondini, type: development of only a single curved tube representing the cochlea and the presence of similar immaturity of the vestibule and canals.

3. Bing-Siebenmann type: underdevelopment of the membranous labyrinth, particularly its sense organ, with a well-formed otic capsule.
4. Scheibe type: malformation restricted to organ of Corti and saccular neuroepithelium.

Reference to the developmental schema given above suggests that: (1) corresponds to (a), (b) and (c) combined; (2) corresponds to (a); and (3) and (4) both correspond to (b).

There are many defects not included within this classification. Suehiro and Sando in 1979[4] listed a large number of congenital lesions and proposed a new and more detailed system based on the presence of structural anomalies of parts of the bony or membranous labyrinth or both. An outline of this classification is given in Table 6.1. An index of those malformations of the inner ear that have been studied in temporal bone specimens, with notes on some of the changes found and an alphabetical list of references, is provided in Table 6.2.

New System

A new system of malformations of the inner ear has arisen as a result of the remarkable access to inner ear structure in the living that has been provided by modern imaging techniques. The structural studies performed by meticulous use of the then standard radiological techniques of polytomography and thin-slice high-resolution computed technology allowed a new classification to be put forward.[5] The availability of computerised scanning and magnetic resonance imaging (MRI) scanning techniques has more recently resulted in the further description of structural anomalies. A practical approach has arisen from these now widespread facilities whereby two broad groups of malformation are recognised:

1. Morphogenetic – those that can be recognised by modern imaging methods.
2. Non-morphogenetic – those that cannot be recognised by modern imaging methods.

Morphogenetic Malformations

Extensive advances in our knowledge of malformations of the temporal bone have taken place in recent years. These have resulted not only through the use of computed tomography and MRI in the living patient, but also as a result of the massive growth in molecular genetics that provides the blueprints for the development of most of these malformations (see below).

Table 6.1. Anatomical classification of malformations of inner ear (after Suehiro and Sando[4])

Inner ear as a whole
Absence and underdevelopment of labyrinth

Cochlea
A. Cochlea in general absent, underdeveloped or anteriorly displaced
B. Osseous cochlea
   1. Osseous cochlea in general deformed
   2. Round window absent, displaced or partitioned by bony bar
   3. Scala tympani underdeveloped
   4. Scala vestibuli absent or underdeveloped
   5. Modiolus absent, underdeveloped or focally thickened
   6. Cochlear aqueduct absent, underdeveloped or widened
C. Membranous cochlea
   1. Cochlear duct in general absent or underdeveloped
   2. Organ of Corti absent or underdeveloped
   3. Tectorial membrane underdeveloped or rolled and covered by single epithelial layer
   4. Spiral limbus partially absent
   5. Stria vascularis absent, deformed, underdeveloped or displaced
   6. Spiral ligament absent, deformed or calcified
   7. Reissner's membrane absent or displaced
   8. Basilar membrane elongated, absent or displaced
   9. Ductus reuniens absent or enlarged

Vestibule
A. Vestibule in general undeveloped
B. Osseous vestibule
   1. Osseous vestibule in general underdeveloped or malformed
   2. Oval window absent, thin or malformed; calcified annular ligament
   3. Vestibular aqueduct underdeveloped or displaced
C. Membranous vestibule
   1. Utricle absent, underdeveloped, large or malformed. Anomalies of macule
   2. Saccule absent, underdeveloped or malformed. Anomalies of macule
   3. Endolymphatic duct and sac including underdevelopment, shortening and widening, and anomalies of utriculoendolymphatic valve

Semicircular canal
A. Semicircular canal in general absent, underdeveloped or enlarged
B. Superior semicircular canal
   1. In general, absence of canal or parts of it
   2. Osseous superior semicircular canal underdeveloped or widened
   3. Membranous superior semicircular canal
   Absence of part or widening of part of it
   Absence or underdeveloped crista
C. Posterior semicircular canal
   1. Posterior semicircular canal in general absent, underdeveloped, displaced superiorly or deformed
   2. Osseous posterior semicircular canal narrow or enlarged
   3. Membranous posterior semicircular canal absent, widened, narrowed or crista malformed
D. Lateral semicircular canal
   1. Lateral semicircular canal in general absent, underdeveloped or malformed
   2. Osseous lateral semicircular canal absent or underdeveloped and widened
   3. Membranous lateral semicircular canal absent, underdeveloped or flat. Crista undeveloped or flat and macula-like

Internal auditory meatus
Absent, underdeveloped, displaced or deformed

Nerves
A. Facial nerve absent, underdeveloped or displaced
B. Eighth nerve
   1. In general absent or underdeveloped
   2. Cochlear nerve absent or displaced
   3. Vestibular nerve absent or displaced

Vessels
Displaced, e.g. crossing perilymphatic space of cochlea

Subarcuate fossa
Absent, underdeveloped, displaced or enlarged

Table 6.2. Index of malformations of inner ear which have been studied in temporal bone section. The subjects are listed in alphabetical order. The second line summarises morphological changes. The index was drawn up with the aid of Suehiro and Sando,[1] Konigsmark and Gorlin[11] and Konigsmark[12] and Internet Grateful Med V2.6.3, National Library of Medicine, http://igm.nlm.nih.gov/

Acrocephalosyndactyly (Apert's syndrome)
    large, open subarcuate fossa (Lindsay et al. 1975)
Alagille's syndrome.
    absence of parts of posterior and anterior semicircular canals (Okuno et al. 1990)
Alport's syndrome
    see Nephritis and sensorineural hearing loss
Anencephaly
    defects of cochlea, vestibule, semicircular canals and internal auditory meatus (Lindsay 1973)
Apert's syndrome
    see Acrocephalosyndactyly
Arachnodactyly (Marfan syndrome)
    bony lip projecting into vestibular aqueduct (Kelemen 1965)
Arnold-Chiari malformation
    defects of cochlea, vestibule and semicircular canals (Altmann 1964)
Atresia auris congenita
    hypoplasia of cochlea, semicircular canals and internal auditory meatus (Altmann 1955)

Bing-Siebenmann defect
    underdevelopment of membranous labyrinth; well-formed bony labyrinth (Siebenmann and Bing 1907)
Bony vestibule
    see Osseous vestibule
Brevicollis (Klippel-Feil syndrome)
    defects of cochlea, vestibule, semicircular canals and internal auditory meatus (Zeitzer and Lindemann 1971)

Campomelic dysplasia
    abnormal cartilagenous and osseous tissues
    abnormality in the globuli interossei
    deformities of the vestibule and semicircular canals (Takahashi et al. 1992)
Cardio-auditory syndrome (Lange-Nielsen Jervell syndrome)
    atrophy of organ of Corti and stria vascularis (Friedmann et al. 1968)
Cervico-oculoacoustic dysplasia (Wildervanck syndrome)
    defects of cochlea, vestibule and semicircular canals (Lindsay 1971)
CHARGE association
    Mondini-type malformation of cochlea
    multiple anomalies of vestibular apparatus (Wright et al. 1986)
    Mondini dysplasia of pars inferior
    complete absence of pars superior (Guyot et al. 1987)
Cholesteatoma, congenital
    defects of cochlea, vestibule and semicircular canals (Peron and Schuknecht 1975)
Cleft palate, micrognathia and glossoptosis (Pierre-Robin syndrome)
    defects of cochlea, vestibule, semicircular canals and internal auditory meatus (Igarashi et al. 1976)
Cloverleaf skull syndrome (Kleeblattschadel syndrome)
    external and middle ear anomalies (Miyata et al. 1988)
Cochlea
    absent (Paparella and El-Fiky 1969)
    absent apical turn (Hvidberg-Hansen and Jorgensen 1968; Wells and Michaels 1982)
    absent hook portion (Sando et al. 1975)
    anterior displacement (Bergstrom et al. 1972; Maniglia et al. 1970)
    deformity (Lindsay 1973; Maniglia et al. 1970)
    underdevelopment (Valvassori et al. 1969; Lindsay 1971)
Cochlear aqueduct
    absent (Altmann 1964)
    hypoplasia (Bergstrom et al. 1972)
    wide (Suehiro and Sando 1979)
    in children (Bachor et al. 1997)
Cochlear duct
    absence (Miglets et al. 1975)
Cochlear implant in Mondini dysplasia
    suppurative labyrinthitis (Susuki et al. 1998)
Common cavity deformity
Cochlear dysplasia and meningitis (Phelps et al. 1994)
Conjoined twin
    absence of inner ear and oval window (Igarashi et al. 1974)
Cornelia de Lange syndrome
    see de Lange syndrome

Table 6.2. (*continued*)

Craniodiaphyseal dysplasia
 hyperostosis middle ear
 narrow and tortuous internal canal (Himi et al. 1993)
Craniofacial dysostosis (Crouzon disease)
 underdeveloped periosteal layer of labyrinth (Baldwin 1968)
Craniometaphyseal dysplasia (Pyle disease)
 narrow internal auditory meatus (Kietzer and Paparella 1969)
Crouzon disease
 see Craniofacial dysostosis

Deafness, congenital, spiny hyperkeratosis and universal alopecia
 defects of tectorial membrane and otolithic membrane (Myers et al. 1971)
De Lange syndrome
 short cochlea
 mesenchyme-filled perilymphatic spaces
 spiral and vestibular ganglion cells misplaced (Sasaki et al. 1996)
Deleted chromosome D syndrome
 hypoplastic cochlear aqueduct (Bergstrom et al. 1972)
Deletion of short arm of chromosome 4 (Wolf-Hirschhorn syndrome)
 depression of cochlear duct and saccule
 malformation of ossicles, absence of oval windows (Iino et al. 1987)
DiGeorge syndrome
 see Third and fourth pharyngeal pouch syndrome
Dominant progressive early-onset sensorineural hearing loss
 hydrops (Gussen 1969)
Down's syndrome
 see Trisomy 21 syndrome

Edward syndrome
 see Trisomy 18 syndrome
Endolymphatic duct
 shortened (Altmann 1964; Lindsay 1971)
 underdeveloped (Altmann 1964)
 wide (Miglets et al. 1975; Sando et al. 1970; Fitch et al. 1976)
Endolymphatic hydrops in children (Bachor and Karmody 1995)

Gargoylism (Hurlism)
 resorption of perichondrial and periosteal layers (Kelemen 1966)
Generalised spiny hyperkeratosis, universal alopecia and congenital sensorineural deafness
 cochleosaccular abnormality of Scheibe type (Myers et al. 1971)
Goitre and profound sensorineural hearing loss (Pendred syndrome)
 defects of cochlea, vestibule and semicircular canals (Hvidberg-Hansen and Jorgensen 1968)
 Mondini defect (Johnsen et al. 1986)
Goldenhar syndrome
 see Ochloauriculovertebral dysplasia
Gonadal dysgenesis (Turner's syndrome)
 Mondini defect in (Windle-Taylor et al. 1982)

Heart disease, congenital
 defects of cochlea, vestibule and semicircular canals (Egami et al. 1979)
Hemifacial microsomia
 see Oculoauriculovertebral syndrome
Hereditary haemorrhagic telangiectasia (Rendu-Osler-Weber disease)
 hypoplasia of vestibular aqueduct and endolymphatic sac (Sando et al. 1976)
Heredopathia atactica polyneuritiformis (Refsum syndrome)
 degeneration of stria vascularis, atrophy of organ of Corti and loss of spiral ganglion cells (Hallpike 1967)
Hurler syndrome
 see Gargoylism
Hydrops
 in dominant progressive early-onset sensorineural hearing loss (Gussen 1969)
Hypophosphatasia
 calcified spiral ligament (Nomura and Mori 1968)

Internal auditory meatus
 absent (Jorgensen et al. 1964)

Table 6.2. (*continued*)

Interoculoiridodermato auditive dysplasia (Waardenburg syndrome)
   absence of organ of Corti and most neurons in spiral ganglion (Fisch 1959)
   loss of spiral and vestibular ganglion cells (Rarey and Davis 1984)
   absence of pigmentation in inner ear and cochleosaccular abnormality (Nakashima et al. 1992)
Interscalar septum
   absent between apical and middle coils (Lindsay 1971, 1973)
   absent between middle and basal coils (Lindsay 1973; Valvassori et al. 1969)

Jervell and Lange-Nielsen syndrome
   see Cardioauditory syndrome

Keratitis, ichthyosis and deafness syndrome
   cochleosaccular abnormality (Tsuzuku et al. 1992)
Klippel-Feil syndrome
   see Brevicollis

Labyrinth
   absent (Igarashi et al. 1974; Jorgensen et al. 1964)
   underdeveloped, thalidomide induced (Jorgensen et al. 1964)
Larsen's syndrome
   poor development of the labyrinth
   dislocation of malleus and incus (Kaga et al. 1991)
Lateral semicircular canal
   absent (Altmann 1964; Zeitzer and Lindemann 1971)
   dilated (Altmann 1964)
   flat crista (Sando et al. 1970, 1975)
   undeveloped crista (Lindsay 1971)
   wide (Lindsay 1973; Igarashi et al. 1977)

Macula of utricle
   small (Lindsay 1971)
Mandibulofacial dysostosis (Treacher Collins syndrome)
   short cochlea, wide aqueduct, large utricle, absent lateral canal (Ruben et al. 1969; Sando et al. 1968)
Marfan syndrome
   see Arachnodactyly
Michel defect
   complete absence of labyrinth
Microstomia, aglossia, agnathia and synotia
   wide cochlear aqueduct and bony lateral canal (Black et al. 1973)
Mid-frequency sensorineural hearing loss
   loss of organ of Corti, atrophic stria vascularis and
   loss of spiral ganglion cells in basal coil (Paparella et al. 1972)
Modiolus
   absent in apical turn (Karmody and Schuknecht 1966)
   absent in apical and middle coils (Valvassori et al. 1969; Beal et al. 1967)
   absence of whole (Zeitzer and Lindemann 1971; Lindsay 1971; Maniglia et al. 1970)
   broad base (Fitch et al. 1976; Lindsay 1971)
Moebius syndrome
   see Congenital facial diplegia
Mondini defect
   in Turner's syndrome (Windle-Taylor et al. 1982)
Mondini-Alexander defect
   see Mondini defect
Mondini defect
   one and a half turns of cochlea (Mondini 1791)
   in trisomy 21 (Bilgin et al. 1996)
Mondini dysplasia with cochlear implant
   suppurative labyrinthitis (Susuki et al. 1998)
Muckle-Wells syndrome
   see Nephritis, urticaria, amyloidosis and sensorineural hearing loss

Nephritis, urticaria, amyloidosis and sensorineural hearing loss (Muckle-Wells syndrome)
   absent organ of Corti and vestibular sensory epithelium; ossification of basilar membrane (Muckle and Wells 1962)
Nephritis and sensorineural hearing loss
   minor defects of cochlea and vestibule (Lindsay 1973)

Table 6.2. (*continued*)

Norrie's disease (oculoacousticocerebral degeneration)
    marked atrophy of stria vascularis
    severe degeneration of hair cells and cochlear neurones
    connective tissue proliferation in spiral ganglion, osseous spiral lamina and walls of membranous vestibular labyrinth (Nadol et al. 1990)

Oculoauriculovertebral dysplasia (Goldenhar's syndrome) (Wells et al. 1983; Sando and Ikeda 1986)
Organ of Corti
    absent (Lindsay 1973)
Osseous spiral lamina
    absent (Lindsay 1973; Zeitzer and Lindemann 1971)
Osseous vestibule
    large (Zeitzer and Lindemann 1971; Lindsay 1971)
    small
Otocephaly
    otic capsule incompletely developed (Hinojosa et al. 1996)
Otopalatodigital syndrome
    defect of the modiolus with wide communication between subarachnoid space of the internal auditory canal and scala vestibuli (Shi et al. 1985)
Oval window
    absent (Igarashi et al. 1974; Wells et al. 1983; Adkins and Gussen 1974a, 1974b)
    malformed (Altmann 1957)

Patau syndrome
    see Trisomy 13–15 syndrome
Pendred syndrome
    see Goitre and profound sensorineural hearing loss
Pierre-Robin syndrome
    see Cleft palate, micrognathia and glossoptosis
Posterior semicircular canal
    absent (Murakami and Schuknecht 1968)
Potter's syndrome (bilateral renal agenesis)
    absence of the organ of Corti
    residual middle ear mesenchyme (Bhaya et al. 1993)
Preauricular pit, branchial fistula and hearing loss
    defects of cochlea, vestibule and semicircular canal (Fitch et al. 1976)
Pyle disease
    see Craniometaphyseal dysplasia

Refsum syndrome
    see Heredopathia atactica polyneuritiformis
Reissner's membrane
    absent (Kelemen 1943)
Rendu-Osler-Weber disease
    see Hereditary haemorrhagic telangiectasia
Retinitis pigmentosa and congenital sensorineural hearing loss (Usher syndrome)
    hypoplasia of organ of Corti and stria vascularis (Siebenmann and Bing 1907; Cremers and Delleman 1988; Shinkawa and Nadol 1986)
Round window
    congenital absence of (Hough 1958)

Saccule
    absent (Zeitzer and Lindemann 1971; Wolff 1964)
    adhesion of wall to macula (Lindsay 1973)
    large (Lindsay 1971; Beal et al. 1967)
    undeveloped (Lindsay 1971)
Saccular macula
    otolithic membrane in fibrous envelope (Myers et al. 1971)
Scala tympani
    undeveloped (Lindsay 1971)
Scala vestibuli
    malformed (Sando et al. 1975)
    underdeveloped (wide)
Scheibe defect
    abnormality of organ of Corti and saccule (Scheibe 1892)
Semicircular canals
    absent (Phelps and Lloyd 1983; Wolff 1964)
    underdeveloped (Valvassori et al. 1969; Lindsay 1971)

Table 6.2. (*continued*)

Sensory radicular neuropathy and progressive sensorineural deafness
    atrophy of stria vascularis and loss of hair cells in organ of Corti (Hallpike 1967)
Sickle cell disease and sensorineural hearing loss
    degeneration of organ of Corti and stria vascularis (ischaemia) (Morgenstein and Manace 1969)
Spiral ligament
    absent in apical and middle coils (Murakami and Schuknecht 1968)
    calcified (Nomura and Mori 1968)
Spiral limbus
    absent (Murakami and Schuknecht 1968)
Stria vascularis
    absent (Lindsay 1971; Paparella and El-Fiky 1969)
    atrophic (Wells and Michaels 1982)
    in membranous labyrinth underdevelopment (Subotic et al. 1997)
Superior semicircular canal
    absent (Zeitzer and Lindemann 1971)
    absent crista (Zeitzer and Lindemann 1971; Bergstrom et al. 1972)
    absent crus commune (Altmann 1964; Fitch et al. 1976)

Tectorial membrane
    rolled and covered by epithelium (Myers et al. 1971; Saito et al. 1974; Ward et al. 1962)
    undevelopment (Beal et al. 1967)
Third and fourth pharyngeal pouch syndrome
    defects of cochlea and lateral semicircular canal and internal auditory meatus.
    Absent oval window (Adkins and Gussen 1974a)
Treacher Collins syndrome
    see Mandibulofacial dysostosis
Trisomy 13–15 syndrome
    defects of cochlea, vestibule, semicircular canals, internal auditory meatus (Sando et al. 1975; Kos et al. 1966)
Trisomy 18 syndrome
    shortened cochlea with decreased spiral ganglion cell population
    vestibular anomalies (Saito et al. 1987)
    defects of cochlea, vestibule, semicircular canals and singular nerve
    retarded ossification of otic capsule and organ of Corti (Chrobok and Simakova 1997)
Trisomy 21 syndrome
    shortened cochlea, vestibular defects, superiorly displaced internal auditory meatus (Igarashi et al. 1977)
    shortened cochlea, Mondini deformity (Bilgin et al. 1996)
Turner's syndrome
    see Gonadal dysgenesis

Usher syndrome
    see Retinitis pigmentosa and congenital sensorineural hearing loss
Utricle
    absent (Zeitzer and Lindemann 1971; Paparella and El-Fiky 1969)
    large (Altmann 1964; Lindsay 1971)

Vater syndrome
    anomalous configuration of lateral semicircular canal
    abnormally high location of the utricle and saccule (Sakai et al. 1986)
Vestibular aqueduct
    bony lip (Kelemen 1965)
    hypoplastic (Lindsay 1971; Egami et al. 1978)
    large (Lindsay 1971; Fitch et al. 1976)

Waardenburg syndrome
    see Interoculoiridodermato auditive dysplasia
Wildervanck syndrome
    see Cervico-oculoacoustic syndrome
Wolf-Hirschhorn syndrome
    see deletion of short arm of chromosome 4

Table 6.2 References
Adkins WY Jr, Gussen R. Temporal bone findings in the third and fourth pharyngeal pouch (DiGeorge) syndrome. Arch Otolaryngol 1974a;100:206–208
Adkins WY Jr, Gussen R. Oval window absence, bony closure of round window and inner ear anomaly. Laryngoscope 1974b;84:1210–1224
Altmann F. Congenital atresia of ear in man and animals. Ann Otol Rhinol Laryngol 1955;64:824–858
Altmann F. The ear in severe malformations of the head. Arch Otolaryngol 1957;66:7–25

Table 6.2. (*continued*)

Altmann F. The inner ear in genetically determined deafness. Report and analysis of 2 new cases. Acta Otolaryngol (Stockh) 1964;187(suppl):1–39

Bachor E, Byahatti S, Karmody CS. The cochlear aqueduct in pediatric temporal bones. Eur Arch Otorhinolaryngol 1997;1(suppl):S34–38

Bachor E, Karmody CS. Endolymphatic hydrops in children. ORL J Otorhinolaryngol Relat Spec 1995;57:129–134

Baldwin JL. Dysostosis craniofacialis of Crouzon (a summary of recent literature and case reports with emphasis on involvement of the ear. Laryngoscope 1968;78:1660–1677

Beal DD, Davey PR, Lindsay JR. Inner ear pathology of congenital deafness. Arch Otolaryngol 1967;85:134–142

Bergstrom L, Hemenway WG, Sando I. Pathological changes in congenital deafness. Laryngoscope 1972;82:1777–1792

Bhaya MH, Schachern P, Morizono T et al. Potter's syndrome: a temporal bone histopathological study. J Otolaryngol 1993;22:195–199

Bilgin H, Kasemsuwan L, Schachern PA et al. Temporal bone study of Down's syndrome. Arch Otolaryngol Head Neck Surg 1996;122:271–275

Black FO, Myers EN, Rorke LB. Aplasia of the first and second branchial arches. Arch Otolaryngol 1973;98:124–128

Chrobok V, Simakova E. Temporal bone findings in trisomy 18 and 21 syndromes. Eur Arch Otorhinolaryngol 1997;254:15–18

Cremers CW, Delleman WJ. Usher's syndrome, temporal bone pathology. Int J Pediatr Otorhinolaryngol 1988;16:23–30

Egami T, Sando I, Black FO. Hypoplasia of the vestibular aqueduct and endolymphatic sac in endolymphatic hydrops. ORL 1978;86:327–339

Egami T, Sando I, Myers EN. Temporal bone anomalies associated with congenital heart disease. Ann Otol Rhinol Laryngol 1979;88:72–78

Fisch L. Deafness as part of an hereditary syndrome. J Laryngol Otol 1959;73:355–382

Fitch N, Lindsay JR, Srolovitz H. The temporal bone in the preauricular pit, cervical fistula, hearing loss syndrome. Ann Otol Rhinol Laryngol 1976;85:268–275

Friedmann I, Froggatt P, Fraser GR. Pathology of the ear in the cardio-auditory syndrome of Lange-Nielsen and Jervell. J Laryngol Otol 1968;82:883–896

Gussen R. Delayed hereditary deafness with cochlear aqueduct obstruction. Arch Otolaryngol 1969;90:429–436

Guyot JP, Gacek RR, DiRaddo P. The temporal bone anomaly in CHARGE association. Arch Otolaryngol Head Neck Surg 1987;113:321–324

Hallpike CS. Observations on the structural basis of two rare varieties of hereditary deafness. In: de Reuch AVS, Knight J (eds) Myotatic, kinesthetic and vestibular mechanisms. CIBA Foundation Symposium. Little Brown, Boston, 1967

Himi T, Igarashi M, Kataura A et al. Temporal bone findings in craniodiaphyseal dysplasia. Auris Nasus Larynx 1993;20:255–261

Hinojosa R, Green JD, Brecht K et al. Otocephalus: histopathology and three-dimensional reconstruction. Otolaryngol Head Neck Surg 1996;114:44–53

Hough JVD. Malformations and anatomical variations seen in the middle ear during the operation for mobilization of the stapes. Laryngoscope 1958;68:1337–1379

Hvidberg-Hansen J, Jorgensen MB. The inner ear in Pendred's syndrome. Acta Otolaryngol (Stockh) 1968;66:129–143

Igarashi M, Singer DB, Alford BR. Middle and inner ear anomalies in a conjoined twin. Laryngoscope 1974;84:1188–1201

Igarashi M, Filippone MV, Alford BR. Temporal bone findings in Pierre-Robin syndrome. Laryngoscope 1976;86:1679–1687

Igarashi M, Takahashi M, Alford BR. Inner ear morphology in Down's syndrome. Acta Otolaryngol (Stockh) 1977;83:175–181

Iino Y, Toriyama M, Sarai Y et al. A histological study of the temporal bones and the nose in Wolf-Hirschhorn syndrome. Arch Otolaryngol Head Neck Surg 1987;113:1325–1329

Johnsen T, Jorgensen MB, Johnsen S. Mondini cochlea in Pendred's syndrome. A histological study. Acta Otolaryngol (Stockh) 1986;102:239–247

Jorgensen MB, Kristensen HK, Buch NH. Thalidomide-induced aplasia of the inner ear. J Laryngol Otol 1964;78:1095–1101

Kaga K, Susuki J, Kimizuka M. Temporal bone pathology of two infants with Larsen's syndrome. Int J Pediatr Otorhinolaryngol 1991;22:257–267

Karmody CS, Schuknecht HF. Deafness in congenital syphilis. Arch Otolaryngol 1966;83:18–27

Kelemen G. Malformation involving external, middle and internal ear, with otosclerotic focus. Arch Otolaryngol 1943;37:183–198

Kelemen G. Marfan's syndrome and hearing organ. Acta Otolaryngol (Stockh) 1965;59:23–32

Kelemen G. Hurler's syndrome and the hearing organ. J Laryngol Otol 1966;80:791–803

Kietzer G, Paparella MM. Otolaryngologic disorders in craniometaphyseal dysplasia. Laryngoscope 1969;79:921–941

Kos A, Schuknecht HF, Singer JD. Temporal bone studies in 13–15 and 18 trisomy syndromes. Arch Otolaryngol 1966;83:439–445

Lindsay JR. Inner ear pathology in congenital deafness. Otolaryngol Clin North Am 1971;4:249–290

Lindsay JR. Profound childhood deafness. Inner ear pathology. Ann Otol Rhinol Laryngol 1973;82(suppl 5):1–121

Lindsay JR, Black FO, Donnelly WH Jr. Acrocephalosyndactly (Apert's syndrome): temporal bone findings. Ann Otol Rhinol Laryngol 1975;84:174–178

Maniglia AJ, Wolff D, Herques AJ. Congenital deafness in 13–15 trisomy syndrome. Arch Otolaryngol 1970;92:181–188

Miglets W, Schuller D, Ruppet E et al. Trisomy 18: a temporal bone report. Arch Otolaryngol 1975;101:433–440

Miyata H, Kato Y, Yoshimura M et al. Temporal bone findings in cloverleaf skull syndrome. Acta Otolaryngol 1988;447(suppl):105–112

Mondini C. Anatomico surdi nati sectio: Die Bononiensi Scientiarum et articum instituto atque academii comentarii, Bononiae 1791;7:419–431

Morgenstein KM, Manace ED. Temporal bone histopathology in sickle cell disease. Laryngoscope 1969;79:2172–2180

Muckle TJ, Wells M. Urticaria, deafness and amyloidosis: a new heredofamilial syndrome. Q J Med 1962;31:235–248

Murakami Y, Schuknecht HF. Unusual congenital anomalies in the inner ear. Arch Otolaryngol 1968;87:335–349

Myers EN, Stool SE, Koblenzer PG. Congenital deafness, spiny hyperkeratosis and universal alopecia. Arch Otolaryngol 1971;93:68–74

Nadol JB Jr, Eavey RD, Liberfarb RM et al. Histopathology of the ears, eyes, and brain in Norrie's disease (oculoacousticocerebral degeneration). Am J Otolaryngol 1990;11:112–124

Nakashima S, Sando I, Takahashi H et al. Temporal bone histopathologic findings of Waardenburg's syndrome: a case report. Laryngoscope 1992;102:563–567

Nomura Y, Mori W. Hypophosphatasia. Histopathology of human temporal bones. J Laryngol Otol 1968;82:1129–1136

Okuno T, Takahashi H, Shibahara Y et al. Temporal bone histopathologic findings in Alagille's syndrome. Arch Otolaryngol Head Neck Surg 1990;116:217–220

Paparella MM, Saguira S, Hoshino T. Familial progressive sensorineural deafness. Arch Otolaryngol 1972;90:44–51

Paparella MM, El-Fiky FM. Mondini's deafness. Arch Otolaryngol 1969;95:134–140

Peron DL, Schuknecht DH. Congenital cholesteatomata with other anomalies. Arch Otolaryngol 1975;101:498–505

Phelps PD, King A, Michaels L. Cochlear dysplasia and meningitis. Am J Otol 1994;15:551–557

Phelps PD, Lloyd GAS. Radiology of the ear. Blackwell Scientific, Oxford, 1983

Rarey KE, Davis LE. Inner ear anomalies in Waardenburg's syndrome associated with Hirschsprung's disease. Int J Pediatr Otorhinolaryngol 1984;8:181–189

Ruben RJ, Toriyama M, Dische MR et al. External and middle ear malformations associated with mandibulo-facial dysostosis and renal abnormalities. A case report. Ann Otol Rhinol Laryngol 1969;78:605–624

Saito H, Okano Y, Furuta M et al. Temporal bone findings in trisomy D. Arch Otolaryngol 1974;100:386–389

Table 6.2. (*continued*)

Saito R, Jurado AB, Inokuchi I et al. Temporal bone histopathology in trisomy 18 syndrome: a report of two cases. Acta Med Okayama 1987;41:125–131

Sakai N, Igarashi M, Miller RH. Temporal bone findings in VATER syndrome. Arch Otolaryngol Head Neck Surg 1986;112:416–419

Sando I, Hemenway WG, Morgan WR. Histopathology of the temporal bones in mandibulofacial dysostosis (Treacher Collins syndrome). Trans Am Acad Ophthalmol Otolaryngol 1968;72:913–924

Sando I, Bergstrom L, Wood RP. Temporal bone findings in trisomy 18 syndrome. Arch Otolaryngol 1970;91:552–559

Sando I, Leiberman A, Bergstrom L. Temporal bone findings in trisomy 13 syndrome. Ann Otol Rhinol Laryngol 1975;84(suppl 21):1–20

Sando I, Holinger LD, Balkany TJ et al. Unilateral endolymphatic hydrops and associated abnormalities. Ann Otol Rhinol Laryngol 1976;85:368–377

Sando I, Ikeda M. Temporal bone histopathologic findings in oculoauriculovertebral dysplasia. Goldenhar's syndrome. Ann Otol Rhinol Laryngol 1986;95:396–400

Sasaki T, Kaga K, Ohira Y et al. Temporal bone and brain stem histopathological findings in Cornelia de Lange syndrome. Int J Pediatr Otorhinolaryngol 1996;36:195–204

Scheibe A. Ein fall von Taubstummheit mit Acusticusatrophie und Bildungsanomalien in hautigen Labyrinth beiderseits. Z Hals Nasen Ohrenheilkd 1892;22:11–23

Shi SR. Temporal bone findings in a case of otopalatodigital syndrome. Arch Otolaryngol 1985;111:119–121

Shinkawa H, Nadol JB Jr. Histopathology of the inner ear in Usher's syndrome as observed by light and electron microscopy. Ann Otol Rhinol Laryngol 1986;95:313–318

Siebenmann F, Bing R. Über den Labyrinth und Hirnbefund bei einem an Retinitis pigmentosa erblindeten Angeboren Taubstummen. Z Hals Nasen Ohrenheilkd 1907;54:265–280

Subotic R, Handzccuk J, Cuk V. Morphological changes of stria vascularis in congenital hearing impairment due to membranous labyrinth underdevelopment. Acta Otolaryngol (Stockh) 1997;117:513–517

Suehiro S, Sando I. Congenital anomalies of the inner ear. Introducing a new classification of labyrinthine anomalies. Ann Otol Rhinol Laryngol 1979;88(suppl 59):1–24

Susuki C, Sando I, Fagan JJ et al. Histopathological features of a cochlear implant and otogenic meningitis in Mondini dysplasia. Arch Otolaryngol Head Neck Surg 1998;124:462–466

Takahashi H, Sando I, Masutani H. Temporal bone histopathological findings in campomelic dysplasia. J Laryngol Otol 1992;106:361–365

Tsuzuku T, Kaga K, Kanematsu S et al. Temporal bone findings in keratitis, ichthyosis, and deafness syndrome. Case report. Ann Otol Rhinol Laryngol 1992;101:413–416

Valvassori GE, Naunton RF, Lindsay JR. Inner ear anomalies, clinical and histopathological considerations. Ann Otol Rhinol Laryngol 1969;78:929–938

Ward PH, Kinney CE, Lindsay JR. Inner ear pathology and congenital deafness. Laryngoscope 1962;72:435–455

Wells M, Michaels L. Congenital abnormalities of the ear in perinatal deaths. Clin Otolaryngol 1982;7:107–119

Wells M, Phelps PD, Michaels L. Oculo-auriculo-vertebral dysplasia. A temporal bone study of a case of Goldenhar's syndrome. J Laryngol Otol 1983;97:689–696

Windle-Taylor PC, Buchanan G, Michaels L. The Mondini defect in Turner's syndrome. A temporal bone report. Clin Otolaryngol 1982;7:75–80

Wolff D. Malformations of the ear. Arch Otolaryngol 1964;79:288–301

Wright CG, Brown OE, Meyerhoff WL et al. Auditory and temporal bone abnormalities in CHARGE association. Ann Otol Rhinol Laryngol 1986;95:480–486

Zeitzer LD, Lindemann RC. Multiple branchial arch anomalies. Case report and temporal bone study. Arch Otolaryngol 1971;93:562–567

The classification of the morphogenetic malformations brought to light by imaging is still in a state of flux, and it must be said that knowledge is incomplete because some of the structural changes described by imaging have not yet been confirmed or clarified by histopathological studies.

Morphogenetic malformations involve the wide range of structural abnormalities noted in Table 6.1. Three of them – diminished cochlear coiling, large endolymphatic duct and sac and modiolar deficiency – have been extensively investigated by imaging methods; the observation of a "gusher" of perilymph or a perilymphatic fistula has also been frequently found in morphogenetic malformations. The presence or absence of these four features in a range of clinically recognised syndromes and dysplastic states is noted in Table 6.3.

Diminished coiling of the cochlea often is detected only by the absence of the interscalar septum between the middle and apical coil, so that

Table 6.3. Changes in the otic capsule in morphogenetic malformations seen at histopathology and/or imaging

Condition	Diminished coiling of cochlea	Large endolymphatic duct and sac	Deficiency of modiolus	Gusher or perilymphatic fistula
Mondini malformation	+ Minor	+	–	–
Large vestibular aqueduct syndrome	–	+	+[6]	+[7]
Pendred syndrome[8]	+ Minor	+	–	–
Common cavity dysplasia[9]	+ Severe	–	+	+
X-linked deafness[10]	–	+/–	+	+
Otopalato-digital syndrome[11]	+ Minor	–	+	–

the upper part of the cochlea lacks a bony framework. This degree of diminution of coiling may be associated with a moderate reduction only of hearing function and is noted in Table 6.3 as "minor". It is associated with the classical Mondini malformation. More severe forms may be found in which the cochlea comprises a single chamber only and this is depicted in Table 6.3 as "severe". The severity of hearing loss in these conditions seems to reflect the severity of defective cochlear coiling.

A dilated endolymphatic duct and sac is present in some conditions. The relationship of this change to hearing loss or vestibular symptoms is not yet understood. The classical Mondini malformation comprised both the diminution of cochlear coiling and the dilated endolymphatic duct.

Deficiency of the modiolus is an important aspect of the structural change in some malformations because it seems to enable a direct communication between the cerebrospinal fluid (CSF)-containing subarachnoid space in the internal auditory canal and the perilymph-containing space of the scala vestibuli, which in turn communicates with the perilymph-containing space of the vestibular cavity. Thus the latter will take on the higher pressure of the CSF. When surgical entry into the vestibule from the middle ear is effected, as in the removal of an ankylosed stapes footplate or the insertion of a cochlear implant, a "gusher" will result. This is the forcible ejection of perilymph/CSF through the opening as a result of the greater pressure of CSF in the vestibule. Another possible result of the deficiency of modiolus and the rise in perilymph pressure that this causes is the erosion of the footplate of the stapes with the eventual production of a perilymphatic fistula from the vestibule into the middle ear through the footplate defect. Since this allows direct communication between the potentially infected middle ear space and the subarachnoid space, attacks of meningitis are likely. Treatment of this lesion to prevent further attacks of meningitis is by removal of the footplate, filling up the vestibule with muscle, and inserting a prosthesis to the incus as in otosclerosis (see Chapter 10).

Examples of these findings in malformations of the inner ear will now be given in the form of two conditions that we have studied.

Pendred Syndrome

The histological changes of Pendred syndrome provide examples of two of the otic capsule changes mentioned in Table 6.3.

Pendred syndrome is an autosomal recessive hereditary disorder characterised by sensorineural hearing loss and goitre. Some recent developments in the genetics of Pendred syndrome are the mapping of the gene to chromosome 7q[12] and the subsequent identification of mutations in a putative ion-transport gene as the molecular basis of Pendred syndrome.[13] Computed tomography and MRI scans show in almost all cases of Pendred syndrome an enlargement of the endolymphatic duct and sac, and deficiency of the interscalar bony septum of the cochlea in many cases.

The patient was a child of 13 years who had been a hypothyroid cretin and deaf from birth. She died suddenly in 1964. At autopsy the cause of death was established to be aspiration of vomited food into the lungs. The thyroid gland showed a nodular colloid goitre.

Pathological changes on both left and right sides show a deficiency of the bony interscalar septum, which comprises only the normal bar of bone between the proximal portion of the basal coil and the adjacent middle coil, the more apical parts of the septum being absent, but the membranous cochlea shows two coils plus a small apical portion (Fig. 6.1). The endolymphatic duct and sac are both grossly dilated (Fig. 6.2).

The records of the above patient were no longer available in the hospital where she had died, but a surviving sister, the only sibling, was traced to another city in the UK. The parents were normally hearing and unrelated to each other. The sister was now aged 40 and had had a severe sensorineural hearing loss since birth. Goitre was first noticed during her teens and she had had a subtotal thyroidectomy at age 35 years. Perchlorate discharge, a diagnostic test for Pendred syndrome, undertaken after discontinuing the thyroxine treatment on which she had been maintained, was in excess of 40% (normal <10%), which is characteristic of Pendred syndrome. Imaging of the temporal bone showed marked dilatation of endolymphatic duct and sac.[8]

"Common Cavity" Dysplasia

In this malformation the name given suggests that the cochlear and vestibular cavities are fused into a single cavity. This is not so either on the basis of the imaging or on study of a single case of this entity that came to post-mortem.

Case 1 was an 18-year-old man with complete absence of hearing in the left ear since birth. An MRI scan, T2 weighted image, of temporal bones, showed the appearances of a common cavity dysplasia on the left in contrast to normal inner ear on the patient's right side (Fig. 6.3). The affected ear indicates an non-coiled cochlea and a separate vestibu-

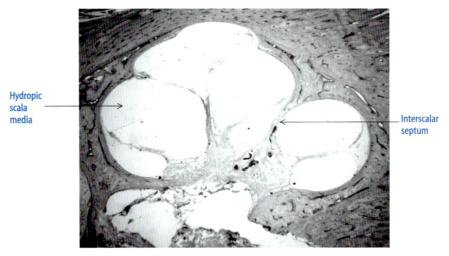

Figure 6.1 There is a deficiency of the bony interscalar septum, which comprises only the normal bar of bone between the proximal portion of the basal coil and the adjacent middle coil, the more apical parts of the septum being absent. The membranous cochlea shows two coils plus a small apical portion. There is hydrops of the scala media

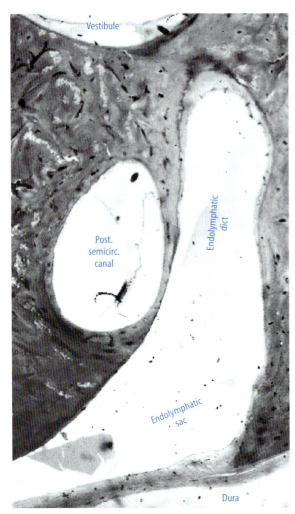

Figure 6.2 Dilated endolymphatic duct and sac in Pendred syndrome[8]

lar cavity. The origin of two semicircular canals from the latter can be clearly made out.

Case 2 was a 3-year-old seen in hospital for severe hearing loss. She was found to be completely deaf except for a small amount of residual hearing in the lower tones. No imaging investigations were done. Five months later she developed pneumococcal meningitis. She recovered but the meningitis recurred 1 month later and she died. At autopsy the features of meningitis were found in the brain.

In the tissues of the temporal bone there was an acute meningitis and acute otitis media. A fistula was present between the anterior portion of the stapes footplate and the subarachnoid space in the

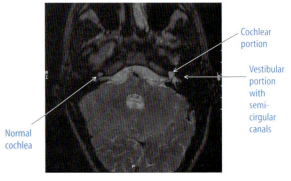

Figure 6.3 Magnetic resonance T2 weighted image of temporal bones in a man of 18 years with no hearing on the left since birth, showing common cavity dysplasia on the left in contrast to normal inner ear on the right

internal auditory canal. There was a gross deficiency in the modiolus, this being represented only by small fragments of modiolar tissue superiorly and inferiorly. The cochlea was not coiled but remnants of basilar membrane, organ of Corti and stria vascularis were found.

The changes are shown diagrammatically in Fig. 6.4. The reason for the fistula in the stapes foot-

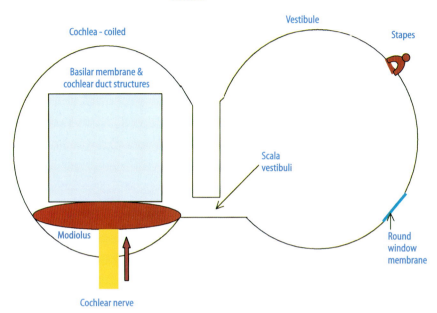

NORMAL

Diagram showing normal arrangement of labyrinthine structures & cochlear nerve
CSF around the cochlear nerve (brown arrow) is blocked from passing into the vestibule by the modiolus.

a

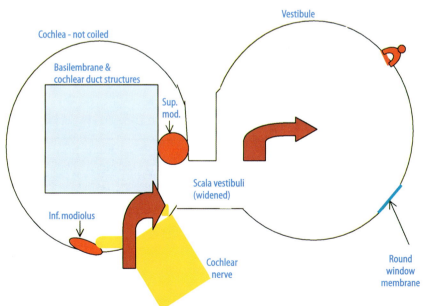

"COMMON CAVITY DYSPLASIA"

In this condition CSF around the cochlear nerve can enter vestibule through the gap in modiolus and exert pressure on the footplate during development, leading to a fistula.

b

Figure 6.4 a Normal arrangement of labyrinthine structures and cochlear nerve. Cerebrospinal fluid around the cochlear nerve (*brown arrow*) is blocked from passing into the vestibule by the modiolus. **b** Common cavity dysplasia. In this condition cerebrospinal fluid around the cochlear nerve can enter the vestibule through the gap in the modiolus and exert pressure on the footplate during development, leading to a fistula

plate is the pressure of CSF onto the stapes through the patency of the modiolus, which normally prevents entry of CSF from the subarachnoid space in the internal canal into the cochlea. Perilymph passes normally from the cochlea to the vestibule via the scala vestibuli.

Non-morphogenetic Malformations

An estimated 80% of neonates with a congenital hearing loss do not have a morphogenetic defect, the inner ear abnormalities being confined to the membranous labyrinth alone. In genetically deaf mice, non-morphogenetic defects have been classified into neuroepithelial and cochleosaccular malformations.[14] A similar grouping of human non-morphogenetic malformations has been suggested.[15] In the neuroepithelial forms the organ of Corti and later spiral ganglion cells and spiral laminar nerve fibres atrophy. An example of this is the condition of Friedreich-like ataxia with sensorineural deafness, in which spiral ganglion nerve cells are absent and there is also a corresponding reduction in the numbers of nerve fibres leading to the organ of Corti. In the cochleosaccular form it is the stria vascularis and sometimes the saccular macula which are defective. An example of this is the cardioauditory syndrome (Jervell and Lange-Nielsen syndrome) in which deposits of periodic acid–Schiff material are seen in the stria vascularis and, clinically, there may be a vestibular anomaly (Fig. 6.5).

It must be admitted, however, that this mouse-based grouping does not adequately explain many non-morphogenetic forms of inner ear malformation.

Aetiology

A great deal of genetic work has been carried out to unravel the genetic aetiology of malformations of the inner ear. Many of them are part of a "disease" or "syndrome" usually associated with other defects. Some of the commoner syndromes associated with hearing loss are listed in Table 6.4 together with their genetic bases.

Table 6.4. Genetic bases of some syndromes of hearing loss

Associated with integumentary system disease
    e.g. interoculoiridodermato auditive dysplasia (Waardenburg syndrome)
    Genes: *PAX 3* on chromosome 2
    MITF on chromosome 3
Associated with eye disease
    e.g. retinitis pigmentosa (Usher's syndrome)
    Genes: seven different genes on chromosomes 1–5 and others
Associated with nervous system disease
    e.g. bilateral vestibular schwannoma, neurofibromatosis 2 (see Chapter 11)
    Gene: on chromosome 22
Associated with renal disease
    e.g. nephritis and sensorineural hearing loss (Alport's disease)
    Genes: *COL 4A5* on X chromosome
    COL 3A3 and *COL 4A4* autosomal recessive
Associated with goitre
    e.g. goitre and profound sensorineural deafness (Pendred syndrome)
    Gene: on chromosome 7q

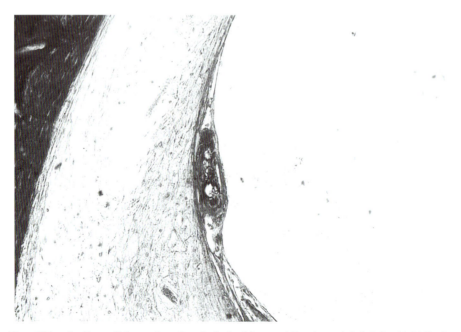

Figure 6.5 Jervell and Lange-Nielsen syndrome. Deposit of red-staining material in stria vascularis. Periodic acid–Schiff stain

Many families of genetic *non-syndromic* hearing losses have also been studied and several genes located. Three recessive genes have been identified, one on chromosome 11q, one on chromosome 13q and one on chromosome 17p. In addition, two genes causing dominant hearing impairment have been located, one on chromosome 1p and another on chromosome 5q.

The number of known genes causing hearing impairment is growing and it is likely that many more will be unravelled in the future. The new knowledge is certain to impact on the diagnosis of disorders of hearing impairment by molecular techniques. It is probable also that this basic genetic information about hearing impairment must lead to a better understanding of the pathogenesis of malformations.

References

1. Zechner G, Altmann F. The temporal bone in Hunter's syndrome (gargoylism). Arch Klin Exp Ohren Nasen Kehlkopfheilkd 1968;192:137–144
2. Fechner G, Moser M. Otosclerosis and mucopolysaccharidosis. Acta Otolaryngol (Stockh) 1987;103:384–386
3. Ormerod F. The pathology of congenital deafness. J Laryngol Otol 1960;74:919–950
4. Suehiro S, Sando I. Congenital anomalies of the inner ear. Introducing a new classification of labyrinthine anomalies. Ann Otol Rhinol Laryngol 1979;88(suppl 59):1–24
5. Jackler RK, Luxford WM, House WF. Congenital malformations of the inner ear: a classification based on embryogenesis. Laryngoscope 1987;97(suppl 40):2–14
6. Lemmerling MM, Mancuso AA, Antonelli PJ et al. Normal modiolus: CT appearance in patients with a large vestibular aqueduct. Radiology 1997;204:213–219
7. Gibson W. Cochlear implantation in children with large vestibular aqueduct syndrome. Am J Otol 1999; 20:183–186
8. Gill H, Michaels L, Phelps PD et al. Histopathological findings suggest the diagnosis in an atypical case of Pendred syndrome. Clin Otolaryngol 1999;24:523–527
9. Graham JM, Michaels L, Phelps PD. Congenital malformations of the cochlea and cochlear implantation in children: review and temporal bone report of common cavity. J Laryngol Otol 2000;114(suppl 25):1–14
10. Talbot JM, Wilson DF. Computed tomographic diagnosis of X-linked congenital mixed deafness, fixation of the stapedial footplate, and perilymphatic gusher. Am J Otol 1994;15:177–182
11. Shi S-R. Temporal bone findings in a case of otopalodigital syndrome. Arch Otolaryngol 1985;111:119–121
12. Coyle B, Coffey R, Armour JAL et al. Pendred syndrome (goitre and sensorineural hearing loss) maps to chromosome 7 in the region containing the nonsyndromic deafness gene, DFNB4. Nature Genetics 1996;12:421–423
13. Everett LA, Glaser B, Beck JC et al. Pendred syndrome is caused by mutations in a putative sulphate transporter gene. Nature Genetics 1997;17:411–422
14. Steel KP, Bock GR. Hereditary inner-ear abnormalities in animals. Arch Otolaryngol Head Neck Surg 1983;109: 22–29
15. Smith RJH, Steel KP, Barkway C et al. A histological study of non-morphogenic forms of hereditary hearing impairment. Arch Otolaryngol Head Neck Surg 1992;118:1085–1094

7 Trauma; Haemorrhage; Ototoxicity

Trauma

Fractures

The temporal bone is affected in the majority of fractures of the base of the skull. Although such lesions are frequent at autopsy, there has hardly been any study of fractures of the temporal bone in pathological material and what knowledge there is has largely been derived from clinical and radiological observations.

It has been found that fractures of the petrous portion of the temporal bone fall within two anatomical groups: longitudinal and transverse. The effects on the cochlea of these two types of lesion are quite different. Longitudinal fractures arise as a result of direct blows to the temporal and parietal areas of the head. The fracture line starts in the squamous portion of the temporal bone, usually involves the external auditory canal, the tympanic membrane and one or more of the ossicles of the middle ear, and ends in the region of the foramen lacerum near the apex of the petrous temporal bone. The cochlea is spared. Transverse fractures are caused by blows to the front or back of the skull producing a sideways tearing effect. The fracture line in these cases passes from the dural membrane on the posteromedial aspect of the petrous temporal, often through the internal auditory meatus to involve the seventh and eighth cranial nerves and then into the cochlea in the region of the basal turn at its posterolateral side. The adjacent vestibule and round and oval windows are also frequently damaged. Thus, in the case of a longitudinal fracture, the hearing loss is usually mild or moderate of the conductive type, which may be helped by surgery. By contrast a transverse fracture, involving as it does both the sensory organ and the afferent nerve derived from it, pro-

duces severe sensorineural deafness from which little improvement is to be expected. A further serious side-effect of transverse fractures is the result of their establishing a communication between the meninges and the middle ear, so that there may be a leak of cerebrospinal fluid, which invariably leads to infection spreading to the meninges. This may cause death if not controlled by antibiotic therapy. Another form of fluid leakage in transverse fractures, that of perilymph, may be associated with symptoms like those of Ménière's disease. The pathological changes in these cases come about from the lowering of perilymph pressure with secondary endolymphatic hydrops. Reissner's membrane is seen to be grossly distended throughout the cochlear duct and the saccule may be dilated (see Chapter 9).

In the temporal bone callus does not form; the union of the two fractured portions is by fibrous tissue, not bone. This type of fracture healing seems to be general in skull fractures and may be related to the immobility of these affected bones.

Small fractures, which may or may not be united by fibrous tissue, are often found in sections of temporal bone at post-mortem in cases with no history of trauma and no symptoms related to the bone damage, which is usually insignificant. These healed fractures are found most frequently between the vestibule or cochlea and the middle ear. Their pathogenesis is uncertain, but it is likely that they are produced at autopsy during removal of the temporal bone.

Microscopic Cochlear Damage in Head Injury

After a head injury a sensorineural type of deafness may develop without any detectable macroscopic damage to the cochlea. The hearing loss is in the higher frequency ranges from 3000 to 8000 Hz. Experimental studies have revealed microscopic cochlear damage following direct head injury.[1] The anaesthetised animals were given a blow to the exposed skull in the midline with a mallet of standard weight. The animals were allowed to recover and then tested audiometrically until they were killed some weeks after the trauma had been inflicted. All animals had hearing losses at least between 3000 and 8000 Hz, and some had even more widespread damage. The cochleae of all the animals were examined histologically by serial section. A constant change was found to be a loss of outer hair cells in the upper basal coil region. In some animals damage was more marked and in a few there was a complete disappearance of internal and external hair cells in some areas. Nerve fibres and ganglion cells were correspondingly reduced in these areas.

Blast and Gunshot Injury

Peripheral damage to the ear, particularly rupture of the tympanic membrane, is the most striking result of explosive blast and gunshot injury (see Chapter 3); however, permanent damage to the internal ear and its hearing mechanism is also a likely sequel. In the experimental study of such and other types of injury to the hair cells of the cochlea, a particularly valuable technique has been examination of surface preparations of the spiral organ. The effects of blast and gunshot injury fall initially on the outer hair cells of the basal coil. When this type of trauma is particularly severe, outer hair cells in long stretches of the cochlea may be destroyed and the supporting cells in these areas may become disrupted.

Sound Wave Injury

Sound waves of high intensity damage the cochlea. Again on pathological examination there is destruction of hair cells. The earliest changes affect isolated outer hair cells. As the intensity of the sound is increased, large groups of outer hair cells perish and their supporting cells are lost with them. The basal coil is once more the main centre for outer hair cell loss. These findings have been obtained mainly in animal experiments, but there is a little material from human pathology replicating the same pattern of injury.

"Stimulation Deafness"

The changes in the inner ear following the trauma of direct blows to the head, of explosive blasts and of high-intensity sound waves, which together produce a condition that may be designated as "stimulation" deafness[2] all seem to be directed particularly to the outer hair cells of the basal coil. Inner hair cells and higher cochlear coils may be affected by greater degrees of these insults to the inner ear. Although there have been a number of studies of stimulation deafness to determine its pathogenesis, the mechanism of hair cell damage is not understood.

Haemorrhage

Haemorrhage into the cochlea may occur from trauma to the temporal bone, as a result of a blood dyscrasia, or blood may enter the cochlea or vestibule from haemorrhage into a neighbouring structure. There is experimental evidence that blood may enter the scala tympani from haemorrhage in the subarachnoid space through the cochlear aqueduct. There seems indeed to be a flow of this blood from the scala tympani of the basal coil with time upwards to the apex, following which it may move into the scala vestibuli.[3] Following intracranial operations or other causes of intracranial haemorrhage, such as ruptured aneurysm of the circle of Willis or intracerebral haemorrhage caused by blood dyscrasias such as thrombocytopenic purpura, blood can spread into the perilymphatic spaces of the inner ear through the cochlear aqueduct.[3]

Fibrosis of the blood remaining in the cochlear or vestibular spaces after haemorrhage has been observed in the following circumstances:

1. After surgery for vestibular schwannoma[4] or craniotomy.[5]
2. Following the haemorrhage caused by leukaemia.[6]

The fibrosis may be seen as a fine web of fibroblasts across the cavity of the scala tympani or the perilymph space of a semicircular canal. Residua of the haemorrhage in the form of red blood cells may be seen in fibrous web (Fig. 7.1).

Haemorrhage in the Inner Ear in Very Low Birth Weight Infants

Sensorineural Hearing Loss in Very Low Birth Weight Infants

Very low birth weight infants are known to be at an increased risk of sensorineural hearing loss. There has been little post-mortem study on those infants, who do not survive to ascertain the possible pathological basis for the hearing loss. In cases of neonatal

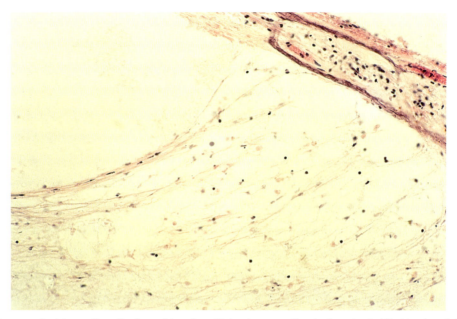

Figure 7.1 Repair process of scala tympani 3 months after craniotomy for vestibular schwannoma. There is a fine network of fibroblasts bounded from the empty cavity of the scala tympani by a membrane formed by several layers of these cells. Remains of red cells can be identified between the fibroblasts. Note basilar membrane in upper right hand corner

hyperbilirubinaemia it is well known that the cochlear nucleus may be damaged by the toxic effect of unconjugated bilirubin. The use of anti-D prophylaxis has greatly reduced the incidence of this complication, however.

In a study of the cochlear hair cells at autopsy of five preterm infants by scanning electron microscopy, one of them was found to have an almost complete loss of *inner* hair cells throughout the cochlea[7] (Fig. 7.2). A post-mortem study using histology of the temporal bones was carried out on the cochleas of 12 preterm infants who had failed a hearing test using auditory brainstem-evoked responses. Five of these cases showed inner hair cell loss. In three of these it was unaccompanied by outer hair cell loss.[8] Inner hair cell loss has been thought to be very rare and the aetiology of this lesion is of importance in order to be able to prevent sensorineural hearing loss in infants born prematurely.

Inner Ear Haemorrhage

Attention has been drawn to the possibility that haemorrhage into the cochlea around the time of birth may be a cause of this deafness. In the scanning electron microscope study mentioned above[7] a blood clot was present in the scalae vestibulae and tympani, which might have been related to the inner hair cell loss. In another study of 12 of 49 premature neonates at post-mortem, haemorrhage was observed within the eighth nerve.[9] This was always composed of bright red blood, which had exuded at the apex of the fundus within the cochlear division of the nerve. In three cases the vestibular division of the eighth cranial nerve was also affected by haemorrhage. Histological examination showed the haemorrhage to be of fresh blood only, with no hemosiderin (Fig. 7.3). The haemorrhage in these cases is probably the result of anoxia, like the frequently concomitant intracranial haemorrhage of the newborn, especially if premature. So haemorrhage into the inner ear is common in very low birth weight infants, but evidence is still lacking that this may have any connection with the sensorineural hearing loss that these infants suffer.

Ototoxic Damage to the Inner Ear

Ototoxic injury to the inner ear has been observed with a variety of drugs. There are five classes of substances, the ototoxicity of which has been carefully investigated clinically and experimentally because they are so frequently used in practice: (1) aminoglycoside antibiotics, (2) loop diuretics, (3) salicylates, (4) quinine and (5) cytotoxic drugs used in the treatment of malignant disease.

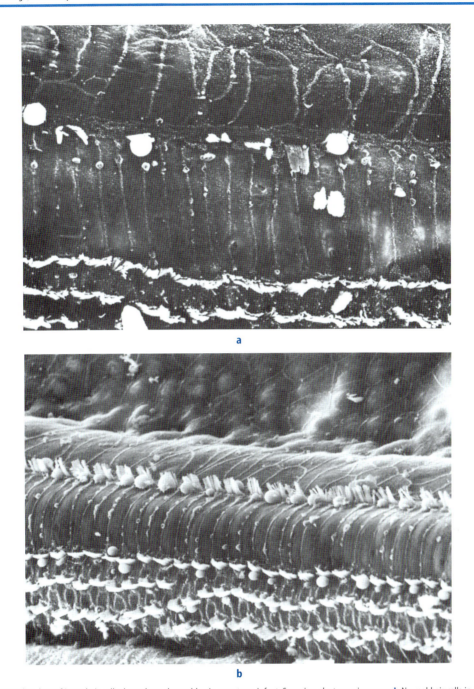

Figure 7.2 a Complete loss of inner hair cells throughout the cochlea in a preterm infant. Scanning electron microscopy. **b** Normal hair cells in an infant with Potter's syndrome for comparison[7]

Pathogenesis

Aminoglycoside Antibiotics

Aminoglycoside antibiotics are in common clinical use in the treatment of a variety of infections. The following members of this group have all been found to be associated with ototoxic effects on the inner ear: streptomycin, kanamycin, gentamycin, tobramycin, viomycin and amikacin.

The aminoglycosides produce toxic effects on the renal tubules as well as the inner ear. Excretion is mainly by glomerular filtration. Disturbance of renal

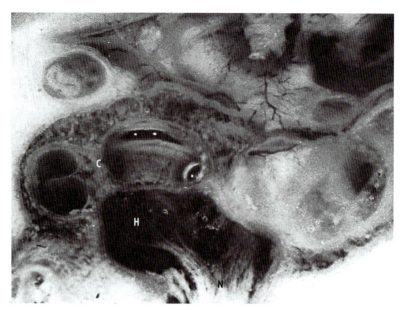

Figure 7.3 Microsliced specimen of temporal bone showing haemorrhage (*H*) into fundus of internal auditory meatus of premature infant. *C*, cochlea; *N*, eighth cranial nerve

function may lead to impaired excretion of the drug. The raised blood levels so produced will increase the tendency for the drug to cause ototoxicity. It would seem from numerous animal studies that the ototoxicity of aminoglycosides is the result of a direct effect of the drug on the sensory cells of the cochlea and vestibule. To reach these cells it is likely that there is passage from the bloodstream into the endolymph via the stria vascularis or spiral lamina. High levels of streptomycin in the subarachnoid space were noted during the early days of therapy for tuberculous meningitis to be particularly likely to result in ototoxicity. This suggests that there is transport of the substance to the perilymph via the cochlear aqueduct in such cases.

Experimentally, in a wide variety of mammalian species, including guinea-pigs, cats, chinchillas and monkeys, the ototoxic effects of aminoglycoside antibiotics have been shown to occur in the hair cells of the organ of Corti, in the maculae of the utricle and saccule and in the ampulla of the semicircular canals. In the hair cells of the organ of Corti the lesion produced in the early stages is one of degeneration and death of the outer hair cells principally in the basal coil. In the later stages inner hair cells, supporting cells and nerve elements may also be involved. A sequence of hair cell destruction has been observed in many experiments in the following order of decreasing susceptibility: third row outer hair cells, second row outer hair cells, first row outer hair cells and finally inner hair cells. At a later stage in experimental studies the spiral ganglion cells are noted to become degenerate.

Human Aminoglycoside Ototoxicity

Table 7.1 records the histopathological findings in the few human cases of ototoxicity due to aminoglycosides which have been studied at post-mortem. Clinical investigations would suggest that aminoglycosides do damage the hair cells, particularly of the basal coil of the cochlea and also some vestibular structures. In all post-mortem studies the outer hair cells throughout the cochlea were found to be destroyed. In most studies it is stated that the inner hair cells were also almost completely lost. These observations are of doubtful validity. It is generally agreed that the hair cells of the cochlea are not well demonstrated in histological sections of the human temporal bone (see Chapter 1). However, the report of Tange and Huizing[14] is based on surface preparation studies of the hair cells of the cochlea in a patient with gentamycin ototoxicity. In this patient most inner and outer hair cells were lost. There is a need for further study of surface preparation of human cases with aminoglycoside ototoxicity, particularly in the early stages of cochlear damage.

In four of the six cases detailed in Table 7.1 there was loss of spiral ganglion nerve cells. Two of these patients were 73 and 68 years old, so that the ganglion cell loss may have been a manifestation of presbyacusis. The other two patients were 48 and 24 years old and it is possible that the ganglion cell loss was a late manifestation of ototoxic change, particularly since the basal coils were involved. Matz and Lerner[17] cite the case of a 29-year-old patient who had a moderate hearing deficit due to ototoxic

Table 7.1. Labyrinthine changes in human aminoglycoside ototoxicity

Authors	Aminoglycoside antibiotic	Destruction of hair cells	Loss of spiral ganglion cells	Vestibular structures
Lindsay et al.[10]	Neomycin	Most IHC	–	N
Matz et al.[11]	Kanamycin	Occ. IHC Most OHC	Basal coil	N
Michaels[12]	Gentamycin	Most IHC Most OHC	Left side	Atrophy of cristae and maculae
Michaels[12]	Gentamycin	Most IHC Most OHC	–	Atrophy of cristae and maculae
Keene et al.[13]	Gentamycin	Most OHC	Basal coil	Vacuolisation hair cells in cristae
Tange and Huizing[14(1)]	Gentamycin	Most IHC Most OHC	Middle and basal coils	Not examined
Pollak and Felix[15]	Neomycin	–	–	–
Sone et al.[16]	Tobramycin (six patients)	Patchy IHC and OHC	Most coils	–

Abbreviations: IHC, inner hair cells; OHC, outer hair cells; N, normal; occ., occasional
[(1)] Surface preparation used to observe hair cells

damage by gentamycin, in whom the spiral ganglion cells were reduced on both sides but the cochlear hair cells were normal in all areas on histological examination. Again the validity of identification of hair cells in histological section must be questioned. Can ototoxic drugs produce direct nerve and ganglion cell damage, leaving hair cells intact? The matter can only be settled by further studies of human temporal bones using surface preparation for hair cell assessment and histological sectioning for spiral ganglion.

A recent study[16] in six patients showed no loss or scattered loss of hair cells, but general degeneration of the spiral ganglion cells was observed. It was suggested that trophic factors (neurotrophins and acidic fibroblast growth factor), known to interact with hair cells and the spiral ganglion, protect the inner ear from damage causing degeneration of ganglion cells without loss of hair cells.

In some temporal bone studies in cases of aminoglycoside ototoxicity there were changes in the sensory epithelium of the maculae and/or cristae. This again is in accordance with clinical findings of vestibular disturbances and with findings in experimental studies of damage to vestibular structures, but much more information is required in human cases on the nature of the change and the particular anatomical sites affected. The sensory epithelia of maculae and cristae are subject to autolytic changes similar to those described in Chapter 1 in the cochlear hair cells, and surface preparation studies of perilymphatic perfused specimens will also be required for post-mortem analysis in these regions. In animals clear-cut changes are seen in macular hair cells after ototoxic damage with aminoglycosides. These involve apoptosis and extrusion, non-inflammatory processes that may allow regenerative processes to take place.[18]

Loop Diuretics

Ethacrynic acid, a loop diuretic, has been associated with ototoxicity. In laboratory animals the first sign

of cochlear damage is in the stria vascularis. The earliest changes are seen by the electron microscope,[19] but later ones become visible by light microscopy. At a further stage of ethacrynic acid experimental ototoxicity, the hair cells of cochlea and vestibular structures are affected. In humans the clinical effects of ototoxicity of ethacrynic acid, like those of aminoglycosides, are both hearing loss and vestibular disturbance.

Studies of histopathological changes in the human temporal bone are few. Outer hair cell damage is present in the basal cochlear turn and in the case of Matz[20] there were oedematous changes in the cells of the stria vascularis in addition to damage to outer hair cells. Vestibular changes were also reported in this case but not in the other two case reports. These vestibular changes took the form of cyst formation in the sensory epithelia of the posterior semicircular canal and the saccular macula. This very small number of observations would indicate that ethacrynic acid ototoxicity in the human has a similar cellular effect to ototoxicity due to aminoglycoside antibiotics, as far as evidence for hair cell damage by histological study can be accepted. In addition there is a little evidence in human material that, as in experimental studies, the stria vascularis may be damaged.

Salicylates

The ototoxic effect of salicylates is well known in clinical practice, but no morphological changes have been noted in experimental animals in cochlear or vestibular structures after salicylate overdose.

Quinine

Sensorineural hearing loss of temporary duration with smaller doses, but permanent with heavier doses, is an important complication of treatment with quinine, the first and oldest drug known to cause deafness. In experimental animals severe degeneration of the organ of Corti, particularly in the basal coil, of cochlear nerves and of stria vascularis has been observed. There have been no human autopsy temporal bone studies.

Cytotoxic Drugs

Nitrogen mustard, an alkylating agent, has been observed to have ototoxic properties when administered by total body perfusion. Experimental animals given carotid perfusion with nitrogen mustard showed loss of both inner and outer hair cells in basal and middle turns of the cochlea. Examination of the cochlea in a human patient with ototoxicity who had been perfused with nitrogen mustard showed shrinkage of the organ of Corti without actual loss of hair cells.[21]

Cisplatin (cis-platinum; cis-dichlorodiammine-platinum) is a cytotoxic drug that is frequently used in the treatment of advanced malignant disease. Ototoxicity is an established side-effect of the use of this drug and the hearing of the patient is tested routinely to monitor its dosage. In guinea-pigs, outer hair cell damage at first, and later inner hair cell damage, was found over the whole length of the cochlea. Definite degenerative changes were seen in the stria vascularis of the animals. Wright et al.,[22]

using scanning electron microscopy in five patients, found degenerative changes in cochlear hair cells in all and in one patient found severe degeneration of the maculae and cristae, which could be correlated with the absence of caloric response seen after chemotherapy in that patient. A cystic degeneration of the stria vascularis was reported in the first edition of the present work[12] (Fig. 7.4). Hinojosa et al.[23] found loss of inner and outer hair cells in the basal turn of the cochlea, degeneration of the stria vascularis and a significant decrease in spiral ganglion cells predominantly in the upper turns.

References

1. Schuknecht HF, Neff WD, Perlman HB. An experimental study of auditory damage following blows to the head. Ann Otol Rhinol Laryngol 1951;60:272–289
2. Paparella MM, Melnick W. Stimulation deafness In: Graham AB (ed) Sensorineural hearing processes and disorders. Little Brown, London, 1967, p 427
3. Walsted A, Garbarsch C, Michaels L. Effect of craniotomy and cerebrospinal fluid loss on the inner ear. An experimental study. Acta Otolaryngol (Stockh) 1994;114:626–631
4. Sidek D, Michaels L, Wright A. Changes in the inner ear in vestibular schwannoma. In: Iurato S, Veldman JE (eds) Progress in human auditory and vestibular histopathology. Kugler Publications, Amsterdam, 1996
5. Graham JM, Ashcroft P Direct measurement of cerebrospinal fluid pressure through the cochlea in a congenitally deaf child with Mondini dysplasia undergoing cochlear implantation. Am J Otol 1999;20:205–208

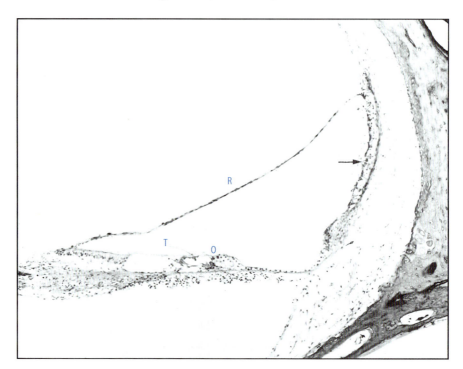

Figure 7.4 Cochlea of 7-year-old boy who died of multiple metastases of neuroblastoma, treated by cis-platinum. There is cystic degeneration of the stria vascularis (*arrow*) and apparent absence of inner and outer hair cells in the organ of Corti (*O*). *R*, Reissner's membrane; *T*, tectorial membrane

6. Smith N, Bain B, Michaels L et al. Atypical Ph negative chronic myeloid leukaemia presenting as sudden profound deafness. J Clin Pathol 1991;44:1033–1034

7. Slack RW, Wright A, Michaels L et al. Inner hair cell loss and intracochlear clot in the preterm infant. Clin Otolaryngol 1986;11:443–446

8. Amatuzzi MG, Northrop C, Liberman MC et al. Selective inner hair cell loss in premature infants and cochlea pathology patterns from NICU autopsies. J Pediatrics, in press

9. Michaels L, Gould SJ, Wells M. The microslicing method in the study of temporal bone changes in the perinatal period: an interim report. Acta Otolaryngol (Stockh) 1985;423(suppl):9–14

10. Lindsay JR, Proctor LR, Work WP. Histopathologic inner ear changes in deafness due to neomycin in a human. Laryngoscope 1960;70:382–392

11. Matz GJ, Wallace TH, Ward PH. The ototoxicity of kanamycin. A comparative histopathological study. Laryngoscope 1965;75:1690–1698

12. Michaels L. Ear, nose and throat histopathology. Springer, London, 1987

13. Keene M, Hawke M, Barber HO et al. Histopathological findings in clinical gentamycin ototoxicity. Arch Otolaryngol 1982;108:65–70

14. Tange RA, Huizing EH. Hearing loss and inner ear changes in a patient suffering from severe gentamycin ototoxicity. Arch Otorhinolaryngol 1980;228:113–121

15. Pollak A, Felix H. Histopathological features of the spiral ganglion and cochlear nerve in temporal bones from three patients with profound hearing loss. Acta Otolaryngol 1985;423(suppl):59–66

16. Sone M, Schachern PA, Paparella MM. Loss of spiral ganglion cells as primary manifestation of aminoglycoside ototoxicity. Hear Res 1998;115:217–223

17. Matz GJ, Lerner SA. Drug ototoxicity. In: Beagley HA (ed) Audiology and audiological medicine, vol 1. Oxford University Press, Oxford, 1981, pp 573–592

18. Li L, Nevill G, Forge A. Two modes of hair cell loss from the vestibular sensory epithelia of the guinea pig inner ear. J Comp Neurol 1995;355:405–417

19. Forge A. The endolymphatic surface of the stria vascularis in the guinea pig and the effects of ethacrynic acid as shown by scanning electron microscopy. Clin Otolaryngol 1980;5:87–95

20. Matz GJ. The ototoxic effects of ethacrynic acid in man and animals. Laryngoscope 1976;86:1065–1086

21. Schuknecht HF. The pathology of several disorders of the inner ear which cause vertigo. South Med J 1964;57:1161–1167

22. Wright CG, Schaefer SD. Inner ear histopathology in patients treated with cis-platinum. Laryngoscope 1982;92:1408–1413

23. Hinojosa R, Riggs LC, Strauss M et al. Temporal bone histopathology of cisplatin ototoxicity. Am J Otol 1995;16:731–740

8 Infections of the Inner Ear

Infection of the inner ear may be produced by viruses, bacteria, treponemes or fungi.

Viral Infections

Infecting viruses could reach the inner ear in the following ways:

1. Via the bloodstream.
2. Via the nerves.
3. From the middle ear.
4. Along the meninges.

There are four viral infections that are thought to reach the labyrinth by the bloodstream: cytomegalovirus infection, measles, mumps and rubella. The virus of herpes zoster oticus (the varicella zoster virus) enters the inner ear along the seventh and eighth cranial nerves.

Cytomegalovirus (CMV) Infection

Cytomegaloviruses are DNA-containing members of the herpes virus group. General infection is frequent, an intrauterine source often being incriminated.

Neonatal and Congenital Infection

The developing human ear has been thought to be particularly susceptible to CMV infection[1] and the virus has been incriminated on clinical and virological grounds as the most common cause of congenital hearing loss.[2] A total of six neonatal temporal bones has been described in which CMV inclusion-bearing cells were present in the inner ear; all of the cases had generalised cytomegalic inclusion disease.[3,4,5,6] In these infant inner ears the endolabyrinth was mainly involved (Fig. 8.1). A further case of congenital CMV infection of the inner ear has been described in a 14-year-old male who died of the sequelae of congenital CMV infection.[7] Endolymphatic hydrops was observed in the basal turn of the cochlear duct, strial atrophy and a loss of cochlear hair cells along the entire length of the basilar membrane. Vestibular neuroepithelial regions were degenerated and fibrosis was seen within the vestibular perilymphatic tissue spaces, suggesting prior labyrinthitis within the perilymph compartment in addition to the more typical pattern of endolabyrinthitis associated with human CMV infection. Distention of the saccular membrane was evident. In both cochlear and vestibular tissues, there were isolated regions of calcification. There were no typical inclusions of CMV.

CMV in AIDS

CMV infection is commonly seen in patients with AIDS. Thirty-nine per cent of patients with AIDS are found to have a hearing loss of sensorineural type.[8] In a study of the temporal bones at autopsy of 25 patients, CMV infection was identified in the inner ears of five patients by the presence of the characteristic inclusions. The inclusions were found in the vestibular nerve in the internal canal (Fig. 8.2), in the stria and in the saccule (Fig. 8.3), utricle and lateral semicircular duct.[9] It is likely, therefore, that the hearing loss in patients with AIDS is due to cochlear CMV infection.

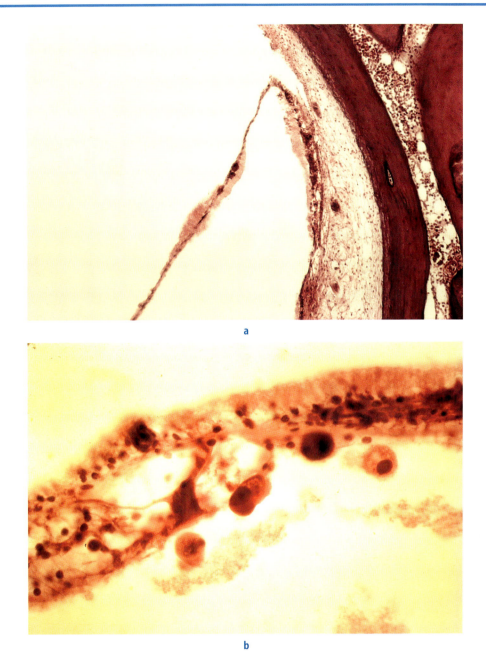

Figure 8.1 Congenital cytomegalovirus infection of the scala media of the cochlea in a low-birthweight infant. **a** Enlarged (infected) cells in Reissner's membrane. **b** Higher power view of infected cells in region of organ of Corti showing markedly enlarged and hyperchromatic nuclei (Courtesy of Dr. G.L. Davis)

Measles

Measles is caused by an RNA myxovirus, in which the main lesions are in the upper respiratory tract and lymphoid tissue. Involvement of the inner ear is rare. In two of the very few reported cases with pathological study the cochlea was involved.[10] In one of these there was severe loss of nerve fibres and spiral ganglion cells associated with atrophy of the organ of Corti. Both cases showed adhesions of Reissner's membrane. A case of labyrinthitis due to measles has been described in which there were two projecting nodules of inflammatory cells in the wall of the utricle.[11]

Mumps

Mumps is caused by an RNA virus, which usually attacks the salivary glands and sometimes the testes,

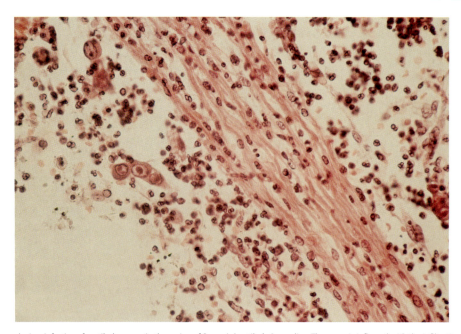

Figure 8.2 Cytomegalovirus infection of vestibular nerve in the region of Scarpa's (vestibular) ganglion. The nerve is inflamed with the infiltration of neutrophils, lymphocytes and plasma cells. Four enlarged cells (three to left of centre, the fourth on the far right) with purplish inclusions, each surrounded by a pale halo, features characteristic of cytomegalovirus infection, can be identified. Autopsy finding in a patient with AIDS

ovaries or pancreas. Sensorineural hearing loss is a well-known complication. In the temporal bone of such a case[12] there was atrophy of most of the basal coil of the cochlea, with corresponding nerve fibre and spiral ganglion cell loss.

Rubella

Maternal rubella is an important factor in the genesis of congenital sensorineural hearing loss. The virus is an RNA one. Some temporal bones have been examined, mainly of premature or young infants. A fairly uniform finding was partial collapse of Reissner's membrane with adherence to the stria vascularis and organ of Corti. The tectorial membrane was rolled up. The stria vascularis was usually atrophic, often with cystic areas, and in two cases there were inflammatory collections at the upper end near the junction with Reissner's membrane and adherent to it[13] (Fig. 8.4). The organ of Corti was mainly normal. Collapse of the saccule has been observed in some cases.[14]

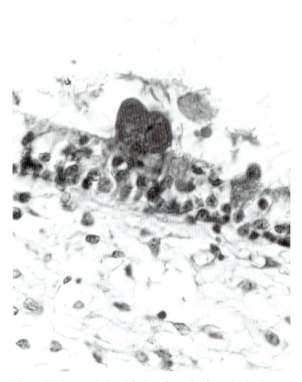

Figure 8.3 Cytomegalovirus infection of macule of saccule showing two enlarged cells with intranuclear inclusions and perinuclear halos. Autopsy finding in a patient with AIDS

Herpes Zoster

In herpes zoster auris (Ramsay Hunt syndrome), the virus (the DNA herpes varicella virus) enters the inner ear along the seventh and eighth cranial nerves, presumably from nerve ganglia, where it lies

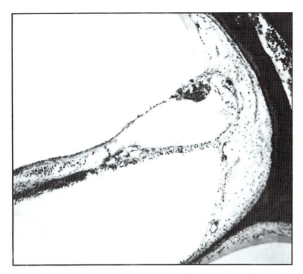

Figure 8.4 Cochlea of newborn with rubella infection showing inflammatory focus at junction of stria vascularis with Reissner's membrane (case reported by Friedmann and Wright[13])

dormant until there is a change in the immunological status of the patient. In the five histopathological studies previously described, there were extensive pathological changes, mainly in the two nerves serving in the transmission of the virus. In the case of Blackley et al.[15] there were extensive lymphocytic infiltrates in the nerves, modiolus and skin of the external auditory meatus. Varicella zoster has also been detected in the cytoplasm and nuclei of inflammatory cells of the middle ear in two cases of the Ramsay Hunt syndrome by an immunofluorescence method.[16] Herpes varicella-zoster viral (VZV) DNA has been identified, using the polymerase chain reaction (PCR), in archival celloidin-embedded temporal bone sections from two patients who clinically had Ramsay Hunt syndrome (herpes zoster oticus).[17] The herpes zoster virus was found both in the geniculate ganglion of the side with facial paralysis and in a cutaneous recrudescence in both patients. One of the patients had had a sudden hearing loss and was found to have VZV genomic DNA in sections from the affected side containing the spiral ganglion, Scarpa's ganglion, organ of Corti and macula of the saccule.

Bell's Palsy

A condition possibly due to viral infection in the inner ear is that of Bell's palsy, which is manifested clinically as a peripheral facial paralysis. The suggestion has been made, with some virological support, that this condition is the result of infection with herpes simplex virus, type 1. There have been a very small number of reports of temporal bone studies from patients with Bell's palsy. The report of Fowler[18] deals with a patient who died 14 days after the onset of facial paralysis. There was evidence of degeneration of the myelin sheaths and axis cylinders throughout the course of the nerve in the temporal bone. There were fresh haemorrhages in and around the facial nerve, but no evidence of inflammation. In two cases of Bell's palsy studied by the present authors, serial sections of the temporal bones both showed the following histological findings. In the genu region there appeared to be constriction of the facial nerve by inflammatory tissue, which formed a sheath around it and encroached on its interior. The adjacent bone showed foci of resorption with abundant osteoclasts (Fig. 8.5). The geniculate ganglion was infiltrated by lymphocytes. In some places the affected facial nerve appeared severely oedematous and nerve cells were shrunken and showed an eosinophilic cytoplasm. The descending part of the facial nerve presented swelling and vacuolation of myelin sheaths with some loss of axis cylinders. These findings are compatible with geniculate ganglionitis. In one of these cases, herpes simplex viral type 1 was demonstrated in archival paraffin-embedded sections of the affected geniculate ganglion by carrying out PCR followed by electrophoresis on agarose gel.[19]

Bacterial Infections

Petrositis

Bacterial infections of the inner ear may involve both the petrous bone itself and the labyrinthine structures within it. Bacterial infection of the petrous bone is frequently derived by extension from middle ear infection. There are four possible routes by which infection may extend from the middle ear into the petrous bone:

1. Via air cells. Mastoid air cells frequently extend in the temporal bone as far as the apical region. It is possible, therefore, that infection to the petrous apex may extend from the middle ear by the medium of infection of air cells.
2. As direct spread of the inflammatory process by bone necrosis (osteitis).
3. By extension through the bone marrow of the petrous bone (osteomyelitis).
4. Along vessels and nerves.

In addition to inflammatory infiltration the pathological process of petrositis comprises three main changes in the bone tissue, all of which may be seen simultaneously: (1) bone necrosis, (2) bone

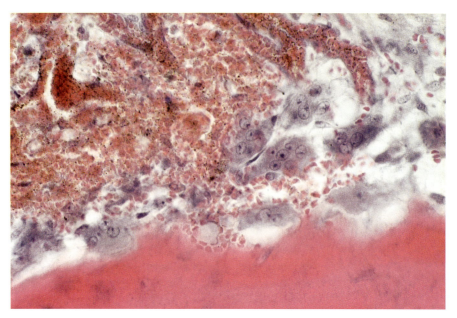

Figure 8.5 Region of interface between geniculate ganglion and adjacent bone in a case of Bell's palsy. There are numerous osteoclasts with Howship's lacunae. The nerve shows congestion and lymphocytic infiltrate. Autopsy findings

erosion, (3) new bone formation. It should be noted that these three processes are frequently seen in the bony wall of the middle ear in many cases of otitis media in which extensive petrositis has not taken place (see Chapter 3). The inflammatory changes that accompany the bony ones may be "acute", i.e. with an exudate largely of neutrophils, or "chronic", i.e. with one of lymphocytes, plasma cells, histiocytes and fibroblasts forming fibrous tissue. These two forms of inflammatory infiltrate are often found in the same ear in the very variegated pathological picture of otitis media when the whole temporal bone is examined in sections (see Chapter 3).

Petrositis is of great importance because involvement of the labyrinth, nerves, artery, veins, meninges and cerebral tissue embedded in and surrounding the petrous bone may each cause serious symptoms, and perhaps death:

1. Extension to the labyrinth may lead to labyrinthitis with destruction of the organs of hearing and balance.
2. Important nerves may be damaged. The facial nerve is at risk early. Involvement of the trigeminal ganglion and the sixth cranial nerve lead to "Gradenigo's syndrome". Extension to the jugular foramen region by the inflammatory process may cause palsy of the ninth, tenth and eleventh cranial nerves ("jugular foramen syndrome").
3. The wall of the internal carotid artery may become inflamed and this may lead to thrombosis of the vessel.

4. Similarly the lateral sinus may become thrombosed and this and/or extension of the thrombus to the superior sagittal sinus may be associated with the somewhat arcane syndrome of otitic hydrocephalus.
5. Spread of the infection to the immediately adjacent cranial structures will lead to meningitis and cerebral abscess.

It should be pointed out that patients with diabetes mellitus are especially prone to develop an extension of otitis media as outlined above. A concept of "malignant otitis externa" has grown up in regard to diabetics in whom, because of the presence of external otitis, which frequently coexists with otitis media, it is postulated that the infection (usually by *Pseudomonas aeruginosa*) spreads from the ear canal to the petrous apex under the temporal bone. It is likely that spread of infection in these cases is from otitis media as described above (see Chapter 2).

Labyrinthitis

Otitic

The source of labyrinthitis is, in many instances, otitis media, as with petrositis. Infection may enter the labyrinth by penetrating the oval or the round window. An infected air cell may rupture into the labyrinthine system at some point of its complex periphery. Occasionally damage to bone by the inflammation may produce a fistula between the middle ear and the labyrinth, usually in the lateral semicircular canal because this is the nearest vulnerable point to the middle ear. The latter complication takes place in most cases when a cholesteatoma is present, which has the effect of stimulating the inflammatory process.

Meningitic

There is another possible source of infection of the labyrinth – the meninges – and the two ducts that join them, the cochlear aqueduct and the internal auditory meatus, may convey infection from meningitic lesions into the labyrinth. Sensorineural hearing loss is an important sequel of acute bacterial meningitis. It seems likely from a study of 41 human temporal bones in cases of acute bacterial meningitis, that the origin of the hearing loss is labyrinthitis produced by the spread of bacteria from the infected meninges through both the cochlear modiolus and cochlear aqueduct.[20] Although the cochlea was the site of labyrinthitis in approximately one-half of the temporal bones in this study, the sensory and neural structures of this structure appeared intact in the majority of specimens, indicating the possibility of preventing or reversing sensorineural hearing loss by therapeutic intervention. Eosinophilic staining of inner ear fluids without the presence of inflammatory cells (so-called "serous" or "toxic" labyrinthitis) was often seen, usually within the vestibular system. Spiral ganglion cells were severely degenerated in 12% of bones, suggesting that subsequent cochlear implantation may not be successful in this group.[20]

In suppurative labyrinthitis the perilymph spaces display usually a massive exudate of neutrophils (Fig. 8.6). If the process extends to the endolymphatic spaces there is concomitant destruction of membranous structures and irreparable damage to sensory epithelia.

Healing is at first by fibrosis, but later osseous repair is frequent, leading to a condition of "labyrinthitis ossificans". In this condition the spaces of the bony labyrinth are filled in by a newer bone, which appears in striking contrast with the normal bone surrounding the bony labyrinth (Fig. 8.7).

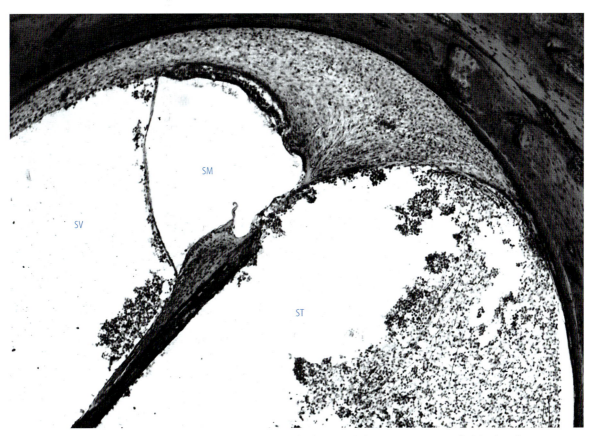

Figure 8.6 Suppurative labyrinthitis. The scala vestibuli (*SV*) and scala tympani (*ST*) contain numerous pus cells. *SM,* scala media

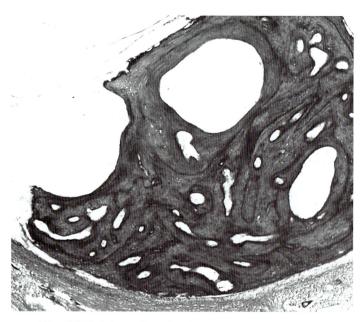

Figure 8.7 Labyrinthitis ossificans. The scala tympani is occupied by new bone.

Syphilis

Syphilis has not been fully eradicated by penicillin treatment; the incidence may, in fact, be rising. Sensorineural hearing loss is common in all forms of acquired syphilis. In secondary syphilis the pathological changes of the labyrinth seem to be part of lymphocytic meningitis.[21] In tertiary syphilis the pathological changes are similar to those of late congenital syphilis described below. Hearing loss is also an important feature of congenital syphilis, forming one of the constituents of Hutchinson's triad (interstitial keratitis, deformed incisor teeth and deafness). More than one-third of patients with congenital syphilis develop deafness.[22] In infantile congenital syphilis the labyrinthine symptoms are an insignificant aspect of a widespread and often fatal illness.

Late Congenital Syphilis

"Late congenital syphilis is essentially a bone disease of the ear". This quotation from Mayer and Fraser[23] gives the key to the most important aspect of the complex pathological processes which account for the lesions of congenital syphilis. The osseous nature of the disease is emphasised by the site of infection with treponemes (*Treponema pallidum*) found in the temporal bone at autopsy in a 48-year-old man with congenital syphilis.[24] The spirochaetes were seen within the bone surrounding the cochlear duct and semicircular canals. There was in most places no inflammatory reaction to the organisms. Syphilis of the temporal bone is not related to inflammation of the middle ear mucosa, unlike petrositis (see above) or the rare cases of tuberculous involvement of the bony labyrinth.

The bony lesions of congenital syphilis assume two forms: (1) gummatous involvement of bone marrow and periosteum and (2) diffuse periostitis.

The former is seen most frequently external to the bony cochlea. Gummata are foci of epithelioid cells, occasional giant cells of Langhans type, lymphocytes and plasma cells, frequently arranged around blood vessels. They widen the bone marrow spaces by bone destruction in the region around the bony cochlea and vestibule and in relation to the outer periosteum of the petrous bone. These inflammatory foci enlarge and spread centrally to erode the bony labyrinth. Tongues of inflammatory tissue reach the endosteum in some places. This inflammatory tissue may also involve the vestibular aqueduct and lead to replacement of the endolymphatic duct (see below).[25] Areas of necrotic bone may be seen in the inflammatory tissue. Fibrosis is a prominent component of the lesion. Also new bone formation, both lamellar and woven, contributes to the complex appearances of the pathology of syphilitic osteitis.

In the second form of bony labyrinthine involvement in congenital syphilis, a diffuse periostitis is present. This lesion is seen most often in the semicircular canals. It is characterised by a formation of bony and fibrous tissue, which is continuous with the bony capsule of the semicircular canals and may completely obliterate their lumen.

Although the main emphasis in the pathology of congenital syphilis is on bony lesions, the membranous cochlea always undergoes changes, which are clinically more manifest than those of bone. There is frequently a process of hydrops identical in appearance to that seen in Ménière's disease (see Chapter 9). This affects endolymphatic channels in both cochlea and vestibule and may be severe.[25] In temporal bones from three cases of syphilis with hydrops, all of the bones showed infiltration and obliteration of the endolymphatic duct by round cells, giant cells and fibrous tissue, and this lesion probably was at the root of the hydrops.[26] The organ of Corti is always atrophic in congenital syphilis and the spiral ganglion cells are greatly depleted.

Mycotic Infections

Fungus infections of the inner ear are rare and only a few cases have been reported in temporal bone pathology studies. Mycotic infections are increasing due to the widespread use of immunosuppressive therapy in the treatment of malignant and renal disease. Mucor infection is usually a lesion of nasal origin (see Chapter 13), but Meyerhoff et al[27] described a case in which such an infection reached the inner ear, probably by the bloodstream. Three other cases of inner ear infection by Candida are also described in the same work. The route of infec-

tion in these cases was from the middle ear and meninges. Cryptococcosis is a fungus infection which usually infects the meninges. Igarashi et al.[28] describe a case in which there was extension of infection by the organism Cryptococcus neoformans, from the meninges along the internal auditory meatus and then into the cochlea via the modiolus. Such a progression was clearly present in two cases of AIDS with cryptococcal meningitis that had spread to the labyrinth[9] (Fig. 8.8).

References

1. Stagno S, Reynolds DW, Amos CS et al. Auditory and visual defects resulting from symptomatic and subclinical congenital cytomegaloviral and toxoplasma infections. Pediatrics 1977;59:669–678
2. Hanshaw JP. School failure and deafness after "silent" congenital cytomegalovirus infection. New Eng J Med 1976:295:468–470
3. Myers EN, Stool S. Cytomegalic inclusion disease of the inner ear. Laryngoscope 1968;78:1904–1915
4. Davis GL. Cytomegalovirus in the inner ear: case report and electron microscopic study. Ann Otol 1969;78:1178–1188
5. Davis LE, Johnsson L-G, Kornfeld M. Cytomegalovirus labyrinthitis in an infant: morphological, virological and immunofluorescent studies. J Neuropath Exp Neurol 1981;40:9–19
6. Strauss M. Human cytomegalovirus labyrinthitis. Am J Otolaryngol 1990:11:292–298
7. Rarey KE, Davis LE. Temporal bone histopathology 14 years after cytomegalic inclusion disease: a case study. Laryngoscope 1993;103:904–909
8. Soucek S, Michaels L. The ear in the acquired immunodeficiency syndrome. II. Clinical and audiologic investigation. Am J Otol 1996;17:35–39

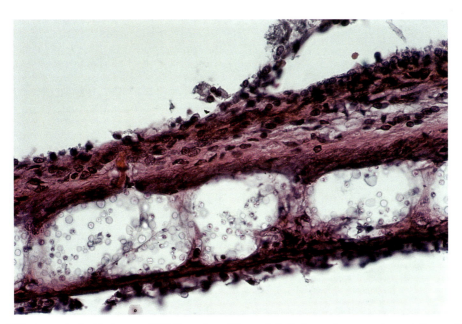

Figure 8.8 Cryptococcosis of cochlea in a case of AIDS. The cryptococci fill spaces in the basilar membrane normally occupied by nerve fibres[29]

9. Michaels L, Soucek S, Liang J. The ear in the acquired immunodeficiency syndrome: I. Temporal bone histopathologic study. Am J Otol 1994;15:515–522

10. Bordley JE, Kapur YP. Histopathologic changes in the temporal bone resulting from measles infection. Arch Otolaryngol 1977;103:162–168

11. Lindsay JR. Histopathology of deafness due to postnatal viral disease. Arch Otolaryngol 1973;98:258–264

12. Smith GA, Gussen R. Inner ear pathologic features following mumps infection. Report of a case in an adult. Arch Otolaryngol 1976;102:108–111

13. Friedmann I, Wright MI. Histopathological changes in the foetal and infantile inner ear caused by maternal rubella. Br Med J 1966;II:20–23

14. Brookhouser PE, Bordley JE. Congenital rubella deafness. Pathology and pathogenesis. Arch Otolaryngol 1973;98:252–257

15. Blackley B, Friedmann I, Wright I. Herpes zoster auris associated with facial nerve palsy and auditory nerve symptoms: a case report with histopathological findings. Acta Otolaryngol 1967;63:533–550

16. Fujiwara Y, Yanagihara N, Kurata T. Middle ear mucosa in Ramsay Hunt syndrome. Ann Otol Rhinol Laryngol 1990;99:359–362

17. Wackym PA. Molecular temporal bone pathology: II. Ramsay Hunt syndrome (herpes zoster oticus). Laryngoscope 1997;107:1165–1175

18. Fowler EP Jr. The pathologic findings in a case of facial paralysis. Trans Am Acad Ophth Otolaryngol 1963;67:187–197

19. Burgess RC, Michaels L, Bale JF et al. Polymerase chain reaction amplification of herpes simplex viral DNA from the geniculate ganglion of a patient with Bell's palsy. Ann Otol Rhinol Laryngol 1994;103:775–779

20. Merchant SN, Gopen Q. A human temporal bone study of acute bacterial meningogenic labyrinthitis. Am J Otol 1996;17:375–385

21. Goodhill V. Syphilis of the ear. A histopathological study. Ann Otol Rhinol Laryngol 1939;48:676–706

22. Karmody CS, Schuknecht HF. Deafness in congenital syphilis. Arch Otolaryngol 1966;83:18–27

23. Mayer O, Fraser JS. Pathological changes in late congenital syphilis. J Laryngol Otol 1936;51:683–714 and 755–778

24. Mack LW, Smith JL, Walter EK et al. Temporal bone treponemes. Arch Otolaryngol 1969;90:11–14

25. Belal A, Linthicum FH. Pathology of congenital syphilitic labyrinthitis. Am J Otolaryngol 1980;1:109–118

26. Linthicum FH Jr, el-Rahman AG. Hydrops due to syphilitic endolymphatic duct obliteration. Laryngoscope 1987; 97:568–574

27. Meyerhoff WL, Paparella MM, Oda M et al. Mycotic infections of the inner ear. Laryngoscope 1979;89: 1725–1734

28. Igarashi M, Weber SC, Alford BR et al. Temporal bone findings in cryptococcal meningitis. Arch Otolaryngol 1975;101:577–583

29. Michaels L. Chapter 80. The ear. In: Damjanov I, Linder J (eds) Anderson's pathology, 10th edn. Mosby Year Book Inc., St. Louis, Missouri, 1996, pp 2876–2900

Ménière's Disease; Pathology of the Vestibular System; Presbycusis

Ménière's Disease

Hydrops and its Causes

Ménière's disease is an affection of both the hearing and balance organs of the inner ear, characterised by episodes of vertigo, hearing loss and tinnitus. Its pathological basis has become firmly established as "hydrops", i.e. distention of the endolymphatic spaces of the labyrinth by fluid. The cause of the hydrops in Ménière's disease is unknown. There are, however, other diseases of known aetiology in which hydrops may be present as a complication. The common feature of these conditions is presence of inflammatory or neoplastic involvement of the perilymphatic spaces. Thus otitis media complicated by perilymphatic labyrinthitis (see Chapter 3), syphilitic involvement of the labyrinth (see Chapter 8), leukaemic deposits in the perilymph spaces or vestibular schwannoma (see Chapter 11) may be associated with hydrops.

It is now well established that idiopathic endolymphatic hydrops may be present in patients who do not have the clinical symptoms of Ménière's.[1,2] The patients who have Ménière's symptoms seem to show a more severe degree of hydrops and a greater number of membrane ruptures (see below) than those without.

Pathological Appearances of Hydrops

The hydrops of Ménière's disease may affect one or both inner ears. In most cases the cochlear duct and saccule are involved, but the utricle and semicircular ducts are usually not. In some cases the cochlear duct alone is hydropic. A rare and debatable form of Ménière's is thought to affect the vestibule, but not the cochlea. Symptoms are those of vertigo, but not hearing loss. Another rare syndrome – Lermoyez's syndrome – in which tinnitus and hearing loss precede an attack of vertigo, has been associated with endolymphatic hydrops limited to the basal turn of the cochlea and the saccule.[3]

In the hydropic cochlear duct, Reissner's membrane, which is elastic, shows a variable degree of bulging. In the most severe cases, the membrane reaches the top of the scala vestibuli and may be in contact with a wide area of cochlear wall (Fig. 9.1). In the apical region it may bulge to such an extent that it fills the helicotrema. In this way the distended scala media may even enter the scala tympani. The saccule swells up from its position on the medial wall of the vestibule and frequently touches the vestibular surface of the footplate of the stapes (Fig. 9.2). The utricle may be compressed in the process. In some cases the swollen saccule may herniate from the vestibule into the semicircular canals. Less frequently the utricle may be distended, sometimes with small infoldings producing a scalloped appearance.

Changes in Walls of Membranous Labyrinth

Changes may be seen in the thin distended membranes of the hydropic endolymphatic spaces. Ruptures may be present, particularly in Reissner's membrane, and the terminal end of the ruptured membrane may be curled up. Such ruptures have been incriminated as possible pathological bases of the fluctuations in pure tone thresholds that patients with Ménière's disease may suffer. It has been sug-

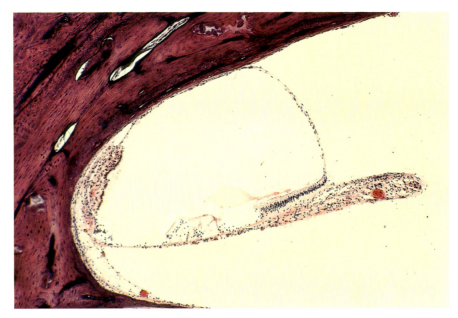

Figure 9.1 Cochlear hydrops in Ménière's disease. The distended Reissner's membrane reaches the top of the scala vestibuli. Note that, although the general structure of the organ of Corti is normal, the hair cells cannot be detected. This may be the result of the changes of Ménière's disease, but post-mortem autolysis cannot be ruled out

gested that the flooding of the perilymph with endolymph with its high potassium level may inhibit the bioelectric activity of the cochlea.[4] It is likely, however, that many of these ruptures are artefactual. They may be found in non-hydropic labyrinths. They are often multiple in the same membranous labyrinth. Outpouchings are often seen in which dilatation of part of the wall of the membranous labyrinth takes place and a lining is present here that is thinner than elsewhere. These outpouchings have

been explained as healed ruptures, but, because of their regular features, it is more likely that they are simply areas of increased distension of parts of the labyrinthine wall, which are normally thinner. Fibrous tissue may be present in cases of Ménière's hydrops external to the endolymphatic space in the scala vestibuli and in the vestibule deep to the footplate of the stapes. It is possible that the foci of connective tissue in these two situations are reactions to the irritation produced by repeated distension and subsidence of the adjacent cochlear duct and saccule respectively.

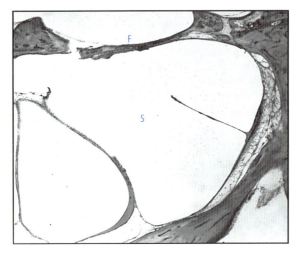

Figure 9.2 Hydrops in Ménière's disease involving vestibule. The saccule (*S*) is distended to such a degree that it lines the base of the footplate (*F*) of the stapes, which is artefactually fractured. A thin membrane, possibly the result of rupture, projects into the saccule

Changes in Vestibular Aqueduct and Endolymphatic Duct

While hydrops involving the scala media and saccule is accepted by all as a basic feature of the pathology of Ménière's disease, there is no such unanimity with regard to the alterations in the endolymphatic duct and its surrounding vestibular aqueduct. There have been many descriptions of obstructive or potentially obstructive lesions of these structures associated with Ménière's disease whereby restriction of the flow of endolymph may have caused the hydrops. The following list gives a brief indication of the lesions discussed at length in the literature:

1. Fibrosis (Fig. 9.3).
2. Metastatic breast carcinoma.
3. Decreased vascularity.

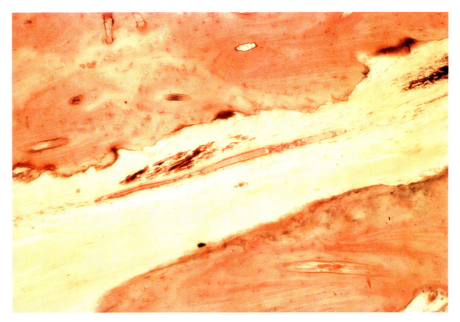

Figure 9.3 Fibrosis of vestibular aqueduct in a case of Ménière's disease. The endolymphatic duct is constricted to a narrow canal

4. Partial atresia of the intermediate portion of the vestibular aqueduct with decreased amounts of endolymphatic duct tissue.

5. Irregularity of the osseous wall of the vestibular aqueduct, sometimes with blockage of the orifice of the vestibule.

6. Blockage of the vestibular aqueduct by syphilitic microgummata – "perivascular round cell infiltrations".

7. The neoplasm, low-grade adenocarcinoma of the endolymphatic sac may give rise to Ménière's-like symptoms in parts of its course (see Chapter 11).

8. Developmentally narrowed endolymphatic duct and vestibular aqueduct as shown by histological measurements of post-mortem specimens and magnetic resonance scanning in living patients.

In contrast to these observations it must be pointed out that careful studies of some Ménière's hydropic temporal bones have shown no changes whatever in the endolymphatic duct or vestibular aqueduct.

Changes in the Sensory Epithelia of the Labyrinth

Alterations of the sensory cells of the organ of Corti have been described in Ménière's, but it is still not clear whether these changes actually exist in the living patient or whether they are the result of post-mortem autolysis or even the effects of acid used in decalcification of the temporal bone (see Chapter 1). The possibility that some of the changes may be artefactual has been ignored in some reports. Changes in the hair cells, particularly in the apical region, have been described and associated with low-frequency hearing loss.[4] Atrophy of the macula of the saccule may also be found, which does not appear to be artefactual (Fig. 9.4).

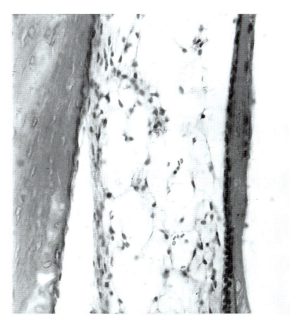

Figure 9.4 Atrophy of sensory cells of part of saccular macula in Ménière's hydrops in *right part of the figure*

Relationship of Symptoms to Pathological Changes

Image analysis of the areas in histological section of the cochlear duct (corresponding to volume in the whole structure) has been carried out in two studies and related to the hearing loss. In the study of Antoli-Candela[5] the area of the cochlear duct was significantly increased in relation to the degree of hearing loss. Losses of over 70 dB showed a particularly high degree of hydropic expansion. In the study of Fraysse et al.,[6] a similar relationship was found between cochlear duct size and the total average hearing loss. There was also a correlation of those dimensions with the duration of the disease: the longer the history of symptoms, the more pronounced the cochlear duct dilatation. A relationship also seemed to be present between (1) the amount of dilatation of vestibular structures and (2) the response to caloric tests and the presence of positional nystagmus, but this was less definite than the cochlear duct/hearing loss association.

Pathogenesis

Ablation of the endolymphatic sac in guinea-pigs results in endolymphatic hydrops within 3 months. In cats the same result can only be attained with survival times of 6 months to 3 years.[7] In humans, operations for drainage of endolymph into the subarachnoid space are sometimes of value in the treatment of Ménière's disease. These facts and the data regarding endolymphatic duct obstruction given above suggest that obstruction of the endolymphatic duct may indeed play a part in the pathogenesis of Ménière's disease.

Pathology of the Vestibular System

The pathology of the vestibular system in man has been even less adequately investigated than that of the auditory one. The following account considers conditions the pathological bases of which have been established by direct observation at autopsy or surgery; affections such as "vestibular neuronitis (or neuritis)", in which the possible structural changes have been only guessed at from the clinical symptoms, are not considered. Further details of some of the conditions are given elsewhere in Part A of this work.

Malformations

A wide variety of malformations may affect the vestibular structures and semicircular canals (see Chapter 6).

Ageing Changes

Changes comparable to those in the cochlea in presbycusis (see below) have been described for the vestibular structures. With advancing age there is degeneration of the saccular macula and, to a lesser degree, of the utricular macula. Type 1 cells are more prone to disappear than type 2 cells.[8] These changes are accompanied by a loss of otoconia. Epithelial cysts have been seen in the sensory epithelium of the posterior and superior ampullary cristae in advanced old age.[9] There does not appear to be a reduction of vestibular ganglion cell numbers in old age comparable to that seen in the spiral ganglion.[10]

Trauma

Fractures may involve the vestibular system. Surgical operations may be complicated by accidental penetration of the vestibule or semicircular canals. The production of a fistula from the lateral semicircular canals, by design, into the middle ear was part of the now-abandoned operation of fenestration for otosclerosis. This procedure was replaced by stapedectomy; a fistula may occur from the vestibule into the middle ear as a complication of this operation.

Ototoxicity

Part of the damage produced by aminoglycoside antibiotics such as gentamycin may be to the sensory epithelium of the cristae and maculae (see Chapter 7).

Virus Infection

In measles, rubella and cytomegalovirus infection changes have been observed in the utricle and saccule (see Chapter 8).

Bacterial Infection

Bacterial infection may involve the vestibular system as part of labyrinthitis. In most bacterial infections, spread occurs from the middle ear via the oval window (see Chapter 8). A direct fistula resulting from the bone erosion of otitis media may take place leading into the lateral semicircular canal, particularly in the presence of cholesteatoma (see Chapter 3).

Syphilis

The diffuse periostitic form of syphilis has a special tendency to involve the semicircular canals, and the lumina of the canals may be completely obliterated by bone and fibrous tissue (see Chapter 8).

Bone Diseases

Paget's disease frequently involves the bony vestibule and semicircular canals to a severe degree and as a result clinical symptoms referable to this system are likely to occur. Otosclerosis, although frequently present in relation to the bony wall of the vestibule, rarely involves the membranous structures of the vestibular system so that vestibular symptoms are rare in this condition (see Chapter 10).

Hydrops

Hydrops of the saccule, which sometimes extends to the utricle, is the major pathological feature of Ménière's disease (see above). Saccular hydrops may also be a manifestation of syphilitic and bacterial inflammation involving the labyrinth (see Chapter 8).

Atelectasis

A process of collapse of the walls of the ampullae and utricle termed vestibular atelectasis was described in 1988.[11] The clinical histories and temporal bone studies support the existence of a primary type with a paroxysmal or insidious onset, and a secondary type that occurs in association with other inner ear disorders. The principal clinical symptom was described as chronic unsteadiness, precipitated or aggravated by head movement, and sometimes associated with short episodes of spinning vertigo. It was presumed that the collapsed membranes interfere with the motion mechanics of the cupulae and otolithic membranes. This description may explain some of the obscure clinical cases of vertigo arising from vestibular dysfunction, but

the existence of vestibular atelectasis as a pathological entity has not yet been confirmed.

Positional Vertigo

Positional vertigo is a condition in which vertigo is induced in the patient by alteration in the position of the head. Since nystagmus is used clinically as an objective test of this condition, the term "positional nystagmus" is often preferred.

A temporal bone study of a patient who suffered a bout of severe vertigo without deafness, followed by the features of positional vertigo showed atrophy of the superior division of the vestibular nerve, utricle and crista of the lateral semicircular canal.[12] The authors attributed these changes to occlusion of a vessel supplying the vestibular labyrinth, but pathological change in such a vessel was not actually observed.

A temporal bone study of two cases of positional vertigo revealed degeneration of the macula of the utricle and of the cristae of the lateral and superior semicircular canals and of the superior vestibular nerve.[13,14] In these two cases the changes were also attributed to atherosclerosis of supplying arteries, although such changes were not actually seen in the temporal bone sections.

In 1969 Schuknecht described the temporal bone findings in two cases of positional vertigo.[15] Attached to the posterior surface of the cupula of the left posterior semicircular canal in each of the cases was a basophilically stained homogeneous deposit measuring 300 μm in one case and 350 μm in the other, in their greatest diameters. On the basis of these cases, Schuknecht has built up an explanation of the symptomatology of positional vertigo. He postulates that the calcific material derived from otoconia in a degenerated utricular macula will descend by gravity along the endolymph and form on the crista of the posterior semicircular canal, the lowest region of the labyrinthine sensory epithelium. Schuknecht suggested that such a mechanism was responsible for the positional vertigo in the three other cases described above even though cupulolithiasis was not described in the serial sections.

This ingenious theory has attracted much interest and the term "cupulolithiasis" is nowadays frequently used as a synonym for positional vertigo. Surgical operations on the posterior semicircular canal in cases of positional vertigo have been devised and are claimed to be successful. No further autopsy studies of positional vertigo have been described since Schuknecht's 1969 paper, but there is recent support of the concept of cupulolithiasis with the discovery of particles within the posterior semicircular canal in eight of the patients in a study of 26 posterior canals during the operation for the relief of positional vertigo. This was contrasted with the absence of particles in the same canal when patients without the symptoms of positional vertigo were tested during removal of vestibular schwannoma or labyrinthectomy.[16] The particulate material identified in the posterior semicircular canals had the ultrastructural appearance of degenerated otoconia.

Neoplasms

The most important neoplasm of the vestibular system is schwannoma of the vestibular division of the eighth cranial nerve (acoustic neuroma). This does not usually invade the vestibule, but may do so in cases of neurofibromatosis 2 (see Chapter 11). The saccule and utricle show an exudate of proteinaceous fluid in the presence of a schwannoma of the internal auditory meatus. Vestibular schwannoma is discussed in Chapter 11. Other primary neoplasms of the vestibular system are rare; the recently described low-grade adenocarcinoma of the endolymphatic sac is also described in Chapter 11. Metastatic deposits are unusual; invasion of the vestibular system from the internal auditory meatus by way of the vestibular nerve may occur in metastatic neoplasm or in carcinoma of the middle ear (see Chapter 5).

Presbycusis

Presbycusis is a term in current use to denote the hearing loss in aged people that cannot be ascribed to any known cause other than old age.

Clinical and Audiological Features

The deafness has the features of a sensorineural hearing loss and it has been debated whether the disability lies in the hair cells of the cochlea, in other parts of the cochlea, particularly the spiral ganglion cells, the cochlear nerve or the stria vascularis, or in the parts of the brain such as the brainstem that innervate the cochlea. In a study of brainstem-evoked responses in patients with presbycusis, changes of a degree suggestive of any participation of brainstem cells in the hearing loss were not found.[17] Schuknecht and his co-workers have detected morphological and audiological evidence of involvement of four regions of the cochlea in four

different forms of presbycusis. In addition a fifth form of presbycusis associated with hypothetically diminished qualities of the cochlear duct and a sixth comprising a mixture of the other five have been added.[18] So the six types of presbycusis presented by Schuknecht and accepted by many as a valid summary of the pathological basis of presbycusis, are:

1. Sensory, loss of organ of Corti hair cells.
2. Neural, loss of spiral ganglion cells and nerve fibres.
3. Strial, loss of stria vascularis cells.
4. Cochlear conductive, diminution of conductivity of basilar membrane.
5. Cochlear duct, alterations in the physical characteristics of the cochlear duct.
6. Mixed, any mixture of the other five.

Pure tone audiometry has been the usual means of testing the hearing in presbycusis. Soucek et al. found in a study of extratympanic electrocochleograms in geriatric patients that the cochlear nerves were functioning adequately in all cases. These findings suggested that, contrary to the elaborate schema presented above, it was the hair cells in which the primary deficit of the hearing loss of the elderly people was to be sought.[17]

Pathological Appearances

Investigations by Histological Section

In most investigations of the pathological basis of presbycusis, histological sections were used. In some of these investigations hair cells were incriminated as showing pathological changes.[19,20] Statements about the appearances of these cells in histological section must be regarded with caution, however, since they are very liable to undergo post-mortem autolysis. Moreover, representation of the functionally most important part of the hair cells – the stereocilia – in a histological section is very small, even when adequately fixed. Clear-cut losses in the spiral ganglion cells and the nerve fibres derived from them are, however, well documented[20,21,22,23,24] (Fig. 9.5). Careful analysis of the cochlear nuclear cells in the brainstem has also shown some loss in presbycusis.[25] It is difficult to accept nerve cell atrophy as the basis of a universal defect and it seems more likely that there is some more fundamental disturbance giving rise to it. Atrophy of the stria vascularis has been stated to be the pathological basis of presbycusis in some subjects.[26] Like the hair cells, the stria is subject to post-mortem

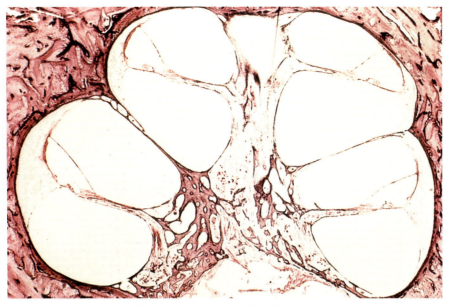

Figure 9.5 Cochlea from a patient with presbycusis showing marked loss of spiral ganglion cells, situated in the modiolus

change, as a result of which the appearances may resemble atrophy. Vascular thickening in the cochlea has been incriminated by some, but its importance has been difficult to assess.[22,27]

Surface Preparation Appearances

It seems to us that to study adequately possible hair cell damage as the basis of presbycusis in the human it is necessary to use surface preparations, in view of the certainty of confusion of the ever-present autolysis with real damage to these structures. The studies of Bredberg[28] and of Johnsson and Hawkins[29] give strong evidence based on surface preparation observations to incriminate hair cells as the primary site of the defect. A detailed study of surface preparations from perfused cochleas of patients in a geriatric unit was made in the department of one of the authors. The preparations had all been stained for light microscopy by the method described in Chapter 1. Two major pathological changes were present: (1) atrophy of the outer hair cells and (2) giant stereociliary degeneration in some of those outer hair cells that survived.[17]

A severe degree of loss of outer hair cells was present in all coils of all cochleas from the elderly patients. Approximate estimates of hair cell losses showed that the inner hair cells had sustained little loss, the first row of outer hair cells had a greater loss, the second row loss was even greater and in the third row, hair cells were very scanty or absent (Fig. 9.6). In addition there was a complete loss of all

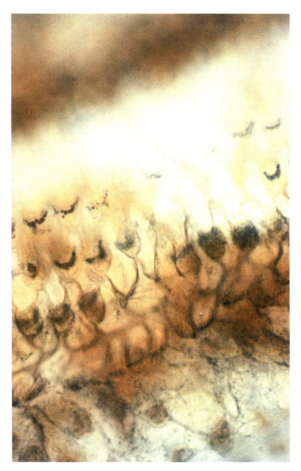

Figure 9.6 Loss of hair cells from three rows of outer hair cells in the basal coil of the cochlea of a patient with presbycusis. Surface preparation, stained with Alcian blue and osmic acid

hair cells of all rows, inner and outer, at the extreme lower end of the basal coil in every elderly cochlea.

The other change was the presence of enormously lengthened and thickened stereocilia emanating from some surviving hair cells. These giant structures were found to measure as much as 60 μm in length. They overlapped many cells in the organ of Corti and sometimes covered the tunnel of Corti. The thickening in some places could be seen to be due to adhesion of hairs to each other as longitudinal lines were identified within an enlarged stereocilium. Giant stereocilia were found only in the outer hair cells of middle and apical coils, not in the outer hair cells of the basal coil (although loss of hair cells was just as advanced in this coil) (Fig. 9.7). Giant stereociliary degeneration was present to a mild degree in the inner hair cell layer of the basal, middle and apical coils.

Relationship of Surface Preparation Changes to Functional Findings

The loss of outer hair cells throughout the cochlea may be the cause of the general hearing disability shown by Soucek et al.[17] to be present at all frequencies. The exacerbation of hearing loss in the higher tones found by these and other workers using audiometry is explained by the short segment at the lower end of the basal coil with complete atrophy of both inner and outer hair cells.

Pathogenesis

It is possible that giant stereociliary degeneration is a stage in the dissolution of the outer hair cells in the apical and middle coils. In the basal coil the stereocilia are normally different, being shorter than in the other two coils. It may be that the changes preliminary to the death of outer cells of the basal coil do not include a giant stereociliary phase or that this phase is too short-lived in those cells to be identified by histological examination. Giant stereocilia have been seen with the scanning electron microscope in human cochleas by Wright in people as young as 20 years of age.[30] Bredberg has shown that hair cells begin to disappear from an early age.[28] Perhaps giant stereociliary degeneration is an alteration that is slowly taking place throughout life, resulting eventually in presbycusis, for it is not until the later years have been reached that hair cells will have been lost to a sufficient extent to produce significant deafness.

Molecular Biology of Presbycusis

Mitochondria in the cytoplasm contain a set of genes that contribute to the phenotype of the individual. It is the mother only whose genotype is inherited. The membrane hypothesis of ageing proposes an association between reactive oxygen metabolites and the ageing process, the former

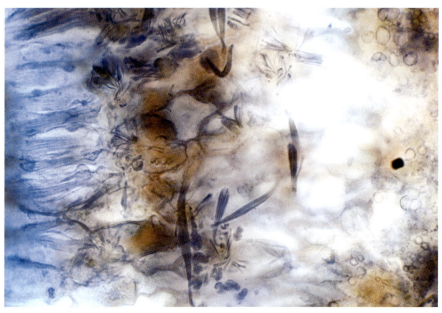

Figure 9.7 Surface preparation from middle coil of cochlea in a 76-year-old woman. Outer hair cells show giant stereocilia, some of which have longitudinal lines. Many hair cells are missing. Stained with Alcian blue and osmic acid

leading to damage to mitochondrial DNA, resulting in cellular dysfunction and eventually death.[31] A form of mitochondrial DNA damage, that of deletion of mtDNA 4977 bp, has been discovered, which accumulates in human tissues, especially those of neural and muscular type, with increasing age.[32] Using the polymerase chain reaction on celloidin-embedded archival sections of human cochleas to determine deletion of the mtDNA 4977 bp in that structure, it has been found that 14 of 17 patients with sensorineural hearing loss, mainly associated with ageing, exhibited such deletion, while only eight of 17 patients with normal hearing exhibited the same deletion.[33] Thus this 4977 bp mitochondrial deletion may cause presbycusis.

References

1. Rauch SN, Merchant SN, Thedinger BA. Ménière's syndrome and endolymphatic hydrops. Double-blind temporal bone study. Ann Otol Rhinol Laryngol 1989; 98:873–883
2. Sperling NM, Paparella MM, Yoon TH et al. Symptomatic versus asymptomatic endolymphatic hydrops: a histologic comparison. Laryngoscope 1993;103:277–285
3. Xenellis JE, Linthicum FH, Galey FR. Lermoyez's syndrome: histopathologic report of a case. Ann Otol Rhinol Laryngol 1990;99:307–309
4. Schuknecht HF. Pathology of the ear, 2nd edn. Lea & Febiger, Philadelphia, 1993
5. Antoli-Candela F Jr. The histopathology of Ménière's disease. Acta Otolaryngol (Stockh) 1976;340(suppl):5–42
6. Fraysse BG, Alonso A, House WF. Ménière's disease and endolymphatic hydrops. Clinicopathological correlations. Ann Otol Rhinol Laryngol 1980;8(suppl 76):2–22
7. Schuknecht HF, Northrop C, Igarashi M. Cochlear pathology after destruction of the endolymphatic sac in the cat. Acta Otolaryngol (Stockh) 1968;65:479–487
8. Gleeson M, Felix H. A comparative study of the effect of age on the human cochlear and vestibular neuroepithelia. Acta Ororolaryngol (Stockh) 1987;436(suppl):103–109
9. Rosenhall U. Epithelial cysts in the human vestibular apparatus. J Laryngol Otol 1974;88:105–112
10. Fleischer K. Histologische und audiometrische Studien über den altersbedingten Struktur und Funktionswandel des Innenohres. Archiv Ohren-usw Heilk u Z Hals-usw Heilk 1956;170:142–167
11. Merchant SN, Schuknecht HF. Vestibular atelectasis. Ann Otol Rhinol Laryngol 1988;97:565–576
12. Lindsay JR, Hemenway WG. Postural vertigo due to unilateral sudden partial loss of vestibular function. Ann Otol 1956;65:692–706
13. Dix MR, Hallpike CS. The pathology, symptomatology and diagnosis of certain common disorders of the vestibular system. Ann Otol Rhinol Laryngol 1952;61:987–1016
14. Cawthorne TE, Hallpike CS. A study of the clinical features and pathological changes within the temporal bones, brain stem and cerebellum of an early case of positional nystagmus of the so-called benign paroxysmal type. Acta Otolaryngol (Stockh) 1957;48:89–105
15. Schuknecht HF. Cupolithiasis. Arch Otolaryngol 1969;90:765–778
16. Welling DB, Parnes LS, O'Brien B et al. Particulate matter in the posterior semicircular canal. Laryngoscope 1997;107:90–94
17. Soucek S, Michaels L, Frohlich A. Evidence for hair cell degeneration as the primary lesion in hearing loss of the elderly. J Otolaryngol 1986;15:175–183
18. Schuknecht HF, Gacek MR. Cochlear pathology in presbycusis. Ann Otol Rhinol Laryngol 1993;102:1–16
19. Schuknecht HF. Presbycusis. Laryngoscope 1955;65:402–419
20. Suga F, Lindsay JR. Histopathological observations of presbycusis. Ann Otol Rhinol Laryngol 1976;85:169–183
21. Guild SR, Crowe SJ, Bunch CC et al. Correlations of differences in the density of innervation of the organ of Corti with differences in the acuity of hearing, including evidence as to the location in the human cochlea of the receptors for certain tones. Acta Otolaryngol (Stockh) 1931;15:269–308
22. von Fieandt H, Saxen A. Pathologie und Klinik der Altersschwerhörigkeit. Acta Otolaryngol (Stockh) 1937;23(suppl):5–85
23. Fleischer K. Das alternende Ohr: morphologische Aspekte. HNO Berlin 1972;20:103–107
24. Hansen CC, Reske-Nielsen E. Pathological studies in presbycusis. Arch Otolaryngol 1965;82:115–132
25. Arnesen AR. Presbycusis – loss of neurons in the human cochlear nuclei. J Laryngol Otol 1982;96:503–511
26. Schuknecht HF. Further observations on the pathology of presbycusis. Arch Otolaryngol 1964;80:369–382
27. Johnsson LG, Hawkins JE Jr. Vascular changes in the human ear associated with aging. Ann Otol Rhinol Laryngol 1972;81:179–193
28. Bredberg G. Cellular patterns and nerve supply of the human organ of Corti. Acta Otolaryngol (Stockh) 1965;236(suppl):1–135
29. Johnsson LG, Hawkins JE. Sensory and neural degeneration with aging, as seen in microdissection of the human inner ear. Ann Otol Rhinol Laryngol 1972;81:1–15
30. Wright A. Giant cilia in the human organ of Corti. Clin Otolaryngol 1982;7:193–199
31. Seidman MD, Bai U, Khan MJ et al. Mitochondrial DNA deletions associated with aging and presbycusis. Arch Otolaryngol Head Neck Surg 1997;123:1039–1045
32. Lee HC, Pang CY, Hsu HS et al. Differential accumulations of 4,977 bp deletion in mitochondrial DNA of various tissues in human ageing. Biochim Biophys Acta 1994;1226:37–43
33. Bai U, Seidman MD, Hinojosa R et al. Mitochondrial DNA deletions associated with aging and possibly presbycusis: a human archival temporal bone study. Am J Otol 1997;18:449–453

10 Bony Abnormalities

Paget's disease

Paget's disease (osteitis deformans) is a common condition affecting particularly the skull, pelvis, vertebral column and femur in people over 40 years of age. The cause is not yet certain, but the presence in many cases of paramyxovirus-like structures seen within osteoclasts has prompted the suggestion that Paget's disease may be of viral aetiology and the measles virus and canine distemper viruses have been under scrutiny as candidates. The pathological change is one of active bone formation proceeding alongside active bone destruction. The affected bones are enlarged, porous and deformed. Microscopically, bone formation is seen in trabeculae of bone with a lining of numerous osteoblasts. A mosaic appearance is formed by the frequent successive deposition of bone, cessation of deposition resulting in thin, blue "cement lines", followed again by resumption of deposition and its cessation, and so production of further cement lines. Bone destruction is shown by the presence of numerous, large osteoclastic giant cells with Howship's lacunae. Areas of chronic inflammatory exudate intermixed with the bone are common (Fig. 10.1).

The pathology of involvement of the temporal bone by Paget's disease has been well studied.[1,2] The petrous apex, the mastoid and the bony part of the Eustachian tube are most frequently affected. The periosteal part of the bony labyrinth is the first to undergo pagetoid changes. The endochondral layer is also affected in many cases but the endosteal layer and modiolus infrequently (Fig. 10.1). The internal auditory meatus may show protruberances of pagetoid tissue into its lumen. In a few cases the stapes may be tethered by pagetoid change of its footplate.[1,2] Calcification of the annulus fibrosis is cited as another cause of such fixation. Involvement of other ossicles is unusual. An alternative means of ossicular fixation may be involvement of the malleus by pagetoid tissue in the epitympanum.[1] Fissure fractures, occurring during life, are more frequent in the temporal bone of patients with Paget's disease. The round window niche may be narrowed by the bony overgrowth. The sensorineural hearing loss that patients with Paget's disease may experience is probably caused by encroachment on the membranous cochlea.

Patients with Paget's disease are predisposed to neoplasms of bone, particularly osteosarcoma and fibrosarcoma. A spindle cell sarcoma of the temporal bone has been described.[2] Cases of a benign neuromatous lesion of the cochlea associated with Paget's disease of the temporal bone are also on record (see Chapter 11).

Osteogenesis Imperfecta

Osteogenesis imperfecta is a general bone disease with a triad of clinical features: multiple fractures, blue sclerae and conductive hearing loss. There is a congenital recessive form, which is often rapidly fatal, and a tardive one in adults, which is inherited as a Mendelian dominant and is more benign. Mutations of type I collagen genes have been established as the underlying cause leading to a general disturbance in the development of collagen, hence the thin (blue) sclerae as well as poorly formed bone tissue.

The pathology is well seen in the long bones where resorption of cartilage in the development of bone is normal, but the bony trabeculae themselves are poorly formed. In the temporal bone the bony

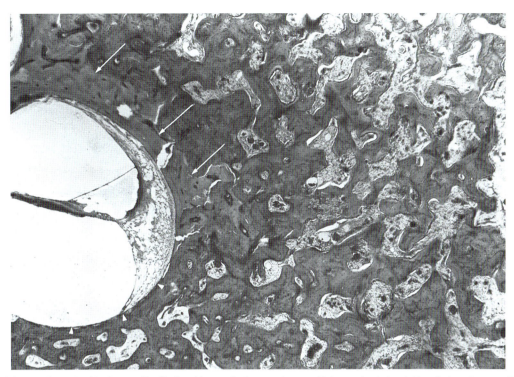

Figure 10.1 Paget's disease involving bony cochlea. The line of demarcation between the pagetoid tissue and endochondral bone is shown by *arrows*. The *arrowheads* indicate where pagetoid tissue has reached the endosteum

labyrinth is sometimes deficient in bone.[3] In the temporal bone of an infant with the congenital recessive form of osteogenesis imperfecta, X-ray of the bony labyrinth showed a sharply defined, sieve-like pattern of the highly calcified but poorly collagenised trabeculae of endochondral bone. Histological examination indicated scanty periosteal and endosteal bony trabeculae (Fig. 10.2). The ossicles in the tardive form are very thin and subject to fractures. The stapes footplate is also frequently fixed. The disturbance in lamellar bone formation can lead to extreme thinness, dehiscence, and non-union of the stapedial superstructure with the footplate or thickening with fixation of the footplate. The nature of the bony tissue causing fixation is problematical. It has been suggested that osteogenesis imperfecta can be associated with otosclerosis so that the fixation is indeed otosclerotic.[4] Otosclerosis, like osteogenesis imperfecta, may indeed be part of a general connective tissue disturbance.[5] Indeed, some cases of clinical otosclerosis may be related to mutations within the *COL1A1* gene that are similar to those found in mild forms of osteogenesis imperfecta.[6]

Osteopetrosis

Osteopetrosis (often known as marble bone disease) is a rare disease of bone, in which there is a failure to

absorb calcified cartilage and primitive bone due to deficient activity of osteoclasts. A relatively benign form, inherited as a dominant, presents in adults, and a malignant one, inherited as a recessive, in infants and young children. The patients with the benign form often survive to old age and present prominent otological symptoms.

The intermediate, endochondral portion of the otic capsule is swollen and appears as an exaggerated thickened form of the normal state. Globuli ossei composed of groups of calcified cartilage cells are normally present in this region (see Chapter 1), and in osteopetrosis they are greatly increased in number and are arranged into a markedly thickened zone (Fig. 10.3). The periosteal bone is normal. The organ of Corti is usually normal, but in a few cases has been said to be atrophied. The ossicles are of fetal shape and filled with unabsorbed, calcified cartilage. The canals for the seventh and eighth cranial nerves are greatly narrowed by the expanded cartilaginous and bony tissue and these changes are probably responsible for the characteristic symptoms of facial palsy and hearing loss, respectively.[7,8,9]

Achondroplasia

In achondroplasia, which is an inherited congenital disorder, there is a deficiency of growth of cartilage

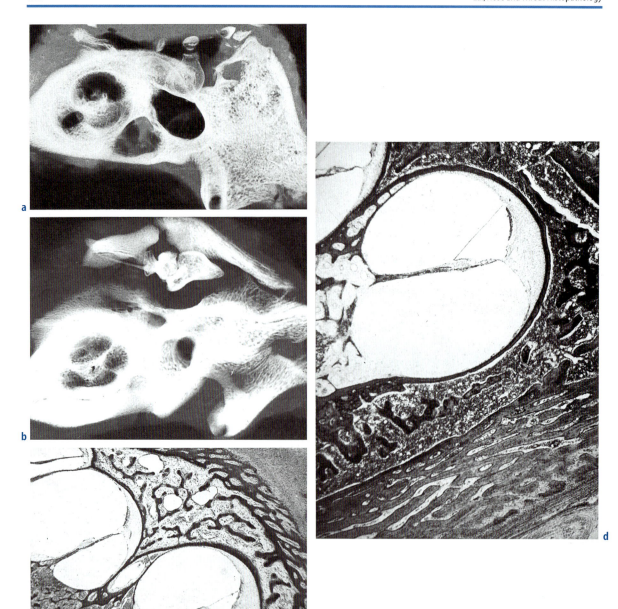

Figure 10.2 Osteogenesis imperfecta in cochlea of a stillborn infant of 26 weeks' gestation. **a** X-ray of microsliced temporal bone. There is a sieve-like appearance of most of the bone due to thinness of bony trabeculae. **b** X-ray of cochlea of normal 26-week gestation fetus showing coarser bone. **c** Section of cochlea showing thin and cellular periosteal layer. Bony trabeculae are thin and highly calcified. **d** Section of normal fetus at 26 weeks' gestation for comparison

so that the patient becomes a dwarf with stunted growth of the long bones, but there is normal growth of bones formed in membrane. Hearing loss of conductive and sensorineural type is frequent. Computed tomography scans in achondroplasiacs have shown relative "rotation" of the cochlea and other temporal bone structures, but this probably does not account for the hearing loss.[10] The temporal bone histology in such an achodroplasiac was described as showing a normal endochondral layer, but thickened middle and periosteal layers com-

posed of dense thick trabeculae without globuli ossei.[11]

Otosclerosis

Prevalence

Otosclerosis is a common focal lesion of the otic capsule, which is found principally in relation to the

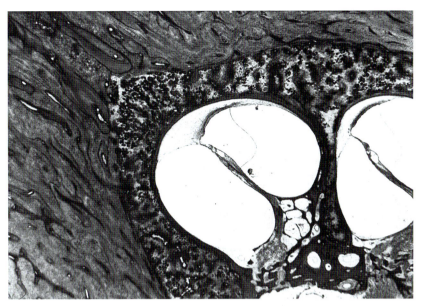

Figure 10.3 Osteopetrosis involving bony cochlea. The endochondral layer is enlarged and globuli ossei are excessively basophilic (Courtesy of Dr. V.J. Hyams)

cochlea and footplate of the stapes. "Histological otosclerosis" refers to a disease process without clinical symptoms or manifestations that can be discovered only by routine sectioning of the temporal bone at autopsy. "Clinical otosclerosis" concerns the presence of otosclerosis at a site where it causes conductive hearing loss, usually by interfering with the motion of the stapes. The mean prevalence of histological otosclerosis has been estimated from temporal bone studies at 8.3%.[12] According to Guild,[13] 15% of temporal bones with histological otosclerosis demonstrate ankylosis of the stapedio-vestibular articulation: hence $8.3 \times 15/100 = 1.2\%$ of all temporal bones studied could by such extrapolation be considered as having clinical otosclerosis. The figure derived from actual clinical studies of large populations is 0.3%.[14] It is likely that the temporal bones studied by Guild and others are biased towards greater numbers of cases of otosclerosis by the fact that a large proportion of the patients had been investigated during life for otologic conditions. In a study that was not so biased, consisting of unselected consecutive autopsied patients in one hospital,[15] 2.5% of 236 temporal bones showed otosclerosis, with an extrapolated figure for clinical otosclerosis of 0.37%. This correlates well with the clinically derived figure of 0.3%.[14]

Aetiology

Otosclerosis seems to have some features of a hereditary disease, but its genetics still remain incompletely elucidated. There is a histological similarity between otosclerosis and Paget's disease of bone. Because of the finding of measles-like virus particles in Paget's disease of bone osteoclasts (see above), a search for a similar connection has been made in otosclerosis. Ultrastructural and immunohistochemical evidence has indeed been found for measles virus in otosclerotic tissue. Using a method for isolation and identification of both DNA and RNA sequences in archival human temporal bone specimens with the polymerase chain reaction technique, a 115-base-pair sequence of the measles nucleocapsid gene has been identified in eight of 11 different temporal bone specimens with histologic evidence of otosclerosis. None of nine control specimens without histologic evidence of otosclerosis were positive.[16] It thus seems likely that otosclerosis is associated with the measles virus, possibly through the intermediary of an immune reaction.

Gross Appearances

Otosclerosis usually affects both ears symmetrically. The disease process is probably confined to the temporal bone. In cases with prominent otosclerotic involvement of the otic capsule, the lesion may be seen as a smooth prominence of the promontory. The stapes is sometimes fixed. The pink swelling of the otosclerotic focus may sometimes even be detected clinically through a particularly transparent tympanic membrane.

In microsliced temporal bones showing otosclerosis, the focus appears well demarcated and pink. Blood vessels are prominent and evenly distributed.

X-rays of temporal bone specimens show the well-defined lesion as a patch of mottled translucency (Fig. 10.4).

Microscopic Appearances

The histological characteristic of otosclerosis is the presence of trabeculae of new bone, mostly of the woven type (Figs 10.5 and 10.6). This contrasts with the well-developed bone under the outer periosteum, the endochondral middle layer and the endosteal layer of the otic capsule (see Chapter 1), a sharply demarcated edge between normal otosclerotic bone being a prominent feature. The pathological bony tissue has a variable appearance, with areas of differing cellularity. In most places osteoblasts are very abundant within the woven

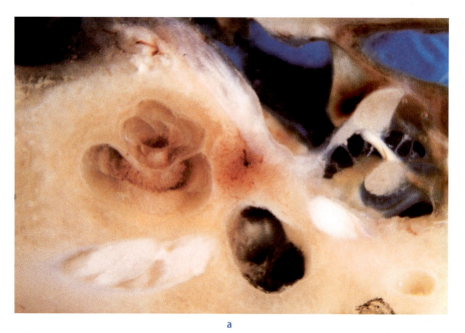

a

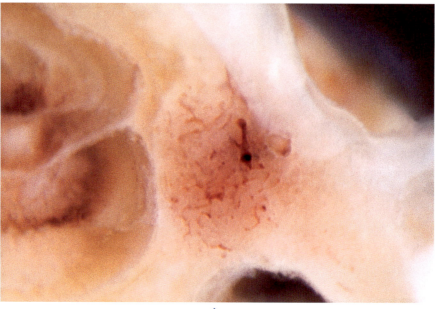

b

Figure 10.4 Otosclerosis. **a** Microsliced temporal bone showing oval vascular-appearing focus of otosclerosis to right of cochlea. Note vestibule below it and stapes and facial nerve to right. **b** Higher power of focus of otosclerosis. **c** X-ray of microslice shown in **a** and **b**. The otosclerotic focus (*O*) appears as a mottled, translucent area. *C*, cochlea; *S*, stapes. *Arrowheads* indicate fissula ante fenestram

(Figure 10.4 c, see opposite)

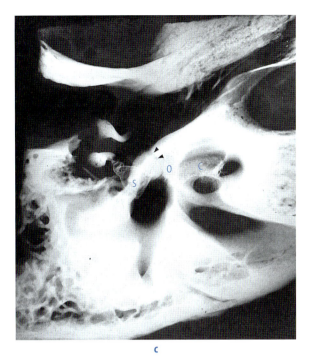

c
Figure 10.4 c

active (more cellular and more vascular) and inactive (less cellular and less vascular) otosclerotic foci may be recognised.[17]

The commonest site for the formation of otosclerotic foci is the bone anterior to the oval window. The fissula ante fenestram, a normally appearing slit connecting middle ear with vestibule, is present in the same region (Fig. 10.4), but the significance of this relationship is still not understood. Cartilaginous rests are also normal in this area and may be seen nearby. Otosclerotic foci may also be seen in the bone near the round window membrane, in the inferior part of the cochlear capsule or in the bone around the semicircular canals.

Otosclerotic involvement of the stapes footplate leading to functional fixation of the stapes may occur in two ways:

1. There may be actual participation by the stapes footplate in the formation of otosclerotic bone so that the otic capsular focus of pathological bone is continuous with the former, the annulus fibrosis being obliterated (Fig. 10.7). Involvement of the oval window takes place at any point of its circumference, or indeed around most of it. The process may also occasionally be associated with similar alterations in the lower parts of the stapedial crura.

2. Frequently the footplate is not affected by the otosclerotic process, but the bone surrounding it proliferates to such an extent that the oval window is distorted and narrowed. Fibrous

bone. Osteoclasts may be present and are accompanied by evidence of bone resorption. Marrow spaces contain prominent blood vessels and connective tissue. In a few places the bone may be more mature and less cellular, and even lamellar bone may be found. In these areas marrow spaces are small. Thus

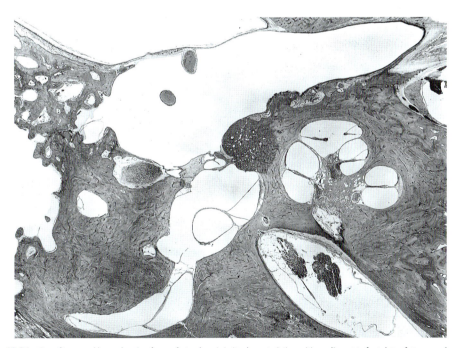

Figure 10.5 Section of temporal bone showing focus of otosclerosis in its characteristic position adjacent to footplate of stapes and vestibule

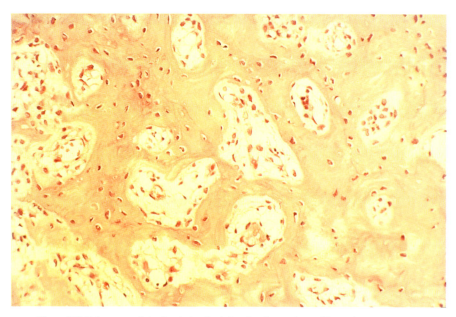

Figure 10.6 Higher power of otosclerosis showing trabeculae of woven bone with vascular marrow spaces

thickening of the annulus fibrosis may be prominent. The otosclerotic focus may also encroach on the round window, narrowing it in the same fashion.

Otosclerotic bone frequently reaches the endosteum of the cochlear capsule. In some cases it may lead to a fibrous reaction deep to the spiral ligament. Overgrowth of otosclerotic bone may, rarely, cause distortion of the cochlear contours and even affect the modiolus and lead to spontaneous fractures of the modiolar septa.[18]

An entity of "otospongiosis" is often referred to by radiologists implying a more vascular, less bony lesion. Looking at temporal bone sections, "otospongiotic" and "otosclerotic" lesions are found side by side in both active and inactive lesions[19] so that whether it is an "otospongiotic" or "otosclerotic" lesion appears to have no relation to the activity of the condition.

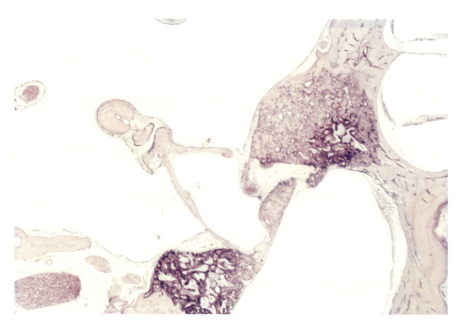

Figure 10.7 Focus of otosclerosis involving the anterior part of the footplate. A smaller one is involving the posterior part of the footplate

Hearing Loss in Relation to Otosclerotic Foci

By far the commonest form of hearing loss in otosclerosis can be accounted for by oval window fixation as described above, and is conductive in type. Depression of sound waves derived from air conduction also occurs following obstruction of the round window by otosclerosis. It is likely that otosclerotic involvement of the cochlea may lead to sensorineural hearing loss – "cochlear otosclerosis".

References

1. Davies DG. Paget's disease of the temporal bone. A clinical and histopathological survey. Acta Otolaryngol (Scand) 1968;242(suppl):1–47
2. Nager GT. Paget's disease of the temporal bone. Ann Otol Rhinol Laryngol 1975;84(suppl 22):3–32
3. Igarashi M, King AI, Schwenzfeier CW et al. Inner ear pathology in osteogenesis imperfecta congenita. J Laryngol Otol 1980;94:697–705
4. Dieler R, Muller J, Helms J. Stapes surgery in osteogenesis imperfecta patients. Eur Arch Otorhinolaryngol 1997;254:120–127
5. Arslan M, Ricci V. Histochemical investigations of otosclerosis with special regard to collagen disease. J Laryngol Otol 1963;77:365–373
6. McKenna MJ, Kristiansen AG, Bartley ML et al. Association of COL1A1 and otosclerosis: evidence for a shared genetic etiology with mild osteogenesis imperfecta.. Am J Otol 1998;19:604–610
7. Milroy CM, Michaels L. Temporal bone pathology of adult-type osteopetrosis. Arch Otolaryngol Head Neck Surg 1990;116:79–84
8. Myers EN, Stool S. The temporal bone in osteopetrosis. Arch Otolaryng 1969;89:460–469
9. Hamersma H. Ostepetrosis (marble bone disease) of the temporal bone. Laryngoscope 1970;80:1518–1539
10. Cobb SR, Shohat M, Mehringer CM et al. CT of the temporal bone in achondroplasia. Am J Neuroradiol 1988;9:1195–1199
11. Schuknecht HF. Pathology of the ear. Harvard University Press, Cambridge Mass, 1974
12. Altmann F, Glasgold A, Mcduff JP. The incidence of otosclerosis as related to race and sex. Ann Otol Rhinol Laryngol 1967;76:377–392
13. Guild SR. Histologic otosclerosis. Ann Otol Rhinol Laryngol 1944;53:246–267
14. Causse JR, Causse JB. Otospongiosis as a genetic disease. Early detection, medical management and prevention. Am J Otol 1984;5:211–223
15. Declau F, Van Spaendonck M, Timmermans JP et al. Prevalence of otosclerosis in an unselected series of temporal bones (in preparation) Am J Otol in press
16. McKenna MJ, Kristiansen AG, Haines J. Polymerase chain reaction amplification of a measles virus sequence from human temporal bone sections with active otosclerosis. Am J Otol 1996;17:827–830
17. Nager GT. Histopathology of otosclerosis. Arch Otolaryngol 1969;89:157–179
18. Nager GT. Sensorineural deafness and otosclerosis. Ann Otol Rhinol Laryngol 1966;75:481–511
19. Parahy C, Linthicum FH Jr. Otosclerosis and otospongiosis: clinical and histological comparisons. Laryngoscope 1984;94:508–512

11 Neoplasms of the Inner Ear

Primary

The cellular constituents of the inner ear, apart from bone are, for the most part, fully differentiated non-mitotic structures – nerve cells and sensory epithelia – so that neoplasms would not be expected to arise in them. Primary neoplasms are indeed rare except for vestibular schwannoma.

Internal Auditory Canal and Cerebellopontine Angle Tumours

Tumours occurring in the internal auditory canal are the solitary vestibular schwannoma, the bilateral vestibular schwannoma (neurofibromatosis 2), the latter usually accompanied in this situation by neoplasm-like masses of meningioma and neurofibroma. Primary meningiomas and lipomas also are seen in this region. Tumours of the internal auditory canal on enlargement extend into the cranial cavity, filling the cerebellopontine angle.

Vestibular Schwannoma (Acoustic Neuroma)

The neoplasm is stated to arise most commonly at the glial–neurilemmal junction of the eighth nerve, which is usually within the internal auditory meatus (see Chapter 1). When seen at surgery or autopsy, however, vestibular schwannoma in most cases is found to occupy a much greater part of the nerve. Usually it is the vestibular division of the nerve that is affected; in a few the cochlear division is the source of the neoplasm (Fig. 11.1). Growth takes place from origin, both centrally onto the cerebellopontine angle, and distally along the canal. A case has been described in which the acoustic neuroma arose from the intravestibular portion of the nerve.[1] Nager reported a small schwannoma arising in the cochlea of a case of Paget's disease affecting the temporal bone and a similar case with both lesions is in the Institute of Laryngology and Otology temporal bone collection[2] (see Chapter 10). Vestibular schwannoma is usually unilateral but may be bilateral (see below). In a large series 129 cases were unilateral and 11 bilateral.[3]

Clinical Features

Vestibular schwannoma arises on the eighth cranial nerve. The neoplasm may grow slowly for years without causing symptoms and may be first diagnosed only at post-mortem where it has been found in about one in 220 consecutive adults.[4] Although it arises on the vestibular branch of the eighth cranial nerve, hearing loss and tinnitus are early symptoms produced by involvement of the cochlear division of the nerve; in the later stages vertigo and abnormal caloric and electronystagmographic responses develop from damage to the vestibular division itself.

Gross Appearance

The neoplasm is of variable size and of round or oval shape. Small tumours either do not widen the canal at all or produce only a small indentation in the bone. The larger tumours often have a mushroom shape with two components, the stalk – an elongated part in the canal – and an expanded part in the region of the cerebellopontine angle. The bone of the internal auditory canal is widened funnelwise as the neoplasm grows (Fig. 11.1). The tumour surface is smooth and lobulated. The cut surface is yellowish, often with areas of haemorrhage and cysts. The vestibular division of the eighth nerve may be identified on the surface of the tumour.

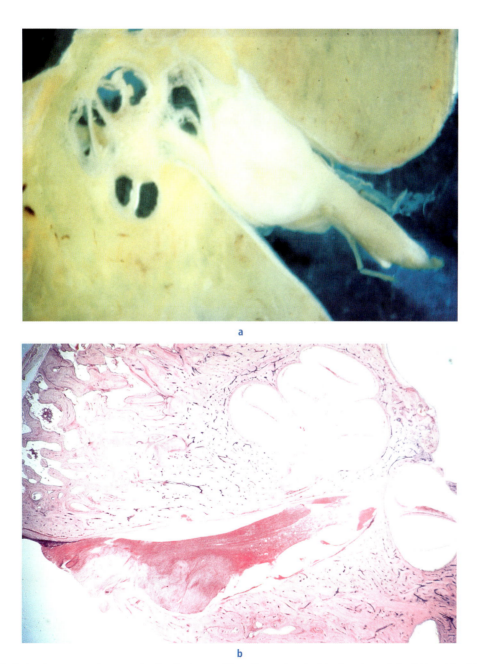

a

b

Figure 11.1 Vestibular schwannoma. **a** Appearance in microsliced temporal bone. The neoplasm is arising from the vestibular division of the eighth nerve and compressing the cochlear division. Note the granular deposit lining the cochlea. **b** Small vestibular schwannoma. It is arising from the vestibular division of the eighth nerve in the region of the glial neurilemmal junction and causing a small indentation only of the bony wall of the internal canal. There is exudate in the vestibule, but not in the cochlea. **c** Section of acoustic neuroma from a case with bilateral neurofibromatosis 2. This tumour was invading the vestibule. This area shows Antoni A appearances and Verocay bodies. There is no more atypical change than may be seen in unilateral acoustic neuroma. **d** Another part of the neoplasm seen in **c** to show Antoni B area

(Figure 11.1c and d, see overleaf)

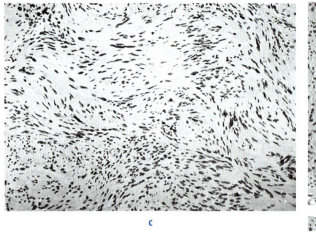

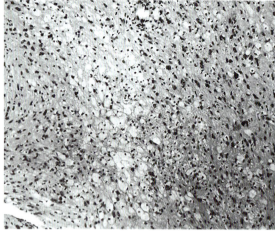

Figure 11.1 c,d

Histological Findings

Acoustic neuroma has the features of a neoplasm of schwann cells showing Antoni A and Antoni B areas. Antoni A areas display spindle cells closely packed together with palisading of nuclei. Verocay bodies, which may be present in the Antoni A areas, are whorled formations of palisaded tumour cells resembling tactile corpuscles. The spindle cells of the tumour may lack palisading and Verocay bodies, however. The degree of cellularity of the neoplasm can be high or low. The spindle cells frequently are moderately pleomorphic, but mitotic figures are rare. The presence of pleomorphism does not denote a malignant tendency. Antoni B areas, probably a degenerate form of the Antoni A pattern, show a loose reticular pattern, sometimes with histiocytic proliferation. Thrombosis and necrosis may be present in some parts of the neoplasm. A mild degree of invasion of modiolus or vestibule along cochlear or vestibular nerve branches may be present even in solitary vestibular schwannomas. Granular or homogeneous fluid exudate is usually present in the perilymphatic spaces of the cochlea and vestibule. This may arise as a result of pressure by the neoplasm on veins draining the cochlea and vestibule in the internal auditory meatus. Hydrops of the endolymphatic system may occur and in larger tumours there is atrophy of spiral ganglion cells and nerve fibres in the basilar membrane.[5]

Electron Microscopy

The ultrastructure of acoustic neuroma is characterised by the presence of Schwann cells in both Antoni A and B areas. These cells have a network of thin, interdigitating processes covered by a fine basal lamina in all areas.

Biologic Behaviour

The tumour is benign and usually grows slowly. Serious symptoms and even death may occur, however, due to damage to cerebral structures if the neoplasm grows to a large size.

Neurofibromatosis 2 (Bilateral Vestibular Schwannoma)

Bilateral vestibular schwannoma acoustic neuroma (neurofibromatosis 2, NF2), unlike neurofibromatosis 1 (von Recklinghausen's disease), is not associated with large numbers of cutaneous neurofibromas and cafe-au-lait spots, but the temporal bone locality of the neural tumour and its bilaterality are inherited as an autosomal dominant trait. This condition has been related to a gene localised near the centre of the long arm of chromosome 22.[6] At autopsy of cases of NF2, neural neoplasms are present in both eighth nerves and other central nerves. There are often many small schwannomas and collections of cells of neurofibromatous and meningiomatous appearance growing on cranial nerves and on the meninges in the vicinity of the vestibular schwannomas and sometimes even intermixed with them. The NF2 tumours are histologically similar to those of the single tumours except that the former have more Verocay bodies and more foci of high cellularity.[7] The NF2 tumours are more invasive, however, tending to infiltrate the cochlea and vestibule more deeply.

Immunohistochemistry

As with all schwannomas the strongest and most consistent immunohistochemical reaction is the positivity displayed when staining with a polyclonal antibody against S100 protein is carried out. The vimentin marker is also usually positive. These findings are common to both unilateral vestibular schwannoma and the schwannomas of NF2. Glial fibrillary acidic protein and neurone-specific enolase markers are also sometimes positive; the tumours are consistently negative for CD34.

Antibody against Ki-67 (MIB-1 in paraffin sections) has been utilised in a number of investigations to determine whether the degree of positivity with this proliferation marker can be related to the clinical activity of the tumour. So far studies have shown that there is no correlation between Ki-67 marker reactivity and tumour size or recurrence numbers in cases of solitary vestibular schwannoma,[8] but that the degree of labelling with the proliferation marker is higher in cases of NF2 that in those of solitary vestibular schwannoma.[9]

Meningioma

Meningiomas are usually intracranial masses. They arise from arachnoid villi, which are small protrusions of the arachnoid membranes into the venous sinuses. Arachnoid villi may be found in parts of the temporal bone, including the inner ear, and on occasion meningiomas may arise from these structures as primary neoplasms of the inner ear region. The most likely position for a primary inner ear meningioma is in the wall of the internal auditory meatus, where arachnoid villi are normally frequent. The histological appearances of a meningioma are those of a tumour with a whorled arrangement of cells: meningotheliomatous if the tumour cells appear epithelioid, psammomatous if calcification of the whorled masses is prominent and fibroblastic if the tumour cells resemble fibroblasts (Fig. 11.2). Meningiomas as well as acoustic neuromas may appear in the inner ear in the neurofibromatosis 2 syndrome. The meningioma is a slowly growing tumour of the temporal bone, which has had a reputation for complete benignity. In the temporal bone, however, it has a strong propensity for local recurrence and invasion (see Chapter 5).

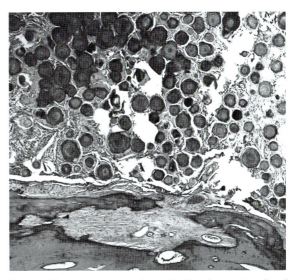

Figure 11.2 Psammomatous meningioma arising from the posterior surface of the temporal bone in a case of neurofibromatosis 2

Lipoma

Lipomas of the internal auditory canal and cerebellopontine angle are rare tumours that may be confused clinically with the much commoner vestibular schwannoma. On magnetic resonance imaging (MRI), however, this tumour displays characteristics of adipose tissue rather than those of schwannoma. There may be erosion of the walls of the internal auditory canal as with vestibular schwannoma, and lipoma may be grossly similar to the latter at operation. Since the seventh and eighth cranial nerves or their branches (Fig. 11.3) may pass through the lesion and their integrity be damaged by removal of the tumour, it is recommended that diagnosis be made whenever the possibility of this neoplasm is suspected by intraoperative examination of frozen sections. If a diagnosis of lipoma is made in this way it should not be resected, since its further growth does not constitute a threat to vital structures.[10]

Apex of Petrous Temporal Bone and Cerebellopontine Angle Tumours

A variety of neoplasms and tumour-like lesions may present at the apex of the petrous temporal bone. These include the following: jugular paraganglioma (see above), jugular foramen schwannoma arising usually from the vagus nerve, low-grade adenocarcinoma of probable endolymphatic sac origin and the tumour-like entities of cholesteatoma (epidermoid cyst) and cholesterol granuloma. Such lesions, on enlargement, may extend into the cerebellopontine angle.

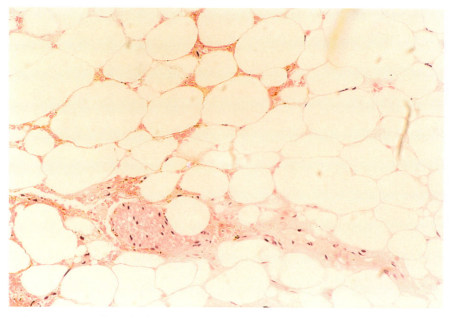

Figure 11.3 Lipoma of internal auditory canal. Note nerve branch passing through adipose tissue near the bottom

Low-grade Adenocarcinoma of Probable Endolymphatic Sac

There is evidence of the existence of a rare epithelial neoplasm of the endolymphatic system, mainly in the endolymphatic sac.[11–13] Although of benign glandular histological appearance and of slow growth, the neoplasm seems to have considerable invasive capacity and therefore the term "low-grade adenocarcinoma of probable endolymphatic sac origin" has been applied (Heffner's tumour). Some cases have presented bilateral neoplasms of the same type and some have been associated also with von Hippel-Lindau disease.[14]

The course of the tumour's growth may extend over many years. Tinnitus or vertigo, similar or identical to the symptoms of Ménière's disease, are present in about one-third of patients. It is presumed that early obstruction of the endolymphatic sac leads to hydrops of the endolymphatic system of the labyrinth and so to the Ménière's symptoms. Imaging reveals a lytic temporal bone lesion, appearing to originate from the region between the internal auditory canal and sigmoid sinus (which is the approximate position of the endolymphatic sac). There is usually prominent extension into the posterior cranial cavity and invasion of the middle ear (Fig. 11.4).

In most cases the tumour has a papillary–glandular appearance, the papillary proliferation being lined by a single row of low cuboidal cells. The vascular nature of the papillae in some cases has given the tumour a histological resemblance to choroid plexus papilloma. In some cases the tumour also shows areas of dilated glands containing secretion that has some resemblance to colloid and under these circumstances the lesion may resemble papillary adenocarcinoma of the thyroid (Fig. 11.5). Such thyroid-like areas may even dominate the histological pattern. A few cases show a clear cell predomi-

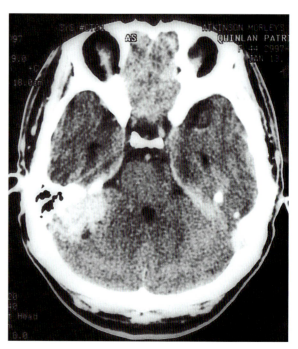

Figure 11.4 Low-grade adenocarcinoma of probable endolymphatic sac origin. Computerised tomogram showing involvement of left petrous temporal bone by large neoplasm

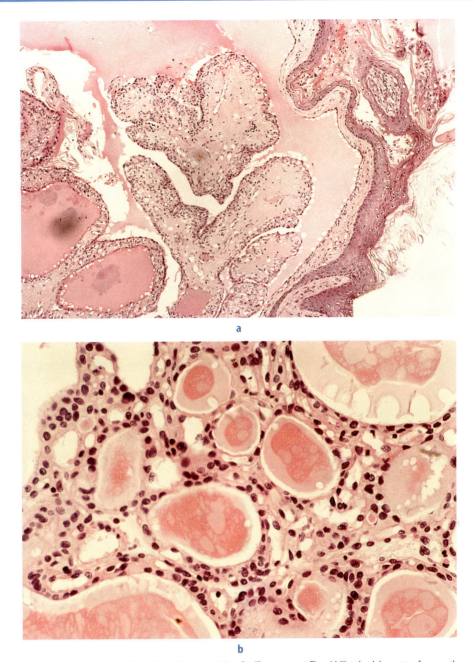

a

b

Figure 11.5 Low-grade adenocarcinoma of probable endolymphatic sac origin. **a** Papillary pattern. **b** Thyroid-like glandular pattern from another area of the same

nance resembling carcinoma of the kidney. On immunohistochemistry the epithelial cells of this neoplasm contain antigens of cytokeratins. Some tumours contain glial fibrillary acidic protein. Thyroglobulin is always absent.

It seems possible that the so-called "aggressive papillary middle ear tumour"[15] (see Chapter 5) may be low-grade adenocarcinoma of endolymphatic sac with extension of neoplasm to the middle ear. In a described case the lumen of the endolymphatic sac

appeared tumour-free at surgery (although the wall of that structure was involved). This feature, together with the rather non-specific ultrastructural and immunohistochemical features found in that case, provoked the authors to contend that the origin of that tumour was from the mucosa of the pneumatic spaces (middle ear) surrounding the jugular bulb rather than from the endolymphatic sac.[16]

The histological appearances of low-grade adenocarcinomas of probable endolymphatic sac origin are indeed in keeping with the normal histological structure of the endolymphatic sac, which is lined by a papillary columnar epithelial layer. The development of the endolymphatic sac is characterised by a stage in which the epithelium is closely associated with a network of capillaries to give rise to the "endolymphatic glomerulus".[17,18] This may account for an appearance similar to that of the choroid plexus papilloma displayed by some of the low-grade adenocarcinomas of the endolymphatic sac.

Tumour-like Lesions

Cholesteatoma (Epidermoid Cyst)

This lesion usually presents with symptoms relating to its involvement of the seventh and eighth cranial nerves in the cerebellopontine angle.[19] The histological appearance is similar to that of middle ear cholesteatoma (see Chapter 3). It is probably of congenital origin, but no cell rest has been discovered from which it might arise.

Cholesterol Granuloma

A lesion of the petrous apex with the typical features of cholesterol granuloma, as seen in the middle ear and mastoid in chronic otitis media (see Chapter 3), is being revealed by MRI scan in recent years with increasing frequency. At operation it appears cystic, the contents being altered blood, and cholesterol clefts with a foreign-body giant-cell reaction.

Microscopic examination shows non-specific granulation tissue and hemosiderin deposits in its wall. It is believed to result from an inflammatory response to an obstruction of the pneumatised air cells at the apex of the temporal bone. Haemorrhage into the air cells breaks down to hemosiderin and cholesterol with a foreign-body reaction and progressive granuloma formation. As the process develops, bone is eroded by this expansile lesion, often involving the petrous apex, the cerebellopontine angle and the middle ear.[20,21]

Directly Invading

There are two routes by which tumours invading from outside may reach the inner ear:

1. The first route is directly through the petrous bone. It is rare for tumours invading by this route to reach the membranous labyrinth. The otic capsule seems to provide a particularly strong barrier against invasion. Neoplasms that may enter the inner ear by this bony route are jugular paraganglioma and squamous carcinoma. Jugular paraganglioma arises from paraganglia situated in the wall of the jugular bulb (see Chapters 1 and 5) and then invades the temporal bone. The pathway of invasion by this tumour usually bypasses the cochlea and vestibule, traversing rapidly the floor of the middle ear. Squamous carcinoma originating in the middle ear soon erodes the thin bony plate on the anterior wall separating the Eustachian tube from the carotid canal (Chapter 5). Superficial invasion of the bone around the middle ear takes place, but the otic capsule is not invaded directly until a late stage in the disease.

2. The other route is into the internal auditory meatus, proceeding to the lateral end of the meatus and then through the foramina in the anteroinferior part of the cribriform plate alongside the filaments of the cochlear nerves, arriving by this route at the modiolus and even into the osseous spiral lamina. The vestibule appears to be more resistant to invasion by a similar mechanism, perhaps because there are fewer foramina communicating with the internal auditory meatus. Squamous carcinoma originating from the middle ear may invade in this fashion as well as by the mode described above. Infecting bacteria and fungi may reach the basilar membrane of the cochlea by the same route (see Chapter 7) and this may be a route for the spread of neoplasms from the meninges (Fig. 11.4).

Metastatic

The temporal bone is frequently the site of blood-borne metastasis for carcinomas originating in the following organs: breast, kidney, lung, stomach, larynx, prostate and thyroid. The internal auditory meatus is a common location for such growth. Once deposited, the further spread into the cochlea may take place by the route outlined above (see Chapter 5).

Leukaemia

Leukaemia may involve the inner ear in several ways. The most important is haemorrhage into the membranous spaces, to which leukaemic patients

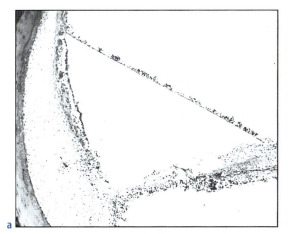
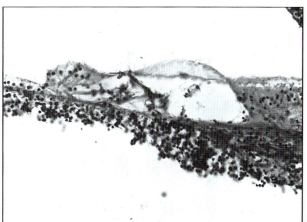

Figure 11.6 a Cochlea in chronic lymphatic leukaemia. Numerous lymphoid cells are present in the scala vestibuli adjacent to Reissner's membrane, in the scala tympani adjacent to the basilar membrane and in the spiral ligament. **b** Higher power of **a** showing lymphoid cells in scala tympani in relation to basilar membrane and organ of Corti

are particularly prone. The haemorrhage may be into the perilymphatic spaces alone or into both perilymphatic and endolymphatic spaces. If the patient survives a massive intracochlear leukaemic haemorrhage for several months, the organ of Corti and spiral ganglion will become severely degenerated and connective tissue and new bone will grow into the scalae (see Chapter 7). Another type of involvement may occur in chronic lymphocytic leukaemia, in the form of severe leukaemic infiltration of the perilymphatic spaces of the cochlea. The leukaemic cells are probably conveyed from the cerebrospinal fluid via the cochlear aqueduct (Fig. 11.6).

Malignant Lymphoma, Lymphoplasmacytic Type (Waldenstrom's Macroglobulinaemia)

Malignant lymphoma of the lymphoplasmacytic type is a modern term for Waldenstrom's macroglobulinaemia. It is a primary dyscrasia of B-type lymphoid cells in which an excess of monoclonal macroglobulin of the IgM variety is produced. Hearing loss and vertigo are present in some patients and are probably related to increased blood viscosity. In one such case coming to post-mortem, histological examination of the temporal bone showed complete disruption of the labyrinth by haemorrhage.[22]

References

1. Wanamaker WH. Acoustic neuroma: primary arising in the vestibule. Laryngoscope 1972;82:1040–1044
2. Nager GT. Paget's disease of the temporal bone. Ann Otol Rhinol Laryngol 1975;84(suppl 22):3–32
3. Erickson LS, Sorenson GD, McGavran MH. A review of 140 acoustic neurinomas (neurilemmoma). Laryngoscope 1965; 75:601–627
4. Leonard J, Talbot M. Asymptomatic acoustic neurilemmoma. Arch Otolaryngol 1970;91:117–124
5. Sidek D, Michaels L, Wright A. Changes in the inner ear in vestibular schwannoma. In: Iurato S, Veldman JE (eds) Progress in human auditory and vestibular histopathology. Kugler Publications, Amsterdam, 1996, pp 95–101
6. Wertelecki W, Rouleau GA, Superneau MD et al. Neurofibromatosis 2: clinical linkage studies of a large kindred. N Engl J Med 1988;5:278–283
7. Sobel RA. Vestibular (acoustic) schwannomas: histologic features in neurofibromatosis 2 and in unilateral cases. J Neuropathol Exper Neurol 1993;52:106–113
8. Chen JM, Houle S, Ang LC et al. A study of vestibular schwannomas using positron emission tomography and monoclonal antibody Ki-67. Am J Otol 1998; 19:840–845
9. Aguiar PH, Tatagiba M, Samii M et al. The comparison between the growth fraction of bilateral vestibular schwannomas in neurofibromatosis 2 (NF2) and unilateral vestibular schwannomas using the monoclonal antibody MIB 1. Acta Neurochir (Wien) 1995;134:40–45
10. Singh SP, Cottingham SL, Slone W et al. Lipomas of the internal auditory canal. Archiv Pathol Lab Med 1996;120:681–683
11. Gussen R. Meniere's disease: new temporal bone findings in two cases. Laryngoscope 1971;81:1695–1707
12. Hassard AD, Boudreau SF, Cron CC. Adenoma of the endolymphatic sac. J Otolaryngol 1984;13:213–216
13. Heffner DK. Low-grade adenocarcinoma of probable endolymphatic sac origin. A clinicopathologic study of 20 cases. Cancer 1989;64:2292–2302
14. Poe DE, Tarlov EC, Thomas CB et al. Aggressive papillary tumours of temporal bone. Otolaryngol Head Neck Surg 1993;108:80–86
15. Gaffey MJ, Mills ES, Fechner RE et al. Aggressive papillary middle-ear tumour. A clinico-pathologic entity distinct from middle-ear adenoma. Am J Surg Pathol 1988; 12:790–797
16. Pollak A, Bohmer A, Spycher M et al. Are papillary adenomas endolymphatic sac tumours? Ann Otol Rhinol Laryngol 1995;104:613–619
17. Kronenberg J, Leventon G. Histology of the endolymphatic sac of the rat ear and its relationship to surrounding blood

vessels: the "endolymphatic glomerulus". Am J Otol 1986;7:130–133

18. Kronenberg J, Rickenbacher J. The vascular pattern of the endolymphatic sac in the human embryo. Am J Otol 1986;7:326–329

19. de Souza CE, Sperling NM, da Costa SS et al. Congenital cholesteatomas of the cerebellopontine angle. Am J Otol 1989;10:358–363

20. Henick DH, Feghali JG. Bilateral cholesterol granuloma: an unusual presentation as an intradural mass. J Otolaryngol 1994;23:15–18

21. Amedee RG, Marks HW, Lyons GD. Cholesterol granuloma of the petrous apex. Am J Otol 1987;8:48–55

22. Wells M, Michaels L, Wells DG. Otolaryngeal disturbances in Waldenstrim's macroglobulinaemia. Clin Otolaryngol 1977;2:327–338

B

The Nose and Paranasal Sinuses

12 The Normal Nose and Paranasal Sinuses

Development

The development of the inner structure of the nose and paranasal sinuses is initiated by the formation in the second month of an ectodermal thickening, the olfactory placode, on each side. These are each placed above and medial to a maxillary swelling, which has been formed above a mandibular swelling, the four swellings, two maxillary and two mandibular (the latter of which soon fuse to form the lower jaw) being arranged around a primordial mouth cleft. Medial to each olfactory placode a swelling is formed, the medial nasal fold. The fusion of the two medial nasal folds gives rise to the frontonasal process, a precursor of the external nose and nasal septum. Lateral to each olfactory placode, a lateral nasal process on each side forms the groove between the nose and the eye. The groove between the maxillary process and the lateral nasal fold on each side gives rise to the nasolacrimal duct.

The olfactory placode forms a pit, which sinks deeper and eventually joins posteriorly with the oral cavity. The pit of the nasal cavity produces ledges on its lateral wall, which are each eventually supported by a bony skeleton to produce the turbinates. Paranasal sinuses bud off the main nasal cavity (Fig. 12.1).

The process of lateral budding from the main olfactory placode to form the paranasal sinuses has been described as "asymmetric dichotomy". The early formation of developing buds shows a stage in which the free edge of the offshoot is filled with indeterminate epithelial cells. These stages in the early development of the paranasal sinuses are said to be mirrored in the tumour known as inverted papilloma (see Chapter 15), possibly indicating the primordial nature of the growth in these neoplasms.[1]

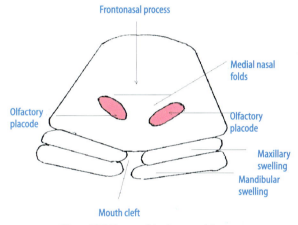

Figure 12.1 Diagram of development of the nose

Receptors for smell are borne on special ectodermal cells, which come to lie in the medial and lateral walls of the upper nasal cavity. These cells give rise to olfactory nerve fibres, which grow up into the olfactory bulb to synapse with nerve fibres in the cranial cavity, through the skeletal base of the skull, which is at first cartilaginous and later bony. The perforated cartilage, becoming bone later, is the cribriform plate.

Anatomy

A working knowledge of the gross structure of the nose and paranasal sinuses can be obtained by a consideration of three aspects and their relationships: the nasal septum, the maxilla and the lateral wall.

Septum

The nasal septum (Fig. 12.2) is composed of two bones: the vomer situated posteriorly and the perpendicular plate of the ethmoid with which the vomer articulates anteriorly. Below the perpendicular plate the vomer articulates with the septal cartilage, which extends anteriorly to the tip of the nose. The septal cartilage is attached to the lateral nasal cartilage on each side and the latter articulates with the lateral wing of the greater alar cartilage, which forms the outer wall of the ala nasi, the flared expansion of the nostril. The septal cartilage is covered by skin on its inferior border and this firm external base, which separates the two nostrils, is known as the columella. Thus cartilage tissue received in the pathological laboratory in a biopsy specimen can be derived not only from the septal cartilage, but also from smaller cartilages, which form the skeletal framework of the external nose. Posteriorly the vomer and perpendicular plate of the ethmoid articulate with the bone on the anterior wall of the sphenoid sinus above. Inferiorly they fit on the upper surface of the hard palate.

Arising laterally from the perpendicular plate of the ethmoid and passing across the roof of the nose on each side to the lateral mass of the ethmoid is the cribriform plate. Filaments of olfactory nerve pass from the olfactory epithelium through the small canaliculi of the cribriform plate of the ethmoid to reach the olfactory bulb in the cranial cavity directly above.

Maxilla

The body of the maxilla encloses the maxillary sinus. Frontal, zygomatic, alveolar and palatal processes come from the body of the maxilla. The frontal process articulates with the nasal bone, which forms the bony external skeleton of the nose in its upper part. The zygomatic process forms part of the boundary of the orbit. The alveolar process gives origin to the teeth of the upper jaw. The roots of the first and second upper molar teeth and sometimes other teeth are close to the mucosa of the maxillary sinus. The palatine process contributes to the anterior part of the hard palate; the posterior part is formed by the horizontal plate of the palatine bone.

Lateral Wall

The lateral wall of the nose (Fig. 12.3) is the site of origin of most of the pathological processes that

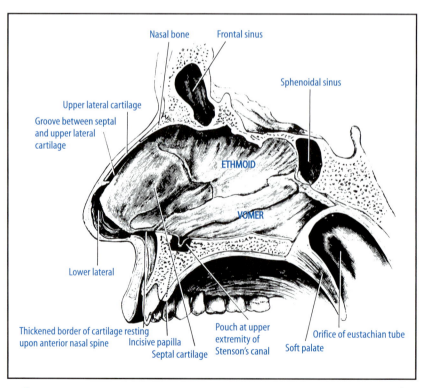

Figure 12.2 Nasal septum and related structures. Structures related to teeth are not mentioned in the text[3]

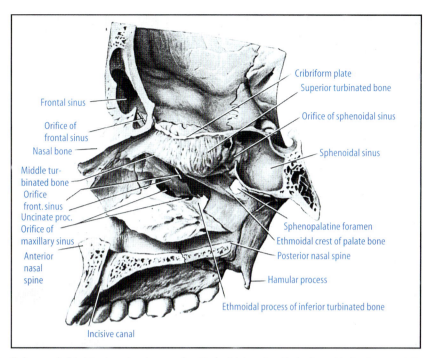

Figure 12.3 Lateral wall of nose and related structures. A probe passes from the frontal sinus along the frontonasal duct and emerges in the nasal cavity above the middle turbinate bone (Wording is as in the original, and "turbinated" is used for turbinate)[a]

affect the nose. The anatomical structure of this region will, therefore, be described in some detail. The bony structure is composed of the nasal bone in front; behind this is the ethmoid, which gives rise to the small superior turbinate and larger middle turbinate. Behind the ethmoid the bony lateral nasal wall is composed of the sphenoid, within which is the sphenoid sinus. The occipital bone is the most posterior, forming the roof of the nasopharynx. The maxilla also participates in the lateral wall of the nose anteriorly, linking the nasal bone to the ethmoid and the palatine bone is posterior, linking the ethmoid to the sphenoid. At the junction of palatine and sphenoid bones lies the sphenopalatine foramen, through which pass all the nerves and blood vessels supplying the nasal mucosa. The inferior turbinate is a separate bone in its own right. Between the middle and inferior turbinate is a gap in the bony lateral wall known as the maxillary hiatus. This is covered by a membrane and also parts of the palatine, ethmoid and lacrimal bones overlap it. In this region, behind the middle turbinate, lies the ethmoid bulla, which is produced by ethmoid air cells that bulge into this region. There are many other air cells within the ethmoid bone. Some open into the superior meatus (above the superior turbinate); others open into the middle meatus (between the middle and inferior turbinates) in the region of the ethmoid bulla. The hiatus semilunaris is a deep gutter lying between the bulging

ethmoid bulla above and the unciform process below. The latter is a hook-like process of the ethmoid bone. The anterior end of the hiatus semilunaris is known as the infundibulum. The region of the middle meatus above and anterior to this is known as the frontal recess. The frontonasal duct, which discharges secretions from the frontal sinus, opens into the frontal recess. The various openings into the lateral wall of the nose and their origins are listed in Table 12.1.

Histology

The vestibule, the anterior chamber of the nasal cavity, is lined by an internal extension of the integument of the external nose including a keratinising stratified squamous epithelial surface and an underlying dermis containing hair follicles, sebaceous and sweat glands. The degree of posterior extension of the vestibule varies with physiological conditions, races and individuals. The average depth is between 1 and 2 cm from the external rim of the nares. As the mucocutaneous junction (limen nasi) representing the anterior limits of the inner nasal cavity proper is approached, there is a gradual diminution and disappearance of the adnexa.

The nasal cavities are normally lined by ciliated, pseudostratified columnar epithelium designated as

Table 12.1. Openings in the lateral wall of the nose

Origin in paranasal sinuses	Position
Frontal sinus	Frontal recess of middle meatus
Sphenoid sinus	Sphenoethmoid recess (behind superior turbinate)
Ethmoid "sinus" (about 10 ethmoid cells)	
Posterior	Superior meatus
Middle	Ethmoid bulla in middle meatus
Anterior	In hiatus semilunaris of middle meatus
Maxillary sinus	In hiatus semilunaris near posterior end Accessory opening posterior to latter
Sphenopalatine foramen	Posterior to middle turbinate
Nasolacrimal duct	Beneath inferior turbinate

the "Schneiderian membrane" to emphasise its origin from the ectoderm, as contrasted with a similar-appearing epithelium of the larynx and lower respiratory tract, which is of endodermal origin. In the sinuses this epithelium is lower and sometimes of a simple cuboidal type containing a few goblet cells. The tissue of the nasal cavity between bone and airway surface varies in thickness, being most pronounced over the inferior, medial and lateral portions of the middle and inferior turbinates, which represent the nasal surface most prominently exposed to inspired air. Immediately beneath the nasal cavity epithelium is a thin uniform zone of fibro-elastic tissue, the lamina propria. More deeply to this is a layer containing seromucinous glands and distinctive vascular structures; the glandular elements are situated more superficially. The majority of the blood vessels in the vascular tissue of the nasal cavity are capable of marked variation in luminal capacity (nasal "erectile" tissue) (Fig. 12.4). This normal vascular pattern is, in its abundance, sometimes mistaken by pathologists for neoplasms such as haemangioma or angiofibroma. The paranasal sinus linings also contain some seromucinous glands, particularly near their ostia, but these are many fewer than in the nasal cavity. No prominent vascular network is present in the sinuses, the usual finding being only a thin submucosal fibrous layer adjacent to the periosteum.

The turbinate bones are scroll-like bony plates covered by mucosa, glandular and vascular tissue. The surface of the turbinate bones is irregular and frequently shows thin formations of osteoid, indicating recent bony deposition.

Olfactory Epithelium

Olfactory epithelium is normally found in the superoposterior portion of each nasal cavity and is said to occupy an area of about 1.5 cm². Occasional patches

are also said to be present on areas of the turbinates. The olfactory epithelium is composed of elongated sustentacular (supporting) cells, small basal cells and olfactory neural cells. The latter are bipolar structures with swellings protruding from their mucosal surfaces forming the olfactory vesicles. The latter give rise to cilia, which project into the overlying mucous blanket. The central processes pass via the cribriform plate, as nerve fibres lacking myelin sheaths, and Schwann cells, to the olfactory bulb. A fourth type of cell, known as a microvillar cell, which shows marked projections of microvilli from the surface, has also been described in the olfactory epithelium. Small, simple, serous-like glands – Bowman's glands – are located in the olfactory mucosa and their ducts open onto the surface (Fig. 12.5). The columnar sustentacular cells rest on the basilar membrane and seem to act as supporting cells. The innermost polygonal basal cells perform as reserve replacements for both the sustentacular cells and the olfactory neural cells. It may be of importance with regard to the pathogenesis of olfactory neuroblastomas (see Chapter 18) that the olfactory epithelium is in a state of constant turnover and regenerates after damage, unlike any other peripheral nerve cell.

Examination at Autopsy

The nose and paranasal sinuses are an extensive system of bones and air-containing spaces near the face. It is important to preserve the external appearances of this area after autopsy. Access to the deeper parts of the nose and to the paranasal sinuses can be obtained through the base of the skull after the brain has been removed, but a satisfactory view of the cavities is difficult to obtain in this way. The olfactory epithelial area and ethmoid air cells can be inspected by removing the cribriform plate of the ethmoid and the adjacent anterior fossa. The lower parts of the nose require a wider exposure; it is necessary to remove the eyeballs and orbital contents as well as the bone of the anterior fossa. The maxillary antrum may be opened at this stage through the floor of the orbit. The sphenoid sinuses are conveniently inspected also in their position just posterior to the ethmoid cells. The frontal sinuses can be opened in the lower vault of the skull.

Inspection by Coronal Saw-cut

A simple, effective way for examining the nasopharynx, the nose and the maxillary sinuses has been

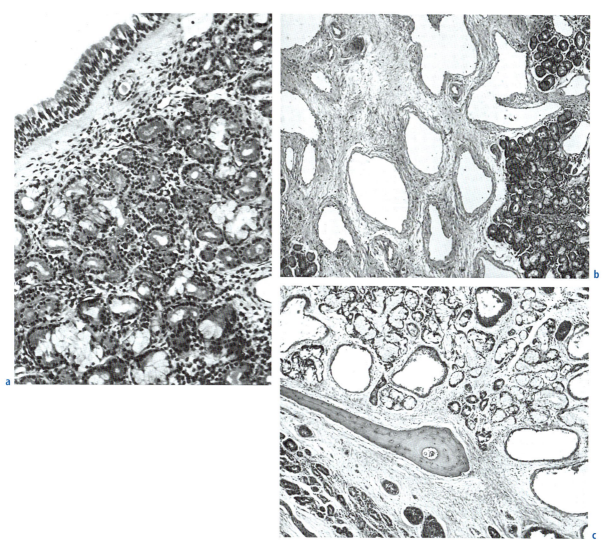

Figure 12.4 Normal histology of the nose. **a** Pseudostratified columnar epithelium, beneath which are the lamina propria and seromucinous glands. **b** Deeper part of lining showing seromucinous glands and vascular tissue. **c** Section of middle turbinate showing seromucinous glands, blood vessels of venous plexus and thin plate of bone with expanded tip

devised. After removing the skull cap and brain, a coronal saw-cut is made right through the whole width of the base of the skull. This cut must be in front of the vertebral bodies, but behind the condyle of the mandible. A line joining the external auditory meatuses on each side satisfactorily achieves this position. The saw-cut exposes the superior wall of the nasopharynx. After cutting the soft tissues on each side as far as necessary, the anterior part of the base of the skull falls forward. The nose and sinuses can then be examined through the nasopharynx. For reconstruction, the two parts of the base separated by the coronal cut, together with the vault, fit together well.

Examination of Surgical Specimens

Surgical removal of the maxilla, ethmoid cells and lateral wall of the nose is carried out for malignant disease, usually squamous cell carcinoma, but occasionally adenocarcinoma, malignant melanoma or some other form of neoplasm.

The operation for tumours situated in the maxillary sinus is usually that of a hemimaxillectomy (Fig. 12.6). If the tumour is situated in the roof of the maxillary sinus the palatal part of the maxilla is usually left in situ, but if the orbital floor is involved, an orbital exenteration is carried out in continuity with the specimen. If the tumour involves the floor

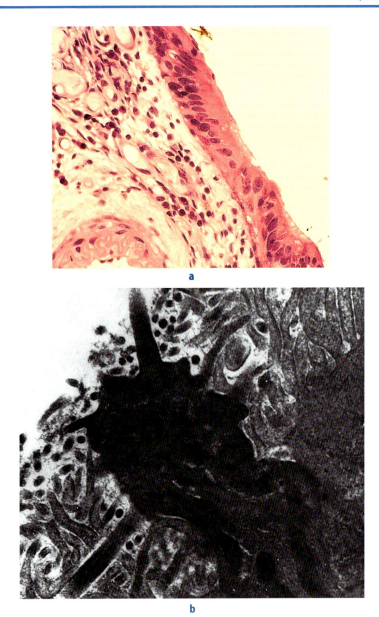

Figure 12.5 Olfactory epithelium. **a** Light micrograph with underlying arteriole. Spindle cells are probably nerve filaments, and there are also numerous plasma cells and lymphocytes. **b** Electron micrograph showing an olfactory neural cell with projecting vesicle, which is bearing cilia. The deep process from this cell is passing downwards to become a nerve fibre. The adjacent sustentacular cells show numerous microvilli on the surface. Guinea-pig preparation, original magnification × 39 000

of the maxillary sinus only, the orbital contents can be saved, but the palatal part of the maxilla is usually removed.

The specimen is first oriented anatomically by locating such structures as the lower orbital wall and the alveolar and zygomatic processes of the maxilla. The resection margins in the region of the tumour are painted with India ink and blocks are taken from them as well as from the tumour proper, to determine whether resection has been complete.

For pathological examination the specimen is best sliced coronally at right angles to the orbital floor and palatal bone (Fig. 12.6). The pterygoid area posterior to the maxillary sinus may have been removed at the same time, and to assess the possibility of spread to this region, the posterior part of this specimen should be sliced horizontally. Further details of the examination of specimens from the nose and paranasal sinuses may be obtained from the manual by Slootweg and de Groot.[2]

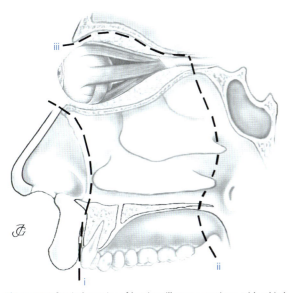

Figure 12.6 Surgical margins of hemimaxillectomy specimen with orbital exenteration indicated by dashed lines i, ii, iii in diagram of lateral wall of nose and orbit.[2]

References

1. Stammberger H. Neue Aspekte zur Genese des invertierten Papilloms. [In German] Laryngol Rhinol Otol 1983;62:422–426

2. Slootweg PJ, de Groot JAM. Surgical pathological anatomy of head and neck specimens. A manual for the dissection of surgical specimens from the upper aerodigestive tract. Springer, London, 1999

3. Sobotta J, McMurrich JP (eds) Atlas and text-book of human anatomy, vol 1. Urban and Schwarzenberg, Baltimore, 1911, p 78, Fig. 102

4. Hensman A. The nose. In: Morris H (ed) A treatise on human anatomy by various authors, part 2. W and A Churchill, London, pp 889–897, Fig. 515

13 Infections

A large number of infectious agents have been identified in the nose, including bacteria, viruses, fungi and protozoa. The relationship of the infecting agents to pathological changes may be summarised under three headings:

1. Colonisation.
2. Transmission.
3. Association with local inflammatory change.

Colonisation is defined as the presence of a microorganism without a host response. The nasal vestibule frequently harbours *Staphylococcus aureus* from an early age. Although no nasal disease is produced, the organisms are capable of infecting other parts of the body or other individuals with ensuing pyogenic inflammatory reactions. In a study of nasal colonisation in 64 patients with AIDS or AIDS-related complex, 35 (55%) were nasal carriers of *S. aureus*, compared with 18 (28%) of 64 control patients.[1] The greatly raised carriage rate of this organism in the nose may contribute to the high incidence of intravenous catheter-related *S. aureus* infections in this population.

Viral infections are not usually in this group. They are as a rule connected with a pathological response and when this has subsided the virus can no longer be detected.

Transmission of microorganisms through the nose is important in the infection of the lower respiratory tract by inward spread, or in the infection of other parts of the body and of other individuals by outward spread. The latter may occur by hand transmission, by large moisture droplets or by aerosols.[2]

The important infections of the nose in which local and pathological changes take place are listed in Table 13.1.

Table 13.1. Infections of the nose and paranasal sinuses

Infection	Causative agent
Bacterial (and related)	
Cellulitis	*Staphylococcus aureus*
Scleroma	*Klebsiella rhinoscleromatis*
Leprosy	*Mycobacterium leprae*
Tuberculosis	*Mycobacterium tuberculosis*
Sinusitis	Various aerobic organisms
	Anaerobic streptococci and bacteroides
Nasopharyngitis in infants	*Streptococcus pyogenes*
Diphtheria	*Corynebacterium diphtheriae*
Glanders	*Pfeiferella mallei*
Syphilis	*Treponema pallidum*
Fungal	
Aspergillosis	*Aspergillus* sp.
Zygomycosis:	
Subcutaneous	*Conidiobolus coronatus*
Rhinocerebral	*Rhizopus oryzae* (mucor)
Rhinosporidiosis	*Rhinosporidium seeberi*
Blastomycosis	*Blastomyces dermatidis*
Paracoccidioidomycosis	
(South American blastomycosis)	*Blastomyces brasiliensis*
Cryptococcosis	*Cryptococcus neoformans*
Coccidioidomycosis	*Coccidioides immitis*
Protozoal	
Leishmaniasis	*Leishmania* sp.
Viral	
Mucocutaneous herpes	Herpes simplex virus
Chickenpox, herpes zoster	Varicella zoster virus
Pharyngoconjunctival fever	Adenovirus
Influenza	Influenza virus
Common cold	Rhino-, corona, parainfluenza, respiratory, syncytial, adeno- and influenza viruses

Acute Inflammation

The nose and paranasal sinuses represent a system of mucosa-lined spaces, which are in free communication with each other. Pathological changes, particularly those of neoplasia and inflammation, spread easily throughout the system. Thus nose and paranasal sinuses are often simultaneously involved, although in some cases the main impact seems to fall on one particular region.

Acute Rhinitis

Acute inflammation of the nose (the common cold) is the commonest affection of the human race. It is caused by several viruses, of which rhinoviruses are the most frequent. The pathological features are those of acute inflammation with oedema, hypersecretion by seromucinous glands and desquamation of respiratory epithelium. The inflammation is short-lived and rapidly followed by regeneration of epithelium.

Acute Sinusitis

The most frequent cause of acute inflammation of any of the sinuses is the common cold, the resulting mucosal oedema from which produces obstruction of the ostium. Lack of drainage of the secretion produced within that sinus then exacerbates the already existent infection. Bacterial infection, particularly by *Haemophilus influenzae, Streptococcus pneumoniae, S. aureus* and *Streptococcus pyogenes* is the most frequent basis for the acute inflammation at this stage. In the case of the maxillary sinus, infection can reach the mucosa directly from a periapical abscess of upper jaw teeth. The pathological changes of acute inflammation may go on to suppuration with pus in the lumen of the antrum.

Atopic (Allergic) Rhinitis

Atopic rhinitis is part of an hereditary syndrome, the other manifestations of which include atopic eczema, rhinitis and asthma. In the nasal condition (hay fever) large particles of allergens, usually grass pollen, lodge in the nasal mucosa where they combine with reaginic antibodies of IgE class, which are bound to mast cells. The latter become degranulated and release histamine into the surrounding tissue, giving rise to the characteristic symptoms of watery rhinorrhoea and nasal obstruction. The molecular basis of the changes that take place in allergic rhinitis have been worked out in detail.[3]

Histological examination of the mucosa in atopic rhinitis shows large numbers of eosinophils beneath the epithelium. In some cases the mast cells are increased in number. In the early stages the basement membrane is destroyed but later it is reduplicated or thickened. Plasma cells are usually also abundant. The respiratory epithelium shows goblet cell hyperplasia.

Chronic Non-specific Rhinitis

Hypertrophic Type

A chronic inflammation of the nose may develop following acute rhinitis. Frequently there is also an atopic aspect to the inflammation (see above). There follows a marked swelling of the nasal mucosa, which leads to nasal airway obstruction. The anterior end of the middle turbinate and the inferior edge and posterior end of the inferior turbinate are particularly swollen. The raspberry-like protrusion at the anterior end of the middle turbinate is sometimes removed surgically and pathological changes of chronic rhinitis may be observed in the specimen. There is some hypertrophy of goblet cells and seromucinous glands. The vascular tissue is engorged and there is a chronic inflammatory exudate. The turbinate bone shows evidence of new bone formation.

Atrophic Type (Ozaena)

In another form of chronic rhinitis there is atrophy of mucosal and submucosal nasal elements. An unpleasant odour is produced by secondary bacterial inflammation. Ozaena is now a rare condition. The organism, *Klebsiella ozaenae*, has frequently been isolated from cases of atrophic rhinitis, but it is doubtful whether it is causally significant. The skeleton of the nose participates in the atrophic process of the nasal passages. There is widespread squamous metaplasia and disappearance of seromucinous glands. Treatment is carried out by closing off the nasal cavity at the vestibule surgically for a period of more than a year, following which the nasal mucosa may slowly return to normal. It seems possible that such improvement is related to absence of air flow through the nose. It has been shown, similarly, that after laryngectomy (when inspiration is through a tracheostomy) nasal mucosa becomes free from inflammation and recovers from squamous metaplastic change even on the middle turbinate.[4]

Atrophic rhinitis (ozaena) is a widespread disease of pigs, which is caused by a specific organism, the toxigenic strains of *Pasteurella multocida*. The infection is supported by nutritional factors and especially by *Bordetella bronchiseptica* infection, a common infection of the respiratory tract in these animals.

Chronic Sinusitis

Inflammation of the sinuses may persist after an acute phase and become chronic. The bacteriology of chronic sinusitis frequently differs from the acute type of disease. Anaerobic infection is common; anaerobic streptococci, anaerobic corynebacteria, bacteroides species and *Veillonella* have been cultured from chronic paranasal sinus inflammation.[5] Histologically neutrophils usually persist in the inflammatory exudate. They are frequently accompanied by plasma cells and lymphocytes and fibroblasts with variable degrees of fibrosis. New bone formation, often extensive, may be present in the superficial part of the bony wall of the sinus. Granulation tissue may be seen.

In some cases, particularly in the second and third decades, the chronic inflammation involving the maxillary antrum may be accompanied by severe mucosal oedema and the development of nasal and paranasal sinus polyps.

Some cases of chronic sinusitis, "non-suppurative sinusitis", are characterised by a widespread infiltra-tion of the sinus mucosa with lymphocytes and plasma cells accompanied by lymphoid follicles in various stages of development (Fig. 13.1). The term "plasma cell granuloma" has also been applied to chronic inflammatory lesions of the sinuses with a dense plasma cell infiltrate. Russell bodies may be numerous in this condition. The presence of these grape-like eosinophilic clusters in relation to plasma cells and accompanying infiltration by lymphocytes and other inflammatory cells helps to separate this condition from plasmacytoma (see Chapter 22).

Bacterial Infections

Diphtheria

Diphtheria is an acute mucosal inflammation of the pharynx, tonsils and soft palate caused by *Corynebacterium diphtheriae*. The nose is also sometimes affected and may rarely be the sole site of the disease. The nasal mucosa in this condition is covered by a false membrane, a dull greyish-yellow layer of tissue, which may be easily peeled off. The membrane is composed of fibrin, neutrophils, necrotic epithelium and diphtheria bacilli (see also Chapter 26).

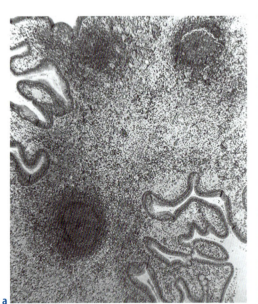
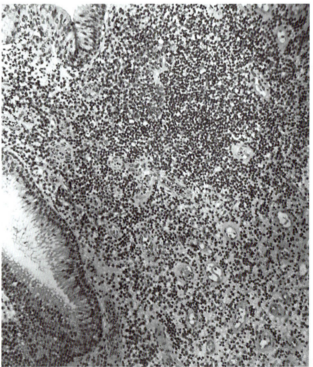

Figure 13.1 a Non-suppurative maxillary sinusitis. There is a chronic inflammation of the sinus mucosa with lymphoid follicles showing germinal centres. **b** Higher power of **a** showing infiltration with plasma cells and lymphocytes

Glanders

Glanders is an infection of horses and other equine animals, which is caused by *Pseudomonas mallei*. It has been transmitted to humans, where it results in nodular foci within the nasal mucosa. In the early stages these are composed of neutrophils with prominent central areas of basophilic detritus resulting from the process of apoptosis. Later the inflammatory reaction becomes a chronic one with epithelioid cells and occasional giant cells.

Scleroma

Scleroma (often termed "rhinoscleroma") is a chronic inflammatory condition in which large deforming masses of tissue distend the nasal cavity. The disease derives its name from the tendency that the inflammatory lesions have to undergo fibrosis, forming "scleromatous" nodules. Scleroma is a chronic, progressive, granulomatous infection of the upper airways caused by the bacterium *Klebsiella rhinoscleromatis*. Although most cases occur in developing countries where it seems mainly to affect impoverished people, predominantly in rural areas, recent immigration patterns have led to an increasing number of patients with rhinoscleroma in the USA.[6]

The disease has not been produced experimentally by inoculation of *K. rhinoscleromatis* into the noses of experimental animals, but lesions histologically similar to human scleroma may be produced in the bronchi of mice by inoculation of these organisms into the upper respiratory tract.[7,8]

Gross Appearances

In fully developed scleroma there are large, firm intramucosal masses with a coarsely granular surface. These lead to external expansion of the nose, particularly in the cartilaginous part. Scleromatous nodules may also be present under the skin adjacent to the nose (Fig. 13.2). The cut surface of the affected tissue is pale grey. A progression of the gross changes of the disease from a "rhinitic" stage, through an "infiltrative" stage to the nodular one is recognised.

Microscopic Appearances

The lesion is a thickening of nasal mucosa, which usually retains its covering of respiratory epithelium; squamous metaplasia is surprisingly unusual in scleroma but is shown in Figure 13.2. The inflammatory exudate, which characterises the lesion, is a pleomorphic one. Plasma cells are prominent and Russell bodies are numerous. The specific cell of the lesion is the Mikulicz cell, which is present in variable numbers. Sometimes large sheets of such cells are present, but frequently they are scattered singly in the exudate. The Mikulicz cell is large cell with clear cytoplasm containing bacilli, *K. rhinoscleromatis*. The intracytoplasmic organisms are difficult to identify in conventionally stained sections, but may be displayed by silver impregnation stains, such as the Warthin-Starry stain, by Giemsa or by specific immunological fluorescence methods. Sometimes the bacilli cannot be detected in 4 μm thick paraffin sections. However, 1 μm thick plastic sections will usually reveal the organisms in the Mikulicz cells (Fig. 13.2). Fibrosis is variable in amount and can be very extensive in older lesions. Neutrophils and occasional eosinophils are also seen as part of the inflammatory exudate.

Immunological Basis

The abundance of plasma cells with Russell bodies would suggest a high level of humoral immunity in reaction to *K. rhinoscleromatis*. At the same time the large numbers of bacilli, lying apparently intact within macrophages, indicate deficient cell-mediated immunity against that organism.

Tuberculosis

Tuberculosis of the nose, apart from lupus vulgaris, a lesion of the skin of the nose, is a rare condition that is almost always associated with tuberculosis of the lungs. The gross manifestations are those of partially confluent ulcers of various sizes found mainly on the anterior part of the septum, the inferior turbinate or the choanal region. Microscopically the characteristic features of tuberculosis are usually present, with epithelioid granulomas showing Langhans giant cells and extensive caseation. Acid-alcohol-fast bacilli are often found in the granulomata.

In cases of tuberculosis of the nose affecting the nares, the histological appearances of granulomatous change may be so overshadowed by a pseudo-epitheliomatous reaction of squamous epithelium that a diagnosis of squamous cell carcinoma may be considered.

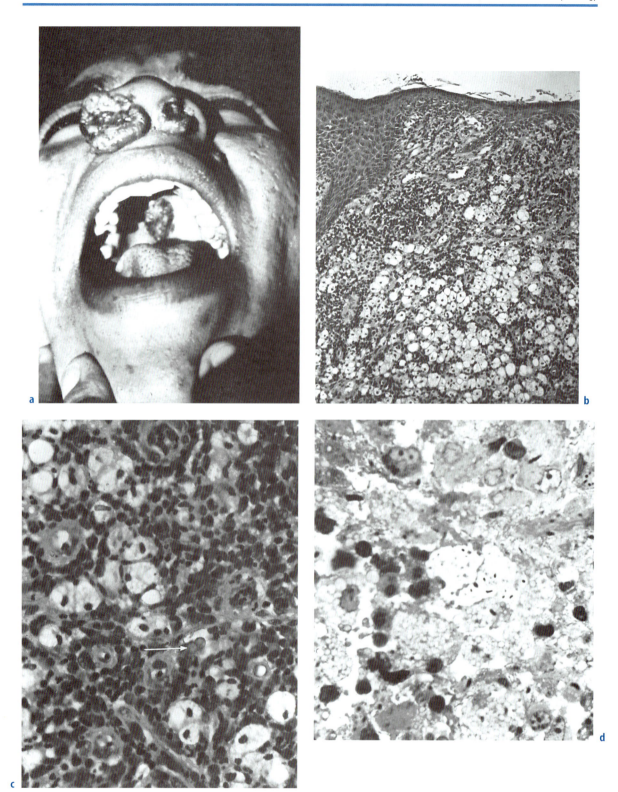

Figure 13.2 Rhinoscleroma. **a** Advanced disease with large intramucosal masses protruding from both nostrils and through the hard palate. The nose is widely expanded. (Courtesy of Dr. D.A. Alfaro.) **b** The exudate contains large numbers of pale Mikulicz cells and numerous plasma cells in the mucosa. The overlying squamous epithelium, which has been produced by metaplasia from respiratory epithelium, is slightly hyperplastic. **c** Higher power to show Mikulicz cells and plasma cells with some Russell bodies (*arrow*). **d** Section of rhinoscleromatous tissue embedded in Araldite and cut at 1 μm. Some of the Mikulicz cells reveal rod-shaped organisms. Toluidine blue

Sarcoidosis

Clinical Diagnosis

Sarcoidosis is a disorder that may affect any part of the body, but most frequently the lymph nodes, liver, spleen, lungs, skin, eyes and small bones of hand and feet. It is characterised histologically by the presence of epithelioid cell tubercles without caseation, which are converted into hyaline fibrous tissue. Sarcoidosis is a clinical diagnosis made on the presence of the characteristic histological features together with certain clinical, radiological and biochemical features. Implicit in the diagnosis is the exclusion of any accepted basis for the epithelioid tubercles, such tuberculosis, fungal infection and Wegener's. The Kveim test (injection of filtered extract of spleen from a case of sarcoidosis into the skin, which, in positive cases, leads to a tuberculoid granuloma in the skin) is no longer used because of the danger of transmission of infection. Sarcoidosis affects the nose fairly frequently. Most patients have extra-pulmonary sarcoidosis involving multiple organs as well as the nose, but in some the disease is isolated to the nose.

Gross Appearances

Sarcoid lesions may affect the nose in three anatomical situations, producing three different forms of gross appearance. Lesions in these situations may occur together in the same patient.

Involvement of the skin of the nose by sarcoid lesions may be present. A particularly disfiguring form of this type of sarcoidosis is lupus pernio, in which deep granulomatous plaques occupy the full thickness of the dermis on the nose, cheeks or ears. The nose is bulbous and red or violet in colour.

The nasal bones may be occupied by sarcoid lesions in a fashion similar to that seen in the small bones of the hands and feet in the same condition. The bridge of the nose is swollen in these cases.

The most common but clinically often the least conspicuous form of nasal involvement is that of the nasal mucosa, which is erythematous, oedematous, friable and hypertrophied.

Microscopic Appearances

The characteristic change is one of rather uniform tubercles composed of groups of epithelioid cells with no caseation (although a limited degree of central necrosis is often present). Foreign body or Langhans-type giant cells are usually present and may contain a variety of crystalline, calcified or other inclusions. Fibrosis of the tubercle takes place around the periphery and grows to involve the whole of it. Later stages may be seen as a group of uniform round, hyaline fibrous masses (Fig. 13.3).

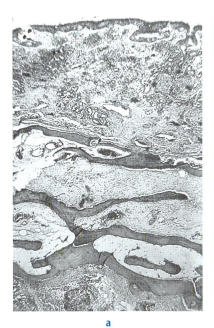
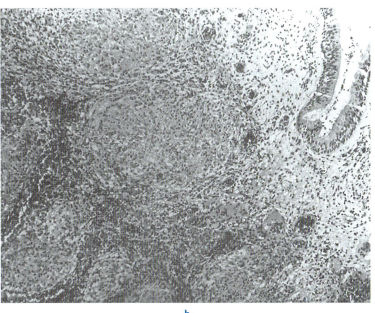

a   b

Figure 13.3 a Sarcoid granulomas of the inferior turbinate part of the nose. Small, round tubercles are seen on each side of the inferior turbinate bone. **b** Higher power of sarcoid granulomas from **a**. The lesions at higher power are seen to be composed of epithelioid cells and occasional giant cells with surrounding lymphocytes. Note duct of mucous gland at *upper right*

Non-sarcoid Granulomas

It is important to note that the above features of the histology of sarcoidosis are non-specific. The diagnosis is essentially a clinical one. Tuberculoid granulomas are seen quite frequently in the nasal mucosa in which the characteristic histological features of sarcoid lesions are present, but in which investigation yields no systemic evidence of sarcoidosis and the patient does not develop clinical sarcoidosis subsequently. Such granulomatous foci usually present minor clinical disturbance or none and the lesions regress in the course of time, even without treatment.

Leprosy

Leprosy is an infective disease of the skin, the mucosa of the upper respiratory tract and the peripheral nervous system caused by *Mycobacterium leprae*. A spectrum of the disease exists between lepromatous leprosy, in which numerous mycobacteria are present, and tuberculoid leprosy, with few organisms. The difference between these forms is based on the immunological relationship of the host to the organism, the lepromatous form representing a state of low cell-mediated immunity and the tuberculoid a high one. An intermediate form called "borderline" develops in patients whose cellular resistance lies between the two major types.

The involvement of the nasal mucosa in leprosy has been recognised to be an important source of infection. The paranasal sinuses, particularly the ethmoids, are now known to be frequently infected and are thought to act as a reservoir for and constant source of reinfection to the nasal mucosa.[9]

Gross Appearances

The gross changes of the nasal disease are most commonly seen as a nodular thickening of the mucous membrane. Perforation of the cartilaginous septum may occur.

Microscopic Appearances

The lepromatous lesion consists in its active stage of a mucosal thickening containing macrophages, many of which appear as large foam cells (Virchow's cells). These contain the acid-fast bacilli of *Mycobacterium leprae* in large numbers. The organisms also appear in round, basophilic structures known as globi, which represent degenerated macrophages. A "clear

zone", in which no inflammatory infiltrate is present, may separate the lepromatous infiltrate from the epithelium of the nose (Fig. 13.4).

In tuberculoid leprosy the lesion resembles that of sarcoidosis and extends up to the epithelium without a clear zone. Leprosy bacilli are very few in this form.

In a study of 20 cases of leprosy affecting the nose, ten were in the lepromatous phase and ten in the tuberculoid phase. Seromucinous glands showed cystic dilatation and hyperplasia.[10]

Syphilis

Syphilis is a venereally acquired infective condition caused by the spirochaete *Treponema pallidum*. The nose may also be affected in the congenital form. Treatment with penicillin has greatly reduced the incidence of nasal syphilis. The following is a summary of the pathological lesions of nasal syphilis as they once were seen.

Primary

A primary chancre has been known to occur on the septum anteriorly. The nasal mucosa was said to be diffusely oedematous. A chancre may also be seen on the skin of the nasal vestibule.

Secondary

Fissures in the vestibule and nasal obstruction have been described as features of this stage.

Tertiary

Two forms have been seen, diffuse and localised. In the diffuse form there is marked swelling leading to necrosis of bone and soft tissue. In the healed phase of this condition there is marked deformity by the fibrosis and destruction (saddle nose). The maxillae are small, resulting in a shallow depression of the central part of the face and a high-arched palate. In the localised form a solitary gumma is followed by destruction, particularly perforation of the nasal septum.

Congenital

In the newborn, syphilis of the nose has been associated with a diffuse inflammation. In the form of con-

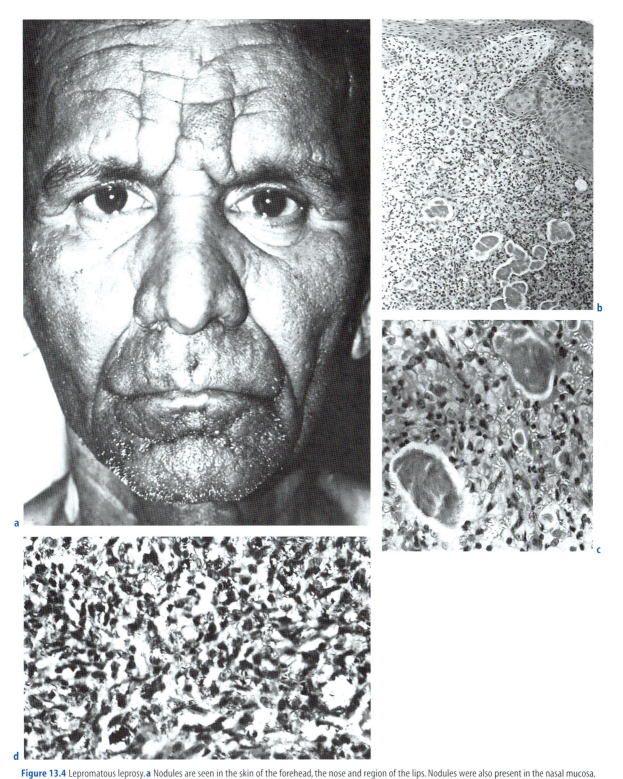

Figure 13.4 Lepromatous leprosy. **a** Nodules are seen in the skin of the forehead, the nose and region of the lips. Nodules were also present in the nasal mucosa.
b Section of nodule in nasal mucosa from same case as **a**. The epithelium, which is metaplastic to squamous, is somewhat hyperplastic. The lamina propria is filled
with foam cells and large darkly staining areas (basophilic in the original). These are larger in this case than the globi often found in lepromatous leprosy, which are
degenerated macrophages. **c** Higher power view of part of **b** showing foam cells and large basophilic areas. **d** Acid-fast stain of tissue shown in **b** and **c**. There are
vast numbers of non-beaded acid-fast bacilli situated both discretely and in clumps. Wade-Fite stain (Courtesy of Dr. S. Lucas)

genital syphilis occurring later in life the changes are similar to the diffuse form of acquired tertiary syphilis.

Microscopic Appearances

In the primary and secondary stages spirochaetes are often numerous. In the tertiary stage the organisms are very rare in the tissues. The histological appearances are of chronic inflammation of nonspecific type. In the tertiary phase there is a prominent endarteritis and plasma cells and macrophages are present around the blood vessels. Gummatous necrosis similar to the caseation of tuberculosis may be present.

Mycotic Infections

The majority of mycotic infections of the nose and paranasal sinuses fall into one of five clinical groups:

1. An allergic reaction to fungi characterised by the accumulation of large amounts of inspissated mucus and necrotic eosinophils (allergic fungal sinusitis).
2. A "fungus ball", usually of aspergilli in the maxillary antrum accompanied only by a low-grade inflammation.
3. A slowly progressive disease process with much fibrosis involving the nasal and paranasal sinus mucosa and spreading externally into the subcutaneous tissues of the side of the nose and orbit (subcutaneous zygomycosis). This lesion is caused by a zygomycete, *Conidiobolus coronatus*.
4. A fulminating disease, usually in diabetics, which spreads rapidly from the nose to the base of skull and brain (rhinocerebral zygmycosis or mucormycosis). This mycosis is caused by another zygomycete, *Rhizopus oryzae*.
5. A chronic granulomatous lesion of the nasal and conjunctival mucosae containing vast numbers of the sporangia of the fungus *Rhinosporidium seeberi* (rhinosporidiosis).

The other mycotic infections of the nose are rare, the literature consisting of a few case reports only for each entity.

Fungi can usually be found in the diseased tissues on histological examination, and the type of the causal organism can in most cases be reasonably inferred. It is helpful, however, if the fungus can be cultured in the laboratory from fresh tissue so that the diagnosis and treatment may be carried out in as accurate a fashion as possible.

Allergic Fungal Sinusitis

Allergic fungal sinusitis is now the commonest form of fungal infection to be diagnosed in the nose and paranasal sinuses. The condition was hardly known until Katzenstein et al. formally described in 1981 an allergic response to fungi in the paranasal sinuses similar to that of allergic bronchopulmonary aspergillosis[11] although it had been previously mentioned in the literature on at least two occasions.[12,13]

Types of Infecting Fungus

Assuming that *Aspergillus* species alone were the causative organisms, the condition was first called "allergic aspergillus sinusitis". It subsequently became apparent that *Aspergillus* species were not the only fungi to be associated with these changes. Black or brown pigmented fungi of a group known as *Dematiaceae* and non-aspergillus, non-dematiaceous fungi have also been incriminated.[14] The condition was, therefore, renamed "allergic fungal sinusitis" (AFS), although it is recognised that the nasal cavity may be also affected by the disease process.

Clinical Features and Sites of Involvement

The condition may present with nasal obstruction together with evidence of infection of the maxillary, ethmoid, sphenoid or frontal sinuses. In some cases evidence of extension of the disease through the wall of the sinus may be found, resulting in symptoms such as proptosis produced by extension to the orbit from the ethmoid sinuses, a soft tissue mass on the cheek produced by extension from the maxillary sinus externally and cerebral symptoms produced by extension from a frontal sinus lesion into the cranial cavity.

Imaging Changes[15]

There is either generalised or unilateral loss of translucence in the sinuses and in the nasal cavity due to associated nasal polyps, accompanied in a typical case by the following triad of appearances due to the presence of inspissated mucus containing necrotic inflammatory cells and fungi:

1. Areas of high attenuation on computerised tomography (CT), surrounded by a thin zone of low attenuation.

2. Low signal on magnetic resonance from the inspissated mucus, especially on T2-weighted sequences, surrounded by a thin peripheral zone of strong enhancement when Gadolinium is administered, consistent with tissue of high vascularity, and corresponding exactly to the zone of low attenuation surrounding the areas of high attenuation found on CT. The thin zones of strong enhancement may cross the lumina of affected sinuses and probably represent acute inflammation on the luminal side of infected glands (see below).

3. Bone changes: expansion of sinus contents leading to widening of bony walls or erosion of bony walls of sinuses.

Gross Appearances

The changes identified by the surgeon are the presence of soft cheesy, grey-green mucoid material filling the lumen of affected sinuses. Bony walls of sinuses may be thinned and expanded by the material and in some places eroded by the pressure of the enclosed material, so that the contents herniate through into tissues outside the sinus.

Microscopic Appearances

The mucoid material in the sinuses is composed of inspissated mucus showing a periphery of darkly staining cellular material, mainly necrotic eosinophils with occasional Charcot-Leyden crystals, hexagonal eosinophilic crystalline structures formed from eosinophils. Septate, branching fungal hyphae, are demonstrated towards the centre of the mass of mucin by the methenamine silver or periodic acid–Schiff stain. The numbers of fungal elements are variable, often being present in large numbers, but sometimes sparse. The fungi show a variety of forms comprising in some wide, in others narrow hyphae. Lobulated granules may be present.[16] Fungal infection can also be observed within ducts or acini of seromucinous glands. The gland/duct involved is expanded by the infective agents together with necrotic eosinophils and mucin.

The tissue covering the infected inspissated mucus, comprising the lining mucosa and submucosa of the nose or paranasal sinus, shows the appearances of allergic inflammatory change with two forms of alteration:

1. In many areas the predominant change is loss of seromucinous glands with severe oedema, together with a moderate basement membrane thickening and eosinophil infiltration. These lesions are sufficiently marked in some places to be identified as allergic type nasal polyps (see Chapter 14).

2. In other areas there are patches of an intense inflammatory change. Such an alteration may be present around the periphery of an expanded gland containing infected mucus or be present in the mucosa or submucosa deep to the lining of the sinus or nasal cavity. The lining epithelium over the inspissated mucus frequently shows areas of severe goblet cell hyperplasia. In some areas it is multilayered with swelling of epithelial cells. Basement membrane thickening is marked and the collagen of this process merges with that of newly formed fibrous tissue that may be found in the mucosa or submucosa. There is an intense infiltrate of eosinophils and plasma cells, in some places showing necrosis. This is accompanied by severe congestion of capillaries and the presence of newly formed blood vessels, notably venules. In some areas this intense inflammation is present over a wide area of subepithelial tissue (Fig. 13.5). Areas of fibrosis are present; these sometimes take the form of a large submucosal fibrous nodule. Stages of transformation may be identified in the tissue, ranging from early infection of the lumen of the gland, through intense allergic-type inflammation of the tissues around the gland, to fibrosis around the gland with eventually a fibrous nodule replacing the gland. Bony trabeculae may be present in the biopsy material. When they are adjacent to the severe inflammatory change, evidence of new bone formation and/or bone erosion can be identified. Appearances suggesting penetration of an attenuated bony septum by vascular inflammatory tissue, fibrous tissue and infected mucus may occasionally be seen.

Pathogenesis

Aspergillus fungal species are known to be present in indoor as well as outdoor air and can colonise the mucosa of the respiratory tract. Little is known in this regard about the dematiacious and non-dematiacious fungi that can also give rise to AFS, but it is likely that they too can colonise the respiratory tract. The early stages of the disease process may be a growth of the fungi in the nasal cavity, in the lumina of paranasal sinuses or in the ducts or acini of seromucinous glands.

The organisms are always found within the spaces of sinus lumena or ducts or acini of seromucinous

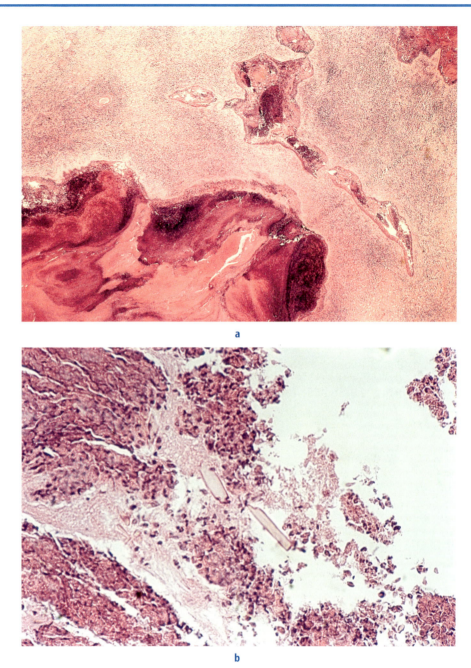

Figure 13.5 Allergic fungal sinusitis. **a** Low-power view of inspissated mucus in distended submucous glands. The dark-staining material is composed of necrotic inflammatory cells, mainly eosinophils. Note thickened epithelium lining glands and dense inflammatory exudate in tissue deep to glands. **b** Necrotic inflammatory cells in inspissated mucus with Charcot Leyden crystals. **c** Dense inflammatory exudate, mainly eosinophils, in tissue surrounding inspissated mucus. Note thickened basement membrane. **d** Branching fungal hyphae in inspissated mucus. Grocott methenamine silver stain.

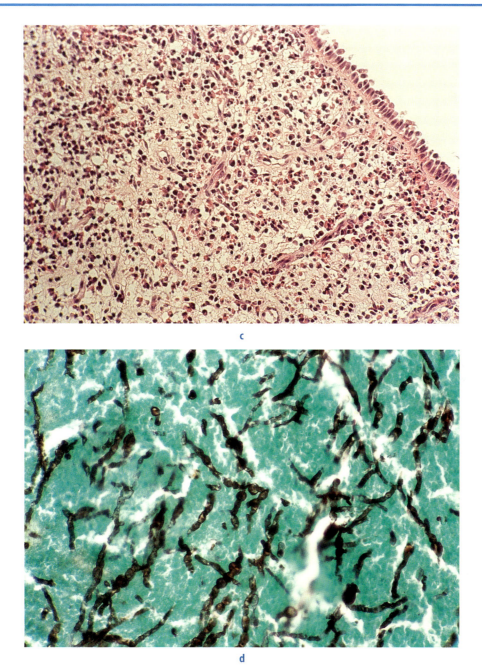

c

d

glands. They are never seen in the tissues. This observation enhances the strong evidence that is already available by systemic immunological tests that AFS is a hypersensitivity response that is triggered by antigen from the infecting fungus.[17] The local immunological mechanism for the pathogenesis of AFS has not yet been studied, but it is presumably based on alterations similar to, but more intense than, those that are known to take place in allergic rhinitis. A soluble fungal allergen presumably passes in through the epithelium and is processed by antigen-presenting cells in the mucosa and then T helper cells, which stimulate B cells to produce high levels of specific antifungal IgE and IgG. Degranulation of mast cells or basophils then occurs from the combination on their surfaces of specific IgE and IgG with fungal antigen. This produces the release of histamine and other spasmogens, the main effect of which is to increase mucous secretion and also to release cytokines, which amplify the inflammatory response in the tissues and activate and accumulate eosinophils.

The mucous secretion in AFS is a conspicuous part of the pathological process. The cells that produce the mucin, presumably under stimulation from the spasmogens released by degranulation of mast cells and basophils, are the hyperplastic goblet cells lining the cavities in which the fungi are harboured: those of the nasal cavity, paranasal sinuses and glands and ducts in the submucosa of these structures. It is likely, because in many cases large numbers of fungi are observed in the mucus, that this material provides ample nutrients for the growth of the fungi, so enhancing the cycle of hyperimmune reactivity.

The other major change, probably stimulated by cytokines released by the degranulation of mast cells, is the intense inflammatory change that takes place in the subepithelial tissues around the inspissated mucus. The mechanism of bone erosion is suggested vascular zone penetrating the sinus wall that is seen on imaging (see above). It seems likely that the erosion of bone is the result of the secretion of substances from the vascular inflammatory tissue in a similar fashion to that of the erosion of ossicular and middle ear wall bone that frequently takes place in cholesteatoma (see Chapter 3) with substances including proteases,[18] cytokines such as tissue necrosis factor (TNF)-alpha[19] and metalloproteinases[20] being derived from the inflammatory tissue that accompanies the cholesteatoma.

Aspergillosis

In most cases of nasal infection with this fungus type the infecting species is *Aspergillus fumigatus*.

Clinical Types

The infection is manifested in five different forms:

1. *Aspergillus* infection as the basis for allergic aspergillus sinusitis (see above).
2. A non-invasive form, the fungus ball, which usually affects the maxillary sinus. The patient has clinical features of a sinus affection such as rhinorrhoea, nasal obstruction and pain, and the sinus is opaque to X-rays. The outlook is excellent, the disease responding well to drainage of the sinus. This lesion takes the form of a soft mass of variable colour, which lies within the lumen or is attached to the side wall of the antrum. Histologically it is a tangled mycelium of aspergilli with a thin coating of inflammatory cells containing neutrophils, lymphocytes and multinucleate giant cells. The fungi are only faintly stained in haematoxylin and eosin sections and the material may be mistaken for mucus. Special fungus stains, particularly Gomori's methenamine silver and periodic acid–Schiff, reveal the hyphae (Fig. 13.6), which characteristically are septate and branch at an acute angle of about 45°. The fungal balls of the paranasal sinuses frequently contain short, bizarrely shaped hyphae. Conidiophores are not seen in the tissues. It is possible that a large proportion of cases of this type of aspergillosis may result from the penetration into the maxillary sinus of zinc-oxide-eugenol paste used in root canal-filling of teeth.[21] Soluble zinc oxide has been shown to promote the growth of tested *Aspergillus* species, the effect diminishing with decreasing concentration.[22]

3. In the rare invasive form of aspergillosis of the nose and paranasal sinuses, the disease develops in patients with an obvious immune deficiency. Pain may be severe and an enlarging mass develops in the orbit, nose or cheek region. In this condition the infection and inflammatory reaction extend beyond the bony walls of the sinuses and may involve the subcutaneous tissues of the cheek and adjacent orbit. Histologically a granulomatous inflammatory reaction represents the major part of the lesion and is composed of giant cells, histiocytes, neutrophils and eosinophils with much fibrosis. The aspergilli are mainly to be found in the cytoplasm of the giant cells.

4. In a recently described form occurring in cases of well-controlled type 2 diabetes mellitus, there was a prolonged illness with proptosis resulting from fungal expansion out of ethmoid sinus infection into the orbit. Cavernous sinus invasion and death resulted.[23]

5. An acute and destructive form of aspergillosis with a fulminating course of *Aspergillus* infection invading into the cranial cavity from the paranasal sinuses is rarely seen in patients with lowered immunological status, including diabetes mellitus. Histologically necrosis accompanies the invading organisms but there is little or no inflammatory reaction[24] (Fig. 13.7).

Infection by Zygomycetes

Zygomycetes represent a class of fungi within the phylum of *Zygomycota*. They are characterised by a

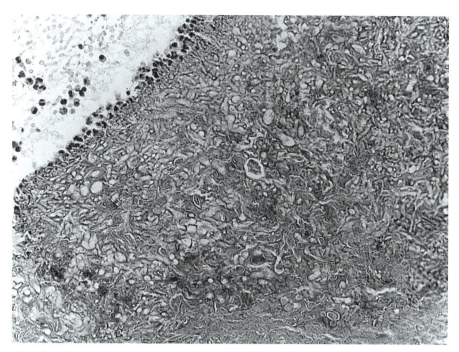

Figure 13.6 Aspergillosis of maxillary antrum. From "fungus ball". The aspergillus is seen as a tangled mass of branching septate hyphae. Necrotic inflammatory cells, especially neutrophils are seen *above left*. Periodic acid–Schiff stain

sparsely septate mycelium and spores borne in sporangia. Two orders of fungi of this class contain representatives, which produce important infections of the nose and paranasal sinuses: the *Entomophthorales* and the *Mucorales*. The disease patterns produced by these two forms of fungi are entirely different and may be classified as: (1) rhinofacial zygomycosis produced by the species *Conidiobolus coronatus* and (2) rhinocerebral zygomycosis caused by *Rhizopus oryzae*.

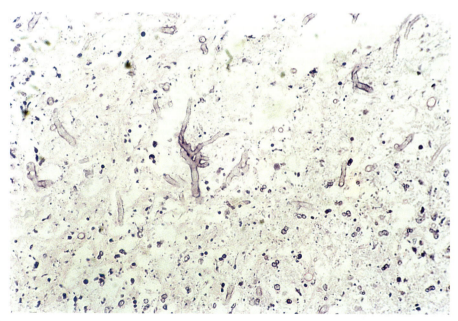

Figure 13.7 Fulminant aspergillus sinusitis from a patient with diabetes mellitus. There are numerous fungal hyphae branching at about 45° (*Aspergillus* sp.) accompanied by severe tissue necrosis, but no inflammatory cells

Rhinofacial Zygomycosis

Geographical Distribution

Patients with this mycosis have been reported from tropical regions in Africa, Asia and South America.[25]

Clinical Features

The infection commences in the nose and paranasal sinuses and then spreads into adjacent tissues of the face and orbit. The progress of the disease is slow. Eventually a large disfiguring mass is formed, which involves the nose, face and eyelids.

Gross Appearances

Pale grey, hard tissue involves the mucosa of the nose and paranasal sinuses and widely infiltrates the tissues of the face and orbit.

Microscopic Appearances

The pathological tissue shows granulomatous inflammation with foreign body giant cells, histiocytes, neutrophils and eosinophils. Fibroblasts and collagen are abundant. Fungal elements may be found only after a careful search. They are short, poorly stained hyphae with thin walls. The fungi,

Conidiobolus coronatus, may show irregular branching and very occasional septae. In many cases, but not all, the fungal fragments are embedded in an eosinophilic material. This lesion is known as the Splendore-Hoeppli reaction. It is found in the tissues surrounding a number of fungal agents and it probably represents an antigen–antibody reaction. The fungi in this condition are seen most clearly in haematoxylin- and eosin-stained sections because the eosinophil material around the hyphae stands out in marked contrast to the clear empty hyphae (Fig. 13.8).

Rhinocerebral Zygomycosis (Mucormycosis)

Clinical Features

Rhinocerebral zygomycosis is a fulminating infection which, classically has occurred in uncontrolled, acidotic diabetics, but is now being described as complicating other immunosuppressive conditions such as leukaemia or after the use of drugs necessary to maintain solid organ or bone marrow graft viability.[26] The nasal turbinates and paranasal sinuses, including the sphenoid sinus, are the first sites of the disease, which rapidly spreads to involve the meninges and brain. Severe headache, chills and fever are prominent symptoms. Neurological features such as ophthalmoplegia are present at an advanced stage of the disease.

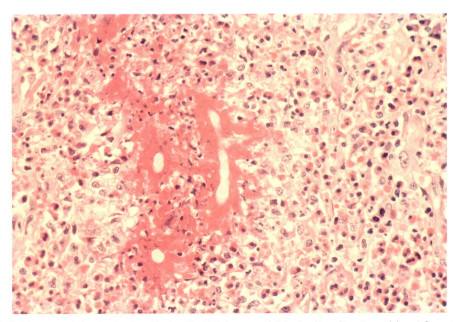

Figure 13.8 Rhinofacial zygomycosis showing clear fungal hyphae (*Conidiobolus coronata*), Splendore-Hoeppli reaction and dense inflammatory exudate with large numbers of eosinophils

Gross Appearances

The bones of the nose show extensive necrosis and abscesses. The palatal bones may be affected, as well as the lateral wall of the nose, maxilla and base of skull.

Microscopic Appearances

Extensive necrosis and diffuse infiltration with polymorphonuclear neutrophils are characteristic features of the condition. Thrombosis due to invasion of blood vessels by the fungus is frequent and infarction is often prominent. The hyphae, *Rhizopus oryzae* of the class Mucorales, are broad, show infrequent septae and have non-parallel sides. They are often basophilic and stain deeply with haematoxylin (Fig. 13.9). Sporangia are seen on rare occasions.

Rhinosporidiosis

Rhinosporidiosis is a chronic disease of the nose and conjunctiva characterised by the formation of persistent polyps caused by a fungus *Rhinosporidium seeberi*, which has not yet been cultured on artificial media. The disease is seen in many countries, but most cases have been identified in the Indian subcontinent and Sri Lanka.

Transmission

The condition is also frequently seen in horses, cows and mules and transmission of the infection is thought to take place by contact with stagnant water in which infected animals have watered.

Gross Appearances

The lesions are rough, corrugated polyps affecting the nasal mucosa and sometimes the conjunctivae. The polyps may be single or multiple and pedunculated or sessile.

Microscopic Appearances

The organism starts its life cycle in the tissues as a parasite measuring 6–8 μm. It then grows by repeated division into a sporangium measuring 200–300 μm, which contains thousands of spores. The latter develop independently after rupture of the sporangium. The tissue reaction is a chronic inflammatory one with numbers of giant cells of Langhans type in reaction to the sporangia. An acute reaction may be present after rupture of the sporangia. A prominent pseudo-epitheliomatous reaction of the overlying squamous epithelium may be present (Fig. 13.10).

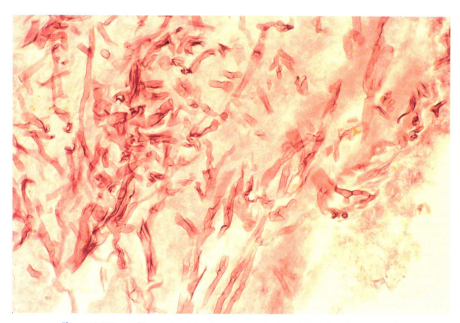

Figure 13.9 Mucor of the nasal wall showing numerous hyphae, which stain with haematoxylin

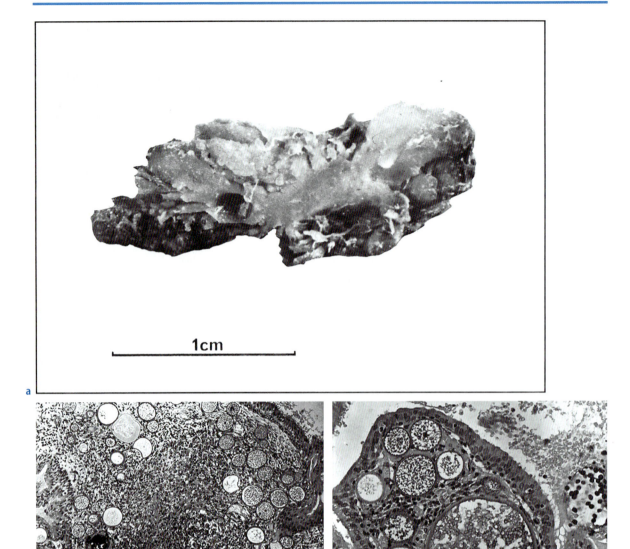

Figure 13.10 Rhinosporidiosis. **a** Cut surface of tissue removed from nose at biopsy, composed of irregular, polypoid mucosa, which is yellowish in the original. **b** Rhinosporidiosis showing numerous sporangia in nasal mucosa with giant cell and lymphocytic reaction. A patch of the epithelium has undergone squamous metaplasia. **c** Sporangia in nasal mucosa situated beneath epithelium. Each contains numerous spores. Spores from a ruptured sporangium lie loosely on the right

Aetiology

The inability for the fungus-like structures to be cultured has suggested alternative explanations for the origin of this disease. In a recent study the cyanobacterium *Microcystis aeruginosa* has been isolated from the water of ponds and river in which patients with rhinosporidiosis had been bathing.

Both large cells and nanocytes, a colourless small-cell stage of *Microcystis aeruginosa*, were recognised inside the round bodies of rhinosporidiosis by light and electron microscopy. It was suggested that this cyanobacterium is the causative agent of this disease.[27] We are unable to find any confirmation of this idea at the time of writing.

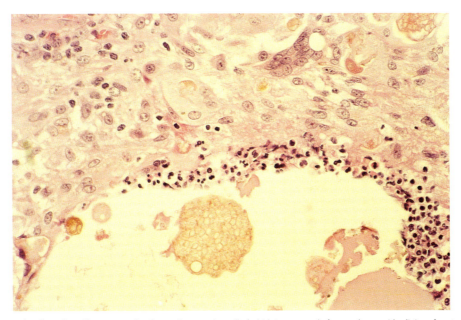

Figure 13.11 Microspherulosis of maxillary antrum showing cystic space, the wall of which is composed of macrophages with a lining of neutrophils. Within the space a brown-staining sac containing spherules is present

Myospherulosis

Myospherulosis (Fig. 13.11) is not a fungus infection, but represents the development of sac-like structures containing globules, which occur in the paranasal sinuses and are associated with a foreign body reaction. Such a lesion was first reported in skeletal muscles, and so was named "myospherulosis". It has been seen most frequently since then in the paranasal sinuses.

Microscopically the lesions in myospherulosis are characterised by the presence of closely arranged spaces in the submucosa giving a "Swiss cheese" appearance. Within the spaces are sac-like structures containing spherules. The sacs range in size from 20 to 120 μm and show slightly refractile outer walls. They are often surrounded by foreign body giant cells and chronic inflammatory cells. The spherules are 5–7 μm in diameter and have a brown to brownish-black colour when viewed in haematoxylin- and eosin-stained sections (Fig. 13.11).

The origin of the lesion has been explained by contact of lipid-containing materials such as petrolatum-based ointments and gauzes with blood during surgery, as a result of which brown "endobodies" resulting from degenerated erythroctes are formed within membranes of lipid.[28]

Protozoal Infections

Leishmaniasis is an infection caused by a protozoon of the genus *Leishmania*. Three distinct clinico-pathological entities exist: (1) tropical sore, (2) mucocutaneous leishmaniasis and (3) disseminated anergic cutaneous leishmaniasis. The nose may be affected in the mucocutaneous form. Leishmania organisms are transmitted from the blood of the infected patients by blood-sucking sand flies. The protozoa multiply in the midgut of the flies and at subsequent biting excursions the organisms are deposited into the next victims.

Mucocutaneous leishmaniasis begins as a tropical sore on the face. This heals slowly, but years after the commencement of the primary infection, a nodular and destructive lesion forms on the nasal septum, which may later be destroyed anteriorly with considerable disfigurement of the nose.

Histological examination of the affected nasal tissue shows hyperplasia of squamous epithelium in relation to a granulomatous process composed of epithelioid cells, lymphocytes and plasma cells, with occasional Langhans giant cells. The parasites are best demonstrated by Giemsa staining. They are not stained with the periodic–Schiff stain. They are situated within the cytoplasm of histiocytes, where they may be detected as round or ovoid structures 1.5–3 μm in diameter. They have a large nucleus and a rod-shaped kinetoplast.

HIV Infection and AIDS

In the immunocompromised host, particularly with AIDS, a wide range of uncommon pathogens have been documented as causing rhinosinusitis. They include: unusual bacterial organisms such as *Pseudomonas aeruginosa*, mycobacteria such as *Mycobacterium avium intracellulare*, fungi such as *Aspergillis* and viral infections such as those caused by Cytomegalovirus.[29] Parasitic rhinosinusitis caused by protozoa such as *Microsporidium, Cryptosporidium* and *Acanthamoeba* species have also been described.[30]

References

1. Raviglione MC, Mariuz P, Pablos-Mendez A et al. High *Staphylococcus aureus* nasal carriage rate in patients with acquired immunodeficiency syndrome or AIDS-related complex. Am J Infect Control 1990;18:64–69

2. Gwaltney JM, Hayden FG. Chapter 16. The nose and infection. In: Proctor DF, Anderson IB (eds) The nose: upper airway physiology and the atmospheric environment. Elsevier, Amsterdam, 1982, pp 399–422

3. Naclerio R. Clinical manifestations of the release of histamine and other inflammatory mediators. J Allergy Clin Immunol 1999;103:S382–385

4. Dixon FW, Hoerr NL, McCall JW. Nasal mucosa in laryngectomised patients. Ann Otol Rhin Laryngol 1949;58:535–547

5. Frederick J, Braude AI. Anerobic infection of the paranasal sinuses. New Engl J Med 1974;290:135–137

6. Andraca R, Edson RS, Kern EB. Rhinoscleroma: a growing concern in the United States? Mayo Clinic experience. Mayo Clin Proc 1993;68:1151–1157

7. Alfaro DA, Michaels L. The pathology of human and experimental scleroma (rhinoscleroma). Rev Inst Invest Med 1980;9:125–140

8. Toppozada H, Gaafar H. Experimental inoculation of *Klebsiella rhinoscleromatis* bacilli in albino mice. J Otorhinolaryngol Relat Spec 1987;49:214–217

9. Srinivasan S, Nehru VI, Mann SB et al. Study of ethmoid sinus involvement in multibacillary leprosy. J Laryng Otol 1998;112:1038–1041

10. Yassin A, El Shennawy M, El Enany G et al. Leprosy of the upper respiratory tract. A clinical, bacteriological, histopathological and histochemical study of twenty cases. J Laryngol Otol 1975;89:505–511

11. Katzenstein AA, Sale SR, Greenberger PA. Pathologic findings in allergic aspergillus sinusitis. A newly recognized form of sinusitis. Am J Surg Pathol 1983;7:439–443

12. Young CN, Swart JG, Ackerman D et al. Nasal obstruction caused by *Drechlera hawaiiensis*. J Laryngol Otol 1978;92:137–143

13. Millar JW, Johnston A, Lamb D. Allergic aspergillosis of the maxillary sinus. Thorax 1981;36:710 (abstract)

14. Torres C, El-Naggar AK, Sim SJ et al. Allergic fungal sinusitis. A clinicopathologic study of 16 cases. Human Pathol 1996;27:793–799

15. Michaels L, Lloyd G, Phelps P. Origin and spread of allergic fungal disease of the nose and paranasal sinuses. Clin Otolaryngol, in press

16. Goodman NL, Roberts GD. Laboratory diagnosis. In: Ajello L, Hay RJ (eds) Topley & Wilson's microbiology and microbial infections, 9th edn. Vol 4. Medical mycology. Arnold, London, 1998, pp 75–88

17. Manning SC, Holman M. Further evidence for allergic pathophysiology in allergic fungal sinusitis. Laryngoscope 1998;108:1485–1496

18. Abramson M., Huang, CC. Localization of collagenase in human middle ear cholesteatoma. Laryngoscope 1977;87:771–791

19. Amar MS, Wishahi HF, Zakhary MM. Clinical and biochemical studies of bone destruction in cholesteatoma. J Laryngol Otol 1996;110:534–549

20. Schönermark M, Mester B, Kempf HG et al. Expression of matrix-metalloproteinases and their inhibitors in human cholesteatomas. Acta Otolaryngol 1996;116:451–456

21. De Foer C, Fossion E, Vaillant JM. Sinus aspergillosis. J Craniomaxillofac Surg 1990;18:33–40

22. Willinger B, Beck-Mannagetta J, Hirschl AM et al. Influence of zinc oxide on Aspergillus species: a possible cause of local, non-invasive aspergillosis of the maxillary sinus. Mycoses 1996;39:361–366

23. deShazo RD, O'Brien M, Chapin K et al. A new classification and diagnostic criteria for invasive fungal sinusitis. Arch Otolaryngol Head Neck Surg 1997;123:1181–1188

24. Milroy CM, Blanshard JD, Lucas S et al. Aspergillosis of the nose and paranasal sinuses. J Clin Path 1989;42:123–127

25. Costa AR, Porto E, Pegas JR et al. Rhinofacial zygomycosis caused by *Conidiobolus coronatus*. A case report. Mycopathologia 1991;115:1–8

26. Nussbaum ES, Hall WA. Rhinocerebral mucormycosis: changing patterns of disease. Surg Neurol 1994;41:152–156

27. Ahluwalia KB, Maheshwari N, Deka RC. Rhinosporidiosis: a study that resolves etiologic controversies. Am J Rhinol 1997;11:479–483

28. Kakizaki H, Shimada K. Experimental study of the cause of myospherulosis. Am J Clin Pathol 1993;99:249–256.

29. Rombaux P, Bertrand B, Eloy P. Sinusitis in the immunocompromised host. Acta Otorhinolaryngol Belg 1997;51:305–313

30. Dunand VA, Hammer SM, Rossi R et al. Parasitic sinusitis and otitis in patients infected with human immunodeficiency virus: report of five cases and review. Clin Infect Dis 1997;25:267–272

14 Non-infective Inflammatory Conditions

Nasal and Paranasal Polyposis

Swelling and polyposis of the mucosa of the nose and paranasal sinuses are produced in many different pathological conditions, both benign and malignant. Histological investigation is essential for accurate diagnosis.

By far the commonest form of nasal polyposis is a chronic oedematous swelling of the mucosa and submucosa, which leads to nasal obstruction.

Pathogenesis

The pathogenesis of nasal polyps is poorly understood and is still not entirely elucidated. Theories proposed during the last decades have included autonomic dysfunction of nasal mucosal blood vessels, allergy, inflammation, bacterial and viral infections. There is some evidence for a genetic predisposition and certain conditions such as immune deficiency, ciliary dyskinesia and aspirin hypersensitivity are associated with nasal polyposis. Circulating and tissue-dwelling subsets of lymphocytes and different cytokines, chemokines included, are local effectors and regulate the complex inflammatory process in the nasal mucosa occurring in nasal polyposis. There is, however, no substantial evidence that allergy causes nasal polyps, nor that the accumulation of eosinophils observed in most polyps is related to allergy. Nasal polyps may show different histological features, but the type of polyp with an oedematous stroma and numerous eosinophils is by far the most common. Nasal polyps occur more commonly in men and are found in all racial groups. The incidence of nasal polyps in the normal population is about 1%, in cystic fibrosis it is 15–20%, while it is as many as 25–30% in Kartagener's syndrome.[1,2]

Gross Appearances

The majority of nasal polyps present a soft, lobular, grey to pink translucent appearance measuring up to 3 cm in diameter. The cut surface is moist and pale pink. A stalk, produced by pulling on the mucosa during removal, is sometimes present. The antrochoanal polyp, a separate entity, is usually found in children. It originates from the mucosa of the maxillary sinus, extrudes through the ostium into the nasal cavity and, because of its size, bulges backwards through the posterior choana into the nasopharynx.

Microscopic Appearances

There is marked oedema of connective tissue with prominent lymphatic dilatation. In some cases the stroma resembles myxoid tissue with markedly oedematous fibrillar deposition and fibrocytes. The respiratory epithelium reveals intense goblet cell hyperplasia and mucinous glands are similarly active. The epithelial basement membrane is markedly thickened. Eosinophils, plasma cells and other inflammatory cells infiltrate the subepithelial tissue in variable, frequently large numbers. Collections of large histiocytic cells in the deeper part of the polyp are common. The stroma may appear fibrous. This feature, in conjunction with the presence of numerous blood vessels, may arouse suspicion of a possible diagnosis of juvenile angiofibroma. Irritation of the surface of

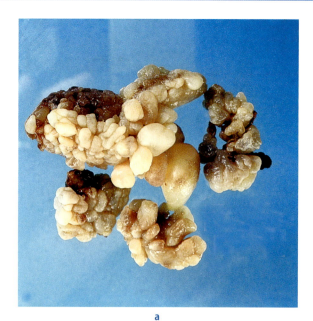

a

b

Figure 14.1 Nasal polyps. **a** Gross appearance of group of polyps showing smooth, shiny, somewhat lobulated surface with "corn-on-cob" formation. **b** There is severe goblet cell hyperplasia. The basement membrane is thickened. Numerous eosinophils and plasma cells are present in the lamina propria. **c** Adenomatous appearance of mucous gland hyperplasia. **d** Case of cystic fibrosis. There is dilatation of most of the ducts by eosinophilic secretion and a chronic inflammatory infiltration. This is not diagnostic for nasal polyps in cystic fibrosis, since such an appearance may also sometimes be found in nasal polyps unassociated with that disease

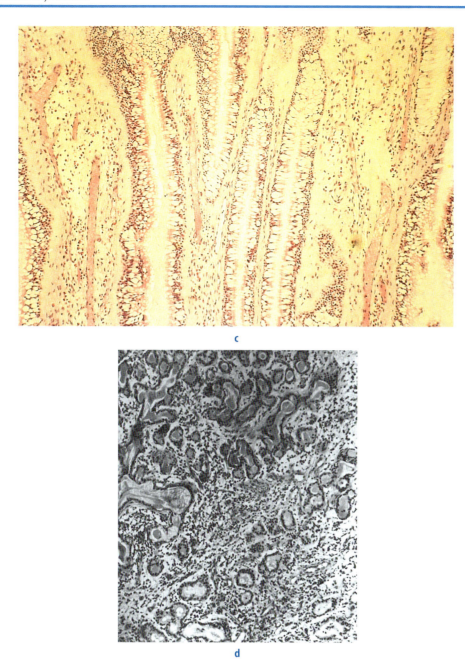

c

d

the polyp frequently gives rise to squamous meta-plasia of the lining epithelium. In some nasal polyps there is a mucous glandular hyperplasia suggesting an adenomatous neoplasm (Fig. 14.1). Rarely, benign metaplastic cartilage or bone has been identified in otherwise benign inflammatory polyps.

Antrochoanal polyps show chronic inflammation only, without the eosinophil infiltrate seen in most other nasal polyps.

Significance of Eosinophilia

The mechanisms causing the accumulation of eosinophils, their functional activities and resolution are at present largely unknown. The inflammatory infiltrate consists not only of numerous eosinophils, but also of a considerable amount of lymphocytes, mast cells, plasma cells, and macrophage-like CD68-positive cells. Ligation of Fas (or CD95, the recently discovered so-called "death receptor") by anti-Fas antibodies or its specific ligand rapidly induces apoptosis in numerous cells, both in vitro and in vivo. For example, certain cytotoxic T cells kill their targets in a calcium-independent manner via activation of Fas. It has been shown that the Fas receptor is frequently expressed on eosinophils within sinonasal polyps. Furthermore the eosinophils signal to macrophages their ongoing apoptosis while within polyps by switching membrane-bound phosphatidylserine molecules, detectable by their binding to Annexin-V. The apoptosis of eosinophils was evaluated by TUNEL and combined with double-staining techniques; their phagocytosis by CD68-positive macrophage-like cells was clearly visualised.[3] Thus the resolution of eosinophils in sinonasal polyps does not appear to be a simple matter of exfoliation or extrusion, but an active process in which the eosinophils signal their ongoing death and are phagocytosed within the polyps.

Nasal Polyposis with Stromal Atypia

Polyposis with stromal atypia is occasionally seen in otherwise typical nasal polyps, mainly in young patients. Microscopically stromal cells of varying sizes are seen in groups or scattered singly.[4,5] The atypical cells are characterised by large hyperchromatic, sometimes multilobulated nuclei with nucleoli which are sometimes multiple and by cytoplasm that is granular or vesicular. The overall appearances of the cells often suggest large fibroblasts (Fig. 14.2). Mitotic activity is absent. There are no cytoplasmic cross-striations and glycogen content is minimal. These appearances and the absence of destruction of nasal or paranasal structures should distinguish this benign process from an embryonal rhabdomyosarcoma, with which it is most often confused. Sinonasal spindle cell carcinoma, although very rare, and malignant melanoma, may also appear as polypoid lesions with scattered, atypical stroma-like cells, but here as well as in rhabdomyosarcoma, immunohistochemistry will help to distinguish the neoplastic cells from reactive fibroblasts in a polyp with stromal atypia.

We have observed the presence of groups of small cells with multiple nuclei in the stroma of nasal polyps; these cells have, likewise, no malignant significance (Fig. 14.2). Adult skeletal muscle cells may be occasionally found in polyps that are otherwise typical (Fig. 14.2). Such appearances should not be confused with teratocarcinoma (see Chapter 22).

Inspissated Mucus

Inspissated mucus represents a collection of impacted mucus and cellular debris in the nose or the paranasal sinuses. This change is a feature of allergic fungal sinusitis and it is likely that the majority of lesions of this type are produced as an allergic reaction to fungus infection (see Chapter 13).

Nasal Polyposis and the Immotile-Cilia Syndrome

The cilia of the nasal respiratory epithelium are responsible for the movement of the mucous stream in which embedded bacteria, dust and other particulate matter are conveyed towards the nasopharynx for ultimate ingestion. Failure of ciliary activity is likely to lead to infection and inflammatory changes in the nose and sinuses. In one such condition, cilia are congenitally defective in their ultrastructure; this has been described as the immotile-cilia syndrome.[6]

Ultrastructure of Normal Cilia

The normal cilium shows on cross-section a pair of separate microtubules in the centre and a peripheral row of nine paired "figure of eight" microtubules (Fig. 14.3). This is a configuration that is common to all flagellum-like structures in both plants and animals. Radial spokes project from a central sheath around the central pair of microtubules and join the peripheral doublets. The latter doublets are also joined together by circularly arranged links composed of nexin. Two short diverging arms project clockwise from each doublet towards the next.[6] It has been shown by biochemical "dissection" of the arms from the doublets that they consist of a protein called dynein, which exhibits adenosine triphosphatase activity, important in the movement of the cilia.

Kartagener's Syndrome

Kartagener in 1933 described a syndrome which included the following features: (1) complete transposition of the viscera, (2) bronchiectasis and (3) nasal polyposis resulting from chronic rhinosinusi-

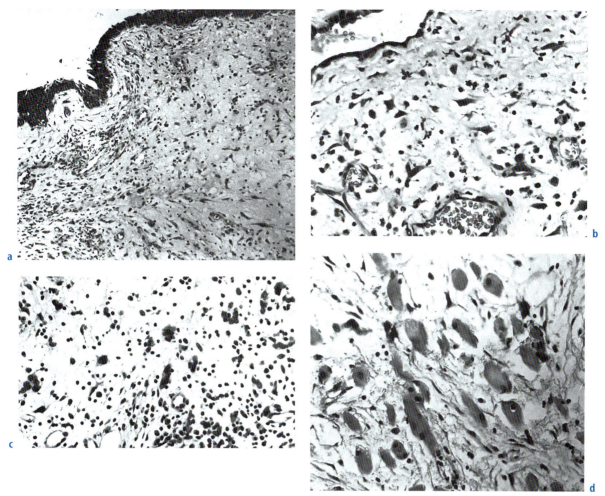

Figure 14.2 Atypical cells in nasal polyps. **a** Nasal polyposis with stromal atypia. Numerous elongated, atypical cells are present in the stroma. **b** Under higher power the atypical cells show large, hyperchromatic, occasionally multilobed nuclei, without mitotic activity. Some appear to line a vessel. **c** Small, compact multinucleate cells in stroma of nasal polyp. **d** Skeletal muscle fibres in stroma of nasal polyp

tis.[7] It was subsequently noted that males with the syndrome were infertile.[8] Absence of dynein arms in the spermatozoa of patients with this syndrome was noted by Afzelius.[9] These cells were immobile. In Kartagener's syndrome the cilia of bronchial and nasal epithelium have also been shown to lack dynein arms.[6] The siblings of patients with Kartagener's syndrome may have the changes of nasal polyposis only, and a family of siblings with nasal polyposis but neither transposition of the viscera nor bronchiectasis, lacked dynein arms in the nasal cilia.[10] Thus a basic feature present in all of these patients is the ciliary defect and it has been suggested that the term immotile-cilia syndrome should be used rather than the eponym.[6] Another cilial deficiency has been observed in a sibship of

patients with sinusitis. Here the radial spokes between the central tubules and the outer doublets were absent.[11] One of the patients also had situs inversus. Some patients with the immotile-cilia syndrome have also been found to have normal ciliary ultrastructure.

Pathological Appearances

The changes in the nose and paranasal sinuses are those of chronic inflammation with polyposis of the mucosa. Histological examination of the upper respiratory mucosa shows normal goblet cells and seromucinous glands, but inflammatory changes are extensive. In polyps in patients with Kartagener's

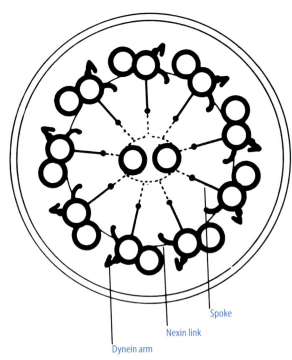

Spoke

Nexin link

Dynein arm

Figure 14.3 Diagram of ultrastructural configuration on cross-section of normal cilium. For description see text (Courtesy of Eliasson et al.[6])

syndrome, and also in those with cystic fibrosis, neutrophils constitute the prevailing inflammatory infiltrate, although eosinophils are present in a significant number.

Ultrastructural examination reveals absent dynein arms or absent radial spokes in cilia. In addition an irregular internal organisation of other constituents of the cilia and megacilia may be found, in which there are many axonemes (internal structures each derived normally from a single cilium). Areas denuded of epithelium may be present in some parts of the nasal mucosa. It is also important to examine the ciliary activity of the fresh epithelium by direct microscopy. Such abnormalities as are present should be quantified since up to 10% of cilia showing the·above defects may be found in individuals without the clinical features of the syndrome.[12]

Granuloma Following Local Steroid Injections

Intranasal injection of prednisolone acetate has been recommended as treatment particularly for long-standing and recurrent nasal oedema that is refractory to other forms of treatment. Foreign body granulomas have been found in nasal tissues removed subsequently from patients so treated.

These lesions show finely granular amorphous masses bordered by palisaded histiocytes, foreign body type giant cells and foamy histiocytes. Particles of birefringent crystalline material, probably the remains of the injected steroid material, are found in the granuloma.[13] The granulomatous foci closely resemble rheumatoid nodules. Lesions of this type are said to develop as rapidly as within 2 days after injection.

Inflammation Following Nasal Cocaine Abuse

Cases have been described of a severe necrotising inflammation following extensive intranasal abuse of cocaine. Grossly there is necrosis and atrophy of the inferior and middle nasal turbinates bilaterally, prominent naso- and oropharyngeal ulcers and nasal septal as well as hard palate perforations. Microscopically focal areas of acute and chronic inflammation with necrosis are seen, but vasculitis is minimal and granuloma is not present. The diagnosis may be mistaken for Wegener's granulomatosis and a serum falsely positive for anti-neutrophil cytoplasmic antibody may enhance this impression.[14]

Cholesterol Granuloma

Cholesterol granuloma is frequently encountered in the nose and paranasal sinuses, particularly in the maxillary antrum. Occasionally it may affect the frontal sinus. There is clinical and radiological evidence of maxillary sinus disease and an operation is carried out to exclude a neoplastic condition. The antrum is found to be occupied by a bluish swelling of the mucosa, sometimes thought to be a cyst. Histologically the changes are similar to those of cholesterol granuloma of the middle ear (see Chapter 3), i.e. haemorrhage, haemosiderin mainly in histiocytes and extensive cholesterol clefts with foreign body type giant cell reaction (Fig. 14.4). In some cases when the tip of the cannula has entered the granuloma, examination of the sinus washings may reveal the characteristically notched crystals of cholesterol. These crystals float on the surface of the washings in a centrifuged specimen (Fig. 14.4).

The cause of this common condition is not known. It seems likely that, as with cholesterol granuloma of the middle ear (see Chapter 3), haemorrhage into the mucosa of the sinus is the basic lesion.

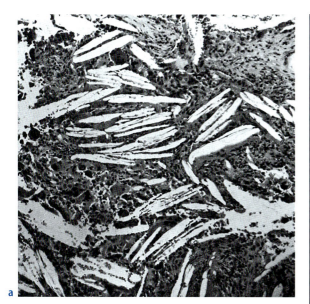
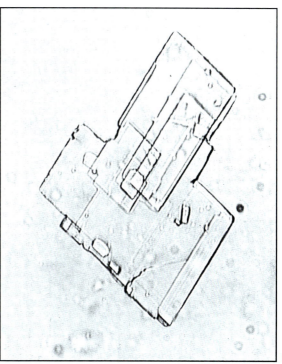

Figure 14.4 a Cholesterol granuloma of maxillary antrum. There are numerous clefts with foreign body giant cells. **b** Crystals removed from surface of fluid in a centrifuged specimen of antral washings from a case of cholesterol granuloma of the maxillary antrum. Note notched edges of crystals, typical of cholesterol. Wet preparation

Rhinitis Caseosa

A rare condition of the nasal cavity is described in which there is a foul-smelling discharge composed histologically of cholesterol crystals with a granulomatous and acute inflammatory change (Fig. 14.5). This condition, which is known as rhinitis caseosa, also shows a haemorrhagic basis for the cholesterol granuloma, like similar lesions in the sinuses and middle ear (see above and Chapter 3).

Granuloma Pyogenicum

Granuloma pyogenicum is a swelling made up of thin-walled blood vessels, which is frequently seen in the nose. It is often difficult to decide whether it is a true haemangioma or an inflammatory reaction (for which the designation granuloma pyogenicum would be more appropriate). Even "haemangioma" – a neoplasm – is inaccurate, since it would seem to be more in the nature of a growth anomaly. Nevertheless, this lesion will be considered with vascular neoplasms of the nose (see Chapter 19).

Organising Haematoma

A mass of organising haemorrhage in the nose has sometimes been mistaken for a malignant neoplasm of blood vessels. It follows intranasal bleeding, when a clot forms either within the mucosa or adhering to its surface. Organisation by granulation tissue then takes place.

Grossly a sessile vascular or pale mass is present, usually on the lateral wall, and biopsy may be carried out with the impression that it is a neoplasm. A large mass frequently develops and it may be removed with a clinical diagnosis of a vascular neoplasm. The cut surface shows deep red and greyish foci. Histologically there are extensive areas of irregular blood vessels often lined by bizarre endothelial cells, which may be mistaken for a malignant vascular neoplasm (Fig. 14.6). Fibroblasts are numerous and fibrosis may be extensive. Large areas of fresh or partially degenerated blood, which is becoming organised by granulation tissue, are also present.

The source of the intranasal haemorrhage may, indeed, be a neoplasm such as an angiofibroma of the nasopharynx. Biopsy material may be taken

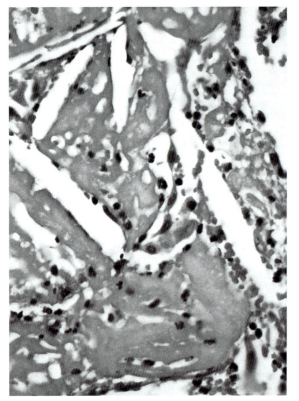

Figure 14.5 Rhinitis caseosa. Section of the material discharged from the nose consists of cholesterol crystals with histiocytic and acute inflammatory reaction. There is also evidence of haemorrhage (Courtesy of Dr. V. J. Hyams)

from the organising haematoma alone so that no evidence of the underlying neoplasm would be seen in the biopsy.

Giant Cell Granulomatous Lesions

A lesion of the nose and sinuses presenting numerous, multinucleated giant cells in a stroma of mesenchymal, often spindle, cells may fall into one of four separate groups:

1. Benign giant cell tumour or granuloma. It is questionable whether this condition is a true neoplasm; probably it is an entity similar to that seen most frequently in the lower jaw, termed giant cell reparative granuloma (Fig. 14.7).
2. The giant cell lesion associated with hyperparathyroidism, often referred to as brown tumour on account of its frequently haemorrhagic basis.
3. An active neoplasm with locally aggressive and sometimes metastatic activity similar to the giant cell tumour of long bones.
4. Oncogenic osteomalacia – a syndrome of hypophosphataemia and osteomalacia associated with a neoplasm containing osteoclast-like giant cells. The nasal cavity is the second commonest site for the neoplasm.

The first three conditions may be difficult to distinguish from one another histologically. The fourth, while usually displaying numerous giant cells, has a very vascular stroma of more primitive-appearing round cells. Any of them may be found in the nose or the maxilla, filling the cavity of the antrum or invading the floor of the orbit. The sphenoid and ethmoid sinuses are sometimes also involved. The benign giant cell tumour is usually seen below the

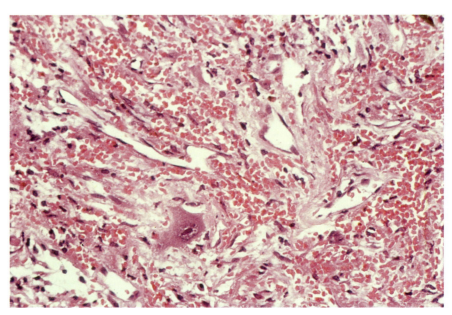

Figure 14.6 Organising haematoma of nasal cavity showing haemorrhage and numerous small thin-walled blood vessels with some atypical endothelial cells

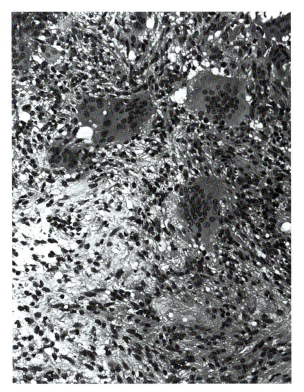

Figure 14.7 Giant cell reparative granuloma involving upper jaw. As well as giant cells there are numbers of fibroblasts and some collagen

age of 40. The malignant one presents at a later age. A diagnosis based on histological criteria alone may prove difficult. Haemorrhage, chronic inflammatory cells and haemosiderin are often, but not always, prominent in giant cell reparative granuloma. In all cases of nasal tumours showing uniformly distributed giant cells in a cellular fibroblastic stroma, it is essential to exclude hyperparathyroidism by clinical examination and serum calcium estimation. Secondary hyperparathyroidism (usually caused by renal failure), as well as the primary variety, may lead to osseous maxillary giant cell lesions. Oncogenic osteomalacia can be suspected in the presence of low blood phosphate and clinicoradiologic features of osteomalacia.[15] The osteomalacia disappears when the neoplasm is removed.[16]

Wegener's Granulomatosis

Definition

Wegener's granulomatosis is a systemic inflammatory condition affecting the nose (often with the paranasal sinuses), lung and kidneys in all cases and other organs in some cases. Typically, the respiratory tract has necrotising granulomas with vasculitis,

whereas the kidneys and skin have vasculitis only. Nearly any organ can, however, be affected and ocular lesions such as sclerouveitis, keratitis, cornoscleral ulceration, and also pseudotumour of the orbit, are present in a rather high proportion of cases. Hearing loss is another less frequent feature of Wegener's granulomatosis, recurrent otitis media being the most common manifestation of involvement of the ear. Carrington and Liebow[17] have suggested that a limited form may affect the lungs only. The relationship of this entity to the systemic variety is not clear and the possibility of involvement of the nasal passages alone has still not been clarified. In the light of present knowledge we would suggest that only those cases in which the kidney is involved as well as the nose should be accepted as Wegener's granulomatosis. We do not think that it is justifiable to treat a patient with cytotoxic drugs unless the full-blown clinical picture of Wegener's granulomatosis with a positive antineutrophil cytoplasmic antibody test is present, however suggestive of that diagnosis the nasal changes may be.

Gross Appearances

In the nose and sinuses there is marked thickening of the mucosa by oedema and accumulation of pus in the maxillary antrum. A rather extensive nasal swelling is usually present and later ulceration with crusting. This crusting is diffuse, large, greenish, bloody and usually foul smelling. The granulomatous tissue may at later stages cause stenosis. Partial destruction of bony confines may be present, but the inflammatory process rarely, if ever, erodes through palate or face. Extranasal deformities occur but facial destruction is usually limited to saddle deformity of the nose, contrary to the more ulcerative and destructive lesions caused by nasal lymphomas.

In the lungs the lesions take the form of sharply circumscribed inflammatory masses in the parenchyma. Sometimes haemorrhagic infarcts caused by thrombosed, arteritic vessels are present.

Kidneys are enlarged and show fine punctate haemorrhages and infarcts of the cortex.

Microscopic Appearances

In the lungs two sorts of lesion are seen without necessarily any causal relationship of one to the other:

1. Areas of destructive necrosis in the parenchyma, resembling caseation. These are of variable size and are usually surrounded by an inflammatory reaction composed of lymphocytes, plasma cells, eosinophils and polymor-

phonuclear leucocytes. Fibroblasts may be prominent around the edge of the lesion, but epithelioid cells are not present. Giant cells are usually prominent in the exudate. They may be of foreign body, Langhans or both types.

2. Vasculitis involving small arteries and veins. The vessels are affected by an acute necrotising inflammatory process, sometimes with mural fibrin infiltration and thrombosis.

Wegener's granulomatosis in the nose shows a gangrene-like crust which covers an area of ulcera-

tion. Deep, and often repeated, biopsies from this area are usually necessary in order to obtain tissue with the microscopic hallmarks of Wegener's granulomatosis. There are three main histological features to be seen (Fig. 14.8):

1. Pyogenic granulation tissue covered with a gangrene-like crust.

2. Granulomas of epithelioid type. These granulomas tend to be rather few and are larger and more irregular than those seen in sarcoidosis or tuberculosis. The granulomas may contain

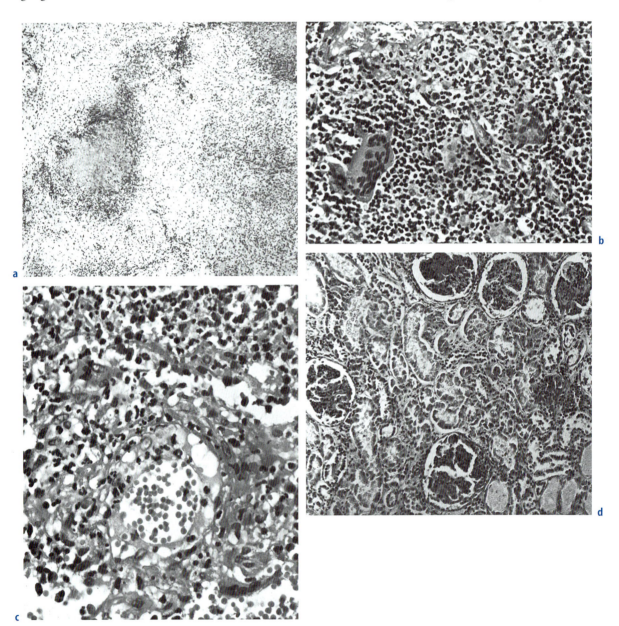

Figure 14.8 Wegener's granulomatosis. **a** Nasal biopsy showing foci of necrosis and inflammation. **b** Nasal biopsy showing giant cells and acute inflammatory infiltration with some eosinophils. **c** Vasculitis in nasal biopsy. Some of the inflammatory cells are eosinophils. **d** Kidney at post-mortem showing segmental deposition of fibrin and necrosis in glomeruli accompanied by crescents.

microabscesses or fibrinoid necrosis, but can also be non-necrotic. In cases of microabscesses blastomycosis has to be ruled out. Multinucleated giant cells are few but invariably present.

3. Vasculitis is mandatory for the morphological diagnosis of Wegener's granulomatosis. The vascular changes are most easily found between the granulation tissue and the overlying crust. Features of vasculitis, or obliterated vessels, can also be seen near the granulomas, which is not the case in tuberculosis.

There are numerous eosinophils in the admixed inflammatory infiltrate and areas of tissue necrosis.

The characteristic feature of the renal changes in Wegener's granulomatosis is one of segmental necrotising glomerulonephritis. This lesion is generally focal. There is evidence of glomerular thrombosis, with or without necrosis. Weiss and Crissman[18] failed to demonstrate evidence of an immune complex pathogenesis for this condition in the renal glomeruli and suggested that glomerular thrombosis and necrosis are the prime findings.

Serum autoantibodies against neutrophils (c-ANCA test) have been found to be fairly specific for Wegener's granulomatosis and are now used extensively in clinical diagnosis

Natural History

Until the last few decades, Wegener's granulomatosis ran a fulminant course with death taking place within 2 years. Cytotoxic drug therapy has proved a highly effective remedy and the disease process can now be completely controlled.[19]

Midline Granuloma

Synonyms

Midline granuloma is a clinical term with several synonyms: Stewart's granuloma, non-healing granuloma, granuloma gangrenescens and lethal granuloma.

Stewart's Report

In midline granuloma a relentlessly progressive ulceration of the nose and adjacent deeper tissues is said to take place. The condition, if untreated, is said to end fatally. The pathological changes are those of non-specific chronic inflammation.

The concept of an entity with these features is derived from a report by Stewart in 1933 in which ten cases with a severe ulcerating condition of the nose were described in detail.[20] Only two of these cases appear to have been directly observed by Stewart himself. Six of the case histories were taken from the literature going back as long as 36 years. Stewart admitted that the condition is rare and cited a long list of known disease entities that should be excluded before the diagnosis of lethal granulomatous ulceration is made. One of these was "malignancy". Yet in three of the ten cases a histological examination of the nasal tissues was reported by eminent pathologists as (1) "atypical spheroidal carcinoma", (2) "sarcoma" and (3) "Hodgkin's lymphadenoma". In spite of this and the relentlessly ulcerating behaviour of the lesion in most of the cases, Stewart labelled the lesion, which he felt was a single entity, "granulomatosis".

Ulcerating Lesions Produced by Lymphoma

A heterogenous group of lesions of the upper respiratory tract can produce extensive midline ulceration (Table 14.1). These include infections, neoplasms and vasculitides. The commonest of the

Table 14.1. Conditions that may be associated with severe ulceration of the nose

Blood dyscrasia	Agranulocytosis
Bacterial and related infections	Osteomyelitis of facial and cranial bones Rhinoscleroma Tuberculosis Sarcoidosis Lepromatous leprosy Syphilis Actinomycosis
Fungal and protozoal infections	Histoplasmosis Blastomycosis Sporotrichosis Leishmaniasis
Vasculitides and defects of vascular innervation	Churg-Strauss syndrome Wegener's granulomatosis Trophic post-encephalitic ulceration
Tumour-like conditions	Giant cell reparative granuloma Inflammatory pseudotumour
Neoplasms	Squamous cell carcinoma Adenocarcinoma Lymphoma Langerhans cell histiocytosis Undifferentiated carcinoma of nasopharynx involving nasal septum
Self-inflicted	Factitious ulceration

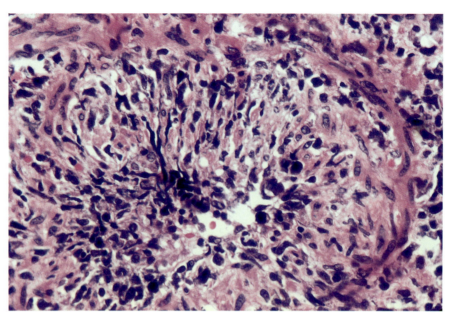

Figure 14.9 T-cell lymphoma of nose invading an artery. There is necrosis of many cells

neoplasms that produce such ulceration are characterised by malignant lymphocytic or histiocytic proliferation. Polymorphic reticulosis (midline malignant reticulosis, lymphomatoid granulomatosis) is the term used in the latest World Health Organisation Classification.[21] It is now certain that this entity is a peripheral (extranodal) malignant lymphoma, usually of T cell origin in Europe and of T/Natural Killer cell lineage in certain parts of Asia and China.[22] Sinonasal peripheral malignant lymphoma is histologically characterised by an abundant atypical lymphoproliferative element, never seen in Wegener's granulomatosis. These infiltrates of polymorphic and atypical cells tend to be arranged in a necrotising, angioinfiltrative growth pattern (Fig. 14.9). They are found in the submucosa and the overlying surface epithelium is always ulcerated. The infiltrates are indeed polymorphic, consisting of plasma cells, histiocytes, eosinophils (but less eosinophils than in Wegener's granulomatosis) and atypical, rather small lymphocytes and immunoblasts with mitoses. The perivascular (and intravascular) distribution of these cells can easily be misinterpreted as representing vasculitis. Granulomas and giant cells are not present. Thrombosis, however, is a common finding. The presence of atypical cells, necrosis, and the angioinfiltrative growth pattern gives the clue to the diagnosis. The T cell phenotype is confirmed by immunohistochemistry. Systemic involvement is common as the disease progresses in untreated cases.

True histiocytic lymphoma is very rare in the sinonasal tract. The cells, derived from the mono-cyte-macrophage system, have lobated or oval nuclei with multiple nucleoli. There is abundant cytoplasm and well-defined cell margins.

Conventional malignant lymphomas, non-Hodgkin and Hodgkin's lymphoma (see Chapter 22), are far from rare, and in some series they constitute the most common non-epithelial malignant tumour of the nose.[23] However, conventional malignant lymphomas much less frequently cause the destructive clinical picture of midline granuloma than does the sinonasal peripheral malignant lymphoma.

Diagnosis of Ulcerating Conditions of the Nose

As emphasised above, we do not believe that midline granuloma exists as a pathological entity. Lymphoma is only one of the many pathological conditions that may give rise to ulceration of the nose (Table 14.1). To categorise an ulcerating nose as "midline granuloma" is a disservice to the patient. Patients with nasal ulceration should be carefully investigated by the standard clinical, laboratory and radiological methods. Biopsy sections should be examined with care for evidence of lymphoma and other neoplastic conditions. If chronic inflammation only is found the pathologist should admit that no specific diagnosis can be made. In a few cases ulceration may continue in the absence of diagnostic features in the biopsy. Under these conditions further biopsy material should be obtained.

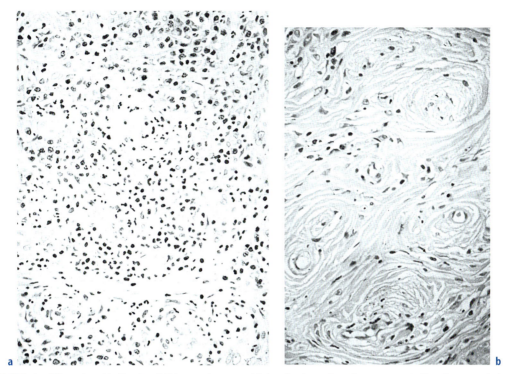

Figure 14.10 Eosinophilic angiocentric fibrosis. **a** Cellular area from a nasal lesion showing perivascular arrangement of lymphocytes and plasma cells. **b** Another area of the lesion in **a** showing "onion-skin" deposits of perivascular fibrosis. There are eosinophils among the collagenous cells

Eosinophilic Angiocentric Fibrosis

A lesion of the nasal septum and lateral nasal wall has recently been described, which bears some histological relationship to granuloma faciale and to angiolymphoid hyperplasia (see Chapter 2). In this condition there are "onion-skin" deposits of perivascular fibrosis with numerous eosinophils[24] (Fig. 14.10). Plasma cells and lymphocytes, mainly of T cell type, are present in large numbers in the early stages.[25] The aetiological basis is unknown, but complete surgical excision of the affected tissue appears to be curative. In one of the cases of Roberts and McCann, there was granuloma faciale of the skin on the side of the nose. One patient presented with a mucosal lesion of the same type in the laryngeal subglottic mucosa.

References

1. Davidsson Å. Allergic rhinitis and nasal polyposis. A clinical study with emphasis on lymphocytes, cytokines and the chemokine RANTES. Medical Dissertation, Gothenburg University, Akademitryck AB Edsbruk, Sweden, 1995
2. Settipane GA, Lund VJ, Bernstein JM et al. (eds) Nasal polyps: epidemiology, pathogenesis and treatment. OceanSide Publications, Inc., Providence, Rhode Island, USA, 1997
3. Davidsson Å, Andersson A, Hellquist HB. Apoptosis and phagocytosis of tissue dwelling eosinophils in sinonasal polyps. Laryngoscope, in press
4. Compagno J, Hyams VJ. Nasal polyposis with atypical stroma. Arch Pathol Lab Med 1976;100:224–226
5. Hellquist HB. Histopathology of nasal polyps. Allergy Asthma 1996;17:237–242
6. Eliasson R, Mossberg B, Camner P et al. The immotile-cilia syndrome. A congenital ciliary abormality as an etiologic factor in chronic airway infections and male sterility. N Engl J Med 1977;297:1–6
7. Kartagener M. Zur Pathogenese der Bronchiektasien; Bronchiektasien bei Situs viscerum inversus. Beitr Klin Tuberk 1933;83:489–501
8. Arge E. Transposition of the viscera and sterility in men. Lancet 1960;I:412–414
9. Afzelius BA, Eliasson R, Johnsen O et al. Lack of dynein arms in immotile human spermatozoa. J Cell Biol 1975;66:225–232
10. Elverland HH. Kartagener's syndrome – a reappraisal. Acta Otolaryngol (Stockh) 1979;360(suppl):129–130
11. Sturgess JM, Chao J, Wong J et al. Cilia with defective radial spokes: a cause of human respiratory disease. N Engl J Med 1979;300:53–56
12. Smallman LA, Gregory J. Ultrastructural abnormalities of cilia in the human respiratory tract. Hum Pathol 1986;17:848–55
13. Wolff M. Granulomas in nasal mucous membranes following local steroid injections. Am J Clin Pathol 1974;62:775–782
14. Sittel C, Eckel HE. Nasal cocaine abuse presenting as a central facial destructive granuloma. Eur Arch Otorhinolaryngol 1998;255:446–447
15. Gonzalez-Compta X, Manos-Pujol M, Foglia-Fernandez M et al. Oncogenic osteomalacia: case report and review of head

and neck associated tumours. J Laryngol Otol 1998;112:389–392

16. Weidner N. Review and update: oncogenic osteomalacia-rickets. Ultrastructural Pathology 1991;15:317–333

17. Carrington CB, Liebow AA. Pulmonary veno-occlusive disease. Hum Pathol 1970;1:322–324

18. Weiss MA, Crissman JD. Renal biopsy findings in Wegener's granulomatosis: segmental necrotizing glomerulonephritis with glomerular thrombosis. Hum Pathol 1984;15:943–956

19. Fauci AS, Haynes BF, Katz P et al. Wegener's granulomatosis: prospective clinical and therapeutical experience with 85 patients for 21 years. Ann Intern Med 1983;98:76–85

20. Stewart JP. Progressive lethal granulomatous ulceration of the nose. J Laryngol Otol 1933;48:657–701

21. Shanmugaratnam K, Sobin LH. Histological typing of tumours of the upper respiratory tract and ear. WHO International Histological Classification of Tumours, 2nd edn. Springer-Verlag, Berlin, Heidelberg, New York, 1991

22. Jaffe ES, Chan JKC, Su I-J et al. Report of the workshop on nasal and related extranodal angiocentric T/Natural Killer cell lymphomas. Am J Surg Pathol 1996;20:103–111

23. Fu Y-S, Perzin KH. Nonepithelial tumours of the nasal cavity, paranasal sinuses and nasopharynx. A clinicopathologic study. X. Malignant lymphomas. Cancer 1979;43:611–621

24. Roberts PF, McCann BG. Eosinophilic angiocentric fibrosis of the upper respiratory tract: a mucosal variant of granuloma faciale? A report of three cases. Histopathology 1985;9:1217–1225

25. Altemani AM, Pilch BZ, Sakano E et al. Eosinophilic angiocentric fibrosis of the nasal cavity. Mod Pathol 1997;10:391–393

15 Papilloma

Papilloma of the Nasal Vestibule and Nostril

In the vestibule and nostril, papillomas are usually stratified squamous arising on the skin surface. Rarely do they recur after simple removal, and malignant transformation is seldom a problem. Abnormal hyperplastic changes of the epithelium are frequent, but if similar criteria of assessment for possible cancerous or precancerous change are used to those applied in other stratified squamous epithelia (see Chapter 34), a diagnosis of malignancy will be unusual.

Papilloma of the Nasal Cavity and Paranasal Sinuses

Three histological types of papilloma of the nose and paranasal sinuses have been described:

1. Everted squamous papilloma is similar to the wart-like squamous-cell lesion seen frequently in other parts of the upper respiratory tract.
2. Inverted papilloma is characterised by epithelial cell groups within the substance of polyps.
3. Cylindric cell papilloma is composed of papillae lined by columnar epithelium.

Although the histological differences between everted and inverted papilloma have been well established and were accepted in the earlier literature as indicating three distinct pathologic entities, most of the recent descriptions of nasal papillomas have regarded the three types as a single entity, "papilloma" or "Schneiderian papilloma". In support of the latter concept it is affirmed that some lesions show patterns that are intermediate between the three types and in recurrent cases the pattern may change to that of an alternative type.[1] In a study carried out on a large series of nasal and paranasal sinus papillomas, specimens from the three histological types were examined to establish the histogenesis and specific histological features of each. Using these criteria the samples from each category were further examined to seek possible intermediate forms between the three lesions. It was concluded that there were no intermediate forms between the three types of papilloma.[2] The three types of nasal papilloma will therefore be presented here as separate entities.

Everted Squamous Papilloma

This condition is also known as exophytic squamous or fungiform papilloma.

Site

Everted papillomas are most frequently seen growing from the mucosa of the nasal septum. Occasionally, such a lesion may be found on the lateral wall of the nose, e.g. on the inferior turbinate. The nasal vestibule or nostril are also quite commonly the seat of such lesions. They are always unilateral.

Incidence

There is a marked preponderance of male patients. Patients affected tend to be younger than in the other forms of nasal papilloma.

Gross Appearances

The lesion is a raised, confluent, verrucous excrescence ranging from 1 to 15 mm in diameter. It is always single and attached to the mucosa by a wide base.

Microscopic Appearances

The microscopic appearance of both the septal and vestibular forms of everted nasal papilloma is one of branching fronds of mucosa, each with a connective tissue core, covered by stratified squamous epithelium. The branching of the papillae is often to a second and sometimes to a third level. The stratified squamous epithelium ranges from predominantly basal cell to the differentiated keratinised form (Fig. 15.1). All the lesions of vestibular origin are well differentiated with hyperkeratosis. Mitotic figures are occasionally seen in or near the basal

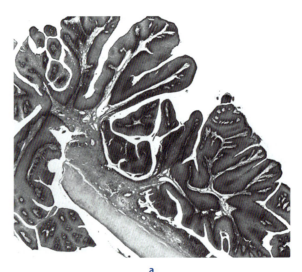

a

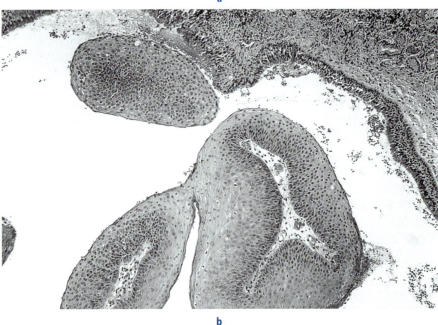

b

Figure 15.1 Everted papilloma of nasal septum. **a** Branching fronds of squamous epithelium arise from the nasal lining. The septal cartilage is present in this specimen. **b** Higher power of **a** showing papillae and respiratory as well as squamous epithelium

layers. Nuclei expressing MIB-1 are present in the basal six layers. Occasional microcysts, some containing mucin globules, may be present. Their maximum diameter is about 50 μm. The contents of the microcysts do not express the macrophage marker PG-M1.

Small zones of respiratory epithelium, either of ciliated or of mucous type, may be seen among the stratified squamous cells of the papillary processes. Koilocytosis (see Chapter 33) is frequently found in the epithelium. Seromucinous glands are numerous in nasal septal papillomas where the underlying submucosa has been sampled. In some of the vestibular papillomas, skin adnexae are seen in the biopsy.

The inwardly structured growth pattern of inverted papillomas or the oncocytic columnar epithelium-lined papillae characteristic of the cylindric cell papilloma are never identified in everted papillomas.

Natural History

Recurrence of everted papilloma is unusual. Malignant change does not occur.

Aetiology

The tendency to classify everted with inverted papillomas of the nose and paranasal sinuses together as a single entity has caused difficulty in interpreting some of the results of investigation of human papilloma virus (HPV) as an aetiologic agent for these conditions. Using in situ hybridisation, some studies have shown a proportion only to be positive for HPV types 6/11, ranging from 16 of 21 cases[3] to three of 19 cases.[4] In some of these series interpretation has been complicated even further by the inclusion of cases showing dysplasia or carcinoma. In three other reports in which the groups of papilloma have, on the contrary, been precisely delineated histologically, the incidence of HPV DNA seems more clear-cut. In an investigation of nine inverted papillomas, three everted papillomas and three cylindric cell papillomas using immunohistochemistry, in situ hybridisation and the polymerase chain reaction for HPV, only the everted papillomas were positive.[5] In a series of nine everted-type nasal septal papillomas concomitant with genital papillomas, eight showed HPV of the 6/11 type.[6] Also, a study of a larger series of sinonasal papillomas, 78 cases, gives strong support that HPV 6/11 may be involved in the pathogenesis of papilloma that are solely of everted type.[7] Accordingly, while there is evidence that the everted type of sinonasal papilloma is related to HPV 6/11 infection, as would be expected from experience with other everted squamous papillomas of the respiratory tract (see Chapter 33), the role of HPV in inverted papilloma remains unclear. It is likely that the preliminary histological identification of the nasal lesion as either everted or inverted papilloma will clarify the interpretation of the results when studies by molecular biologic techniques for HPV and other infective agents are carried out on nasal and paranasal sinus papillomas.

Inverted Papilloma

This condition is also known as Schneiderian, transitional cell or Ringertz papilloma.

Incidence

This is by far the most common type of nasal papilloma. Males predominate by a ratio of five to one. Inverted papillomas are rare in people under 21 years of age.

Site

All lesions are derived from the lateral wall of the nose. In some the ethmoid air cells and maxillary antrum are also involved. Most cases are unilateral; bilateral involvement is occasionally seen.

Gross Appearances

Grossly, inverted papillomas appear as multiple mucosal polyps. A more opaque presentation than regular nasal polyps is often claimed, but it must be emphasised that these lesions can be diagnosed with certainty only by microscopical examination.

Inverted papilloma does not grow in the generally accepted fashion of a "papilloma", a benign epithelial neoplasm producing finger-like or verrucous projections from the epithelial surface, but is essentially a polyp-like lesion with a flat surface and internal epithelial changes.

Microscopic Appearances

The histological changes can be summarised as a patchy, severe squamous metaplasia affecting both the respiratory epithelium of the surface of polypoid protruberances of nasal mucosa and submucosa and of the gland ducts, possibly formed by invagination of surface mucosa within these polyps. The stroma shows oedema with marked infiltration of lymphocytes, plasma cells and macrophages, often with lymphoid follicles, which sometimes feature germinal centres. Eosinophil infiltration is also common.

Seromucinous glands, abundant in the normal nasal submucosa, are absent in these polypoid masses. Gland ducts, often branching, are present in the stroma and are markedly affected by squamous metaplasia. The ducts may be present in moderate numbers only, leaving wide areas of stroma. In other cases the ducts with their attendant metaplasia may be very numerous, leaving a sparse stroma. Dilatation of ducts is frequent. Residual respiratory epithelium of the duct lining can be identified in most cases. It is most frequently ciliated, but goblet cell-type respiratory epithelium is also seen.

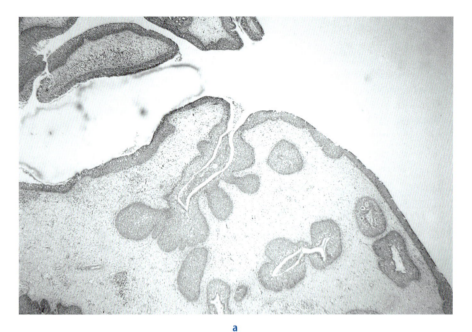

a

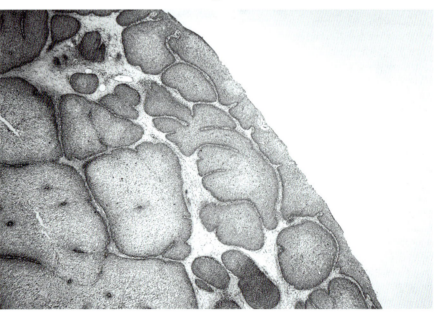

b

Figure 15.2 Inverted papilloma. **a** Squamous metaplasia of a branching duct. **b** More advanced stage of squamous metaplasia showing glycogen formation in stratified squamous epithelium. **c** Zone of squamous metaplasia of a duct showing microcysts. **d** Higher power of **c**

(Figure 15.2 c and d, see opposite)

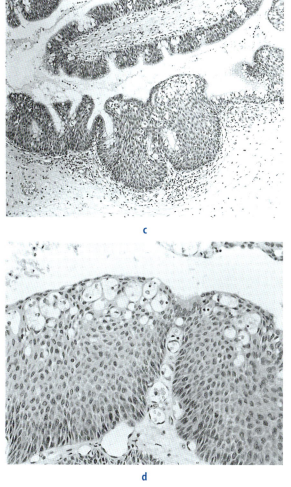

c

d

Figure 15.2 c,d

marked apoptotic activity in the inflammatory cells that accumulate there.

In the region of the microcysts there is an accumulation of basal cells, which focally thickens the deeper portion of the respiratory epithelium. Mitotic figures, often fairly numerous, are present among the proliferated basal cells. Numerous cells in the basal one to three rows show nuclei that express M1B-1.

Adjacent respiratory epithelium without microcysts and basal cell thickening often does not express M1B-1. The proliferated basal cells undergo a progressive epidermoid change with flattening of the superficial cells, the development of intercellular bridges and the formation of surface keratinisation. Keratin squames may fill the lumen of a dilated duct. In some cases glycogen is present in the superficial epidermoid cells. The luminal layer of respiratory epithelium containing microcysts is visible until the squamous metaplastic epithelium, by its growth towards the lumen, eventually replaces it, but leaves the microcysts intact (Fig. 15.2).

No intermediate forms can be recognised between inverted papilloma on the one hand and everted squamous papilloma or cylindric cell papilloma on the other. In sections of inverted papilloma in which there are abundant ducts, the tips of the widened mouths of the ducts sometimes mimic columnar epithelium-lined papillae of cylindric cell papilloma. Similarly, fragmented portions of the walls of ducts may imitate papillae of everted papilloma. Close examination of the whole of the sectioned material in cases with such doubtful areas dispels, however, the possibility that they may be an alternative form of papilloma.

Differential Diagnosis

The histology of a low-grade squamous cell carcinoma of the nose or paranasal sinuses may mimic that of inverted papilloma and cause difficulty in diagnosis. The presence of numerous microcysts in respiratory epithelium in some parts of the material is of value in confirming the diagnosis of inverted papilloma in cases in which most of the metaplastic squamous epithelium shows an advanced stage of epidermoid differentiation. Conversely the absence of any epithelium with microcysts after a careful search of all the biopsy material should cause concern, particularly if the behaviour of the neoplasm has been aggressive, that the diagnosis might be one of low-grade squamous carcinoma (Fig. 15.3). A difficulty that is not overcome by the presence of microcysts is that low-grade squamous carcinoma may be concomitant with inverted papilloma in the same biopsy material.

Phases of the squamous metaplastic process may be observed in different parts of the same specimen, different specimens from the same patient and specimens from different patients. The first phase is the development of numerous microcysts in the respiratory epithelium of both the surface and duct. The microcysts show a maximum diameter of about 30 μm and contain small cells and fragments of degenerated nuclear material. The microcyst contents strongly express PGM-1 (a CD68 macrophage marker that is not expressed by lymphocytes), indicating a composition of macrophages and probably neutrophils in large numbers. Similar cells expressing PGM-1 are also seen in the connective tissue stroma between the ducts. Electron microscopic examination confirms macrophages within microcysts. The cytoplasm of the macrophages contains irregular bodies, some of which appear as myelin figures, others as opaque or granular inclusions. No bacterial or viral organisms are identified. The appearances of the microcyst contents suggest a

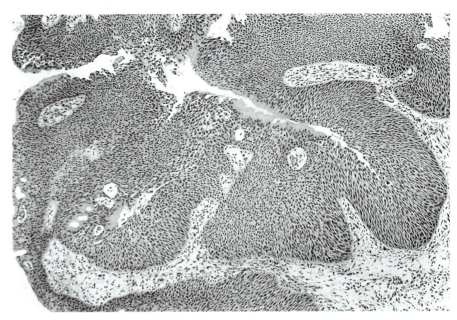

Figure 15.3 Low-grade squamous cell carcinoma of nose and paranasal sinuses. Note the resemblance to inverted papilloma. This neoplasm recurred many times and invaded the base of skull

Lesions of the nose and paranasal sinuses with an inverted papilloma-type histological pattern are distinct from everted papillomas also by their specific site of origin in the lateral wall of the nose and paranasal sinuses, by their strong tendency to recurrence and by their association with a definite incidence of nasal and paranasal sinus malignancy.

Natural History

Inverted papilloma, unlike the everted variety, is a lesion that is subject to recurrence. Complete removal of all of the papilloma-bearing areas at surgery is held by most otolaryngologists to be vital in preventing recurrence. "Development" of carcinoma is very rare, although carcinoma concomitant with inverted papilloma is well recognised (see below).

Histogenesis

The histogenesis of inverted papilloma is usually reported to be one of ingrowth or invagination. It is not possible to determine in the static milieu provided by biopsy material whether the ducts in inverted papilloma are the residua of pre-existing seromucinous glands after atrophy of the terminal acini or whether they are newly formed. It has been suggested that the lesions of inverted papilloma may be the result of squamous metaplasia of pre-existing

ducts.[8] In favour of this concept is the observation that inflammatory nasal polyps also often show loss of seromucinous glands, but gland ducts are retained. Thus the first stage in the development of inverted papilloma may be similar to that of an inflammatory polyp. An interesting suggestion favouring the hypothesis that the duct systems in inverted papilloma are newly formed is the observation that the developing human nasal mucosa shows similar growth patterns to those of inverted papilloma with a system of "asymmetric dichotomy" when developing into the embryonic tissue of the viscerocranium. It was suggested that a built-in tendency to budding of that fashion is lit up in the genesis of inverted papilloma and is responsible for the histological appearance of the inverting papilloma.[9]

Carcinomatous Change

Inverted papilloma has a small but definite association with carcinoma. Carcinoma does not usually develop in the course of the recurrences of inverted papilloma, but may be present in association with the papilloma at the initial presentation. In one series four patients showed the two lesions concomitantly.[10] In another report eight of 112 patients showed carcinoma concomitant with inverted papilloma.[11] The associated malignant neoplasm may be a verrucous carcinoma,[12] but more frequently is a stratified squamous or undifferentiated carcinoma

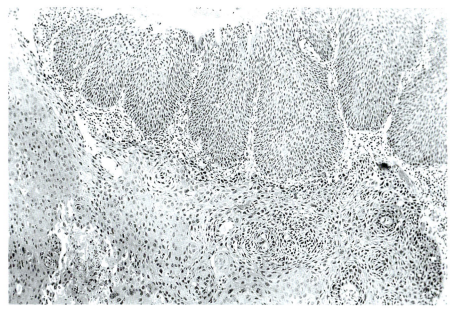

Figure 15.4 Inverted papilloma (*above*) associated with squamous cell carcinoma (*below*)

(Fig. 15.4). Such a malignant association is in contrast to the generally benign behaviour of everted squamous papilloma of the nose.

Aetiology

The difficulty of ascribing an aetiology related to infection with HPV is outlined above. Earlier indications that inverted sinonasal papillomas carry Epstein-Barr virus genomes have not been confirmed.

Cylindric Cell Papilloma

This condition is also known as microcystic papillary adenoma and oncocytic Schneiderian papilloma.

Incidence

Cylindric cell papilloma is less frequent than everted or inverted papilloma. It is found in adults and affects the sexes equally.

Site

Cylindric cell papilloma, in common with inverted papilloma, usually develops in the lateral wall of the nasal cavity and within the maxillary antrum. In some cases it occurs in the maxillary antrum only.

Gross Appearances

Grossly cylindric cell papilloma appears as a diffuse mucosal thickening with a finely granular surface.

Microscopic Appearances

Microscopically cylindric cell papilloma is characterised by thin papillary outgrowths of the nasal mucosa, which often branch to a second or, occasionally, to a third degree. The epithelium is usually deeply crenellated. The glandular appearance that is observed in some areas of this neoplasm is formed by tangential section passing through the region of attachment of the papillary processes to the mucosa. The epithelium is columnar, usually oncocytic. In some cases stunted cilia may be seen on the epithelial surface. Goblet cells are not present. Some individual nuclei of the basal cell layer express M1B-1, but the numbers are fewer than in the metaplastic regions of inverted papilloma and in the basal cells of everted squamous papilloma. Microcysts, often very numerous, containing mucus or nuclear debris are present in the epithelium in each case (Fig. 15.5). The microcysts are larger than the similar structures of inverted papilloma, with a maximum diameter of about 50 μm. Cellular material within microcysts does not express PGM-1 suggesting that it is not composed of macrophages. There is evidence based on the demonstration of secretory component in these cysts by the immunoperoxidase method that they are derived from intracytoplasmic lunina in respiratory epithelial cells rather than goblet cells, since the latter do not produce secretory component.[13] Seromucinous glands and ducts are abundant in the underlying mucosa and submucosa.

No appearances intermediate between this entity and those of inverted and everted papilloma can be identified.

Carcinomatous Change

Like inverted papilloma, the occurrence of cylindric cell papilloma may be related to nasal malignancy,[14]

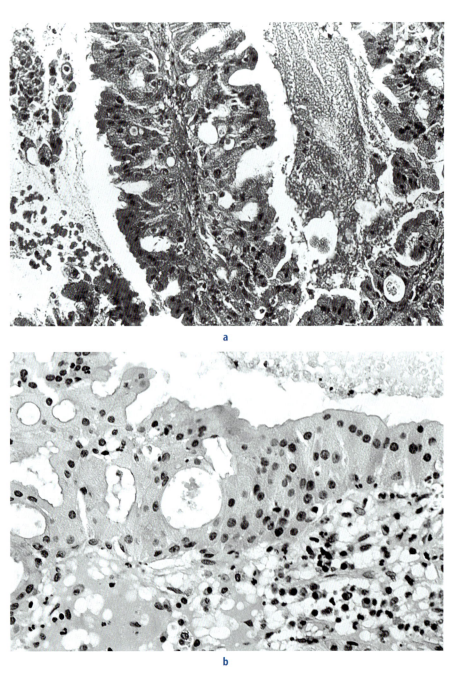

Figure 15.5 Cylindric cell papilloma. **a** Low-power view. **b** High-power view. Note oncocytic epithelium

but the incidence of this form of papilloma is too low to appraise its malignant potential accurately.

References

1. Hyams VJ, Batsakis JG, Michaels L. Tumors of the upper respiratory tract and ear. Atlas of tumor pathology, 2nd series, Fascicle 25. Armed Forces Institute of Pathology, Washington, DC, 1988

2. Michaels L, Young M. Histogenesis of papillomas of the nose and paranasal sinuses. Arch Pathol Lab Med 1995;119:821–826

3. Weber RS, Shillitoe EJ, Robbins KT et al. Prevalence of human papillomavirus in inverted nasal papillomas. Arch Otolaryngol Head Neck Surg 1988;114:23–26

4. Furata Y, Shinohara T, Sano K et al. Molecular pathologic study of human papillomavirus infection in inverted papilloma and squamous cell carcinoma of the nasal cavities and paranasal sinuses. Laryngoscope 1991;10:79–85

5. Judd R, Zaki SR, Coffield LM et al. Sinonasal papillomas and human papillomavirus – human papillomavirus 11 detected in fungiform Schneiderian papillomas by in situ hybridization and the polymerase chain reaction. Human Pathol 1991;22:550–556

6. Fu YS, Hoover L, Franklin M et al. Human papillomavirus identified by nucleic acid hybridization in concomitant nasal and genital papillomas. Laryngoscope 1992;102 :1014–1019

7. Buchwald C, Franzmann MB, Jacobsen GK et al. Human papillomavirus (HPV) in sinonasal papillomas: a study of 78 cases using in situ hybridization and polymerase chain reaction. Laryngoscope 1995;105:66–71

8. Oberman HA. Papillomas of the nose and paranasal sinuses. Am J Clin Pathol 1964;42:245–258

9. Stammberger H. Neue Aspekte zur Genese des Invertierten Papilloms. Laryngol Rhinol Otol (Stuttg) 1983;62:249–255

10. Woodson GE, Robbins KT, Michaels L. Inverted papilloma. Considerations in treatment. Arch Otolaryngol 1985;111:806–811

11. Phillips PP, Gustafson RO, Facer GW. The clinical behavior of inverting papilloma of the nose and paranasal sinuses: report of 112 cases and review of the literature. Laryngoscope 1990;100:468–469

12. Orvidas LJ, Lewis JE, Olsen KD et al. Intranasal verrucous carcinoma: relationship to inverting papilloma and human papillomavirus. Laryngoscope 1999;109:371–375

13. Krisch I, Neuhold N, Krisch K. Demonstration of secretory component, IgA and IgM by the peroxidase-antiperoxidase technique in inverted papillomas of the nasal cavity. Human Pathology 1984;15:915–920

14. Ward BE, Fechner RE, Mills SE. Carcinoma arising in oncocytic Schneiderian papilloma. Am J Surg Pathol 1990;14:364–369

16 Malignant Neoplasms of Surface Epithelium

Squamous Cell Carcinoma of Nasal Vestibule

Squamous cell carcinoma, although rare, is the commonest malignant neoplasm of the nasal vestibule, which is a region covered by modified hair-bearing skin. The other two important malignant neoplasms of the skin, malignant melanoma and basal cell carcinoma, also occur here, but with less frequency.

Incidence

Most of the patients with this neoplasm are males, in the ratio of 4:1, and are over 60 years of age.[1]

Gross Appearances

The lesion is usually situated on the anterior septum and columella where it appears as an irregular, raised, granular and partly ulcerated plaque.

Microscopic Appearances

In most cases the neoplasm is a keratinising, well-differentiated squamous carcinoma. The presence of papillae may cause difficulty in differentiating the tumour from squamous papilloma. As mentioned in Chapter 15, squamous papillomas of the nasal vestibule frequently show epithelial abnormalities and attention should be paid particularly to the overall pattern in diagnosing squamous carcinoma, i.e. irregularity of both rete pegs and papillary for-mations favouring malignancy. If the general pattern is regular, great care is needed in opting for a malignant condition. Keratoacanthoma may also cause some difficulty. Diagnosis of this lesion is based on the presence of a regular cup-shape proliferation of squamous cell epithelium containing keratin.

Spread

Invasion of the skin below the columella, the upper lip and the anterior floor of the nose, including the bone in this situation, is prone to occur. When such invasion takes place, concomitant cervical lymph node metastasis is likely and this can be homolateral or bilateral. The standard treatments of irradiation or surgery are both effective in the early stages of this cancer. A recent study has shown that radiation therapy alone results in a high cure rate of early cases with good cosmesis; patients with large T4 cancers have better results and higher cure rates with radiation and surgery, but more complications.[2]

Squamous Cell Carcinoma of Mucosae

Squamous carcinoma of the mucosae of the nose and paranasal sinuses is a rare neoplasm, but again is the commonest malignant tumour of that region. It probably represents less than 1% of all malignant neoplasms. The mucosae of the nose and paranasal sinuses comprise a freely intercommunicating system of spaces lined by respiratory epithelium. Malignant change tends to affect the mucosae of several parts of the system at the same time; it is unusual for the neoplasm to be confined to one part of the sinonasal system.

Incidence

Squamous cell carcinoma is the most common malignant sinonasal tumour and comprises between 45 and 50% of these malignancies.[3,4] There is a slight male predominance, and although most patients are elderly, sinonasal squamous cell carcinoma may occur in children.

Occupational Relationships

An occupational basis for the origin of squamous carcinoma of the nose and paranasal sinuses has been suggested for boot and shoe industry workers, chromate workers, workers exposed to flour dust and textile workers, but is most certain in relation to workers in the nickel refinery industry. Carcinoma induced in both bronchi and nasal passages in nickel refinery workers is related to industrial handling of nickel carbonyl (NiCo), nickel oxide (NiO), nickel sulphide (NiS) and possibly other nickel-containing substances. The histopathology of nickel carcinogenosis has been particularly well studied in Norway. Ninety-one nickel-exposed workers in Vest Agder, Norway, were submitted to biopsy of the mucosa in the region of the anterior tip of the middle turbinate and the hiatus semilunaris. Varying degrees of atypical change in the epithelium were detected in 72 of the group who had no symptoms and no X-ray changes and one was found to have invasive squamous carcinoma. The other 19 nickel workers had symptoms or X-ray changes: all had atypical change in the epithelium and three had invasive squamous carcinoma.[5,6]

Later studies have confirmed nickel to be carcinogenic, although a weak carcinogen and with a long latency period, but not one as long as for sinonasal adenocarcinoma in patients exposed to hardwood dust[7] (see below). In a later study 100 malignant sinonasal tumours were reported in nickel refinery workers; 48% of these malignancies were squamous cell carcinomas, the others comprising undifferentiated or anaplastic carcinomas.[8] Workers exposed to chromium are known to have a fairly high risk of developing lung carcinoma, and also the risk for sinonasal squamous cell carcinoma appears to be increased. Industrial exposure to organic solvents is well known to have neurotoxic effects, and can damage the nasal olfactory mucosa, but no carcinogenic effect on the sinonasal mucosa has been proven. Tobacco is well known to be a lung carcinogen, and a number of studies also indicate a carcinogenic effect of tobacco use on the sinonasal mucosa. Interestingly, there seems to be a synergistic effect with several other agents. For example, tobacco-smoking workers exposed to nickel, workers exposed to fumes from welding and workers exposed to wood dust show an increased risk for the development of sinonasal squamous cell carcinoma compared with non-smoking workers.

Clinical Features

Although the neoplasm is usually widespread in the nose and paranasal sinuses, a more localised origin is sometimes seen. If this is in the nasal cavity the symptom of nasal obstruction draws early attention to the growth. The neoplasm may originate in some cases only at the anterior tip of the middle turbinate, but almost certainly arises in other cases from a wider field of sinonasal epithelium and it is from that wider area that deeper invasion takes place. Lymph node involvement is infrequent if the neoplasm is confined to the nasal cavity and overall 5-year survival is as high as 56%.[9] In carcinoma confined to the maxillary sinus, on the other hand, the early symptoms of pain and swelling of the cheek are usually attributed to sinusitis and it is often not until the onset of orodental and eye symptoms, produced by spread of the growth to these regions, that the cancerous nature of the illness is manifested. The 5-year cure rate, in unselected series, hardly exceeds 25%.[10]

Gross Appearances

In most cases the growth involves the antral wall of the nose, the maxillary antrum and many of the ethmoid air cells. The frontal and sphenoidal sinuses are rarely affected. Spread of the neoplasm through bone to orbit, cranial cavity, oral cavity and zygoma is frequent. The neoplasm appears as a friable and papillary thickening of the mucosa, often with ulceration of the surface. The maxillary antrum becomes filled with tumour, producing a yellowish-grey mass in that location.

Microscopic Appearances

In 80–85% of cases the neoplasm shows keratinisation, i.e. it is "well" or "moderately well" differentiated. Some well-differentiated but non-keratinising carcinomas have been described as cylindric cell carcinoma or transitional cell carcinoma (see below).

Regions of carcinoma in situ may be seen at the edge of the invasive carcinoma and are sometimes present in biopsy material without invasive carcinoma. Carcinoma in situ may sometimes be seen in inverted papillomas as a manifestation of malignant change (see Chapter 15). Apart from this, carcinoma in situ is rare in the nasal cavity and paranasal sinuses. When present, a careful search for concomitant invasive carcinoma should be carried out (Figs 16.1, 16.2).

Verrucous Squamous Cell Carcinoma

Verrucous squamous carcinoma is rare in the sinonasal tract. It is likely that cases in which biopsy appearances suggest this entity will show less well-differentiated, conventional squamous carcinoma in other parts of the neoplasm (see Chapter 36).

Spindle Cell Carcinoma

Spindle cell carcinoma is a squamous cell carcinoma at the other extreme of the spectrum of differentiation and is also rare in the nose and paranasal sinuses. A definite diagnosis of this entity can only be made if squamous carcinoma in situ or invasive squamous cell carcinoma is present as well as the undifferentiated, malignant spindle cell tissue (Fig. 16.3) (see Chapter 36).

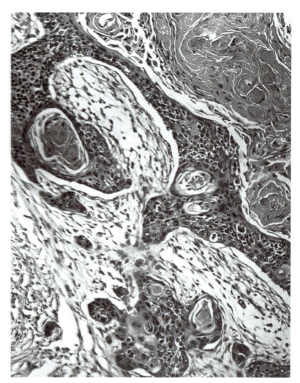

Figure 16.2 Squamous carcinoma of the nose and paranasal sinuses, which is highly keratinising

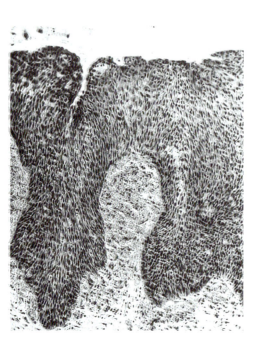

Figure 16.1 Carcinoma in situ of the nasal epithelium. The whole epithelium is replaced by malignant cells and there is hyperplasia without invasion

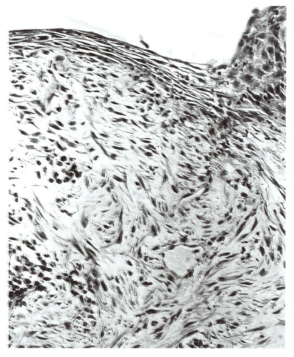

Figure 16.3 Spindle cell carcinoma of the maxillary antrum. The overlying squamous epithelium shows many cells of spindle shape, which seem to give origin to the spindle cells of the underlying tumour

Basaloid Squamous Cell Carcinoma

This a high-grade, aggressive variant of squamous cell carcinoma, morphologically characterised by mixed basaloid and squamous components. This bimorphic carcinoma has a predeliction for the hypopharynx and base of tongue, but is also found in the larynx and oral cavity. Very rarely it has been described in the sinonasal tract, but a recent study reports 14 cases of such an entity.[11] The gross and microscopic appearances of basaloid squamous cell carcinoma are described in Chapter 36.

Spread

Cervical lymph nodes are involved in 17.6% of squamous cell carcinomas of the nose and paranasal sinuses. Disseminated metastases have been found in only 1.6% of all malignant neoplasms in that location.[12]

Cylindric Cell Carcinoma

As mentioned above, the majority of the malignant neoplasms derived from the respiratory epithelium of the nose are of the stratified squamous cell variety. The development of an epidermoid neoplasm in this region is related not only to the tendency that benign respiratory epithelium has to undergo squamous metaplasia, but also to the propensity of the undifferentiated basal cells of respiratory epithelium to produce malignant cells differentiated in an epidermoid direction even without prior benign squamous metaplasia.

There is another malignant neoplasm that is derived from the respiratory epithelium of the nose and paranasal sinuses. This was called cylindric cell carcinoma in the older literature, but designated more recently, with other tumours, as "transitional" carcinoma. The term "transitional epithelium" has been used to designate an upper respiratory epithelium that is intermediate between respiratory and epidermoid epithelium. The carcinomatous form of the latter is a vague expression that has been used to mean a variety of carcinomas with no differentiation. We believe that the use of the designation "transitional" as a description of either non-neoplastic or neoplastic epithelia in this situation is unsatisfactory and that the older term of "cylindric cell" should be restored for the appropriate neoplasms and, indeed, the WHO classification has done this.[13]

Some of the carcinomas of the nose and paranasal sinuses show no differentiation whatsoever and are composed of cells of primitive appearance. In classifying such neoplasms, the nomenclature applicable to tumours of the nasopharynx should be extended to cover tumours of the nose and paranasal sinuses. A carcinoma with a stratified arrangement of well-defined tumour cells, but without keratinisation and without "prickles", is referred to as non-keratinising carcinoma. If the tumour cells have vesicular nuclei and a syncytial rather than pavemented appearance, resembling the corresponding tumour of the nasopharynx, the neoplasm is referred to as undifferentiated (see Chapter 24).

Cylindric cell carcinoma is a neoplasm with characteristic histological appearances. It was well defined in the older literature, which was summarised by Ringertz,[14] who also provided a careful description of his own experience with this cancer. The literature subsequent to Ringertz's account is, however, silent on this entity.

Although the respiratory epithelium of the nose resembles that of the larynx and lower respiratory tract microscopically, its development is from ectoderm, while the latter is derived from entoderm. It would be expected that the nasal (Schneiderian) epithelium would have distinct attributes, particularly in its neoplastic form. Cylindric cell carcinoma is a tumour that is hardly ever found outside the nose and paranasal sinuses.

Incidence

Ringertz[14] gave an age range of 18–80 years with an average of 60 years. Males and females in his series were equally affected.

Site

The site of origin of this neoplasm is similar to that of squamous carcinoma of the nose and paranasal sinuses, i.e. from the lateral wall of the nose, ethmoidal air cells and maxillary antrum. In most cases the origin of the growth is from all three regions.

Clinical Features

The clinical features are similar to those of squamous cell carcinoma of the nose and paranasal sinuses. Ringertz distinguishes two types of clinical onset for this neoplasm. In the first, symptoms suggestive of neoplasm, such as purulent discharge and bleeding, are present from the start. In the second there is a long period of up to 20 years of symptoms suggestive of sinusitis, leading eventually to a clinical picture more typical for a malignant neoplasm of the nose.

Gross Appearances

Cylindric cell carcinoma has a tendency to exophytic growth from the mucosae of the nose and paranasal sinuses, producing protuberant areas with both papillary, i.e. finely corrugated, and polypoid, i.e. smooth-surfaced appearances. Areas recognisable as oedematous nasal polyps may also be seen accompanying neoplastic formations, the latter being rougher and more friable in consistency. The maxillary antrum may be filled with solid yellowish-grey neoplasm. In most cases areas of bone invasion and destruction affecting particularly the maxillary bone are observed.

Microscopic Appearances

The neoplasm is made up of interconnecting ribbons of tumour cells, which, in some parts, appear to be invaginated from the surface epithelium. In some of the latter a double layer enclosing a space (representing the invaginated crypt) can be recognised. Knob-like proliferations into some of the crypts are present. In other areas the invaginations are filled up into solid columns. A further stage in some neoplasms is the confluence of the tumour columns. The stroma, which was external to the invaginations, now appears as isolated zones. In a few cases there is necrosis of tumour cells distant from the stromal zones.

The surface of the tumour shows papillary formations and is covered by malignant cylindric cell epithelium.

The cells of the neoplasm are, for the most part, cylindrical, being set at right angles to the basement membrane on which they rest. Several layers of cells are present, the inner cells (i.e. those furthest from the basement membrane) sometimes being more rounded. The degree of nuclear atypia is variable, ranging from mild to severe. Mitoses are usually scarce. A transition from malignant cylindric cell epithelium to normal epithelium may sometimes be recognised. Foci of malignant squamous metaplasia are frequently present. This may be so widespread that the cylindric cell origin of the neoplastic cells is not recognised and the growth may be considered a squamous cell carcinoma (Fig. 16.4).

Differential Diagnosis

Cylindric cell carcinoma may be difficult to distinguish from:

1. Adenocarcinoma: the origin of double-layered ribbons of non-glandular cells from surface crypts is in favour of cylindric cell carcinoma.

2. Malignant melanoma (non-pigmented): in malignant melanoma the cells are more polygonal, have prominent nucleoli and stain positively for the S-100 protein and HMB-45 antigens using the immunohistochemical staining reaction.

3. Ameloblastoma: this sometimes also involves the nose (see Chapter 22). A correct diagnosis is

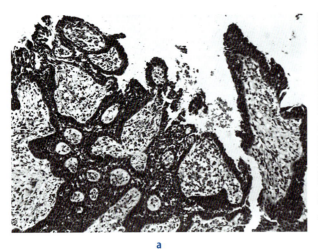
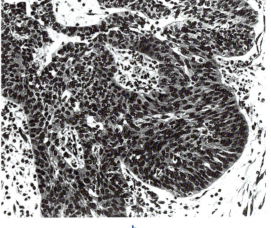

a   b

Figure 16.4 Cylindric cell carcinoma. **a** The surface is covered by malignant cylindric cell epithelium and shows some papillae of this epithelium. The tumour is made up of invaginated ribbons of malignant cylindric cells. **b** Higher power view showing ribbons of tumour lined by cylindric cells aligned at right angles to the basement membrane

made by observation that some of the cell masses in ameloblastoma show an enamel organ-like, plexiform structure of epithelial cells.

4. Squamous cell carcinoma: the difficulty of distinguishing cylindric cell from squamous cell carcinoma has been discussed above.

5. Inverted papilloma of the nose (see Chapter 15): this is the most frequent source of misinterpretation, the invading festoons of growth in the malignant condition being mistaken for the sinus-like inversions of the benign one. In inverted papilloma the heaped-up epithelium which lines the sinus-like structures does not usually show atypical change and zones of normal ciliated epthelium are interspersed.

Spread

Lymph node metastasis to the cervical region is common. A frequent termination of the clinical course is by metastases to the lung and other organs. Metastatic cervical masses produced by this tumour may have a tendency for venous invasion involving the internal jugular vein.

Natural History

The natural history of cylindric cell carcinoma appears to be similar to that of squamous cell carcinoma, but further observation is required to determine possibly distinctive forms of behaviour possessed by this tumour.

References

1. Kagan AR, Nussbaum H, Rao A et al. The management of carcinoma of the nasal vestibule. Head Neck Surg 1981;4:125–128
2. Mendenhall WM, Stringer SP, Cassisi NJ et al. Squamous cell carcinoma of the nasal vestibule. Head Neck 1999;21:385–393
3. Gadeberg CC, Hjelm-Hansen M, Sögaard H et al. Malignant tumors of the paranasal sinuses and nasal cavity. A series of 180 patients. Acta Radiol Oncol 1984;23:181–187
4. Tufano RP, Mokadam NA, Montone KT et al. Malignant tumors of the nose and paranasal sinuses: hospital of the University of Pennsylvania experience 1990–1997. Am J Rhinol 1999;13:117–123
5. Torjussen W, Solberg LA. Clinical and histological investigation of nasal mucosa in nickel workers. Acta Otolaryngol (Stockh) 1976;82:266–267
6. Torjussen W, Haug FM, Olsen A et al. Concentration and distribution of heavy metals in nasal mucosa of nickel-exposed workers and of controls, studied with atomic absorption spectrophotometric analysis and with Timm's sulphide silver method. Acta Otolaryngol (Stockh) 1977;86:449–463
7. Torjussen W, Solberg LA. Clinical and histological investigation of nasal mucosa in nickel workers. Acta Otolaryngol (Stockh) 1976;82:266–267
8. Sunderman FW Jr, Morgan LC, Andersen A et al. Histopathology of sinonasal and lung cancers in nickel refinery workers. Ann Clin Lab Sci 1989;19:44–50
9. Bosch A, Vallecillo L, Frias Z. Cancer of the nasal cavity. Cancer 1976;37:1458–1463
10. Larsson LG, Mårtensson G. Maxillary antral cancers. JAMA 1972;219:342–345
11. Wieneke JA, Thompson LD, Wenig BM. Basaloid squamous cell carcinoma of the sinonasal tract. Cancer 1999;85:841–854
12. Robin PE, Powell DJ. Regional node involvement and distant metastases in carcinoma of the nasal cavity and paranasal sinuses. J Laryngol Otol 1980;94:301–309
13. Shanmugaratnam K. Histological typing of tumors of the upper respiratory tract and ear, 2nd edn. Springer-Verlag, Berlin, 1991
14. Ringertz N. Pathology of malignant tumors arising in the nasal and paranasal cavities and maxilla. Acta Otolaryngol (Stockh) 1938;27(suppl):1–405

17 Non-epidermoid Epithelial Neoplasms

Most cases of carcinoma of the nasal cavity and paranasal sinuses – a rare entity – are of epidermoid type so that the numbers of non-epidermoid carcinomas are very small indeed. Sinonasal adenocarcinomas are primarily of two types, one originating from the surface epithelium and the other from mucosal seromucinous glands (most of the latter being salivary gland adenocarcinomas of different types). The exact incidence of each of these types of sinonasal adenocarcinomas is extremely difficult to access as almost every report on the subject has made no distinction between adenocarcinoma from surface epithelium and seromucinous gland adenocarcinomas (apart from adenoid cystic carcinoma). However, one can estimate sinonasal adenocarcinomas to represent from 6% to 13% of sinonasal malignancies.[1,2]

Sinonasal adenocarcinomas are derived from (1) columnar cells of surface origin, (2) ductal and acinar cells of seromucinous glands or (3) myoepithelial cells associated with the latter (Table 17.1). The latter two cells of origin produce tumours that have a homology with salivary gland neoplasms (see Chapters 40–43). Confusion may arise with well-differentiated primary sinonasal neuroendocrine carcinomas that have a glandular structure (see Chapter 18). On rare occasions adenocarcinomas of the sinonasal tract are metastatic, e.g. from the breast, gastrointestinal tract, lung, kidney, etc., which may also cause diagnostic problems. The sole benign neoplasm of surface respiratory epithelium, the papilloma, has been described in detail in Chapter 15.

Sinonasal Adenocarcinoma

The term adenocarcinoma covers a group of neoplasms composed of glandular structures with a range of patterns. By sinonasal adenocarcinoma is meant an adenocarcinoma that cannot readily be categorised as any type of salivary gland adenocarcinoma (Table 17.1 and Chapter 42). On morphological grounds these tumours can be divided into three major types:[3]

1. Adenocarcinoma – of low-grade and high-grade malignancy.
2. Papillary adenocarcinoma – always low-grade and with typical morphology.
3. Intestinal-type adenocarcinoma (colonic type, mucinous) – always of high-grade malignancy.

Sex and Age Incidence

High-grade adenocarcinomas have a male predominance; the incidence in low-grade tumours tends to

Table 17.1. Non-epidermoid epithelial tumours of the nose and paranasal sinuses

Cells of origin	Neoplasm
Surface columnar	Papilloma Low- and high-grade adenocarcinoma Papillary adenocarcinoma Intestinal-type adenocarcinoma
Seromucinous glands: ductal and acinar cells	Low- and high-grade adenocarcinoma Acinic cell carcinoma Mucoepidermoid carcinoma Basal cell adenoma Oncocytoma
Participation of myoepithelial cells	Adenoid cystic carcinoma Pleomorphic adenoma Myoepithelioma Polymorphous low-grade adenocarcinoma Carcinoma ex pleomorphic adenoma

be similar between the sexes.[4] The peak age is in the sixth and seventh decades, but sinonasal adenocarcinomas are also seen in children.

Site

Adenocarcinomas arise much more frequently in the sinuses than in the nasal cavity. When in the nose they tend to arise high in the nasal cavity and rarely on the septum.

Gross Appearances

In some cases the lesion is exophytic, producing a localised granular swelling, which histologically is usually of a papillary appearance. In others the tumour is deeply infiltrating and grossly represented by a pale grey mass extending widely through the bony walls of the nose and sinuses.

Microscopic Appearances

Adenocarcinoma

Low-grade sinonasal adenocarcinomas are typically composed of uniform small glands lined by regular columnar cells with rare mitotic figures (Fig. 17.1). The columnar cells may be cuboidal in certain areas. The cells have oval or round nuclei, inconspicuous nucleoli and minimal cytological atypia. The glandular elements often show back-to-back patterns, and may show areas with cells having rather eosinophilic cytoplasm. In certain less typical low-grade adenocarcinomas, the structure can be pronounced tubular, or trabecular, microcystic or partly papillary. The degree of cytological atypicism is still minimal, and there are few mitoses. Particularly when the low-grade adenocarcinoma shows a tubular pattern it can be confused with pleomorphic adenoma, and when papillary structures are present, cylindric cell papilloma can be erroneously diagnosed.

High-grade sinonasal adenocarcinomas are more readily diagnosed and confusion with benign tumours is not likely. Microscopically they are similar to the common variety of adenocarcinomas, being composed of irregular glandular structures, with trabeculae or solid sheets of cells. Nuclear atypia and pleomorphism are marked and there are numerous mitotic figures. Hence the morphology is one of adenocarcinoma but without a resemblance to typical colorectal adenocarcinoma (see below).

Papillary Adenocarcinoma

This sinonasal adenocarcinoma of low-grade malignancy has a characteristic appearance. It is typically continuous with the surface epithelium and is composed of complex papillary fronds. There are rather closely packed glandular structures lined by columnar, or pseudostratified, cells with nuclei that tend to be vesicular (Fig. 17.2). The cytoplasm is eosinophilic containing mucin. The tumour is typi-

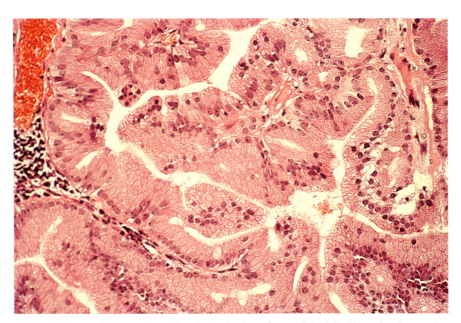

Figure 17.1 Low-grade adenocarcinoma of nasal cavity showing uniform small glands lined by regular columnar cells

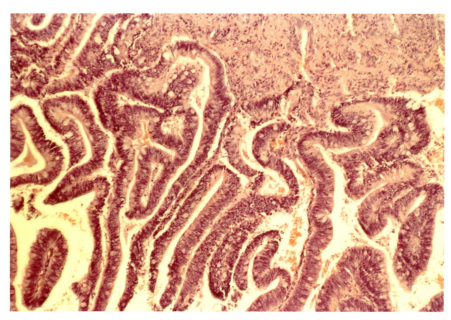

Figure 17.2 Papillary adenocarcinoma of nasal cavity showing closely packed complex papillary fronds

cally superficial but invasion into the mucosa is always seen. Low-grade adenocarcinomas (see above) may have areas with papillary structures, but never show the complexity of the papillae and the typical superficial nature typical of the papillary adenocarcinoma.

Intestinal-type Adenocarcinoma

Intestinal-type, or colonic-type, mucinous, adeno-carcinoma is a tumour with features resembling colorectal carcinoma. It is composed of columnar mucin-secreting cells displaying different growth patterns. The structure can be predominantly papillary, glandular or mucinous. Argentaffin cells and Paneth cells may be present. Often a substantial part of the tumour is occupied by dilated mucin-filled glands, and the resemblance to colorectal adenocarcinoma is striking. The cytologic atypia is pronounced, and there are numerous mitoses as well as frequent areas of necrosis (Fig. 17.3). Intestinal-type sinonasal adenocarcinoma grows aggressively and has a poor prognosis. Naturally the possibility of metastasis from gastrointestinal carcinomas has to be ruled out before the diagnosis of intestinal-type sinonasal adenocarcinoma can be made.

Amplification and/or overexpression of the *c-erbB-2* gene has been described with a prognostic significance in several human adenocarcinomas, breast carcinomas and salivary duct carcinomas in particular. A study of 28 sinonasal intestinal-type adenocarcinomas showed 32% to express the c-

erbB-2 oncoprotein, indicating that activation of the *c-erbB-2* oncogene could be involved in oncogenesis of this particular sinonasal adenocarcinoma.[5]

Atypical Changes in Adjacent Non-neoplastic Epithelium

An alteration described as "cuboidal metaplasia" (a hyperplasia of respiratory epithelium) was reported in the non-neoplastic areas of epithelium, in 19 of 22 woodworkers' adenocarcinomas.[6] Sixteen of these 19 cases showed atypical as well as hyperplastic respiratory epithelium, often in continuity with the tumour. It is possible that these changes may signify the commencement of adenocarcinoma in nasal epithelium.

Relationship to Wood Dust

Early mention of toxic reactions of the respiratory tract to wood dust was made in 1964 at Olomouc, Czechoslovakia. This study was mainly of dermatological conditions, but the authors stated that nasal manifestations, including pronounced coryza and nasal polyps, may also result from heavy wood dust inhalation.[7] In 1967 particles of wood dust were described in relation to centrilobular emphysema in the lungs of woodworkers.[8] An association between occupational exposure to wood dust and adenocarcinoma of the nose and sinuses was first reported from the High Wycombe area of England, where this

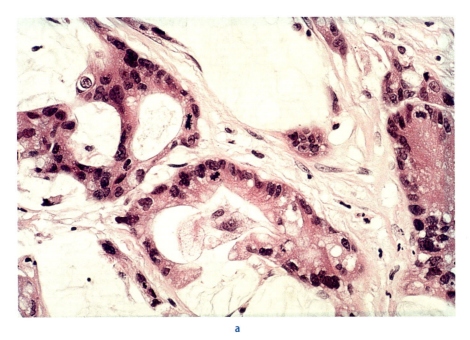

a

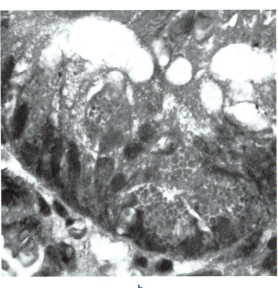

b

Figure 17.3 Intestinal type adenocarcinoma. **a** Columnar mucin-secreting cells form glands in a background of mucus. **b** Cells showing large granules, which are eosinophilic in the original, are present in this nasal tumour. The appearances are suggestive of Paneth cells

disease was found to be 500 times more common among wood furniture workers than in the general population.[9,10] This association has now also been reported from many other countries, all reports agreeing that it is hard wood dust, such as that of beech and oak, rather than soft, such as that of pine, that is carcinogenic and that the characteristic neoplasm seen in the woodworkers is adenocarcinoma.

Both low- and high-grade forms of adenocarcinoma are found in woodworkers; the tumours are all

of the type found in the gastrointestinal tract, with a detailed subgrouping into the following:[11,12]

1. Cylindrical cells with a papillary tubular structure.

2. Alveolar goblet cell carcinomas with much mucus secretion.

3. Carcinomas of the signet ring-type cells.

In a series of 16 patients occupationally exposed to wood dust and with developed sinonasal adenocarcinomas, three mutations were found of the *K-ras* gene (point mutations at codons 12 and 13); all being G:C→A:T mutations, indicating a possible genotoxic agent in wood dust.[13] In a study of a large series of woodworkers' adenocarcinomas, the great majority, 77%, were located in ethmoidal sinuses.[14]

Natural History

The behaviour of adenocarcinoma is closely related to whether it is of low or high grade. Two of the 23 patients with low-grade adenocarcinoma in the series of Heffner et al.[4] died of recurrence and five others had incurable recurrences. In the high-grade group of that series, on the other hand, most of the patients were dead of the neoplasm within 3 years of the date of initial treatment. Metastasis is infrequent in adenocarcinoma of the nose and sinuses; when it occurs it is usually of bloodstream type. Lymph node metastasis is rare.[15]

There have also been attempts to evaluate the prognostic value of further histological typing of intestinal-type adenocarcinoma into well, moderately and poorly differentiated, and mucinous adenocarcinomas. Patients with poorly differentiated and mucinous adenocarcinomas showed a significantly shorter disease-free interval and survival rate.[16]

Pleomorphic Adenoma

Pleomorphic adenoma is a benign neoplasm with a mixed pattern combining epithelial and mesenchymal elements. It is generally believed that the latter stem from myoepithelial cells. While it is the commonest tumour of the parotid gland, it occurs but seldom in the nose and paranasal sinuses.

Incidence

The only large series in world literature has been collected by Compagno and Wong,[17] who reviewed 40 cases of sinonasal pleomorphic adenoma referred to the Armed Forces Institute of Pathology on a consultative basis from 1949 to 1974. The ages of these patients ranged from 3 to 82 years with median and mean both of 42 years. This series comprised 23 females and 17 males, which is in contrast to the more striking female preponderance of pleomorphic adenoma affecting major salivary glands (see Chapter 41).

Site

Most nasal pleomorphic adenomas arise on the septum. Smaller numbers present on the lateral wall of the nose and even more unusual is the presentation of such a tumour in the mucosa of the maxillary antrum.

Gross Appearances

Pleomorphic adenomas are usually well demarcated with smooth, lobulated surfaces. Their cut surfaces are greyish and usually homogeneous with a somewhat translucent appearance.

Microscopic Appearances

Both epithelial and mesenchymal formations of neoplastic cells should be present to allow a definite histological diagnosis of this entity. Epithelium is more prominent in nasal pleomorphic adenomas than in those tumours occurring in major salivary glands. The epithelial structures are mainly regular glands, often with secretion in their lumina. Areas of epidermoid cells are more prominent in nasal pleomorphic adenomas than in those seen elsewhere. The most usual mesenchymal feature in pleomorphic adenomas is the filling of interglandular regions with loosely arranged, short spindle cells that appear to be in contiguity with and of similar structure to epithelial cells lining glands (Fig. 17.4). Mucoid, myxoid and chondroid areas may also be present in which spindle cells of similar appearance are lodged within the particular ground substance. A fibrous

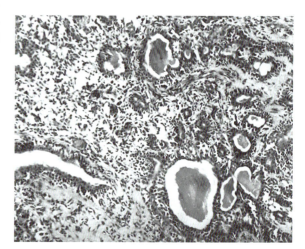

Figure 17.4 Pleomorphic adenoma of the nasal cavity. There are regular glands containing secretion. The interglandular areas show loosely arranged spindle cells that appear to be in contiguity with the cells lining the glands

capsule may sometimes be identified, but is not usually so well defined as in the corresponding tumour of major salivary glands.

Treatment

This benign neoplasm is not expected to show aggressive behaviour. The treatment required is careful and complete excision; radical operative procedures are not indicated. If carefully excised, recurrence is not expected. In the series reported by Compagno and Wong,[17] only 3 of the 31 cases that were followed up for between 1 and 41 years recurred, and in each of these the growth was surgically controlled.

Carcinoma ex Pleomorphic Adenoma and Malignant Mixed Tumour

Carcinoma ex pleomorphic adenoma is an entity in which a malignant epithelial neoplasm, e.g. adenocarcinoma or mucoepidermoid carcinoma, arises in a benign pleomorphic adenoma (see Chapter 42). Malignant mixed tumour, on the other hand, is a lesion in which both epithelial and mesenchymal malignancies develop in a pleomorphic adenoma, and is thus a form of carcinosarcoma. Neither lesion is reported in the nose or paranasal sinuses in the series of Compagno and Wong.[17] We have not seen carcinoma ex pleomorphic adenoma arising in the nose or paranasal sinuses, but have encountered a case of malignant mixed tumour of the maxillary antrum. In this patient there was massive invasion by the neoplasm through the bones of the skull (see Chapter 42).

Oncocytoma

Oncocytoma is a benign epithelial tumour consisting of large cells with granular eosinophilic cytoplasm. The oncocytic nature of the lesion is confirmed on electron microscopy when the cytoplasm of the tumour cells is found to be tightly packed with large, often abnormal, mitochondria.[18] We have seen only a single case of such a lesion in a 70-year-old man. The tumour was situated in the nose, antrum and ethmoid air cells (Fig. 17.5). No recurrence has taken place in more than 15 years of follow-up.

Acinic Cell Carcinoma

Acinic cell carcinoma is unusual in major salivary glands and rare in the nose and paranasal sinuses. In a reported case the tumour arose from the inferior turbinate with no radiological evidence of bone destruction.[19] Histologically there were nests of cells showing acinar and trabecular structure. Most tumour cells contained periodic acid–Schiff-positive, diastase-resistant granules. On transmission electron microscopy these were large and varied in density. The nuclei of the tumour cells were basally placed and formed rows in a regimented fashion. These features are typical of acinic cell carcinoma as seen in major salivary glands (Fig. 17.6). Areas of clear cell appearance due to loss of granules during processing may be found in this neoplasm (see Chapter 42).

Clear Cell Carcinoma

Carcinomas formed by cells of clear cytoplasm, which stain negatively for mucin, are occasionally seen in the nose and paranasal sinuses (Fig. 17.7). Some of these are acinic cell carcinomas with areas where a clear cell appearance is produced as a result of an artefact in processing the tissue. In others periodic acid–Schiff-positive granular cells cannot be found in any part of the neoplasm, so these cases cannot be considered to be acinic cell carcinomas. Glycogen may or may not be present in the clear cytoplasm of the tumour. A locally aggressive behaviour of this lesion with low potential for metastasis is to be expected.

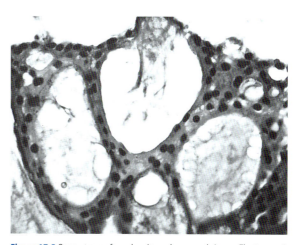

Figure 17.5 Oncocytoma of nasal cavity and paranasal sinuses. The tumour is composed of regular, large cells with granular cytoplasm, eosinophilic in the original

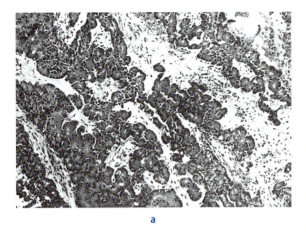
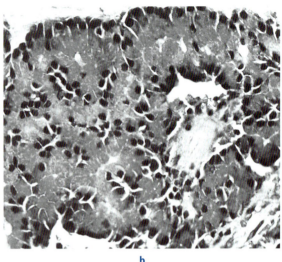

Figure 17.6 Acinic cell carcinoma of nasal cavity. **a** The tumour is composed of small regular acini. **b** Higher power of tumour shown in **a**. The tumour cells contain basophilic granules in their cytoplasm and basally placed nuclei

In each case in which a clear cell carcinoma is seen, the possibility of a metastatic deposit from clear cell carcinoma of the kidney must be considered. The kidney tumour shows cytoplasmic lipid as well as glycogen in the tumour cells and exhibits considerable vascularity (see Chapter 22).

Clear cell tumour, or carcinoma, is not a diagnostic category, but a description of one or several salivary gland neoplasms or tumour-like lesions characterised by a significant population of cells possessing clear cytoplasm (See Chapter 43).

Adenoid Cystic Carcinoma

Adenoid cystic carcinoma is a malignant tumour derived from the salivary-type seromucinous glands of the nose and paranasal sinuses, possibly from the myoepithelial cells of these glands. The malignant nature of the neoplasm has not always been recognised. Designated as a "cylindroma" by Billroth,[20] it was not until the last 30 years that it was realised that this neoplasm had a tendency to relentless recurrence, often over many years, with eventual death of the patient. The term adenoid cystic (or adenocystic) carcinoma has now been universally adopted as being more descriptive of the histological appearance and behaviour of the neoplasm. Confusion with a benign sweat gland neoplasm frequently seen on the scalp, which has also been termed cylindroma, is avoided by calling the malignant lesion adenoid cystic carcinoma (see Chapter 42).

Incidence

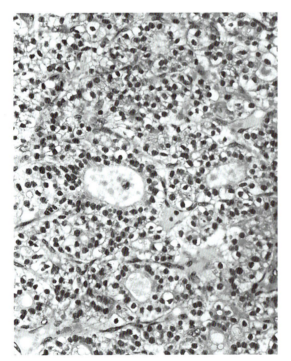

Figure 17.7 Clear cell carcinoma of the nasal cavity. The tumour is composed of fairly regular cells with empty cytoplasm

Adenoid cystic carcinoma is the most common malignant minor salivary gland tumour of the entire upper respiratory tract and constitutes 5–10% of all sinonasal malignancies.[3,21,22] It is most common in the maxillary antra, followed in frequency by the nasal cavity.[23] When occurring in the nasal cavity, adenoid cystic carcinomas (as other nasal salivary gland tumours) are most often located on septum and turbinates. There is a slight preponderance in females, and the majority of adenoid cystic carcinomas occur between 40 and 70 years of age. Occurrence in children and teenagers is very uncommon.

Clinical Features

Facial pain, swelling and nasal obstruction with epistaxis are common forms of presentation. More than 50% of patients have had symptoms for a year or more at presentation. Paraesthesiae or anaesthesia over branches of the fifth cranial nerve, particularly its inframaxillary division, may be prominent.

Imaging Appearances

A soft tissue mass in the paranasal sinuses is frequently observed radiologically. It extends beyond the sinuses with evidence of pressure erosion and destruction of the bony walls. Extension may occur into the clivus, sphenoid sinus and floor of the middle cranial fossa. Perineural spread along the maxillary and mandibular divisions of the trigeminal nerve and involvement of the foramen ovale and foramen rotundum may also be observed.

Gross Appearances

The gross appearances of the neoplasms in the nose and sinuses are not distinctive. The nasal mass may appear polypoid. The maxillary sinus is frequently occupied by grey tumour with evidence of bony invasion.

Microscopic Appearances

The term "cribriform", i.e. having numerous small holes, is descriptive of the most important feature of the variable histology of this neoplasm. It is composed of rather small, regular epithelial cells with uniform nuclei staining darkly and in a homogeneous fashion, and indistinct cytoplasm. Among these cells are many holes, which seem to be punched out without any definite glandular lining. These "pseudocysts" contain amorphous material, which may be eosinophilic or basophilic. It shows histochemical features of connective tissue mucin, such as dissolution of toluidine blue staining after incubation with hyaluronidase. In a few places

columnar epithelium may line acinar structures and the secretions found in these duct-like regions show staining reactions more characteristic of epithelial mucins.

In some parts the small tumour cell masses may appear solid with no cysts. In other areas elongated tubular structures may predominate. These are small and slender, in contrast to the larger masses of the cribriform regions. Attempts have been made to utilise the extent of the solid and tubular patterns for prognostic purposes (see Chapter 42). Masses of tumour cells are often enveloped by pale-staining hyaline zones, giving the neoplasm its characteristic appearance of "cylinders" of cells defined by these outer rims (Figs 17.8 and 17.9). The hyaline material composing these zones stains variably, sometimes positively with periodic acid–Schiff and sometimes positively by acid aniline dyes in a fashion similar to collagen. Laminin and fibronectin – non-collagenous glycoproteins normally associated with basal lamina – have been found to line the periphery of tumour islands and the cystic lumina in most adenoid cystic carcinomas. The loss of immunochemical staining for these substances has been thought to indicate a more aggressive state of the neoplasm.

When examined by the electron microscope the cells lining the pseudocysts do not project microvilli into the space. The glandular cells do show microvilli, on the other hand. The pseudolumina frequently contain a well-defined layer of amorphous material resembling a basal lamina, and collagen, and even elastin, may be found in the spaces. The cells of the neoplasm may show tonofibrils resembling those of squamous cells; bordering cells may contain filamentous bundles indicating a myoepithelial origin.

Spread

Local infiltration, particularly along nerve sheaths, is the most constant means of spread of this neoplasm. In fact infiltration of the neoplasm along perineural spaces is frequently present in histological sections of the neoplasm. Lymph node involvement is infrequent. Bloodstream spread is frequent, however (see Chapter 42).

Natural History

The natural history of adenoid cystic carcinoma is one of repeated recurrences after surgical excision, often continuing over many years until death of the patient.

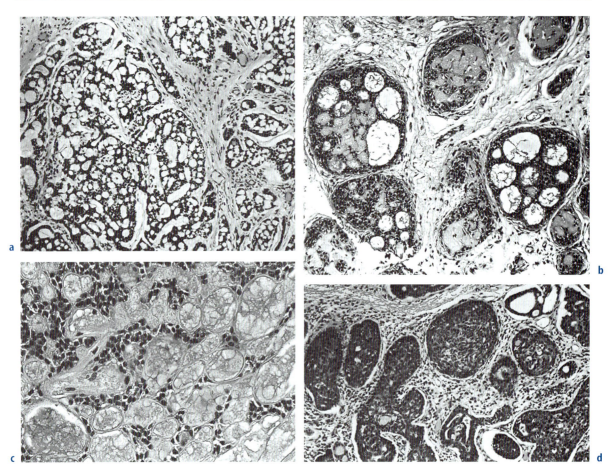

Figure 17.8 Adenoid cystic carcinoma of nasal cavity. **a** In this tumour the cell masses are large with small punched-out spaces (cribriform pattern). **b** This tumour shows less bulky cell masses, but the punched-out mucus-containing spaces are larger than in **a**. **c** "Cylinders" containing globules of mucus with no cellular outline are present in this area (tubular pattern). **d** In this tumour the cell masses are solid with few cysts (solid pattern)

Treatment

In spite of the sombre outlook for this condition, radical surgery, irradiation and sometimes chemotherapy are employed in most cases. The relief of local effects produced by the neoplasm gives validity to these therapeutic endeavours.

Polymorphous Low-grade Adenocarcinoma

Although very rare in the sinonasal tract, it is imperative to be aware of the specific microscopic features of this tumour entity so not to misdiagnose it as adenoid cystic carcinoma. Polymorphous low-grade adenocarcinoma (PLGA) is of low-grade malignancy and does not warrant the aggressive treatment policy necessary in cases of adenoid cystic carcinoma. Polymorphous low-grade adenocarcinoma is described in detail in Chapter 42. Briefly, very bland

cytologic features and a diverse polymorphous growth pattern characterise PLGA, and can in large areas greatly mimic an adenoid cystic carcinoma. Characteristically, PLGA shows a low MIB-1 index and weak bcl-2 staining, contrary to adenoid cystic carcinoma, and these markers can thus be of great help in discriminating the two tumour entities (See Chapter 42).

Mucoepidermoid Carcinoma

Mucoepidermoid carcinoma is a neoplasm of the nose and paranasal sinuses to which very little attention has been paid in the literature. Although it is rare and few studies have been reported, it appears to be more common in the sinuses than in the nasal cavity.

Mucoepidermoid carcinoma is characterised by the presence of epidermoid, mucus-secreting and intermediate cells within the same tumour. Although

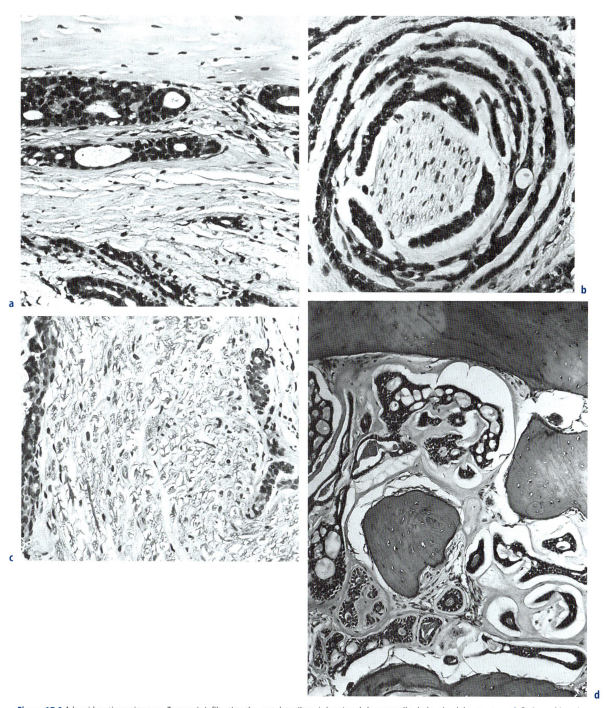

Figure 17.9 Adenoid cystic carcinoma. **a** Tumour is infiltrating the septal cartilage (*above*) and shows small tubular glandular structures. **b** Perineural invasion, which in this neoplasm adopts a concentric pattern around the nerve. **c** Perineural extension associated with swelling and necrosis of nerve fibres. **d** Invasion within the marrow spaces of bone

it has been presumed that this neoplasm is of minor salivary gland origin in the nose and paranasal sinuses, there is evidence of an origin in some cases from surface squamous epithelium. The intimate association of epidermoid and mucous cells is not seen in the nasal neoplasms. It may be that this neoplasm represents a variant of squamous cell carcinoma in this region and its behaviour is in some cases indistinguishable from that tumour (see Chapter 42).

Necrotising Sialometaplasia

Necrotising sialometaplasia rarely affects the major salivary glands and manifests itself most often as an ulcer in the palate (see Chapter 40). It may also be found in the larynx, and occasionally also in the sinonasal tract. The initial lesion may be ischaemia, surgery or trauma of other kind, leading to ulceration and necrosis. The lesion regresses spontaneously, usually in 4–6 weeks, if the initial trauma is removed.

Histologically seromucinous glands show areas of necrosis, involving whole lobules. Other glands show squamous cell metaplasia and it is the presence of these deep masses of epidermoid tissue that give an erroneous impression of malignancy. The lobular architecture of the glands is maintained and careful examination of the cytology of the epidermoid cells reveals their essentially benign character.

References

1. Robin PE, Powell DJ, Stassbie JM. Carcinoma of the nasal cavity and paranasal sinuses: incidence and presentation of different histological types. Clin Otolaryngol 1979;4:431–456
2. Harbo G, Grau C, Bundgaard T et al. Cancer of the nasal cavity and paranasal sinuses. A clinico-pathological study of 277 patients. Acta Oncol 1997;36:45–50
3. Shanmugaratnam K, Sobin LH. Histological typing of tumours of the upper respiratory tract and ear. WHO International Histological Classification of Tumours, 2nd edn. Springer-Verlag, Berlin, 1991
4. Heffner DK, Hyams VJ, Hauck KW et al. Low-grade adenocarcinoma of the nasal cavity and paranasal sinuses. Cancer 1982;50:312–322
5. Gallo O, Franchi A, Fini-Storchi I et al. Prognostic significance of c-erbB-2 oncoprotein expression in intestinal-type adenocarcinoma of the sinonasal tract. Head Neck 1998;20:224–231
6. Wilhelmsson B, Hellquist H, Olofsson J et al. Nasal cuboidal metaplasia with dysplasia. Precursor to adenocarcinoma in wood-dust exposed workers? Acta Otolaryngol (Stockh) 1985;99:641–648
7. Hanslian L, Kadlec K. The products of heat-disintegrated wood (in Czech). Pracovni Lékarství 1964;16:276–282
8. Michaels L. Lung changes in woodworkers. Can Med Assoc J 1967; 96:1150–1155
9. Macbeth R. Malignant disease of the paranasal sinuses. J Laryngol Otol 1965;79:592–612
10. Acheson ED, Cowdell RH, Hadfield E et al. Nasal cancer in woodworkers in the furniture industry. Br Med J 1968;II:587–596
11. Kleinsasser O, Schroeder HG. Pathologie und Klinik der Adenokarzinome der Nase nach Holzstaubexposition. Strahlenther Onkol 1989;165:437–440
12. Franquemont DW, Fechner RE, Mills SE. Histologic classification of sinonasal intestinal-type adenocarcinoma. Am J Surg Pathol 1991;15:368–375
13. Saber AT, Nielsen LR, Dictor M et al. K-ras mutations in sinonasal adenocarcinomas in patients occupationally exposed to wood or leather dust. Cancer Lett 1998, 126:59–65
14. Van den Oever R. Occupational exposure to dust and sinonasal cancer. An analysis of 386 cases reported to the N.C.C.S.F. Cancer Registry. Acta Otorhinolaryngol Belg 1996;50:19–24
15. Klinterberg C, Olofsson J, Hellquist H et al. Adenocarcinoma of the ethmoid sinuses. A review of 28 cases with special reference to wood dust exposure. Cancer 1984;54:482–488
16. Franchi A, Gallo O, Santucchi M. Clinical relevance of the histological classification of sinonasal intestinal-type adenocarcinomas. Hum Pathol 1999;30:1140–1145
17. Compagno J, Wong RT. Intranasal mixed tumours (pleomorphic adenomas). A clinicopathologic study of 40 cases. Am J Clin Pathol 1977;68:213–218
18. Johns ME, Regezi JA, Batsakis JG. Oncocytic neoplasms of salivary glands. An ultrastructural study. Laryngoscope 1977;87:862–871
19. Perzin KH, Cantor JO, Johannessen JV. Acinic cell carcinoma arising in the nasal cavity: report of a case with ultrastructural observations. Cancer 1981;47:1818–1822
20. Billroth T. Beobachtunge über Geschwülste der speicheldresen. Virchows Arch [Pathol Anat Physiol] 1859; 17:357–375
21. Harbo G, Grau C, Bundgaard T et al. Cancer of the nasal cavity and paranasal sinuses. A clinico-pathological study of 277 patients. Acta Oncol 1997;36:45–50
22. Pitman KT, Prokopakis EP, Aydogan B et al.. The role of skull base surgery for the treatment of adenoid cystic carcinoma of the sinonasal tract. Head Neck 1999;21:402–407
23. Da-Quan M, Guang-Yan Y. Tumours of the minor salivary glands. A clinicopathologic study of 243 cases. Acta Otolaryngol (Stockh) 1987;103:325–331

18 Neuroectodermal Tumours

Encephalocele and Glioma

Deposits of cerebral tissue are occasionally seen in the nose. If they are not in direct communication with the brain they are called gliomas. It must be stressed, however, that these lesions are not actually neoplasms of glial tissue, but rather heterotopic brain tissue.

Embryology

The frontal and nasal bones develop anterior to their cartilaginous precursors by intramembranous ossification. A space is present between the newly formed bone and the cartilage. This space in the early stages is occupied by a projection of dura through a bony foramen, the foramen cecum. The latter becomes sealed with further development, but it has been suggested that nasal encephalocele and glioma result from the failure of the foramen cecum to close with consequent protrusion of brain contents. If the communication remains permanently open, the mass is an encephalocele. This is rare. If, however, the communication with brain tissue is cut off, the lesion is known as a glioma[1] (Fig. 18.1).

Clinical Features and Sites

Most nasal gliomas are seen in infants soon after birth. Sixty per cent of the lesions present subcutaneously upon the bridge of the nose, which may be broadened, while 30% are situated high up within the nasal cavity and are seen as smooth, pale polypoid masses. In the other 10% of cases the lesion is both intranasal and extranasal. Rarely heterotopic neural tissue (glioma) may be found in the nose of adults. These are almost always found in the middle turbinate. It is important that imaging investigations be carried out before biopsy to determine whether the heterotopic tissue communicates with the brain, because of the danger of producing meningitis should there be such a connection.

Microscopic Appearances

Nasal glioma is in most cases composed of astrocytes, often the plump gemistocytic form, in a

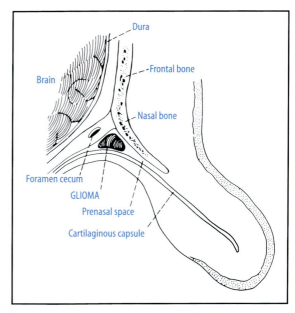

Figure 18.1 Diagram to show possible relation of foramen cecum and other developing nasal structures to glioma[1]

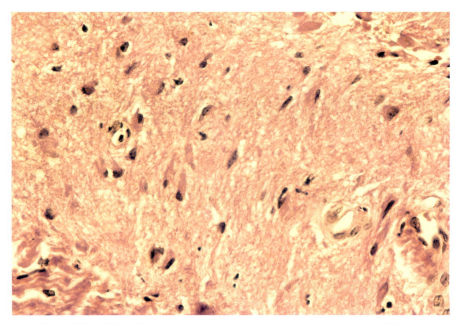

Figure 18.2 Nasal "glioma". The lesion is composed of elongated astrocytes in a background of glial tissue

background of fibrous tissue (Fig. 18.2). In a few cases nerve cells may also be present, although their identification may be difficult because they may be shrunken to a small size. A surface covering of skin or respiratory epithelium is present, depending on the site and size of the glioma. Encephaloceles contain brain, meningeal tissue and sometimes even part of the ventricular system.

Encephalocele and Glioma in the Adult

Glial tissue in the form of a nasal glioma is rare in adults; as mentioned above, the lesion is usually located in the middle turbinate bone. Brain tissue is occasionally found in nasal biopsy material, when it is usually the result of brain herniation following extensive surgical damage to the roof of the nose.

Pituitary Adenoma

Ectopic pituitary adenoma may occasionally be seen in the nasal cavity but most often it represents intranasal extension from a suprasellar tumour rather than an adenoma in ectopic tissue (see Chapter 24). On very rare occasions ectopic pituitary-like cells are found in the walls of the nasal cavity, unconnected with the pharyngeal pituitary, and from these an adenoma could conceivably arise.

Meningioma

Origin

Meningiomas with a histological pattern identical to the intracranial neoplasms are sometimes encountered in the nose. The majority are derived by extension of intracranial meningiomas. Occasionally no intracranial component is detected in a case of nasal meningioma, and it must then be presumed that the lesion is primary in the nose or paranasal sinuses. Such an occurrence can be explained on the basis of an origin from ectopic foci of the cells producing arachnoid villi, which are thought to be the cells of origin of meningioma. Arachnoid villi may be seen in abundance in the neighbourhood of the glial–schwannian junction, particularly of the eighth cranial nerve in the internal auditory meatus (see Chapter 1). This also is an unstable transitional zone where meninges change to endoneurium, and meningiomas may arise from cells producing arachnoid villi in this region. The meningo-endoneural regions of the olfactory nerves which pass through the cribriform plate are less well defined, but it is possible that these may serve similarly as sites of origin for primary intranasal meningioma. In this respect it may be pointed out that the olfactory nerve carries no Schwann cells (see below, neurogenic tumours, and Chapter 12).

Gross Appearances

Meningiomas of the nose may present as nasal polyps. The tumours usually have a firm consistency and may be somewhat granular or fibrous on their cut surfaces.

Microscopic Appearance

Most intranasal meningiomas show a meningothelial or fibroblastic pattern in which tumour cells of epithelial or fibroblastic appearance, respectively, are arranged concentrically around small blood vessels (Fig. 18.3). Both cell appearances may be present in the same meningioma. Psammoma bodies are sometimes seen.

In some cases the tumour displays whorls of dense fibrous tissue over large areas and the lesion may be confused with inflammatory fibrosis. The diagnosis is made by identifying definite concentric whorls of cells as opposed to fibrous tissue only.

Immunohistochemical Findings

Intranasal meningiomas show positivity for neurone-specific enolase and S-100 in most instances, and are almost invariably positive for epithelial membrane antigen. The expression of keratin and vimentin varies, but is usually negative.

Neurogenic Tumours

Neurogenic tumours are probably all derived by proliferation of Schwann cells. There are four varieties:

1. Neurilemmoma.
2. Neurofibroma.
3. Plexiform neurofibroma.
4. Neurogenous sarcoma (malignant schwannoma).

Each of these neoplasms has been identified in the nose and paranasal sinuses, the majority being neurilemmomas. Malignant neurogenic sinonasal tumours are rare, being mainly neurogenic sarcomas.[2]

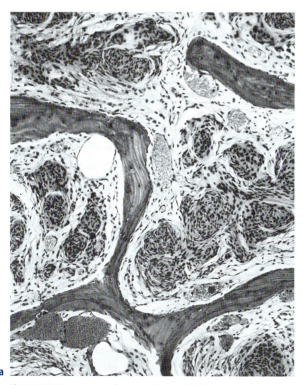
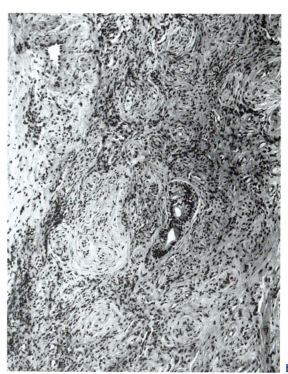

a   b

Figure 18.3 Meningioma in the nose. **a** Meningothelial meningioma in the ethmoid bone. Note whorls of epithelial-like cells. **b** Fibrous meningioma composed of fibrous whorls around small blood vessels. Note duct of nasal gland near centre

Gross Appearances

The lesions are usually discrete, firm masses, often showing cystic degeneration. Although neurilemmomas are frequently attached to a nerve, this is not usually seen in the nasal and sinus neurilemmomas.

Microscopic Appearances

Neurilemmomas show Antoni A areas of palisaded cells, often whorled into Verocay bodies. Antoni B areas are always present in the same tumours, showing looser, reticular, often myxoid parts between the Antoni A areas (see Chapter 11). We have seen three nasal tumours with widespread squamous metaplasia of seromucinous glands, but with a prominent stroma identifiable as schwannoma, the latter being strongly S-100 positive. Neurofibromas are fibrous lesions with frequent nerve fibres traversing the tumour. Plexiform neurofibromas are composed of strands of Schwann cells lying in a loose myxoid stroma. Malignant schwannomas show some of the features of a neurilemmoma such as palisading, but the tumour cells appear malignant.

The characteristic appearance of a sinonasal neurogenic sarcoma is that of a dense fibrosarcoma pattern. Palisading nuclei alternating with poorly cellular areas are often present, but the herring-bone pattern of interlacing fascicles of fibroblasts so typical of fibrosarcoma is not a prominent feature of sinonasal neurogenic sarcoma. Immunohistochemistry is often necessary to distinguish neurogenic sarcoma from malignant fibrous histiocytoma-like tumours (see Chapter 20). Cellular atypia is evident. Sinonasal neurogenic sarcoma arises de novo or as the result of a malignant transformation of a pre-existing neurofibroma, but not from a schwannoma. The term neurogenic sarcoma, or malignant nerve sheath tumour, is therefore to be preferred to malignant schwannoma.[3] A case of malignant sinonasal neurogenic sarcoma with epithelioid features has also been described.[4]

Immunohistochemical Findings

Schwannomas of the nose display the usual striking degree of positivity that these tumours have against S-100 protein antibody wherever they are found (see Chapter 11). A similar but often less strong positivity is found with the other benign neurogenic tumours, but in the case of the malignant ones the reaction with this antigen is variable.

Malignant Melanoma

Incidence

Malignant melanomas, which are tumours arising from melanin-producing cells, are not as unusual in the mucosa of the air and food passages as was previously believed. The greater number (2% of all malignant melanomas) arise in the oral cavity and they constitute approximately 10% of all head and neck melanomas.[5] A very small proportion indeed arise in the nose. In a series of 39 patients with malignant melanoma of the nose and paranasal sinuses, the average age was found to be 61 years, with a range of 17–84 years.[6] More than half of the patients were between 50 and 70 years. Only six patients were black in this American series. In an African series, on the other hand, nasal melanoma was found commonly in African blacks, accounting for 2.6% of all malignant melanomas.[7] A recent study of 25 cases of sinonasal malignant melanomas and a literature meta-analysis (163 cases of sinonasal melanomas) did not confirm a male predominance in the incidence of malignant melanoma reported in reference 6, but rather revealed an equal sex incidence.[8]

Clinical Features

The main symptoms of malignant melanoma are nasal blockage and epistaxis, often accompanied by focal swelling. The neoplasm is in most cases observed in the nasal cavity. It is brownish-grey with a smooth, flat, lacy pattern that looks deceptively benign.

Site

In most cases the tumours arise in the nasal cavity. Occasionally they arise in the maxillary and ethmoid sinuses, and may extend from there into the nasal cavity. The commonest site of origin has been thought to be the septum, followed by the inferior turbinate and then the middle turbinate, corresponding in relative frequency to sites of pigmentation of the normal nasal mucosa in some Ugandan Africans, among whom malignant melanoma of the nose is quite frequent.[7] Other studies also have confirmed the nasal cavity to be the most common location in the sinonasal tract, but it appears now that the lateral walls may be a more frequent site of origin than the nasal septum. For example, a study of 14 primary sinonasal melanomas disclosed 11 cases to be from the lateral part of the nasal cavity, two from the sinuses and in only one case was origin from the nasal septum.[9] Sinonasal mucosal melanomas may also be multifocal, emphasising the possibility of a large, diffuse proliferation of atypical melanocytes in the sinonasal mucosa, an observation that may have therapeutic implications.[10]

Gross Appearances

The tumour may be polypoid but usually presents infiltrating features with evidence of destruction of the bony antral wall. A brownish colouration of the tumour is apparent in approximately two-thirds of the cases.

Microscopic Appearances

Due to the absence of hallmarks analogous to those of the papillary and reticular dermis, Clark's classification of various levels of invasion does not apply to mucosal melanomas. Nor does measurement of the thickness, as proposed by Breslow, although theoretically quite possible to perform, have any practical meaning, as truly radical surgical removal of sinonasal melanomas seldom is possible.

The tumours exhibit cells of variegated appearance including polygonal (epithelioid), spindle-shaped, large and bizarre or small darkly staining cells. The cellular shape is not related to the degree of malignancy. Large eosinophilic nucleoli are often present in the nuclei. High mitotic rate and vascular invasion, absence (or few) of tumour-infiltrating lymphocytes and evidence of regression are features shared by all types of sinonasal melanomas (Fig. 18.4).

The identification of melanin pigment in the tumour cells is important in the light microscopic diagnosis of malignant melanoma of the nose. The pigment identified in conventionally stained sections is negative for haemosiderin and positive by silver staining, such as Fontana's method. The black-staining melanin pigment is bleached with potassium permanganate or hydrogen peroxide solutions. In the majority of cases the tumour cells are heavily pigmented; some are amelanotic, however, and melanin pigment can be identified only by silver staining.

Junctional activity is an important feature of malignant melanoma of the skin, but this change is unusual in the nasal variety of the tumour because, unlike the skin neoplasm, only small amounts of normal epithelium are removed with the tumour. Moreover, the epithelium is frequently ulcerated over the surface of nasal melanoma. Junctional activity is sometimes seen, however, in the epithelium adjacent to the main tumour mass.

Osteocartilaginous differentiation and production of osteocartilaginous structures are rare but well-described features in skin melanomas. A case of nasal mucosal melanoma with bone and osteoid formation, both in primary lesion and lymph node metastasis, has been described.[11]

Immunohistochemistry plays an important role in the diagnosis of sinonasal mucosal melanomas. S-100 protein is almost invariably positive, as are the melanoma marker, HMB-45, and vimentin in most cases, but keratins are negative. Amelanotic tumours almost invariably show HMB-45 positivity, which, together with negativity for neurone-specific enolase, chromogranin, synaptophysin and lymphocyte common antigen, will in most cases distinguish this type of melanoma from olfactory neuroblastoma, small cell undifferentiated carcinoma and lymphoma. The strong HMB-45 positivity in amelanotic small blue cell melanomas is explained by the reaction of this antibody with an oncofetal antigen found in immature melanosomes.[12]

Electron Microscopy

Ultrastructural examination shows ovoid bodies in the cytoplasm of the tumour cells. These bodies, known as melanosomes, which are the precursors of melanin within the cells, possess an internal structure of transversely arranged internal striations (Fig. 18.4).

Spread

Local spread, particularly through the base of the skull to the intracranial fossa, is important in the initial dissemination of this disease. There is a low incidence of cervical lymph node metastasis, but bloodstream metastases are frequent, lungs, brain and skin most commonly showing deposits.

Natural History and Prognosis

A large literature meta-analysis of 163 cases (1977–1995) revealed that the 5-year median survival for all patients was 36 months. Stratification by era (pre-1980 vs post-1980) disclosed that the mean survival has not improved during the last 15 years.[13] Thus the prognosis is poor, in spite of modern advances in imaging and surgical techniques, as well as in adjuvant therapeutics. However, a cumulative

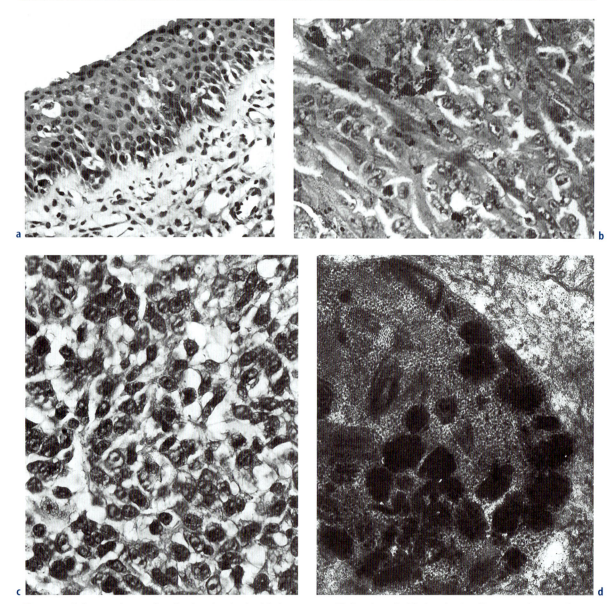

Figure 18.4 Malignant melanoma of nasal cavity. **a** Junctional activity in squamous epithelium (metaplastic) of nasal cavity adjacent to malignant melanoma. Appearances are similar to those in relation to skin melanomas. **b** Pigmented tumour. Note prominent nucleoli, eosinophilic in original, within tumour nuclei. **c** Non-pigmented tumour also showing prominent nucleoli in cells. **d** Electron micrograph showing melanosomes, which have an internal structure of transversely arranged striations

5-year survival rate of 20% has been reported for all head and neck mucosal melanomas, and in fact patients with primary tumours of the nasal cavity had significantly better 5-year survival than do patients with primary melanomas at other sites.[14]

Olfactory Neuroblastoma

Definition

The pathological diagnosis and subclassification of nerve cell tumours of the nose have been uncertain from the time of their original description. A form of nerve cell neoplasm – esthesioneuroepithelioma – which contained rosettes as well as neurocytes and neurofibrils was at first distinguished from esthesioneurocytoma, which did not contain rosettes.[15] It was then suggested that the presence of rosettes or other histological features had no bearing on prognosis, although neuroblasts could be distinguished from neurocytes in the tumours.[16] Other authors could also recognise a single entity only – olfactory neuroblastoma; they felt, however, that a definite diagnosis could be made only in the presence of a prominent intercellular neurofibrillary matrix.[17] In the 1980s a further attempt was once again made to subdivide neoplasms of this type. In this new sub-classification "neuroblastoma" and "neuroen-docrine" forms were distinguished by the presence of neurofibrils and glands respectively.[18] Most authors have stressed the histological similarity of olfactory neuroblastoma to neuroblastoma of sympathetic nervous system origin.

It is still our opinion that there is but a single entity – olfactory neuroblastoma – which does have some differences from neuroblastoma arising elsewhere. The nasal neoplasm displays specific light microscopic features for both tumour cells and stroma, in the presence of which a definite diagnosis can be made; a neurofibrillary matrix is, however, not necessarily present. Olfactory neuroblastoma arises from basal cells of the olfactory neuroepithelium. These cells have a different activity and developmental potential from the primitive cells of the sympathetic nervous system, which give rise to sympathetic neuroblastoma (see below). It should not be surprising, therefore, to find that olfactory neuroblastoma differs from sympathetic neuroblastoma not only in its histological form but also in its age incidence and natural history.

Although the histogenesis is not clearly delineated, its location, histology and immunoprofile suggest that olfactory neuroblastoma is a neural or neuroendocrine neoplasm derived from the olfactory neuroepithelium. Olfactory neuroblastomas are not classical sympathetic neuroblastomas but are related to primitive neuroectodermal tumours. Using modified reverse transcription polymerase chain reaction techniques, it has been shown that the human analogue of the *Drosophila* achaete-scute gene *HASH1* is expressed in olfactory neuroblastomas, while the olfactory marker protein is not. The latter is expressed exclusively in mature olfactory neurones, while *HASH1* is expressed in immature olfactory neurones. This study thus supports the concept that olfactory neuroblastoma is derived from immature olfactory neurones of ectodermal origin.[19] However, demonstration in two putative olfactory neuroblastoma cell lines of the 11;22 chromosomal translocation, seen in Ewing's sarcoma of bone and peripheral neuroectodermal tumours (PNET) of bone and soft tissue, led to the conclusion that olfactory neuroblastoma may be closely related histogenetically to PNET. The overwhelming majority of cases of Ewing's sarcoma and PNET express the protein product MIC-2 (MIC-2 is a cell membrane protein, also recognised as CD99). However, none of the 18 cases of olfactory neuroblastoma reported from John Hopkins Hospital expressed MIC-2, nor did any of the 20 cases from Memorial Sloan-Kettering Cancer Center. Olfactory neuroblastoma is thus still best regarded as a primitive neural tumour and not a member of the PNET family.[20,21]

Origin

As stated above, it seems likely that olfactory neuroblastomas originate from the basal layer of the olfactory neuroepithelium. It has been shown that, unlike nerve cells, this epithelium is constantly renewed, the innermost polygonal basal cells acting as reserve replacements for both the sustentacular and the olfactory neural cells (see Chapter 12). In sections of an olfactory neuroblastoma, we have observed appearances strongly suggestive of an origin of the tumour from the basal cells of the neuroepithelium, with hyperplasia of the latter cells and reduplication of the olfactory neuroepithelium producing structures similar to true rosettes.

Incidence

Olfactory neuroblastoma is a rare tumour occurring over a wide range of ages (from 3 years to 80–90 years of age), but rarely under the age of 10. The median age is approximately 50 years, and there is an apparent peak incidence in the second decade of life and another in the fifth. There is a slight male predominance.[22] The age incidence is thus markedly different from that of adrenal neuroblastoma, which, in most cases, arises in children under 4 years of age. Although a rare tumour, in a large series of 752 sinonasal cancers (French Cancer Centers Group), as many as 64 cases (8.5%) of olfactory neuroblastomas were found, i.e. an incidence similar to that of adenoid cystic carcinoma.[22]

Site

Olfactory neuroblastoma arises high up in the nasal cavity. The tumour may extend into the nearby sinuses. In a series of 27 cases referred to the Armed Forces Institute of Pathology the nasal cavity was also the main site of involvement in every case. In five of these the ethmoid sinuses and in two the maxillary antrum were also involved.[23] There are reports in the literature from the 1960s of olfactory neuroblastomas arising at more outlying extranasal sites such as the nasopharynx, but these cases could now be interpreted as neuroendocrine carcinomas (see below), or metastases from sympathetic neuroblastomas.

Clinical Features and Imaging

The symptoms are those that are common to the majority of neoplasms within the nasal cavity: unilateral nasal obstruction, epistaxis, rhinorrhoea and sinus pain. Extension beyond the nasal cavity and paranasal sinuses is accompanied by specific localising features such as earache from spread to the nasopharynx, with serous otitis media, proptosis and even blindness from orbital involvement. In addition to a nasal mass, cranial nerve palsies and palpable cervical nodes may be found on physical examination. Computerised tomography commonly shows erosion of the cribriform plate by tumour. There may also be bowing of the sinus walls, bone destruction elsewhere and focal calcification within the nasal mass. Magnetic resonance imaging allows a better estimate of tumour spread into surrounding soft-tissue areas, such as the anterior cranial fossa and the retromaxillary space.[24,25]

Gross Appearances

The tumour appears as a fleshy pink mass, which is more opaque than a simple nasal polyp but is sometimes mistaken for the latter. In some patients the olfactory bulbs in the nearby cranial cavity are found to be swollen and completely replaced by neoplasm, which has entered by growth along the olfactory nerves.

Microscopic Appearances

Olfactory neuroblastomas have histological features that enable the pathologist to make an unequivocal diagnosis. In brief these are: (1) well-demarcated lobules of uniform tumour cells and (2) congeries of blood vessels in close apposition to the tumour lobules.

The nasal mucosa and submucosa are expanded in all cases by tumour lobules, which are somewhat round in shape and vary in size from large spheres containing many cells to small groups of some four cells. The lobules are characterised by well-defined edges. In a few cases the neoplasm is composed mainly of wide trabeculae of tumour cells, but the presence of round bulges at their edges reveals a similar lobular configuration. In some areas the neoplasm is formed of anastomosing files a cell or two wide. This appearance is most prominent in recurrences and advanced stages of the tumour growth. Examination of other parts of the neoplasm in those cases will usually show a more typical architecture.

Tumour cells are uniform and rather small. Nuclei are oval and finely granular with uniformly distributed chromatin, without prominent nucleoli. Occasionally in advanced widely invading neoplasms the nuclei may show prominent eosinophilic nucleoli. There is often so little cytoplasm that it is not clearly visible; when observed it is scanty and pink staining. Mitotic figures are seen in some tumours but are never numerous. Nerve cell differentiation is not seen in the primary nasal tumours.

In about half of the tumours, round or oval empty spaces appear in the lobules of tumour cells. These seem to be punched-out and are surrounded by cells which have no special structural alteration. These spaces have been referred to as pseudo-rosettes. True rosettes are characterised by duct-like structures lining the spaces, the cells of which have basally oriented nuclei. Although stressed in some reports in the literature as being frequent in olfactory neuroblastoma, we have seen them but rarely. Dilated gland-like structures lined by cubical epithelium may be present in some cases in close association with tumour cells (see below).

In some lobules of the tumour elongated cells are arranged around the periphery of the lobule. These suggest the possibility of an origin from sustentacular cells and indeed they are positive for S-100 protein antigen (see also below: electron microscopic appearances).

In about one-third of cases the tumour lobules show pink-staining finely fibrillar areas. These occupy a sizeable area, sometimes more than half of the lobule. It seems likely from ultramicroscopic evidence (see below) that such areas are neurofibrils, but satisfactory identification by nerve fibre stains, both immunohistochemical and with silver impregnation, is difficult to achieve.

Stromal vascularisation is a diagnostically important feature of olfactory neuroblastoma. Numerous capillaries and venules, usually in conglomerates, are present in the stroma between tumour lobules and intimately associated with them. The vessels are often embedded in hyaline fibrous tissue. They may indent the lobules of tumour and may appear as vascular islands lying among tumour cells. Areas of amorphous calcification are seen in the stroma of about 15% of cases (Figs 18.5 and 18.6).

Electron Microscopic Appearances

In most cases of "small round cell tumours" (see below) electron microscopy still plays an important role as an adjuvant diagnostic tool, in addition to immunohistochemistry. Electron microscopy of olfactory neuroblastomas shows uniform round nucleated cells with variable amounts of dendritic processes containing dense core granules ranging from 150 to 350 nm in the perikarya and dendritic processes (Fig. 18.6). In some cases also cells with the appearance of sustentacular cells are recognised. The most important electron microscopical differ-

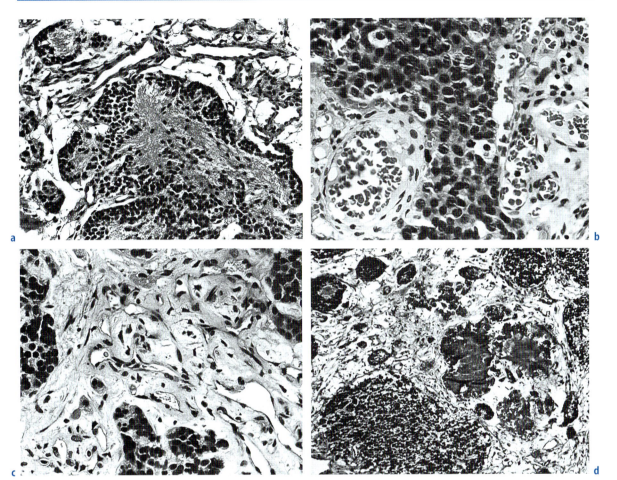

Figure 18.5 Olfactory neuroblastoma. **a** The tumour cells are arranged in lobules of different sizes, with distinct edges. Some of the lobules in this neoplasm have areas, often extensive, of fine fibrils, which stained pale pink in the original. The stroma contains numerous capillaries and venules. **b** Higher power of another tumour showing regular nuclei and moderate amounts of cytoplasm. Some pseudo-rosettes are present in this field. Prominent blood vessels are displayed in the stroma. **c** The blood vessels in the congeries of this tumour are surrounded by hyaline collagenous tissue. **d** Calcification is present between tumour lobules in this case

ence between olfactory neuroblastoma and neuroendocrine carcinoma is the absence of these sustentacular cells in neuroendocrine carcinomas.[26] Microtubules 30 nm thick may also be present. Groups of cell processes may be surrounded by electron-dense material in a fashion similar to that of Schwann cell cytoplasm. The true rosettes have been examined ultrastructurally, with the finding of "olfactory vesicles" and microvilli projecting from the apices of marginal cells. These were interpreted as a neoplastic replication of olfactory neuroepithelium[27] (Table 18.1).

Biochemical and Immunohistochemical Findings

The catecholamine substances dopamine-—hydroxylase, adrenaline and noradrenaline have been

Table 18.1. Features of olfactory neuroblastoma

Light microscopic	Well-demarcated, round lobules of uniform cells
	Pseudorosettes; rarely true rosettes
	Fibrils in tumour cell lobules in some cases
	Large, wide glands in some cases
	Spindle, sustentacular-like cells around some lobules
	Congeries of blood vessels in septae related to tumour lobules
	Stromal calcification in some cases
	Grimelius positive in most cases
Electron microscopic	Neurosecretory granules 150–350 nm in diameter
	Axonal cell processes also showing neurosecretory granules
	Sustentacular cells
Immunohistochemical	Catecholamines positive
	Neuroendocrine markers positive (chromogranin, synaptophysin, NSE, neurofilaments, class III beta-tubulin)
	Cytokeratins usually negative; MIC-2 negative

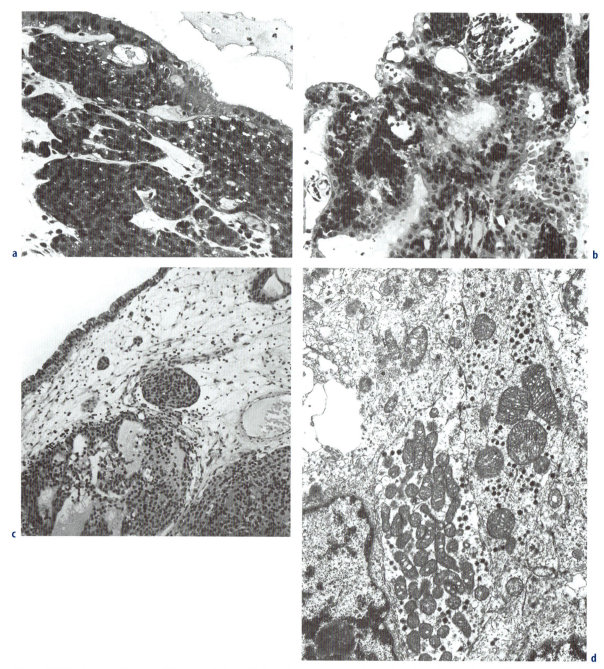

Figure 18.6 Olfactory neuroblastoma. **a** Origin from olfactory epithelium. The tumour cells forming as lobules have direct continuity with the surface epithelial cells stretching across the *top of the figure*. **b** Lobules of cells derived from olfactory epithelium (*upper left*) form glandular lumina. **c** Glandular spaces are present in some of the lobules at *lower left*. **d** Electron micrograph showing elongated processes of cytoplasm containing numerous mitochondria and membrane-bound dense-core granules. Original magnification × 16 000

detected biochemically in olfactory neuroblastomas, albeit at levels far below those in sympathetic neuroblastomas. In three cases of olfactory neuroblastoma, urinary catecholamine levels were found to lie within normal limits before and after surgery.[28] A reduction in urinary vanillylmandelic acid was found in the seven patients in whom it was tested after surgical removal of the nasal tumour, although the pretreatment levels were not significantly elevated above normal.[29]

Olfactory neuroblastomas often stain positively by the Grimelius method for argyrophilia. Catecholamines including both adrenaline and noradrenaline are present, but not to the same

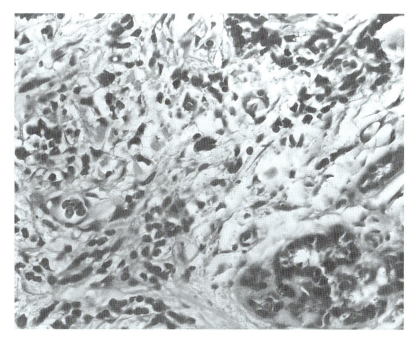

Figure 18.7 Melanotic neuroectodermal tumour of infancy, showing an alveolar arrangement of small dark cells, which are neuroblasts, and larger melanin pigment-containing cells (*bottom right*)

extent as in sympathetic neuroblastomas, and can readily be demonstrated immunohistochemically. Olfactory neuroblastomas are invariably immunoreactive for one or more neuroendocrine marker, such as chromogranin, synaptophysin and neurone-specific enolase. Keratins are usually negative, and the Ewing sarcoma-associated MIC-2 antigen is uniformly negative[30] (Table 18.1).

Spread and Prognosis

Local spread to the ethmoid, sphenoid and maxillary sinuses and, particularly, along the olfactory filaments through the cribriform plate is frequent. Metastasis was formerly reported in about a quarter of the cases, the commonest site being the cervical lymph nodes, followed by lungs and bones in that order. Multidisciplinary management of olfactory neuroblastoma has effected a marked increased survival during the last 20 years, although a completely standard protocol for the management of these lesions has not yet been accepted. A common treatment policy is radical craniofacial surgery for complete bloc resection of the tumour and possibly its olfactory bulb extension, from both the nose and anterior cranial fossa. This is usually combined with preoperative radiotherapy, with or without chemotherapy. With neoadjuvant therapy the overall

5- and 10-year survival rates have been shown to be 81 and 55%, respectively.[31]

Neuroendocrine Carcinoma

The amine precursor uptake and decarboxylation (APUD) system is made up of cells of endocrine origin derived from endodermal epithelium and neuroendocrine cells derived from neuroepithelium. Malignant tumours arising from these cells ("apudomas") are known as endocrine and neuroendocrine carcinomas respectively. Such neoplasms as carcinoid tumour of the small intestine are in the endocrine carcinoma group and medullary carcinoma of the thyroid and neuroblastoma of the adrenal are in the neuroendocrine group. These tumours tend to be argentaffin or argyrophil positive, they often secrete hormones such as ACTH, inappropriately, they always show neuroendocrine granules in their cytoplasm and they display a positive reaction for neurone-specific enolase by the immunoperoxidase method. A variety of histological patterns has been described for these tumours, from solid nests of cells to glandular formations.

A very small number of case reports describing nasal paragangliomas (chemodectomas) can be found in the older literature. However, there are several grounds to believe that these tumours today likely would be interpreted as neuroendocrine carcinomas. The typical histological features of paraganglioma are given in Chapters 5 and 37.

Microscopic Appearances

The spectrum of the neuroendocrine tumours ranges from biologically benign tumours to extremely aggressive highly malignant tumour types. The current classification is similar to that of lung neuroendocrine carcinomas, and based on studies such as those of references 32 and 33. As the nomenclature of the tumours was not homogenous, the classification of the neuroendocrine tumours of different organs has been standardised and correlated with the clinical course of the tumours. The important parameters for this classification can be checked using only careful morphologic examination, with two additions – the determination of the "proliferative rate" using MIB-1 and the actual diagnosis of large cell neuroendocrine carcinoma, for both of which immunohistochemical examination is required. The histological characterisation of the different entities takes into account the degree of atypia, nuclear indentation and compression, tumour cell size, the presence and extent of single cell or mass necrosis, mitotic rate (per ten high power fields (HPF)) and – optionally – the percentage of MIB-1-immunoreactive tumour cells. Based on these factors three different types can be recognised.[34]

I.   Benign or low-grade malignant behaviour: highly differentiated neuroendocrine tumour (typical carcinoid, classical carcinoid).

II. Low-grade malignant behaviour: highly differentiated neuroendocrine carcinoma (atypical carcinoid).

III. High-grade malignant behaviour: small cell or intermediate cell neuroendocrine carcinoma; large cell neuroendocrine carcinoma.

Highly differentiated neuroendocrine tumour (typical carcinoid, classical carcinoid)

The histological growth pattern is either adenoid, solid-trabecular, paragangloid or spindle cell, but this has no influence on the biological behaviour. There is only mild or no atypia. Nuclear molding, single cell necrosis and mass necrosis are not present. The mitotic rate is between none and three per ten HPF, the percentage of MIB-1-reactive cells is always below 1.1 (average 0.6).

Highly differentiated neuroendocrine carcinoma (atypical carcinoid)

The tumour cell nuclei are more variable in size as well as in chromatin pattern; nucleoli can also be present. Nuclear molding does not appear. Single cell necrosis occurs only rarely while necrosis of greater groups or mass necrosis are absent. The numbers of mitoses per ten HPF range from three to ten. The percentage of MIB-1-immunoreactive cells varies considerably; on average it is around 5.1.[35]

Highly malignant neuroendocrine tumours

These are divided into small and intermediate cell, and large cell neuroendocrine carcinomas. Both entities show high-grade atypia; the small and intermediate cell variants show distinct and classical nuclear molding, both entities show extensive necrosis, most often in the form of mass necrosis. Glandular structures may be present, but not to the same extent as in highly differentiated neuroendocrine tumours. The mitotic rate is above ten per ten HPF, the percentage of MIB-1-positive cells averages 27%. The discrimination of large cell neuroendocrine carcinoma from highly differentiated neuroendocrine tumour is generally simple using these criteria. The identification of intermediate cell carcinoma is, according to the definition, based on a tumour cell diameter greater than 33 μm (= three lymphocyte diameters). To distinguish large cell neuroendocrine carcinoma from large cell non-neuroendocrine carcinoma, the expression of at least two neuroendocrine markers is necessary for the former (e.g. neurone-specific enolase, synaptophysin, chromogranin, Phe 5, PGP 9.5 or Leu 7). Alternatively the detection of specific hormone/amine-products by immunohistochemistry is required.

Hence, in the sinonasal tract, one may very occasionally encounter typical and atypical carcinoids. More common, but still rare, are the highly malignant variants, i.e. the small and intermediate cell type and the large cell type of neuroendocrine carcinoma.

Immunohistochemical Findings

Unlike olfactory neuroblastomas, neuroendocrine carcinomas usually stain positively for cytokeratins, e.g. low molecular weight keratins (CAM 5.2) and also AE:AE3. As mentioned above, they should also stain positively for at least two neuroendocrine markers. They are usually negative for S-100 protein and neurofilament stain.[36]

Prognosis

The 5-year survival rate of highly differentiated neuroendocrine tumour is excellent. The prognosis of the small and intermediate cell neuroendocrine carcinoma is poor, although probably not as serious as its lung counterpart, but apparently more aggressive than olfactory neuroblastoma.

Small Round Cell Tumours

Small round cell tumours of the nose and paranasal sinuses often present a problem in differential diagnosis, the solution of which depends not only on a close scrutiny of the morphology in tissue sections but also on the immunohistochemical, electron microscopic and molecular biological findings in biopsy tissue. Olfactory neuroblastoma is frequently high on the list of alternatives in the consideration of tumours in this group. The category of small round cell tumours comprises, apart from olfactory neuroblastoma and small cell neuroendocrine carcinoma, Ewing's sarcoma, PNET and Merkel cell carcinoma. Other tumour categories, e.g. lymphoma and embryonal rhabdomyosarcoma, may also predominantly be composed of small cells. In the head and neck region small round cell tumours are usually found in the larynx, the nose, and occasionally in the salivary glands (see Chapters 37 and 42). Ewing's sarcoma and PNET are dealt with in Chapter 21. Merkel cell carcinoma (cutaneous small cell undifferentiated carcinoma, or neuroendocrine carcinoma) arises in the skin. On rare occasions a recurrent Merkel cell carcinoma may present inside the nose, under the skin and in the mucosa, and thus constitute a diagnostic dilemma if unaware of the previous skin lesion. However, the cells of Merkel cell carcinoma have a characteristic single punctate zone of cytoplasmic immunoreactivity, particularly for cytokeratin 20. This rather characteristic and almost diagnostic, feature of Merkel cell carcinoma is not seen in other small cell carcinomas. The need for different immunohistochemical stainings to separate the different entities is well documented in a study of 69 round cell lesions of the sinonasal tract.[37] The main differential diagnostic criteria of small round cell tumours of the nose are given in Table 18.2. It must be admitted that small cell tumours of the nose are seen from time to time which defy all classification beyond that represented by the term "undifferentiated malignant neoplasm".

Table 18.2. Differential diagnosis of small cell tumours of nose and paranasal sinuses

Neoplasm	Histology	Histochemical and immunohistochemical findings	Electron microscopy
Olfactory neuroblastoma	Compact lobules Vascular stroma	Catecholamines positive Neuroendocrine markers positive	Neurosecretory granules Sustentacular cells
Embryonal rhabdomyosarcoma	Rhabdomyoblasts	Glycogen and desmin positive	Thick and thin filaments
Non-Hodgkin's lymphoma	Usually centroblastic/centrocytic	Common leucocyte antigen and various CDs positive	Not diagnostic
Granulocytic sarcoma	Myeloid cells	Lysozyme and naphthol chloracetate positive	Myeloid cells
Ewing's sarcoma	Perivascular	Vimentin, MIC-2 and glycogen positive	Aggregated glycogen
Mesenchymal chondrosarcoma	Islets of cartilage	Not diagnostic	Characteristic of cartilage
Malignant melanoma	Melanocytes, large eosinophilic nucleoli	Melanin pigment, S-100 and HMB45 positive	Melanosomes
Haemangiopericytoma	Tumour cells around normal vessels	Not diagnostic	Basal lamina around each cell
Undifferentiated carcinoma	Surface origin, "empty" nuclei	Cytokeratins positive	Desmosomes and tonofibrils
Small cell neuroendocrine carcinoma	High-grade atypia, nuclear molding, necrosis, mitoses positive	Neuroendocrine and cytokeratin markers positive	Some epithelial and neuroendocrine features

Melanotic Neuroectodermal Tumour of Infancy (Melanotic Progonoma)

Melanotic neuroectodermal tumour of infancy usually affects the bone of the upper jaw but has also been found in many parts of the body, including the testis and mediastinum. The lesion presents in an infant of either sex, usually within the first year of life. Growth is often very rapid and surgical removal may be required because of difficulty in feeding. The tumour may appear encapsulated and shows a pigmented, often bluish-grey cut surface. Microscopically the lesions consist of two cell populations: (1) cuboidal cells, which contain large amounts of melanin granules in their cytoplasm and (2) small dark cells arranged in an alveolar pattern, which resemble neuroblasts. The neuroblasts are frequently surrounded by the melanocytic cells (Figs 18.7 and 18.8). Ultrastructurally the neuroblasts show secretory granules with eccentric cores suggesting noradrenaline. Melanotic progonoma is thus a rare but well-recognised entity in paediatric pathology, and numerous case reports have been published in the last decade. Recent molecular studies have tried to link melanotic neuroectodermal tumour of infancy to other small cell tumours with well-characterised molecular genetic changes (e.g. *MYCN* gene amplification, deletion of 1p, typical translocations, e.g. t(11;22)(q24;q12). None of the tests performed has yielded positive results, and at present there is no genetic basis to link melanotic prognoma to neuroblastoma, Ewing's sarcoma, PNET or desmoplastic small round cell tumour.[38]

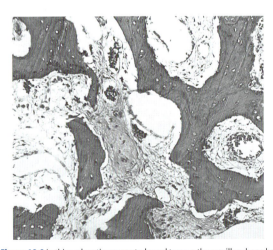

Figure 18.8 In this melanotic neuroectodermal tumour the maxillary bone has become overgrown and trabeculae envelop small groups of neuroblasts

References

1. Katz A, Lewis JS. Nasal gliomas. Arch Otolaryngol 1971;94:351–355
2. Perzin KH, Panyu H, Wechter S. Nonepithelial tumours of the nasal cavity, paranasal sinuses and nasopharynx. XII. Schwann cell tumours (neurilemmoma, neurofibroma, malignant Schwannoma). Cancer 1982;50:2193–2202
3. Hellquist HB, Lundgren J. Neurogenic sarcoma of the sinonasal tract. J Laryngol Otol 1991;105:186–190
4. Fernández PL, Cardesa A, Bombí JA et al. Malignant sinonasal epithelioid schwannoma. Virchows Arch (A) 1993;423:401–405.
5. Gorsky M, Epstein JB. Melanoma arising from the mucosal surfaces of the head and neck. Oral Surg Oral Med Oral Pathol Oral Radiol Endod 1998;86:715–719
6. Holdcraft J, Gallagher JC. Malignant melanomas of the nasal and paranasal sinus mucosae. Ann Otol Rhinol Laryngol 1969;78:5–20
7. Lewis MG, Martin JAM. Malignant melanoma of the nasal cavity in Ugandan Africans. Cancer 1967;20:1699–1705
8. Brandwein MS, Rothstein A, Lawson W et al. Sinonasal melanoma. A clinicopathologic study of 25 cases and literature meta-analysis. Arch Otolaryngol Head Neck Surg 1997;123:290–296
9. Regauer S, Anderhuber W, Richtig E et al. Primary mucosal melanomas of the nasal cavity and paranasal sinuses. A clinicopathological analysis of 14 cases. APMIS 1998; 106:403–410
10. Koppl H, Koppl R, Maier W et al. Recurrent, primary multifocal malignant melanoma of the mucous membrane of the upper respiratory tract. Peculiarities of the in-situ-components [In German]. Pathologie 1999;20:195–199
11. Hoorweg JJ, Loftus BM, Hilgers FJ. Osteoid and bone formation in a nasal mucosal melanoma and its metastasis. Histopathology 1997;31:465–468
12. Regauer S, Anderhuber W, Richtig E et al. Primary mucosal melanomas of the nasal cavity and paranasal sinuses. A clinicopathological analysis of 14 cases. APMIS 1998; 106:403–410
13. Brandwein MS, Rothstein A, Lawson W et al. Sinonasal melanoma. A clinicopathologic study of 25 cases and literature meta-analysis. Arch Otolaryngol Head Neck Surg 199;123:290–296
14. Loree TR, Mullins AP, Spellman J et al. Head and neck mucosal melanoma: a 32-year review. Ear Nose Throat J 1999;78:372–375
15. Mendeloff J. The olfactory neuroepithelial tumours. A review of the literature and report of six additional cases. Cancer 1957;10:944–956
16. Lewis JS, Hutter RVP, Tollefsen HR et al. Nasal tumours of olfactory origin. Arch Otolaryngol 1965;81:169–173
17. Oberman HA, Rice DH. Olfactory neuroblastoma. A clinicopathologic study. Cancer 1976;38:2494–2502
18. Silva EG, Butler JJ, Mackay B et al. Neuroblastomas and neuroendocrine carcinomas of the nasal cavity. A proposed new classification. Cancer 1982;50:2388–2405
19. Carney ME, O'Reilly RC, Sholevar B et al. Expression of the human Achaete-scute 1 gene in olfactory neuroblastoma (esthesioneuroblastoma). J Neurooncol 1995;26:35–43
20. Nelson RS, Perlman EJ, Askin FB. Is esthesioneuroblastoma a peripheral neuroectodermal tumour? Hum Pathol 1995;26:639–641
21. Argani P, Perez-Ordonez B, Xiao H et al. Olfactory neuroblastoma is not related to the Ewing family of tumours: absence of EWS/FLI1 gene fusion and MIC2 expression. Am J Surg Pathol 1998;22:391–398

22. Schwaab G, Lefebvre JL, Julerion M. Cystic adenoid carcinomas (cylindromas) and olfactory esthesio-neuromas of the nasal cavities and paranasal sinuses. Experience of the ORL Group of the National Federation of Cancer Centers [In French]. Neurochirurgie 1997;43:118–120

23. Michaels L, Hyams VJ. Objectivity in the classification of tumours of the nasal epithelium. Postgrad Med J 1975;51:65–707

24. Kairemo KJ, Jekunen AP, Kestila MS et al. Imaging of olfactory neuroblastoma – an analysis of 17 cases. Auris Nasus Larynx 1998;25:173–179

25. Pickuth D, Heywang-Kobrunner SH, Spielmann RP. Computed tomography and magnetic resonance imaging features of olfactory neuroblastoma: an analysis of 22 cases. Clin Otolaryngol 1999;24:457–461

26. Min KW. Usefulness of electron microscopy in the diagnosis of "small" round cell tumours of the sinonasal tract. Ultrastruct Pathol 1995;19:347–363

27. Silva EG, Butler JJ, Mackay B et al. Neuroblastomas and neuroendocrine carcinomas of the nasal cavity. A proposed new classification. Cancer 1982;50:2388–2405

28. Micheau C, Guerinot F, Bohoun C et al. Dopamine-B-hydroxylase and catecholamines in an olfactory esthesioneuroma. Cancer 1975;35:1309–1312

29. Harrison DFN. Surgical pathology of olfactory neuroblastoma. Head Neck Surg 1984;7:60–64

30. Argani P, Perez-Ordonez B, Xiao H et al. Olfactory neuroblastoma is not related to the Ewing family of tumours: absence of EWS/FLI1 gene fusion and MIC2 expression. Am J Surg Pathol 1998;22:391–398

31. Polin RS, Sheehan JP, Chenelle Munoz E et al. The role of preoperative adjuvant treatment in the management of esthesioneuroblastoma: the University of Virginia experience. Neurosurgery 1998;42:1029–1037

32. Gould VER, Linnoila I, Memoli VA et al. Neuroendocrine cells and neuroendocrine neoplasms of the lung. Lab Invest 1983;49:519–539

33. Bonato M, Cerati M, Pagani A et al. Differential diagnostic patterns of lung neuroendocrine tumours. A clinico-pathological and immunohistochemical study of 22 cases. Virchows Arch (A) 1992;420:201–211

34. Capella C, Heitz P, Höfler H et al. Revised classification of neuroendocrine tumours of the lung, pancreas and gut. Virchows Arch 1995;425:547–560

35. Böhm J, Koch S, Gais P et al. Prognostic value of MIB-1 in neuroendocrine tumours of the lung. J Pathol 1996; 178:402–429

36. Perez-Ordonez B, Caruana SM, Huvos AG et al. Small cell neuroendocrine carcinoma of the nasal cavity and paranasal sinuses. Hum Pathol 1998;29:826–832

37. Devaney K, Wenig BM, Abbondanzo SL. Olfactory neuroblastoma and other round cell lesions of the sinonasal region. Mod Pathol 1996;9:658–663

38. Khoddami M, Squire J, Zielenska M et al. Melanotic neuroectodermal tumour of infancy: a molecular genetic study. Pediatr Dev Pathol 1998;1:295–299

19 Vascular Neoplasms; Myogenic Neoplasms

Hereditary Haemorrhagic Telangiectasia (Osler-Weber-Rendu Disease)

This is often called Rendu-Osler-Weber disease and even sometimes Weber-Rendu-Osler disease.

Hereditary haemorrhagic telangiectasia is not a neoplasm but a disease in which groups of dilated vessels are present on the skin and mucosae. These lesions are important because they frequently bleed. The disorder is inherited as an autosomal dominant with evidence of mutant gene on chromosome 9 and perhaps 12. The nose is most commonly affected. Telangiectatic lesions may be seen at the nasal orifice and on the mucosa and, as stated, epistaxis is a common symptom.

The histological appearance is that of a collection of dilated thin-walled blood vessels, which have been shown to be venules on electron microscopy[1] (Fig. 19.1). Haemorrhage takes place onto the surface from blood vessels nearest the epithelium and extravasation of blood into surrounding deeper tissue does not occur.

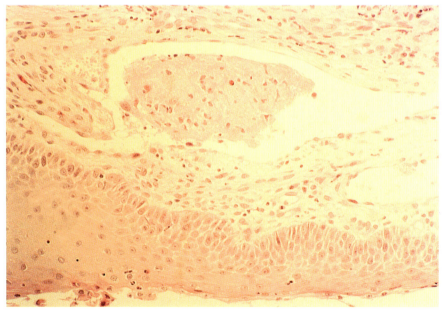

Figure 19.1 Hereditary haemorrhagic telangiectasia. Dilated venules are present near the epithelium of the nasal septum, which is here covered by stratified squamous epithelium

Capillary Haemangioma of Nasal Septum

Capillary haemangioma is a common lesion, which has often been designated "pyogenic granuloma" on the basis of the active inflammatory exudate between the blood vessels. Inflammation is frequent in nasal tumours, particularly if they are polypoid, and so is unlikely to be related to the origin of this condition. We have not been able to separate a "pyogenic" from a "haemangiomatous" form of benign vascular lesion in this situation. The site of the tumour is most frequently the mucosa at the anterior end of the nasal septum. In a series of 30 cases of capillary haemangioma of the nose, seven were also found arising on the turbinates, mostly the inferior turbinate.[2]

Clinical Features and Incidence

Epistaxis is an early symptom and nasal obstruction is frequent. The lesion is not found in children and occurs mostly in the fourth and fifth decades of life. There is an approximately equal sex incidence. Occasionally capillary haemangioma arises on the nasal septum during pregnancy; this form is identical to the conventional capillary haemangioma of the nasal septum and shows a histological appearance similar to that of the "granuloma gravidarum" of the gums.

Gross Appearances

Capillary haemangioma has a characteristic reddish-purple appearance with a smooth surface, which may be somewhat lobulated. The spherical mass usually projects from the mucosal surface and may be polypoid.

Microscopic Appearances

The lesion is composed of capillary channels, which are frequently arranged in small lobules. Larger vessels, often referred to as "feeder" vessels, are situated between the capillary lobules. The capillaries are lined by endothelial cells, which vary in their cytoplasmic content. If the cytoplasm is distended, the lesion may be designated benign haemangioendothelioma by some pathologists. Mitotic figures may be found among these cells, but are not significant as regards recurrence. The epithelial surface of the haemangioma is frequently ulcerated and replaced by a layer of fibrin and polymorphonuclear leucocytes. A variable degree of acute and chronic inflammation is present between the blood vessels. The non-ulcerated epithelium covering the haemangioma often shows squamous metaplasia (Fig. 19.2).

Treatment and Natural History

Surgical removal nearly always produces a cure. Recurrence is rare.

Cavernous Haemangioma

Cavernous haemangioma is a benign neoplasm of blood vessels, which is composed of dilated, thin-walled, blood-filled channels. It has a particular tendency to affect the bones of the nose. Of the five cases reported in one publication,[2] four were in the turbinate bones and one in the wall of the maxillary antrum. We have seen two cases in which the blood-filled channels infiltrated the nasal bones (Fig. 19.3). Microscopically the endothelium-lined spaces are situated in the marrow spaces of the affected bony tissue and may also form a vascular swelling beneath the mucosa.

Angiomatosis

Angiomatosis, sometimes designated "diffuse haemangioma", is a rare condition in which benign-appearing thin-walled blood vessels, often accompanied by fat cells, spread relentlessly throughout a particular area of the body, usually a limb. The tumour, although benign, may lead to death of the patient by its sheer volume. A single case in which a neoplasm of this type filled the maxillary antrum and maxillary bone is described.[2] It required eight operations to produce a remission of growth of 2.5 years at the time of writing.

Haemangiosarcoma

In spite of the high degree of vascularisation that is a feature of the normal nose, malignant neoplasms derived from blood vessels are remarkably rare in this situation. One of the few reported cases is of particular interest as the patient was a worker industrially exposed to vinyl chloride.[3] There is a well-known association between hepatic angiosarcoma and exposure to vinyl chloride monomer. The maxil-

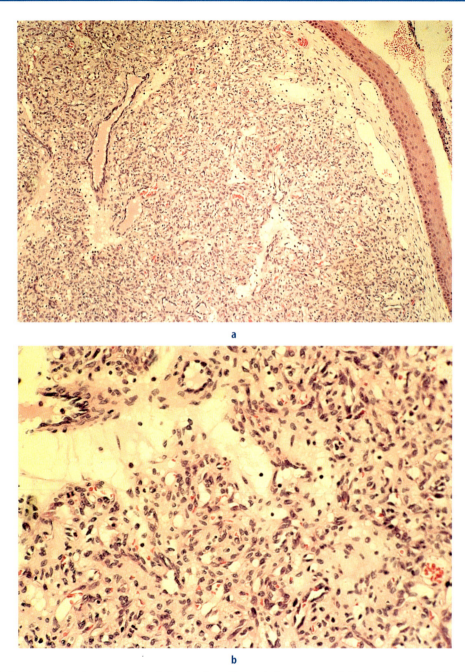

Figure 19.2 Capillary haemangioma (pyogenic granuloma) of nasal septum. **a** The vascular tissue is arranged in lobules, between which lie large "feeder" vessels. There is squamous metaplasia of the overlying nasal epithelium. **b** Higher power view of vessels and inflammatory cells between them

lary antrum is most frequently affected. Microscopically a spectrum of appearances can be recognised, from a well-differentiated angiosarcomatous pattern to a poorly differentiated solid pattern. It is important to ascertain that the actual endothelial cells lining blood vessels have malignant features (Fig. 19.4). These cells usually (but not always) give a positive reaction in their cytoplasm for Factor VIII antigen by the immunoperoxidase method. The few angiosarcomas that do not stain positively by this method are poorly differentiated and are thought to have lost the normal capacity of endothelial cells for producing this antigen. It is possible, as judged by the few literature reports and our own experience, that angiosarcoma of the nose and paranasal sinuses may have a better outlook after

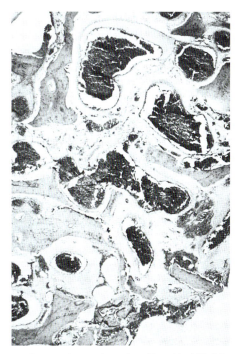

Figure 19.3 Cavernous haemangioma of nasal bone. Blood-filled channels are enclosed by trabeculae of lamellar bone

active therapy than haemangiosarcoma arising in other parts of the head and neck, including the larynx (see Chapter 38).

Systemic Angioendotheliomatosis

Systemic angioendotheliomatosis represents a rare form of malignant neoplasm of blood vessels, which is distinct from haemangiosarcoma. In the latter the neoplasm produces organised blood vessels with a varying degree of differentiation. In systemic angioendotheliomatosis there is an unorganised production of malignant endothelial cells within blood vessels. Most cases have primarily involved the skin, but a case has been described in which the primary lesion first presented in the nasal cavity, but was soon followed by fatal systemic dissemination.[4]

Glomus Tumour

Glomus tumours (glomangiomas) are benign vascular tumours classically located in the subungual region. Extracutaneous glomus tumours are extremely rare. In the head and neck area glomus tumours may occur in the trachea and the sinonasal tract. Only a dozen sinonasal cases have been reported in the literature, most of which have been located in the nasal cavity. The glomus tumour originates in the neuromyoarterial glomus, which is an arteriovenous shunt having a temperature-regulating function. Particularly the subungual glomus tumours have an abundance of nerve fibres and are exquisitely painful. Pain is not a common feature when the tumour is located elsewhere in the skin, but has been described in some of the nasal cases.[5,6]

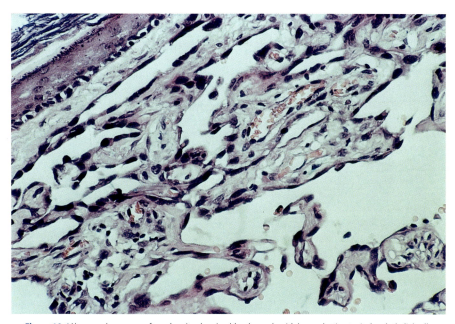

Figure 19.4 Haemangiosarcoma of nasal cavity showing blood vessels with hyperplastic, atypical endothelial cells

The tumours consist of blood vessels that are lined by normal endothelial cells. Microscopically these vessels are seen to be surrounded by solid proliferations of round epithelioid-like cells with almost perfectly round nuclei (Fig. 19.5). Thus the morphological picture may have similarities with haemangiopericytomas, although the nuclei are rounder in a glomus tumour. Immunohistochemistry is of help if in doubt as the cells in glomus tumour stain positively for myosin, and for actin and vimentin, but not for desmin. Haemangiopericytomas do not have myogenous differentiation (see below). Furthermore, axons are present in glomus tumours but not in haemangiopericytomas. Paraganglioma may constitute another differential diagnosis (see Chapter 18).

Sinonasal glomus tumours may be asymptomatic, but usually they present with nasal obstruction

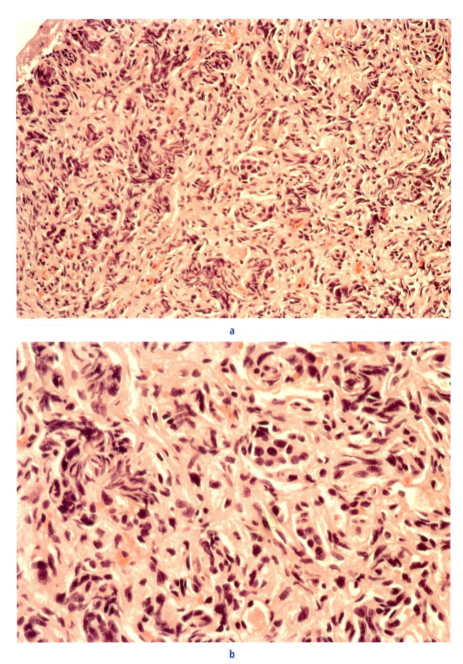

a

b

Figure 19.5 Glomus (glomangioma) of nasal cavity. **a** Numerous blood vessels with groups of epithelioid cells adjacent to them. **b** Higher power view showing detail of epithelioid cells

and/or epistaxis. They are benign and never metastasise. Complete excision normally cures the condition, although an aggressive nasal glomus tumour with multiple local recurrences has been described.[7]

Haemangiopericytoma

Haemangiopericytoma is a neoplasm composed of normal blood vessels surrounded by spindle-shaped or oval tumour cells. On the basis of tissue culture findings, Stout and Murray[8] suggested that the neoplasm was derived from the pericytes of Zimmerman. Since it is still uncertain whether such pericytes exist, the histogenesis of the tumour remains doubtful. Nevertheless, it is a widespread impression among pathologists that, whatever the histogenesis, this is a specific tumour entity conveniently designated by the term haemangiopericytoma. The same histological features seen in haemangioepricytomas may be observed at least focally in diverse neoplasms, e.g. synovial sarcomas, infantile fibrosarcomas, solitary fibrous tumours and malignant fibrous histiocytomas. These neoplasms can be distinguished from each another by specialised pathological techniques, however. Haemangiopericytoma is nowadays "defined" in that context by positive immunoreactivity for vimentin, with or without CD34 and CD57, but it lacks other immunodeterminants of epithelial, neural and myogenous differentiation.[9]

Haemangiopericytoma affecting the nasal cavity and paranasal sinuses is an unusual neoplasm. Compagno and Hyams described 23 cases from the Armed Forces Institute of Pathology.[10]

Incidence

Most often haemangiopericytomas of the nose present in patients of the sixth and seventh decades. There is an equal tendency for the tumour to affect both sexes.

Pathological Appearances

There is no typical gross appearance. The lesions vary with regard to the degree of vascularity that is apparent on the cut surface. Microscopically the vascularity of the neoplasm is apparent in most cases. In some cases the vessels are indistinct on routinely stained sections and it may be helpful to stain the tissue for reticulin, when the uniform and marked vascularity of the neoplasm becomes more apparent. The reticulin stain also serves to demonstrate

that the cells of the tumour are distinct from, and external to the normal endothelium-lined blood vessels. The latter are either capillaries or sinusoidal channels. The cells of the haemangiopericytoma show an oval or elongated nucleus with little atypicism and indistinct cytoplasm. Mitotic rate is low. Fibrosis, diffuse or localised, is present in almost all nasal haemangiopericytomas (Fig. 19.6). The branching stromal vascular pattern with a "staghorn" configuration is often less pronounced in nasal haemangiopericytomas compared with tumours located elsewhere in the body. A unique variant of haemangiopericytoma composed of mature adipocytes and haemangiopericytomatous areas, was recently reported and termed lipomatous haemangiopericytoma. One of the three cases of this possibly distinct pathologic entity was located in the sinonasal area.[11]

Natural History

Haemangiopericytomas of the nose and paranasal sinuses seem to be more benign than their counterparts elsewhere. Recurrence rate is high and rate of metastasis for haemangiopericytomas in general is said to be as high as 50%. The series of Compagno and Hyams showed that in the nose and paranasal sinuses there was a recurrence in only 14% and metastasis in 7%.[10] The low-grade malignancy of sinonasal haemangiopericytomas has been further confirmed by later studies. Although they have a relatively high local recurrence rate, the recurrences tend to be late, and the rate of lymph node metastasis as well as distant metastasis is low.[12] This might be a reflection of early presentation and small tumour mass, and difficulty of complete resection, rather than evidence for having different biological behaviour than haemangiopericytomas located elsewhere in the body.

Myogenic Neoplasms

Leiomyoma

Tumours composed of smooth muscle are rare in the nose. Fu and Perzin[13] described two cases and at that time only one more case had been found in the world literature. Since then only a few more cases have been described. In the two cases described by Fu and Perzin[13] the patients had nasal polyps and the smooth muscle tumour was found incidentally on histological examination among the polyps.

The cells of leiomyoma are spindle shaped with rounded, "cigar-shaped" ends (Fig. 19.7). The cyto-

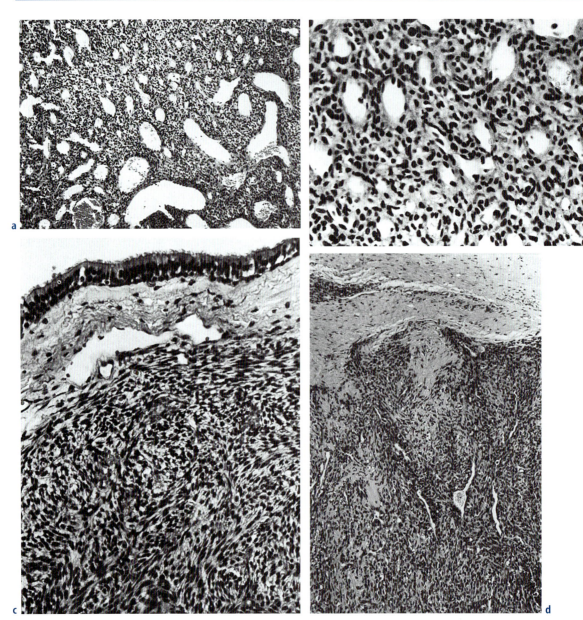

Figure 19.6 Haemangiopericytoma of nasal cavity. **a** The neoplasm is composed of oval cells situated between numerous blood vessels. **b** Higher power of **a** to show oval cells and blood vessels lined by normal endothelial cells. **c** This is composed of spindle-shaped cells. The blood vessels are difficult to detect in some areas. **d** In this neoplasm there are areas of hyaline fibrosis

plasm is eosinophilic and may exhibit longitudinal striations and vacuolation due to accumulation of glycogen. Mitotic figures are rare or absent. Nuclear palisading may be present so that the neoplasm may be mistaken for a neurilemmoma.

Leiomyoma is benign and does not usually recur after resection.

Epithelioid Leiomyoma (Leiomyoblastoma)

Neoplasms of smooth muscle in which the smooth muscle cells display an epithelioid shape, often with vacuolated cytoplasm, have been referred to as leiomyoblastoma. Such neoplasms have occurred mainly in the stomach but are also known at other sites. Most of these tumours are benign and are best known as epithelioid leiomyomas.[14] They are occasionally malignant, in which case the term epithelioid leiomyosarcoma may be applied. The tumours, both benign and malignant, are also often called leiomyoblastomas.

We have studied an epithelioid leiomyoma from the nose in a girl of 5 years. This was a whitish pedunculated mass, which had caused epistaxis and was removed at lateral rhinotomy. The cytoplasm of

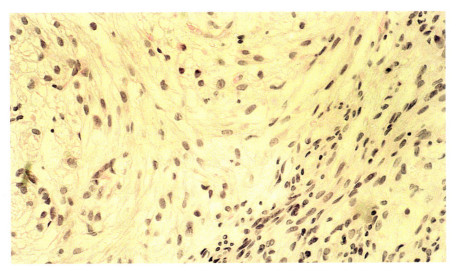

Figure 19.7 Leiomyoma of nose showing regular elongated cells with "cigar-shaped" nuclei

the cells was clear and in places vacuolated due to large amounts of glycogen (Fig. 19.8). Electron microscopy of the tumour cells showed large amounts of glycogen granules, fine fibrils (actin) and pinocytic vesicles. There were two local recurrences of the growth in the first 5 years after resection was carried out. No further recurrence took place.[15]

Immunohistochemistry shows positivity for smooth muscle actin and also desmin, but negativity for keratins, which rules out, for example, a mucinous carcinoma. Epithelioid leiomyoma may show scattered positivity for S-100 protein, which should be kept in mind if liposarcoma is considered as a differential diagnosis. Epithelioid leiomyomas have a very low MIB-1 index, which may help in diagnosis of difficult cases.

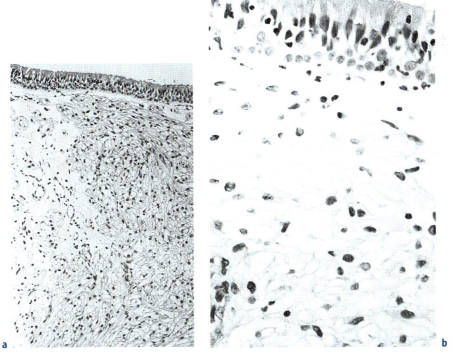

Figure 19.8 Leiomyoblastoma growing in nasal cavity of a 5-year-old girl. **a** Low-power view of tumour showing vacuolated, clear, often elongated cells beneath respiratory epithelium of nose. **b** Higher power view of elongated, clear cells of tumour

Leiomyosarcoma

Malignant tumours of smooth muscle are also unusual in the nose.

Fu and Perzin[13] described six cases of leiomyosarcoma in this situation and 15 years later the only other series of sinonasal leiomyosarcoma was published.[16] This latter report comprised nine cases but also included a review of other reports. To that date 30 cases had been described, so that sinonasal leiomyosarcoma is a rare tumour.

Clinical Features

Compiling the data from these two series the patients were equally distributed between the sexes, with ages ranging from 18 to 86 years (mean 49 years). The most frequent clinical presentation was nasal obstruction unilaterally, but most patients also had epistaxis and pain. In most cases a polypoid mass projected into the lumen of the nose. In approximately half of cases extension to the paranasal sinuses was present. However, upon review of all 30 cases published by 1990, ten patients had the neoplasm confined solely to the nasal cavity.[16]

Pathological Appearances

The histological appearances are similar to those of leiomyoma except that mitotic figures are numerous and the nuclei of the smooth muscle tumour cells exhibit a greater degree of pleomorphism (Fig. 19.9). Thin-walled blood vessels may be prominent in rare areas, causing some confusion with haemangiopericytoma.

Immunohistochemistry shows a similar profile to that described above for leiomyoma, i.e. positivity for smooth muscle actin and desmin but, of course, a much higher MIB-1 index. Cytogenetic analysis has revealed extensive structural and numerical chromosomal aberrations, similar to those of leiomyosarcomas at sites other than the sinonasal tract.[17]

Natural History

The prognosis has improved somewhat since the initial report by Fu and Perzin,[13] and it is today probably best regarded as a locally aggressive tumour with only limited metastatic potential. Complete surgical resection can in many instances be curative. Radiotherapy and chemotherapy do not seem to affect the behaviour of sinonasal leiomyosarcoma.

Neoplasms of Striated Muscle

Rhabdomyoma

Rhabdomyoma and fetal rhabdomyoma occur in the head and neck, particularly in the subcutaneous

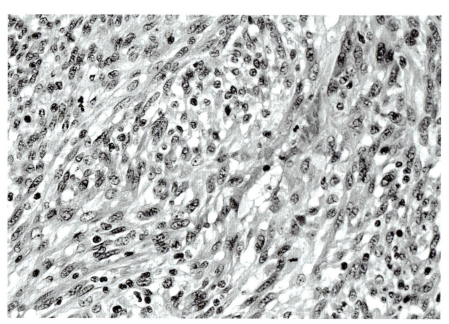

Figure 19.9 Leiomyosarcoma of nose composed of bundles of atypical cells of smooth muscle appearance

tissue and in the larynx (see Chapter 38). Neither rhabdomyoma nor fetal rhabdomyoma occur in the sinonasal tract.

Rhabdomyosarcoma

In children, in contrast to adults, rhabdomyosarcoma is most commonly found in the head and neck area and the urinary tract. Within the head and neck the majority of cases arise from the nasopharynx and the entity is, therefore, described in Chapter 25.

References

1. Menefee MG, Flessa HC, Glueck HI et al. Hereditary hemorrhagic telangiectasia (Osler-Weber-Rendu disease). An electron microscopic study of the vascular lesions before and after therapy with hormones. Arch Otolaryngol 1975; 101:246–251
2. Fu YS, Perzin KH. Non-epithelial tumours of the nasal cavity, paranasal sinuses and nasopharynx: a clinicopathologic study. I. General features and vascular tumours. Cancer 1974;33:1275–1288
3. Williamson IG, Ramsden RT. Angiosarcoma of maxillary antrum – association with vinyl chloride exposure. J Laryngol Otol 1988;102:464–467
4. Wick MR, Banks PM, McDonald TJ. Angioendotheliomatosis of the nose with fatal systemic dissemination. Cancer 1981;48:2510–2517
5. Fleury P, Basset JM, Compere JF et al. Rare tumours of the septum. Eight reported cases [In French]. Ann Otolaryngol Chir Cervicofac 1979;96:767–779
6. Arens C, Dreyer T, Eistert B et al. Glomangioma of the nasal cavity. Case report and literature review. ORL J Otorhinolaryngol Relat Spec 1997;59:179–181
7. Hayes MM, Van de Westhuizen N, Holden GP. Aggressive glomus tumour of the nasal region. Report of a case with multiple local recurrences. Arch Pathol Lab Med 1993;117:649–652
8. Stout AP, Murray MR. Hemangiopericytoma: a vascular tumour featuring Zimmerman's pericytes. Ann Surg 1942;116:26–33
9. Nappi O, Ritter JH, Pettinato G et al. Hemangiopericytoma: histopathological patterns or clinicopathologic entity? Semin Diagn Pathol 1995;12:221–232
10. Compagno J, Hyams VJ. Hemangiopericytoma-like intranasal tumours: a clinicopathological study of 23 cases. Am J Clin Pathol 1976;66:672–683
11. Nielsen GP, Dickersin GR, Provenzal JM et al.. Lipomatous hemangiopericytoma. A histologic, ultrastructural and immunohistochemical study of a unique variant of hemangiopericytoma. Am J Surg Pathol 1995;19:748–756
12. Catalano PJ, Brandwein M, Shah DK et al. Sinonasal hemangiopericytomas: a clinicopathologic and immunohistochemical study of seven cases. Head Neck 1996;18:42–53
13. Fu YS, Perzin KH. Nonepithelial tumours of the nasal cavity, paranasal sinuses, and nasopharynx: a clinicopathologic study. IV. Smooth muscle tumours (leiomyoma, leiomyosarcoma). Cancer 1975;35:1300–1308
14. Enzinger FM, Weiss SW. Soft tissue tumours, 3rd edn. Mosby Year Book Inc., St. Louis, Missouri, 1995
15. Papavasiliou A, Michaels L. Unusual leiomyoma of the nose (leiomyoblastoma): report of a case. J Laryngol Otol 1981; 95:1281–1286
16. Kuruvilla A, Wenig BM, Humphrey DM et al. Leiomyosarcoma of the sinonasal tract. A clinicopathologic study of nine cases. Arch Otolaryngol Head Neck Surg 1990;116:1278–1286
17. Sankary S, Sherwin RN, Malone PS et al. Clonal chromosomal aberrations in a leiomyosarcoma of the sinonasal tract. Cancer Genet Cytogenet 1993;65:21–26

20 Neoplasms of Fibrous Tissue

Fibroma

It is doubtful whether a lesion composed entirely of adult fibrous tissue with collagen and sparse fibrocytes is ever neoplastic; it is usually the end-result of an inflammatory process. Occasionally a fibroblastic form of meningioma may be so poorly cellular as to resemble a fibrous tumour. In such cases the concentrically laminated arrangement of the fibrous tissue may be the only diagnostic feature of meningioma (see Chapter 18). Post-inflammatory fibrous tissue in the nose likewise may present such an arrangement, so it is necessary to search a wider area of the lesion for the presence of more diagnostic cellular whorls of meningioma.

Inflammatory Myofibroblastic Pseudotumour

Definition

Inflammatory myofibroblastic pseudotumour, inflammatory pseudotumour or nodular fasciitis is a locally destructive lesion composed of fibrovascular tissue admixed with chronic inflammatory cells.[1] Fibro-inflammatory pseudotumour is most commonly seen in the urinary bladder, but also in the submucosa of the larynx (see Chapter 38), oral cavity, vagina and endometrium. It is thus, unlike aggressive fibromatosis (see below), not a neoplasm but a reactive submucosal fibroblastic lesion. Caution has to be taken not to misdiagnose this lesion as malignant; confusion particularly with leiomyosarcoma, malignant fibrous histiocytoma and fibrosarcoma may occur.

Pathological Appearances

Inflammatory myofibroblastic pseudotumours have poorly defined margins and involve surrounding structures, often growing into the orbit. They are composed of atypical fibroblasts ("myofibroblasts"), bipolar or stellate in shape, often having bizarre nuclei. The cytoplasm is characteristically basophilic. Mitotic figures are present in sparse numbers, but they are not atypical ones. The fibroblasts are set in a myxoid stroma containing inflammatory cells, particularly primarily lymphocytes and plasma cells and some scattered polymorphonuclear leucocytes. The less-ordered arrangement of the spindle cells, and absence of distinct linear striations in the latter, are two features distinguishing this lesion from a leiomyosarcoma. The cells are usually positive for vimentin but negative for desmin.

Natural History

Inflammatory myofibroblastic pseudotumours tend to involve and grow invasively into the surrounding tissue. Radical surgery is therefore necessary. Recurrences occur and radiotherapy has been given when recurrences could not be controlled surgically.

Solitary Fibrous Tumour

Neoplasms of the nasal cavity and occasionally the maxillary antrum have been described recently, which have a similar appearance to the solitary fibrous tumour of the pleura.[2] The tumours are solid and histologically have a disorganised or "pattern-

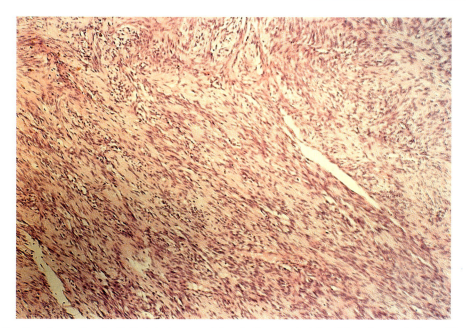

Figure 20.1 Solitary fibrous tumour of nasal cavity. The lesion is composed of a patternless array of spindle cells in a collagenous background. There are numerous prominent vascular channels of different sizes

less" arrangement of spindle cells in a collagenous background and prominent vascular channels of varying size (Fig. 20.1). The lesions lack the characteristic features of other recognised neoplasms that occur in these regions. Immunohistochemically, the tumour cells are diffusely and strongly positive for vimentin and CD34.[2] These lesions are benign.

Aggressive Fibromatosis

Aggressive fibromatosis, or desmoid tumour, is a benign tumour characterised by proliferation of collageneous fibrous tissue (Fig. 20.2). It has a locally infiltrative growth with a tendency to recur but does not metastasise.

The expanding masses of collageneous fibrous tissue can be recognised by the absence of inflammatory cells and a benign appearance of component fibrocytes with abundant collagen. However, at the advancing margins perivascular lymphocytic infiltration is common. The cells have bland cytologic features and often resemble smooth muscle cells. Mitoses are rare.[1]

In one series the fibrous mass was in the maxillary antrum, the maxillary bone or a nasal turbinate bone.[3] Surgical excision even to the extent of partial maxillectomy was required in treating these patients, since all had multiple recurrences. One died of recurrent fibromatosis 18 years following the original resection. In a larger series the maxillary sinus was again the site most frequently involved

and 21% of the patients developed recurrences.[4] In spite of the difficulty of treating some of the above cases, sinonasal aggressive fibromatosis appears to

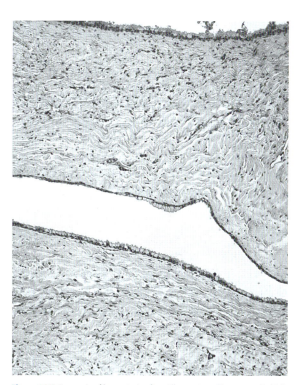

Figure 20.2 Aggressive fibromatosis of maxillary antrum. The mucosa is thickened by wavy bundles of fibrous tissue, which surround a dilated duct

have lower recurrence rates and morbidity than when it arises in many other parts of the body.

Fibrosarcoma

Fibrosarcoma is best defined as a "malignant tumour of fibroblasts that shows no other evidence of cellular differentiation and is capable of recurrence and metastasis".[5] This tumour is rare in the head and neck, but a variety of other lesions have been misdiagnosed as fibrosarcoma, particularly before the era of immunohistochemistry. Only some 30–40 cases of sinonasal fibrosarcoma appear to be have been reported in the literature.

Incidence

There are two series of sinonasal fibrosarcoma reported in the literature, one consisted of 13 patients, the other of 17.[3,6] The ages of these 30 patients at the time of diagnosis ranged from infancy to 77 years, with a mean age of 46 years. Thirteen were males and 17 females.

Clinical Features and Site

The patients presented in most cases with a nasal mass or pain in the cheek. In 13 patients the tumour was confined to the nasal cavity, in eight to the sinuses, and in nine patients the tumour engaged both the nasal cavity and the sinuses.

Pathological Appearances

There is no specific gross appearance, the tumours being composed of homogeneous firm white tissue. Destruction of adjacent bone is an important feature of this neoplasm.

Microscopically there are minor variations, but most fibrosarcomas have in common a rather uniform fascicular growth pattern consisting of fusiform or spindle-shaped cells that vary little in size and shape. The cells have scant cytoplasm, indistinct borders, and are separated by interwoven collagen fibres (Fig. 20.3). The latter is prominently displayed by acid aniline dyes such as Masson's trichrome stain. Mitoses are always present, but bizarre or multinucleated giant cells are rarely a distinctive feature of fibrosarcoma.

The histological grading of fibrosarcoma is mainly based on the degree of cellularity, cellular maturity, mitotic figures, amount of collagen pro-

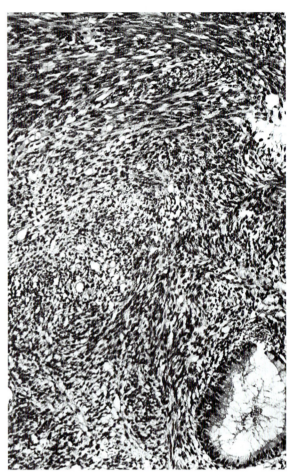

Figure 20.3 Fibrosarcoma of nasal cavity. Interweaving bundles of spindle cells with a little collagen are present in the nasal mucosa. Note surviving gland

duced by the tumour cells and necrosis.[5] There are no sharply defined morphological subdivisions as in, for example, rhabdomyosarcoma. Well-differentiated fibrosarcomas characteristically show the classic herringbone pattern of interlacing fascicles of fibroblasts. In other cases the herringbone pattern may be less distinct yet there is still a uniform, orderly appearance of the spindle cells. Poorly differentiated fibrosarcomas display a less well-orientated pattern, the tumour cells are smaller, there is less collagen and more mitotic figures, and there are areas of necrosis. Reactive new bone formation may be seen at the margin of a fibrosarcoma, as indeed in any other nasal lesions, inflammatory or neoplastic. The cells are immunoreactive for vimentin, but negative for cytokeratins, epithelial membrane antigen and S-100.

Differential Diagnosis

With increased knowledge of connective tissue tumour morphology and employment of immunohistochemistry, neoplasms that were formerly lumped together as fibrosarcomas may now be separated out into other groups, giving greater accuracy in prognosis and effectiveness of treatment. Aggressive fibromatosis can be differentiated by the regular appearance of its fibrocytes and abundant collagen. Osteosarcomas may be mistaken for fibrosarcoma when there is only a small amount of malignant osteoid tissue present.[3] Conversely, a mistake may be made by misinterpretation of invaded normal or reactive bone for tumour bone. Fibrosarcoma may be incorrectly diagnosed as fibrous dysplasia or ossifying fibroma. In both of these conditions (which we usually prefer to lump together as "benign fibro-osseous lesion" – see Chapter 21), trabeculae of bone are intimately associated with the fibrous tissue of the tumour. Leiomyosarcoma may often be identified by the plumper cigar-shaped nuclei and fibrillar cytoplasm of the tumour cells, in contrast to the pointed ends of the nuclei and vesicular cytoplasm of fibroblasts in fibrosarcoma. Fibrous histiocytomas have a more pleomorphic cellular content with histiocytes and giant cells; the growth pattern of fibroblastic areas is storiform (see below). Neurilemmomas and neurofibromas have definite features for identification (see Chapter 18), but malignant schwannomas (neurofibrosarcomas) may be more difficult to recognise, requiring palisading or the juxtaposition of a large nerve for diagnosis. Negative immunostaining for S-100 protein separates fibrosarcoma from spindle cell melanoma, but not necessarily from malignant schwannoma.

Natural History and Treatment

Sinonasal fibrosarcoma is of low-grade malignancy but is notorious for its recurrences, which may eventually kill the patient. A wide resection of the tumour is required. Metastasis of sinonasal fibrosarcoma is unusual but occurs. In the series of Heffner and Gnepp[6] four of the 17 patients died of their disease; three of them had multiple metastases.

Fibrohistiocytic Tumours

Fibrous histiocytoma is a term applied to a wide spectrum of neoplasms, which are formed by both histiocytic and fibroblastic cells. It has been assumed that the cells of origin in these tumours are tissue histiocytes, which could develop into fibroblasts. This is now doubtful. Hence Enzinger and Weiss[5] have suggested the term "fibrohistiocytic

tumours". The nosology of the different forms of neoplasm in this and related groups is difficult. The following is a summary of the classification and main features of fibrohistiocytic tumours propounded by Enzinger and Weiss.[5]

Fibrohistiocytic tumours show both fibroblastic and histiocytic cells. The fibroblasts frequently adopt a storiform pattern. Histiocytes frequently contain lipid and haemosiderin. Lipid-containing multinucleate giant cells – Touton cells – are also frequently seen. Three degrees of neoplastic aggressiveness are recognised on the basis of the histological pattern, cellular atypia and mitotic activity: benign, intermediate and malignant.

Benign Fibrohistiocytic Tumour

Benign fibrohistiocytic tumours are usually found on the skin, and include the common lesions of dermatofibroma and sclerosing angioma, which are always innocent. Deeper forms of tumour in this group occur in the soft tissues; in spite of a benign histological pattern a few have been observed to metastasise. Juvenile xanthogranuloma and reticulohistiocytoma are forms of benign fibrohistiocytic tumour occurring in the skin, which are characterised by large numbers of lipid-containing histiocytes. Xanthomas are collections of histiocytes associated with high levels of serum lipid; they are not neoplasms. Also to be distinguished are lesions such as histoid leprosy, which shows large numbers of organisms of *Mycobacterium leprae* among and within the histiocytes and fibroblasts. Extranodal sinus histiocytosis occurs in the nose and has some features in common with benign fibrohistiocytic tumours. It does not form a tumour mass, however, but infiltrates diffusely the mucosa and submucosa of the nose (see Chapter 22).

Fibrohistiocytic Tumour of Intermediate Malignancy

The term "fibrohistiocytic tumour of intermediate malignancy" refers to a tumour of the skin usually known as dermatofibrosarcoma protuberans, which is more infiltrative than the benign fibrohistiocytic tumours and may even, on occasion, metastasise. Bednár[7] described a melanin-pigmented tumour of the skin, which he regarded as a Schwann cell tumour, but which, apart from pigmentation, had features identical to dermatofibrosarcoma protuberans.

Malignant Fibrohistiocytic Tumour

In malignant fibrohistiocytic tumours (Fig. 20.4) the tumour cells have a decidedly atypical appearance, which, according to Enzinger and Weiss,[5] is a guide to the assessment of malignant potential. The group includes atypical fibroxanthoma of the skin, an actinic-related lesion in aged people, and malignant fibrous histiocytoma. The latter is regarded as the most common soft tissue sarcoma of later life. Malignant appearing as well as Touton giant cells are present in these tumours; the storiform pattern of fibroblasts may still be pronounced. Most of the fibrohistiocytic tumours of the nose fall into this category. Enzinger and Weiss subdivided these neoplasms on a histological basis into five groups:

1. Storiform-pleomorphic: this is variegated, showing a wide range of appearances within the same tumour.
2. Myxoid: at least half of the tumour appears myxoid, the rest showing the ordinary appearances of malignant fibrous histiocytoma.
3. Giant cell: in this type osteoclast-like giant cells are abundant. Osteoid or mature bone is also frequently present.
4. Inflammatory: this type, in which neutrophils and lipid-containing histiocytes are prominent, is usually found in the retroperitoneal region and has been known as retroperitoneal xanthogranuloma. A neoplasm with a similar histology was described in the maxillary sinus of a 23-year-old woman.[8]
5. Angiomatoid. In this form, which is found most commonly in young people, in contrast to the other types of malignant fibrous histiocytoma, the histiocytic cells of the neoplasm are intimately associated with haemorrhagic spaces.

Most malignant fibrous histiocytomas occur in the skeletal muscles of the extremities.

Perzin and Fu described nine cases of fibrous histiocytoma of the nose and paranasal sinuses.[9] Seven of these appear to have been malignant and two benign, judging by the histological descriptions and clinical courses given. Seven of the nine patients were females; ages of patients ranged from 28 to 67 years. Rice et al.[8] described three cases of fibrous histiocytoma of the nose and paranasal sinuses. Two appeared to be in the benign fibrohistiocytic tumour category and one in the xanthogranuloma or inflammatory type of malignant fibrous histiocytic tumour category.

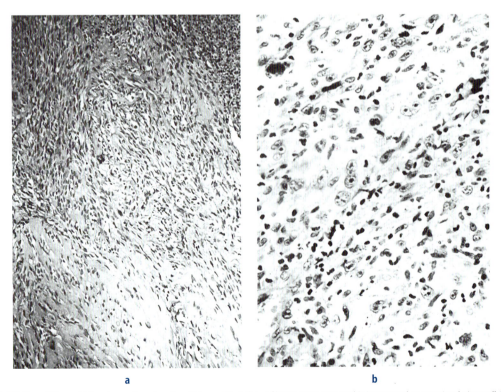

a   b

Figure 20.4 Malignant fibrous histiocytoma of nasal cavity. **a** This neoplasm shows fibrous tissue, tumour histiocytes and an occasional giant cell. **b** Another neoplasm at a higher power showing histiocytes, fibroblasts and giant cells. There is some mitotic activity and nuclear irregularity

Immunohistochemistry

Immunohistochemistry is of limited value and serves primarily as a means of excluding other sarcomas and carcinomas that may resemble malignant fibrous histiocytoma. There is now ample evidence that these tumours are not derived from cells of monocyte or macrophage lineage but rather from fibroblasts. Two histiocytic enzymes, alpha-1-antitrypsin and alpha-1-antichymotrypsin, however, are present in some of the tumours. Such an inconsistent presence can also be found in other sarcomas and carcinomas.

Differential Diagnosis

It may be difficult to distinguish malignant fibrous histiocytoma from other sarcomatous neoplasms such as osteosarcoma, leiomyosarcoma or fibrosarcoma. There is a histological overlap between these neoplasms and it seems reasonable to diagnose the neoplasm according to whichever of the histological features predominates. Spindle cell carcinoma occasionally occurs in the maxillary antrum (see Chapter 16) and closely resembles malignant fibrous histiocytoma. Immunochemical examination for epithelial antigens and electron microscopic examination for desmosomes and tonofibrils may be attempted, but in our experience are frequently negative in spindle cell carcinoma, because of the great dedifferentiation of the neoplasm. Immunochemical detection of

histiocytes for positive identification of fibrous histiocytoma (see above) has been found to be of more value in this connection.

Myxoma

Myxoma is a benign neoplasm that is identified histologically by its infrequent small elongated or stellate cells embedded in a ground substance of mucoid material and reticulin fibres. It occurs principally in muscles and in the extremities, but may also develop in the bones of the jaw, being more common in the lower than in the upper jaw.[10] Upper jaw myxoma is rare (Fig. 20.5). Apart from a few single case reports, the main literature comprises a report of six cases of solely upper jaw myxoma,[11] which included two children and a further report of three cases of upper jaw myxoma comprising only young children aged 13 months, 11 months and 14 months.[12]

Clinical and Imaging Features

Some patients complain of nasal obstruction. In most upper jaw myxomas a mass is identified externally and sometimes within the nasal cavity. Computerised tomography shows the lesion to be well demarcated, occupying part or all of the maxillary antrum and producing expansion of the surrounding bone (Fig. 20.6).

Pathological Appearances

Myxomas are usually described grossly as being gelatinous. Microscopically the tumour is submucosal in the maxillary antrum. It comprises scanty cells showing small dark nuclei with extremely thin cytoplasmic processes, which merge with the reticulin fibres of the stroma to give a stellate appearance. A variable amount of collagen is present. It is sometimes abundant; in such cases the designation of "fibromyxoma" may be applied to the neoplasm, but consideration should then be given to the possibility of a fibrous tumour such as fibromatosis. The stroma is usually abundant, appears mucoid and stains positively with Alcian blue. Blood vessels are very scanty in myxomas. The neoplasm infiltrates between the trabeculae of maxillary bone and also produces bone resorption. Electron micrographic studies of myxomas, albeit from other anatomical sites, have indicated that the myxoma cells have the features of fibroblasts. Immunohistochemical staining gives positive results for vimentin, but desmin,

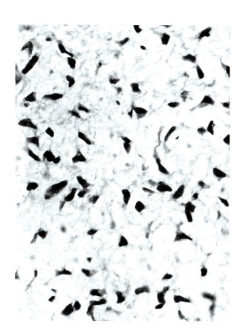

Figure 20.5 Myxoma of maxilla. The small tumour cells show thin cytoplasmic processes, which give them a stellate appearance

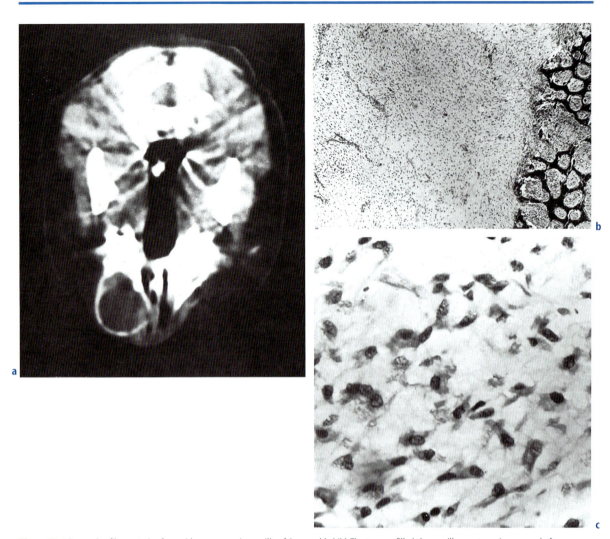

Figure 20.6 Aggressive fibromatosis of myxoid appearance in maxilla of 2-year-old child. The tumour filled the maxillary antrum. It regressed after surgery. **a** Computerised tomogram, axial (i.e. horizontal) section of skull at level of facial swelling showing left antrum expanded by radiolucent mass (*bottom left*), which has expanded its wall to a thin shell. **b** Myxoid tumour encapsulated by wall of woven bone. **c** Higher power showing stellate cells with some nuclear atypicism

myoglobin, smooth muscle actin and S-100 protein antigens are negative.

Differential Diagnosis

Apart from the consideration of a fibrous lesion, such as fibromatosis mentioned above, myxomas of the upper jaw may be confused with Antoni B areas of neurilemmoma. In neurilemmomas, Antoni A areas with palisading and Verocay bodies are usually recognised in non-myxoid parts of the lesion and the neurilemmomas stain strongly positive for S-100 protein. Confusion may exist between myxoma and the myxoid forms of certain sarcomas, notably liposarcoma, embryonal rhabdomyosarcoma, chondrosarcoma and malignant fibrous histiocytoma, which, apart from liposarcoma, do occur in the nose.

They are, however, characterised by a much greater cellularity and atypia than myxomas.

Histogenesis

The origin of this neoplasm is in doubt. Some authors have suggested an odontogenic source, on the basis that in the head and neck it occurs exclusively in the jaws and that it resembles histologically the dental papilla. Others have suggested that it may arise from mesenchymal rests in the alveolar bone.

Treatment

Myxomas are not encapsulated, which probably accounts for the rather high rate of recurrence after curettage that has been experienced. Wide excision is the recommended treatment.

References

1. Shanmugaratnam K, Sobin LH. Histological typing of tumours of the upper respiratory tract and ear. WHO International histological classification of tumours, 2nd edn. Springer-Verlag, Berlin, Heidelberg, 1991

2. Fukunaga M, Ushigome S, Nomura K et al. Solitary fibrous tumour of the nasal cavity and orbit. Pathol-Int 1995;45:952–957

3. Fu YS, Perzin KH. Nonepithelial tumours of the nasal cavity, paranasal sinuses and nasopharynx: a clinicopathologic study. VI. Fibrous tissue tumours (fibroma, fibromatosis, fibrosarcoma). Cancer 1976;37:2912–2928

4. Gnepp DR, Henley J, Weiss S et al. Desmoid fibromatosis of the sinonasal tract and nasopharynx. A clinicopathologic study of 25 cases. Cancer 1996;78:2572–2579

5. Enzinger FM, Weiss SW. Soft tissue tumours, 3rd edn.. Mosby Year Book Inc., St. Louis, Missouri, 1995

6. Heffner DK, Gnepp DR. Sinonasal fibrosarcomas, malignant schwannomas, and "Triton" tumours. A clinicopathologic study of 67 cases. Cancer 1992;70:1089–1101

7. Bednár B. Storiform neurofibromas of skin, pigmented and non-pigmented. Cancer 1957;10:368–376

8. Rice DH, Batsakis JG, Headington JT et al. Fibrous histiocytomas of the nose and paranasal sinuses. Arch Otolaryngol 1974;100:398–401

9. Perzin KH, Fu YS. Non-epithelial tumours of the nasal cavity, paranasal sinuses and nasopharynx: a clinicopathologic study. X1. Fibrous histiocytomas. Cancer 1980; 45:2616–2626

10. Slootweg PJ, Wittkampf ARM. Myxoma of the jaws – an analysis of 15 cases. J Max-fac Surg 1986;14:46–52

11. Fu YS, Perzin KH. Non-epithelial tumours of the nasal cavity, paranasal sinuses and nasopharynx: a clinicopathologic study. VII. Myxomas. Cancer 1977;39:195–203

12. Ang HK, Ramani P, Michaels L. Myxoma of the maxillary antrum in children. Histopathology 1993;23:361–365

21 Neoplasms of Cartilage and Bone

Chondroma

Benign cartilaginous neoplasms of the nose are surprisingly infrequent although hyaline cartilage constitutes the whole anterior part of its framework. Ringertz[1] found only two examples in his series of 391 tumours of the nose and paranasal sinuses. Seven chondromas were found in another review of 256 nasal neoplasms,[2] three being in the nasal septum and four in the nasopharynx. On the other hand in a series in which there was a chondroma arising at the posterior edge of the nasal septum and another in the ethmoids and middle turbinate, it was found, on review of the literature, that 50% of reported tumours arose from the ethmoids and only 17% from the nasal septum.[3] It is indeed a very rare sinonasal tumour.

The ages of the seven patients with nasal chondroma in the series of Fu and Perzin[2] ranged from 10 to 46 years with an average of 26 years.

Grossly the lesions are firm and appear translucent. In a patient whose biopsies we have seen, the cartilaginous deposits were multiple (Fig. 21.1). Microscopically they consist of adult cartilaginous tissue without nuclear atypia. It is likely that some of the cases described in the literature were chondrosarcomas rather than chondromas since some malignant features of the cartilage cells were illustrated.

The treatment of nasal chondroma is surgical excision. There is a definite propensity for recurrence, probably in cases where removal has been incomplete.

Chondroblastoma

Chondroblastoma occurs mainly in people under 20 years of age, and arises usually in the epiphyseal end of long bones (distal femur, proximal tibia and humerus). A few sinonasal cases have been reported.[4] This benign tumour consists of chondroblasts, usually polyhedral but also spindle-shaped. There is

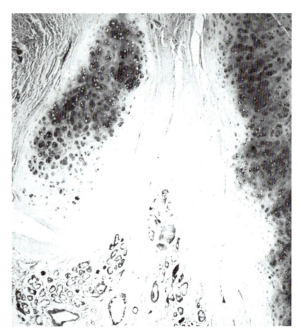

Figure 21.1 Chondroma of nose. The new deposits of cartilage in the nose were multiple in this case. Some were near the glands of the submucosa, as shown in this area.

a chondroid matrix and foci of calcification. The occasional scattered collections of giant cells may lead to confusion with a giant cell tumour. However, the giant cells, which are of osteoclast type, are smaller than those in a giant cell tumour. In a recent study it was demonstrated that the main component of cartilage, type II collagen, is lacking in chondroblastoma. It is thus proposed that chondroblastoma is not a cartilage-forming neoplasm but should be classified as a specific bone-forming neoplasm.[5]

Chondromyxoid fibroma

This rare cartilaginous tumour usually arises in long bones of young adults. Chondromyxoid fibroma of the craniofacial bones are extremely rare and most often involve the mandible and the maxilla. On exceedingly rare occasions it may arise in the paranasal sinuses or in the nasal bone, with extension into the nasal cavity and sinuses.[6,7] Chondromyxoid fibroma shows hypocellular lobules with a myxochondroid appearance, separated by highly cellular tissue composed of giant cells (osteoclasts) and fibroblasts. Although mitotic figures are exceptional, confusion with chondrosarcoma may occur. Also, particularly when involving the clivus, an erroneous diagnosis of chordoma can be made.

Chondrosarcoma

Chondrosarcoma of the nose and paranasal sinuses is a rare condition constituting 3–5% of non-epithelial sinonasal tumours. Some 40 cases arising from the nasal septum have been reported, but most arise in the sinuses.[8] Two large series have been reported,[2,9] consisting of 10 and 12 cases, respectively. The ages of these 22 patients ranged from 15 to 76 years, with an average of 41 years. There were nine males and 13 females. Although exceedingly rare in children, a case of nasal chondrosarcoma in a 5-year-old boy has been reported.

Pathological Appearances

Grossly the tumours were lobulated, firm, grey and glistening on their cut surfaces. Microscopically the appearances met the criteria of Lichtenstein and Jaffe,[10] i.e. the tumour contained too many cells, the cells were too irregular, the nuclei stained too darkly and many were enlarged or giant cells with single, double or multiple nuclei present (Fig. 21.2) (see Chapter 38). Fu and Perzin[2] classified their cases on the basis of resemblance to normal cartilage and number of mitoses as grade 1 (well differentiated), grade 2 (moderately differentiated) and grade 3

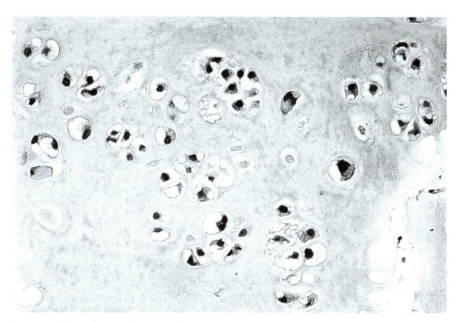

Figure 21.2 Chondrosarcoma of the nasal cavity. Although clearly cartilaginous, this tumour is more cellular than normal cartilage, the nuclei are more darkly staining, larger and more irregular than normal and there are occasional cells with multiple nuclei

(poorly differentiated). Grade 1 showed infrequent and grade 3 numerous mitoses. Only one patient with grade 1 tumour (out of six in this group) died of the disease, this after 18 years of multiple recurrences. Two of the three patients with grade 2 tumours died, as did the single patient with grade 3 neoplasm.

Mesenchymal chondrosarcoma is a rare and highly malignant tumour arising either in bones or in extraosseous sites. Microscopically it shows a biphasic pattern of undifferentiated small round cells and islands of undifferentiated cartilage. It is richly vascularised and failure to find the cartilage islands can lead to a misdiagnosis of haemangiopericytoma (Fig. 21.3). Some cases arising in the maxilla, and involving the sinuses, are reported.[11] Mesenchymal chondrosarcomas are reported to be positive for CD99 (MIC-2), thus mesenchymal chondrosarcoma cannot be distinguished from Ewing's sarcoma and primitive neuroectodermal tumour on the basis of CD99 immunoreactivity.[12]

Differential Diagnosis

Ollier's disease (hereditary multiple exostoses and ecchondromatosis) is the presence of benign growths of cartilage in the metaphyses of several bones. The chondrocytes in these cartilage deposits may present an atypical appearance and in a biopsy may be wrongly interpreted as chondrosarcoma. We have seen one such case, which presented with extensive involvement of the ethmo-sphenoid and skull base, wrongly interpreted as chondrosarcoma, before the onset of long bone lesions (Fig. 21.4).

Natural History

Fu and Perzin[2] reported the 5-year survival of sinonasal chondrosarcoma to be 60%, but Koka et al.[13] showed a 5-year survival of only 36%. The tendency of this neoplasm to recur is said to be related to three factors: (1) position of growth, the posteriorly located tumours having a particularly bad outlook; (2) the presence of tumour in the lines of resection after surgical excision and (3) the degree of dedifferentiation of the growth.[2]

Treatment

Radical surgery is the treatment of choice. Postoperative radiotherapy, with or without chemotherapy, is given only if the excision is incomplete, macroscopically or microscopically.

Osteoma

Osteoid osteoma is a neoplasm usually found in the tibia or fibula. Giant osteoid osteoma, or benign osteoblastoma, is a histologically related entity usually found in the vertebral column. Both are neoplasms of woven bone. A tumour-like lesion of lamellar bone, "true" osteoma, is most frequent in the paranasal sinuses. There is some doubt as to the neoplastic nature of this condition. The density of bone in osteoma of the sinuses is variable. Bone formation in relation to a variety of stimuli is frequent in the paranasal sinuses. It is, therefore, possible that some cases of osteoma may be a hyperplasia of bone reacting to some unknown or indeed known irritant.

Osteomas of the paranasal sinuses were stated to be very common in Egypt, where they were the commonest benign tumour of the nose and paranasal sinuses.[14] Most patients present in the third and fourth decades. Males prevail in all reported series of osteomas of the paranasal sinuses, the ratios of males to females ranging from 1.3:1 to 2.6:1. The lesions occur in the frontal, ethmoid, maxillary and sphenoid sinuses in descending order of frequency.

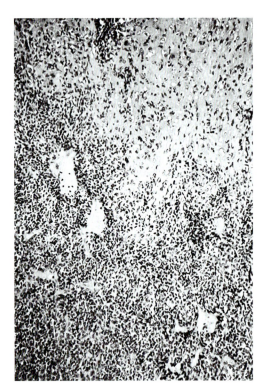

Figure 21.3 Mesenchymal chondrosarcoma of the maxilla. There is an area of malignant cartilage in this field, but most of the tumour shows vascular tissue composed of small malignant cells

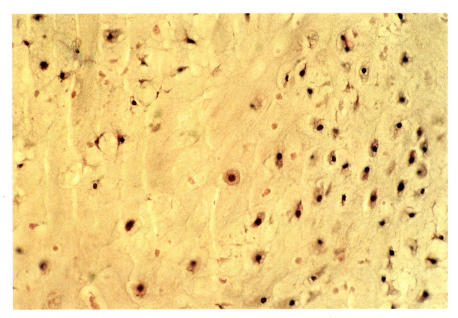

Figure 21.4 Ollier's disease of ethmo-sphenoid region showing atypical chondrocytes

Facial pain or facial asymmetry are the common complaints.[15,16,17] The sinuses frequently undergo secondary infection with suppuration, probably as a result of the occlusion of their ostia by the new bone, with consequent lack of drainage. Osteomas are demonstrable on computerised tomography (CT) scans as clearly defined opacities, which are usually homogeneous. A lobulated edge is frequently observed.

Grossly, osteomas are usually spherical, sometimes lobulated, hard masses of bone. Their density is so great that decalcification by acid in the pathological laboratory may take from 1 to 2 months. Histologically there is variation in the amount of fibrous tissue accompanying the lamellar bone. "Ivory" osteomas usually show very little, while "mature" osteomas show large trabeculae of mature lamellar bone, separated by moderately cellular fibrous tissue[17] (Fig. 21.5). It is difficult to separate mature osteomas from ossifying fibromas with lamellar bone.

The aetiological basis of this condition is not known. A traumatic origin has been implicated in a few cases. The sinuses involved by osteomas are near the junction of the vault of the skull (formed in membrane) and the base of the skull (formed mainly in cartilage); it has been suggested that this is an area of instability of bone formation favouring the development of osteoma.[18] A genetic basis with dominant inheritance is present in a few osteomas. In these cases concomitant colonic polyps are usually present, the association being designated as Gardner's syndrome. The polyps in this syndrome have a pronounced propensity for malignant change.

Giant Cell Tumour

Giant cell tumour, i.e. a tumour composed of large multinucleated osteoclast-like cells and mononuclear cells,[19] is exceedingly rare in the sinonasal region. Most cases have been reported in the sphenoid bone.[20] It should be distinguished from the much more common "brown tumour" of hyper-

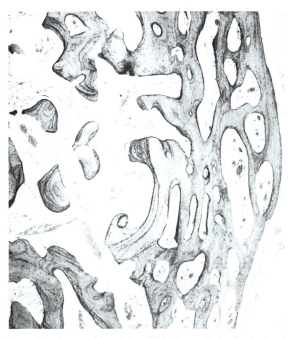

Figure 21.5 Osteoma of frontal sinus. This is a "mature" lesion showing lamellar bone trabeculae and intervening fibrous tissue

parathyroidism, and from giant cell reparative granuloma (see Chapter 14).

Fibrous Dysplasia, Ossifying Fibroma, Benign Fibro-osseous Lesion

Fibrous dysplasia and ossifying fibroma are lesions of bone with well-defined characteristics when they are of odontogenic origin. In the nose and paranasal sinuses, however, a decision as to whether a lesion is fibrous dysplasia or ossifying fibroma is more difficult and other tumours such as benign osteoblastoma and "true" osteoma (see above) may also have to be considered as possible differential diagnoses. Even where some agreement is present, the criteria for the different entities show some overlap in this region. The problem is further compounded by the variable histology that is often found in different parts of the same lesion. We agree with those who acknowledge these difficulties by employing the umbrella term "benign fibro-osseous lesion" for conditions in which we are not capable of giving a more specific diagnosis. Such lesions are particularly likely to be found in children.

Benign Fibro-osseous Lesion

Incidence

Dehner's series[21] consisted of ten females and five males. Their ages ranged from 3 to 15 years, with a mean of 8.6 years.

Clinical Features

Painless swelling of the cheek was present in all cases. Three children had unilateral proptosis and diplopia. Watery rhinorrhoea, which later became purulent, was present in two children and one patient had excessive lacrimation.

Imaging

On X-ray the lesions are circumscribed, fairly homogeneous radiopaque masses, which partially or completely may obliterate the sinuses. A finely granular appearance is sometimes seen of those lesions with a cementifying histological appearance. On CT, ossifying fibromas usually are expansile and circumscribed by a thick bony wall, while on magnetic resonance imaging (MRI), the bony walls often are isointense with grey matter on T1-weighted images and are seen as areas of low density on T2-weighted images. The images of fibrous dysplasia may also vary, and fibro-osseous lesions as such show overlapping radiologic features, emphasising the need of both CT and MRI in the evaluation of these lesions.[22]

Pathological Appearances

Biopsy of benign fibro-osseous lesions of the nose and paranasal sinuses is usually carried out by curettage, so that there is little of significance in the gross appearances of the material removed.

The World Health Organization[19] defined ossifying fibroma as "consisting of spindle-shaped fibroblastic cells usually arranged in a whorled pattern and containing small islands and spicules of metaplastic woven bone and mineralised masses. It may appear encapsulated. Mitosis may be present. The bony spicules may rarely show a lamellar structure peripherally and are frequently rimmed by osteoblasts". Fibrous dysplasia is defined as a "non-encapsulated lesion showing replacement of normal bone by fibrous connective tissue of varying cellularity and containing islands of trabecular or immature non-lamellar metaplastic bone. Osteoblastic rimming is absent or inconspicuous". If there are multiple bony lesions of this type and particularly in the presence of excessive skin pigmentation, the diagnosis of fibrous dysplasia is easily made. The latter features are, however, very rarely present in benign fibro-osseous lesions of the nose and paranasal sinuses. In the absence of such polyostotic and pigmentary features we do not believe that it is possible to decide which of the two names should be assigned to a fibro-osseous lesion in the majority of cases in this region. Thus when faced with a benign neoplasm showing a regular histological pattern of trabeculae of woven bone in a cellular fibrous stroma, we usually designate the condition as benign fibro-osseous lesion (Fig. 21.6). We do not ascribe any significance to the presence or absence of osteoblastic rimming. Lesions of similar appearance and with similar problems of nomenclature are found in the temporal bone (see Chapter 4 and Fig. 4.6).

Juvenile Active Ossifying Fibroma

Juvenile active ossifying fibroma is a form of benign fibro-osseous lesion, which has been carefully analysed by Lent Johnson and his colleagues at the Armed Forces Institute of Pathology in a study

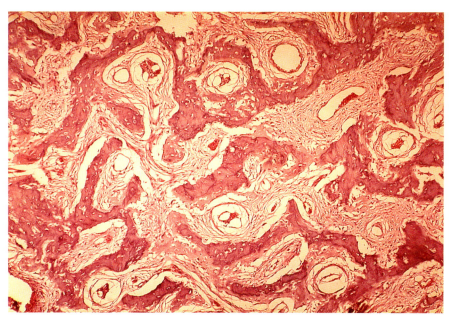

Figure 21.6 Benign fibro-osseous lesion of nose – ossifying fibroma. This lesion consists of trabeculae of mature lamellar bone forming a "Chinese letter" pattern, the elements of which are separated by fibrous tissue

based on the features of 112 cases.[23] This entity has also been referred to as cementifying fibroma, psammo-osteoid fibroma[24] and psammomatoid ossifying fibroma.[25,26] In view of the confusion arising from this multiplicity of terms, we would suggest that the designation "juvenile active ossifying fibroma" (JAOF) replaces the others. "Juvenile active ossifying fibroma" has the advantage of indicating both its relationship to benign fibro-osseous lesion and its tendency to recurrence. The terms "cementifying" and "psammomatoid", although attempting to characterise its histology, have implications, not necessarily valid, of an association of this lesion with other pathological conditions.

Most of these tumours occur in the facial region. Nearly all of the facial lesions arise in the paranasal sinuses, about a third being in the ethmoid turbinate group (ethmoid air cells and turbinate bones pneumatised from ethmoidal air cells) and a third in the supraorbital frontal group (frontal sinus and lateral extension from ethmoid sinus into supraorbital plate). Maxillary lesions constitute about 20%.

The average age at biopsy is 22 years, but the lesion has usually been growing for years when first diagnosed. Patients with these tumours may develop ocular disturbances, particularly proptosis due to orbital involvement, and intracranial extension through the cribriform plate.

Recurrences after surgery occur in 30% of cases. The JAOF that arise in infancy or early childhood tend to be aggressive and spread rapidly despite repeated surgery.

Grossly, lesions are dry, avascular, yellowish-white and crumbly or gritty. Microscopically JAOF show three components:

1. Round bodies with a blue-black-staining centre and a pink-staining osteoid rim. Johnson et al. term these structures "ossicles". Fusion of ossicles can occur to produce elongated woven bone trabeculae.

2. Between the ossicles is a cellular "stroma" composed mainly of nuclei often packed together to suggest a syncytium. On electron microscopy the cells have scant cytoplasm and poorly defined cell membranes. We have found that there is often a marked vascularity in this stroma (Figs. 21.7).

3. Myxomatous areas, which may contain small bluish spheres of cartilage ("chondricles"). The cysts of JAOF are the result of degeneration of the myxoid regions.

Johnson et al. were able to relate the sites of origin, age incidence and histological structure of the growth to the embryogenesis of the facial skeleton. They regard JAOF as a neoplastic product of myxoid tissue, the precursor of cartilage and bone that is particularly prominent in the septa of paranasal sinuses, where it forms the mucoperiosteum between bone and epithelium. The myxoid tissue of JAOF is thought to be derived from this component, which occasionally forms tumours in young children composed only of myxoid tissue[27] (see also

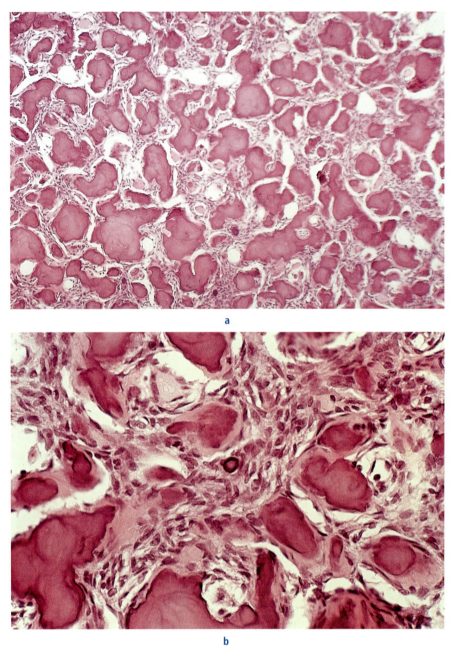

Figure 21.7 Juvenile active ossifying fibroma of the ethmoid sinus with pattern of cementifying fibroma. In this lesion the bony trabeculae are small and round, resembling cementum. **a** Low and **b** higher power views

Chapter 20). In active growth, cellular areas develop from the myxoid tissue and these have their neoplastic component as the stromal cells of the JAOF. Within these cells in the neoplasm an early form of ossification develops, the ossicles, that are so characteristic of these neoplasms. A similar tumour is found in the ramus of the mandible of children between 6 and 12 years, probably originating from the myxomatous tissue of the dental papillae of molar teeth that gives rise to cementum and alveolar bone. Thus the neoplasm seems to replicate the type of bone formation in membrane that is characteristic of the paranasal sinuses and molar teeth.

In a study of the cytogenetics of three cases with this neoplasm, recurring breakpoints were found at Xq26 and 2q33. Two of the tumours showed an identical t(X;2)(q26;q33) reciprocal translocation as the sole abnormality. The third tumour revealed an interstitial insertion of bands 2q24.2q33 into Xq26 as the sole abnormality. This study provides a cytogenetic tumour marker for the identification of this tumour subtype.[28] Tumours similar to JAOF have been reported in long bones[29,30] often with bone cysts of myxoid tissue. The ultrastructure of these lesions is similar to that of JAOF.[30]

Treatment

Most cases of benign fibro-osseous lesion respond well to treatment by a single curettage of the tumour with little tendency to recurrence. The JAOF is more prone to recur, however, as mentioned above.

Osteosarcoma

Although osteosarcoma is rare in the nose and paranasal sinuses, Garrington et al.[31] calculated that about 6.5% of all osteosarcomas arise in the maxilla and mandible. They are at least four times as common in the sinuses than in the nasal cavity.

Incidence

Very large series of sinonasal (maxillary) osteosarcomas are described in the textbook on bone tumours by Unni and Dahlin and from the Armed Forces Institute of Pathology series.[32] Ages ranged from 15 to 50, with a median age of 28 years. There was a sharp peak of incidence in the 20–29 year age group. Cases with this tumour treated at the Royal National Throat, Nose and Ear Hospital, London, showed an even older group of patients ranging from 30 to 69 years, with a mean of 51 and a median of 45 years.[33] Also the 14 patients reported by Koka et al.[34] represented an older age group, the mean being 47 years. Although the Armed Forces cases are weighted towards a lower age group, it is clear that for both of these series the ages of patients with osteosarcomas of the upper jaw are higher than those with osteosarcomas of other sites, which occur mainly in the second decade of life.

The Royal National series showed only two males in a total of seven patients, but the Armed Forces series had a male predominance.

Predisposing Factors

Most osteosarcomas arise de novo but certain conditions have been associated with subsequent development of osteosarcoma, e.g. irradiation treatment, Paget's disease and fibrous dysplasia.[33]

Clinical Features

The main clinical features are those of a visible swelling associated with pain in the upper jaw. Radiological examination shows a mass with evidence of bone destruction and invasion.

Pathological Appearances

The gross features of osteosarcoma are those of an irregularly calcified, destructive tumour. Histologically the neoplasm is composed of sarcoma cells together with foci of malignant osteoid and/or malignant bone (Fig. 21.8). The neoplasm is often less anaplastic than osteosarcoma of long bones and mitoses may not be numerous. Malignant cartilage is frequently present in parts of the growth and may dominate the histological appearances, so that a diagnosis of chondrosarcoma rather than osteosarcoma may be preferred. The distinction is not of serious significance because chondrosarcoma of the upper jaw seems to be just as malignant locally as osteosarcoma,[31] and osteosarcoma of the upper jaw, like chondrosarcoma, rarely metastasises. Fibrosarcoma-like and myxomatous areas may also be prominent in the osteosarcoma. Some osteosarcomas of the maxilla show a marked vascularity with dilated capillary and cavernous vessels.

Spread

Extension of the neoplasm is mainly within the skull. Haematogenous metastasis is much less frequent than with osteogenic sarcoma of long bones.

Natural History

The 5-year survival for osteogenic sarcoma of the maxilla (25%[31]) is stated to be greater than for overall osteogenic sarcoma (18%[35]) . This is also confirmed in the study by Koka et al., which revealed a 5-year survival of 24%.[34]

Treatment

The treatment required is radical surgical excision of the neoplasm. Chemotherapy has been recommended as a useful adjunct.

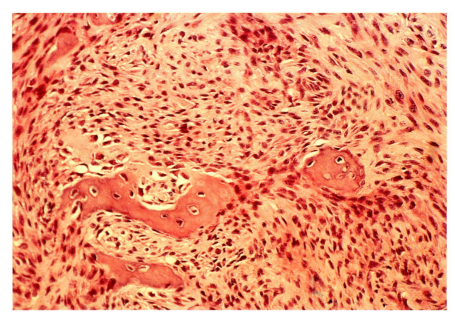

Figure 21.8 Osteosarcoma of nasal cavity. The neoplasm shows spindle cell sarcoma together with woven bone

Ewing's Sarcoma

Ewing's sarcoma of the sinonasal tract is rare and may arise in the maxilla, and on exceedingly rare occasions in the soft tissue of the nose, i.e. as an extraskeletal Ewing's sarcoma.[36,37]

The age incidence of maxillary cases is rather higher than that of Ewing's sarcoma of long bones.[38] Symptoms are those of nasal obstruction, swelling, pain and exophthalmos. On radiological examination the tumour is usually found to infiltrate widely in the maxilla.

Ewing's sarcoma is defined as primitive mesenchymal tumour composed of uniform, small undifferentiated cells. The cells are darkly stained, have scant cytoplasm, which sometimes may be vacuolated. The cells are closely packed in sheets or divided into nests or lobules by fine fibrovascular septa, and usually contain glycogen.[19] There are numerous mitoses and widespread necrosis; focal calcification is common (Fig. 21.9).

Immunohistochemistry and molecular biology are of great help in distinguishing Ewing's sarcoma from other sarcomas and small round cell tumours. Positive immunoreactivity for CD99 (MIC-2) is a hallmark of Ewing's sarcoma; this antigen, however, is also displayed in some other tumours. Recent studies indicate the absence of neural cell adhesion molecules in this tumour, which may be helpful in distinguishing Ewing's sarcoma from rhabdomyosarcoma and other sarcomas that do express this molecule.[39] The reciprocal translocation t(11;22) (q24;q12) is a specific molecular marker for the Ewing's sarcoma family of tumours. Ewing's sarcoma expresses chimeric transcription factors resulting from a fusion of the amino terminus of the *EWS* gene to the carboxyl terminus of one of five ETS proteins. The majority of Ewing's sarcoma express EWS/FLI-1 fusions, some contain variant chimeras such as EWS/ETV-1.[40] Probes localising to 11q24 (FLI-1) and 22q12 (EWS) can be used in an in situ hybridisation assay to evaluate EWS/FL-1 fusion.

The outlook for the patient has been very poor, the neoplasm tending to spread rapidly and widely via the bloodstream and lymphatics, although with modern methods of aggressive chemotherapy this has improved considerably.

References

1. Ringertz N. Pathology of malignant tumours arising in the nasal and paranasal cavities and maxilla. Acta Otolaryngol (Stockh) 1938;27(suppl):1–405
2. Fu YS, Perzin KH. Non-epithelial tumours of the nasal cavity, paranasal sinuses and nasopharynx: a clinicopathologic study. III. Cartilaginous tumours (chondroma, chondrosarcoma). Cancer 1974;34:453–463
3. Kilby D, Ambegoakar AG. The nasal chondroma: two case reports and a survey of the literature. J Laryngol Otol 1977;91:415–426
4. al-Sader MH, Tait R, Leader M. Chondroblastoma – an unusual site in a young female. J Laryngol Otol 1996;110:696–699
5. Aigner T, Loos S, Inwards C et al. Chondroblastoma is an osteoid-forming, but not cartilage-forming neoplasm. J Pathol 1999;189:463–469
6. Koay CB, Freeland AP, Athanasou NA. Chondromyxoid fibroma of the nasal bone with extension into the frontal and ethmoidal sinuses. J Laryngol Otol 1995;109:258–261

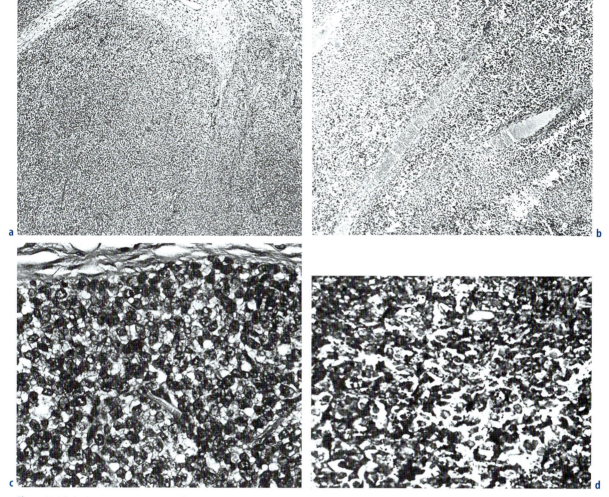

Figure 21.9 Ewing's sarcoma presenting as polyps in nasal cavity in a 14-year-old girl. **a** The tumour is lobulated and is composed of small cells. **b** The tumour cells show a tendency to be deposited around blood vessels. **c** Under higher power the small, round cells of the neoplasm show foamy cytoplasm. **d** The cytoplasm of the tumour cells contains much glycogen, shown as dark material, which is red staining in the original. Periodic acid–Schiff stain

7. Nazeer T, Ro JY, Varma DG et al. Chondromyxoid fibroma of paranasal sinuses: report of two cases presenting with nasal obstruction. Skeletal Radiol 1996;25:779–782

8. Rassekh CH, Nuss DW, Kapadia SB et al. Chondrosarcoma of the nasal septum: skull base imaging and clinicopathologic correlation. Otolaryngol Head Neck Surg 1996;115:29–37

9. Koka V, Vericel R, Lartigau E et al. Sarcomas of nasal cavity and paranasal sinuses: chondrosarcoma, osteosarcoma and fibrosarcoma. J Laryngol Otol 1994;108:947–953

10. Lichtenstein L, Jaffe HL. Chondrosarcoma of bone. Am J Pathol 1943;19:553–589

11. Vencio EF, Reeve CM, Unni KK et al. Mesenchymal chondrosarcoma of the jaw bones: clinicopathologic study of 19 cases. Cancer 1998;82:2350–2355

12. Granter SR, Renshaw AA, Fletcher CD et al. CD99 reactivity in mesenchymal chondrosarcoma. Hum Pathol 1996;27:1273–1276

13. Koka V, Vericel R, Lartigau E et al. Sarcomas of nasal cavity and paranasal sinuses: chondrosarcoma, osteosarcoma and fibrosarcoma. J Laryngol Otol 1994;108:947–953

14. Handousa AB. Primary benign neoplasms of the nose. J Laryngol Otol 1952;66:421–436

15. Samy LL, Mostafa H. Osteomata of the nose and paranasal sinuses with a report of twenty one cases. J Laryngol Otol 1971;85:449–469

16. Atallah N, Jay MM. Osteomas of the paranasal sinuses. J Laryngol Otol 1981;95:291–309

17. Fu YS, Perzin KH. Non-epithelial tumours of the nasal cavity, paranasal sinuses, and nasopharynx: a clinicopathologic study. II. Osseous and fibro-osseous lesions, including osteoma, fibrous dysplasia, ossifying fibroma, osteoblastoma, giant cell tumour, and osteosarcoma. Cancer 1974;33:1289–1305

18. Hallberg OE, Begley JW. Origin and treatment of osteomas of the paranasal sinuses. Arch Otolaryngol 1950;51:750–760

19. Shanmugaratnam K, Sobin LH. Histological typing of tumours of the upper respiratory tract and ear. WHO International histological classification of tumours, 2nd edn. Springer-Verlag, Berlin, Heidelberg, New York, 1991

20. Gupta OP, Samant HC, Bhatia PL et al. Giant cell tumour of the sphenoid bone. Ann Otol Rhinol Laryngol 1975;84:359–363

21. Dehner LP. Tumours of the mandible and maxilla in children. I. Clinicopathologic study of 46 histologically benign lesions. Cancer 1973;31:364–384

22. Wenig BM, Mafee MF, Ghosh L. Fibro-osseous, osseous, and cartilaginous lesions of the orbit and paraorbital region. Correlative clinicopathologic and radiographic features, including the diagnostic role of CT and MR imaging. Radiol Clin North Am 1998;36:1241–1259

23. Johnson LC, Yousefi M, Vinh TN et al. Juvenile active ossifying fibroma. Its nature, dynamics and origin. Acta Otolaryngol (Stockh) 1991;488(suppl):1–40

24. Damjanov I, Maenza RM, Snyder GG et al. Juvenile ossifying fibroma. An ultrastructural study. Cancer 1978;42:2668–2674

25. Margo CE, Ragsdale BD, Perman KI et al. Psammomatoid (juvenile) ossifying fibroma of the orbit. Ophthalmology 1985;92:150–159

26. Slootweg PJ, Panders AK, Nikkels PG. Psammomatoid ossifying fibroma of the paranasal sinuses. An extragnathic variant of cemento-ossifying fibroma. Report of three cases. J Craniomaxillofac Surg 1993;21:294–297

27. Ang HK, Ramani P, Michaels L. Myxoma of the maxillary antrum in children. Histopathol 1993;23:361–365

28. Sawyer JR, Tryka AF, Bell JM et al. Nonrandom chromosome breakpoints at Xq26 and 2q33 characterize cemento-ossifying fibromas of the orbit. Cancer 1995;76:1853–1859

29. Sissons HS, Kanchere PL, Lehman WB. Ossifying fibroma of bone. Bull Hosp Joint Dis 1983;43:1–14

30. Povysil C, Matejovsky Z. Fibro-osseous lesion with calcified spherules (cementifying fibroma-like lesion) of the tibia. Ultrastructural Pathol 1993;17:25–34

31. Garrington GE, Scofield HH, Cornyn J et al. Osteosarcoma of the jaws. Analysis of 56 cases. Cancer 1967;20:377–391

32. Unni KK, Dahlin DC. Bone tumours. General aspects and data on 11,087 cases, 5th edn. Lippincott Williams & Wilkins, Philadelphia, 1996

33. Windle-Taylor PC. Osteosarcoma of the upper jaw. J Maxillofac Surg 1977;5:62–68

34. Koka V, Vericel R, Lartigau E et al. Sarcomas of nasal cavity and paranasal sinuses: chondrosarcoma, osteosarcoma and fibrosarcoma. J Laryngol Otol 1994;108:947–953

35. Arlen M, Higinbotham NL, Huvos AG et al. Radiation-induced sarcoma of bone. Cancer 1971;28:1087–1099

36. Lane S, Ironside JW. Extra-skeletal Ewing's sarcoma of the nasal fossa. J Laryngol Otol 1990;104:570–573

37. Howard DJ, Daniels HA. Ewing's sarcoma of the nose. Ear Nose Throat J 1993;72:277–279

38. Ferlito A. Primary Ewing's sarcoma of the maxilla: a clinico-pathological study of four cases. J Laryngol Otol 1978;92: 1007–1024

39. Molenaar WM, Muntinghe FL. Expression of neural cell adhesion molecules and neurofilament protein isoforms in Ewing's sarcoma of bone and soft tissue sarcomas other than rhabdomyosarcoma. Hum Pathol 1999;30:1207–1212

40. Thompson AD, Teitell MA, Arvand A et al. Divergent Ewing's sarcoma EWS/ETS fusions confer a common tumourigenic phenotype on NIH3T3 cells. Oncogene 1999;18:5506–5513

22 Miscellaneous Conditions

Lymphoma and Plasmacytoma

Lymphoma

Lymphomas have two general forms: Hodgkin's and non-Hodgkin's. We are not aware of a case of Hodgkin's lymphoma having occurred in the nose and paranasal sinuses. In the upper air and food passages the neoplasms considered under the generic term of non-Hodgkin's lymphoma are most commonly seen in the palatine tonsils. Surprisingly, in view of the absence of lymphoid tissue in the normal sinonasal tract, the nose and paranasal sinuses rank second to the tonsils in frequency of occurrence of non-Hodgkin's lymphoma. The incidence of this condition is higher than in the nasopharynx, where lymphoid tissue is normally abundant. The subject of lymphomas of the nose and throat is considered in detail in Chapter 27, apart from extramedullary plasmacytomas, which are dealt with below. Most nasal malignant lymphomas are termed T/NK (T/Natural Killer cell lineage) nasal malignant lymphoma in the new World Health Organization classification. As described in Chapter 14, these lymphomas consist of small, medium or large lymphoid cells with pale cytoplasm and irregular nuclei. The tumours are often angiocentric and even angiodestructive. The immunophenotype is either NK or T cytotoxic with CD8 and TiA1 positivity. Proliferations with coexpression of T and NK markers can be observed.

Extramedullary Plasmacytoma (Malignant Lymphoma, Plasmacytic)

Plasmacytoma is defined as a neoplasm of cells recognisable as plasma cells. In practice it is sometimes difficult to separate plasmacytoma from chronic inflammation. Moreover, plasmacytoma of the sinonasal tract, unlike multiple myeloma, is usually unassociated with paraproteinaemia. Diagnosis is helped, however, by determination of the monoclonality of the plasma cell exudate.

Incidence

A male preponderance has been recorded in sinonasal plasmacytoma.[1,2] In a recently described series of 60 primary nasal malignancies, there were 14 cases of malignant lymphoma (23%) and three plasmacytomas (5%).[3] Thus non-epithelial tumours constitute a considerable proportion of sinonasal malignancies, and plasmacytoma is not exceedingly rare.

Site

Extramedullary plasmacytoma is most commonly found in the upper respiratory tract. Table 22.1 lists the sites at initial presentation in 53 cases of soft tissue extramedullary plasmacytomas of the upper air and food passages seen at the Armed Forces

Table 22.1. Sites of initial presentation in 53 cases of extramedullary plasmacytoma of the upper air and food passages. Armed Forces Institute of Pathology Registry 1940–1980 (cases collected in collaboration with Dr. V.J. Hyams)

Site	Number of cases
Nose and paranasal sinuses	28 (52%)
Nasopharynx	10 (19%)
Pharynx (oropharynx and hypopharynx)	3 (6%)
Tonsil	3 (6%)
Larynx	9 (17%)

Institute of Pathology in Washington D.C. between 1940 and 1980. Cases affecting the nose and paranasal sinuses are more numerous than the total of all the other sites combined. Within the sinonasal tract, the nasal septum, the lateral wall of the nose and the maxillary antrum showed a particularly high incidence.

Clinical Features

The commonest appearance of malignant plasmacytic lymphoma is that of a mass in the soft tissue of the upper air and food passages. Airway obstruction and epistaxis are also frequently present. Proptosis resulting from orbital involvement by an ethmoid mass is sometimes seen, but cranial nerves are rarely affected.[2]

Gross Appearances

In a small proportion of cases, plasmacytoma produces a polypoidal thickening of the mucosa. Mostly there is a grey or pink thickening of the mucosa with underlying invasion of soft tissue or bone.

Microscopic Appearances (Fig. 22.1)

Although plasma cells may be very numerous in non-neoplastic conditions, the histological recognition of the lesion as a neoplasm is usually not difficult. In chronic inflammation plasma cells may be numerous, but there is an admixture of other cells, such as lymphocytes and histiocytes. The hallmark of a plasmacytoma is the presence of large sheets of plasma cells alone, which replace tissue structures and invade locally. Fields of neoplastic plasma cells are generally very broad, being split up only by blood vessels. Sometimes the tumour cells may appear to be adherent to or supported by the blood vessels, and if so an alveolar pattern may be suggested.

The actual identification of a neoplasm as one derived exclusively from plasma cells may sometimes be more difficult. The normal plasma cell has a number of specific features, all of which may be found in cells of well-differentiated plasmacytomas. The small eccentrically situated nucleus, with five to eight deeply basophilic condensations of chromatin regularly arranged around the nuclear membrane in a "cartwheel" fashion, may be found in some plasmacytomas. A lightly stained area (the paranuclear vacuole) may also be identified near the nucleus in some tumour cells. The cytoplasm of the cells is non-granular and basophilic and the high ribonucleoprotein content of the cytoplasm may be confirmed by the Unna-Pappenheim stain, which usually produces a red (pyroninophil) reaction. Even the feature of normal plasma cells that is of greatest ultrastructural significance – the abundant arrays of endoplasmic reticulin – may sometimes be seen in plasmacytomas by the light microscope as small dilated vesicles. Russell bodies may be present in extramedullary plasmacytomas, in spite of statements sometimes made to the contrary. We have seen them in 13% of plasmacytomas of the upper respiratory tract, sometimes in large numbers. They may also be found in metastatic deposits of the plasmacytoma as well as in the primary.

Some 20% of plasmacytomas are accompanied by deposits of amyloid. The presence of amyloid in a plasmacytoma of the upper respiratory tract gives no indication of its malignant potential. The amyloid may be found only in the primary plasmacytoma and not in the metastases. The amyloid tends to be deposited around blood vessels, and to show concentrically laminated masses similar to the deposits of primary amyloid of the larynx[4] (see Chapter 31). Russell bodies and amyloid have not been found in the same neoplasm.

Natural History

The most comprehensive account of the natural history of extramedullary plasmacytomas has been given by Wiltshaw[1] in her analysis both of the cases under treatment at the Royal Marsden Hospital, London, and those collected from the world literature. Nineteen per cent of all patients developed secondaries in bone, but these were single rather than multiple and were distributed in a random fashion throughout the skeleton. Bone marrow involvement was infrequent. In 18% of all cases of extramedullary plasmacytoma collected by Wiltshaw, there was lymph node spread, but in one-third of these it went no further than the lymph nodes draining the primary lesion. Other sites of spread

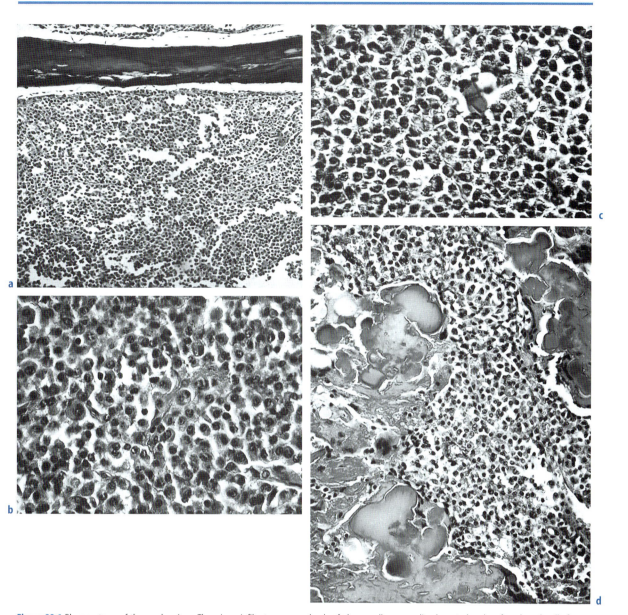

Figure 22.1 Plasmacytoma of the nasal cavity. **a** There is an infiltrate composed only of plasma cells surrounding bony trabeculum from lateral wall of nose. **b** Higher power of another tumour showing cartwheel nuclear chromatin pattern and subnuclear vacuole in some cells. **c** Russell bodies slightly above and to right of centre in infiltrate of neoplastic plasma cells. **d** Amyloid forming large ovoid masses in tumour. The pattern of deposition is similar to primary amyloid deposit (see Chapter 31)

from extramedullary plasmacytoma were the skin, subcutaneous tissue, liver, lungs and pleura and the gastrointestinal tract. Among the Royal Marsden cases, Wiltshaw computed a 10-year survival rate of more than 50%. Renal failure does not seem to have been a feature in the world literature. In approximately half of all cases, further development of the plasmacytoma is to be expected, according to Wiltshaw's findings, but the pattern of spread is to local lymph nodes, random solitary bone sites and deposits in soft tissues, a pattern quite unlike that of

multiple myeloma. Survivals of 15 years without recurrence after treatment by irradiation or surgery are quite common, and cases are seen with long survival even after local recurrence of the tumour.

Immunoglobulin Secretion

Elevation of serum immunoglobulin or the presence of urinary Bence-Jones protein is seen very rarely on presentation of this neoplasm. In Wiltshaw's Royal

Marsden series, about 10% of all patients subsequently developed paraproteinaemia. This was always in the advanced stage of the disease, presumably as a result of the presence of a large mass of immunoglobulin-secreting neoplasm.

By using the immunoperoxidase staining method on paraffin-embedded formalin-fixed sections of extramedullary plasmacytoma, it can be discerned that, like multiple myeloma, this tumour secretes immunoglobulin in a monoclonal fashion. The heavy chain produced is always IgG and the light chains may be either κ or λ. The finding of monoclonal immunoglobulin is useful in deciding whether a particular collection of plasma cells is a plasmacytoma rather than an inflammatory infiltrate, and also in identifying an undiagnosed tumour as a plasmacytoma.

Treatment

Radiotherapy is the treatment of choice and long-term follow-up is necessary. The overall 10-year survival is about 50%.[5] Occasionally local removal of a polypoid neoplasm may be indicated.

Plasma Cell Granuloma

Plasma cell granuloma is not a neoplasm but a chronic inflammatory lesion with heavy plasma cell infiltration. It is usually seen in the mucosa of paranasal sinuses in association with longstanding severe chronic sinusitis. Lymphoid tissue with lymph follicles are seen and also a great number of mature, typical plasma cells. So-called Mott's cells, which have distended cytoplasm filled with eosinophilic globules, i.e. Russell bodies, are present. Immunostaining for immunoglobulins will demonstrate a polyclonal plasma cell population. There are no abnormalities of protein metabolism, nor any bone marrow involvement.

Plasma cell granuloma has to be distinguished from extramedullary plasmacytoma.

Langerhans Cell Histiocytosis (Histiocytosis X)

Langerhans cell histiocytosis is a solitary or multifocal, non-neoplastic proliferative disease of cells of the dendritic cell lineage, closely resembling activated Langerhans cells. The Langerhans cell is characterised by being a dendritic cell that is immunopositive for CD1 and ultrastructurally shows Birbeck granules. The aetiology and pathogenesis of this disease remains unknown, although recently it has been proposed that Langerhans cell histiocytosis is caused by dysregulation of the E-cadherin-beta-catenin cascade.[6] Langerhans cell histiocytosis includes eosinophilic granuloma, Hand-Schuller-Christian disease and Letter-Siwe disease. In the ear, nose and throat region the disease process affects mainly the temporal bone, and the pathological changes that characterise this condition are described in Chapter 4.

More rarely the bones of the nose and paranasal sinuses are involved in this disease process.

Extranodal Sinus Histiocytosis (Sinus Histiocytosis with Massive Lymphadenopathy, Rosai-Dorfman Disease)

Sinus histiocytosis with massive lymphadenopathy was described in 1969 by Rosai and Dorfman.[7] In this condition, in which the lymph nodes affected were usually in the cervical region, general symptoms such as weight loss were stated to be frequent. The histological appearances of the lymph nodes are those of heavy deposition of histiocytic cells in sinuses of lymph nodes. Phagocytosis of lymphocytes by those cells is frequent. In addition, deposits of plasma cells appear in the lymph nodes close to the histiocytes. Extranodal involvement occurs in 30–40% of cases, most often in the head and neck region.[8]

Foucar et al.[9] described deposits of sinus histiocytosis extranodally in the ear, nose and throat region. Deposits of sinus histiocytosis were encountered in 16 patients, most frequently in the nasal mucosa, but salivary gland, pharyngeal, paranasal sinus, tonsillar and tracheal infiltrations were also seen. The course of the disease was one of chronic involvement of the affected part, persisting for a variable period up to 12 years, with eventual disappearance of the lesion. Antibiotics, cytotoxic drugs and steroids had no effect on the condition. Surgical excision resulted in a complete cure in some cases. In others recurrence followed such excision.

The changes in the head and neck involve the mucosa of the upper respiratory tract in most cases (Fig. 22.2). The gross appearances are those of a pale grey or light yellow thickening of the mucosa. In one case in which the subglottic mucosa was primarily affected, the resultant narrowing of the airway was

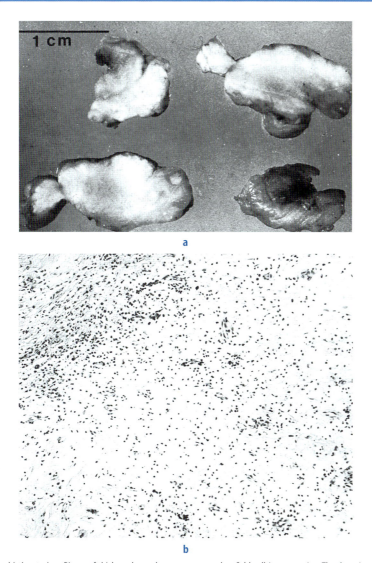

Figure 22.2 Extranodal sinus histiocytosis. **a** Pieces of thickened antral mucosa removed at Caldwell-Luc operation. The deposit was yellowish in the original. **b** Section of antral tissue seen in **a** showing large foam cells in mucosa and submucosa and some plasma cells. **c** In this case the larynx is thickened in the subglottic region. Note large deposit of pale grey material in mucosa and submucosa, with marked narrowing of the airway. Transverse slice of laryngectomy specimen, magnified to approximately twice actual size. **d** Histology of subglottic infiltrate from **c** showing foamy histiocytes and plasma cells

(Figure 22.2 c and d, see overleaf)

so severe that laryngectomy became necessary. Histologically the infiltrate consists of foamy histiocytes and plasma cells with numerous Russell bodies in some areas. Phagocytosis of lymphocytes is not prominent. The histiocytes, with or without obvious engulfment of lymphocytes, express intensively the S-100 protein and, in addition, a variety of macrophage-associated antigens.

In addition to the mucosal involvement, cervical lymph nodes may also be greatly enlarged by sinus histiocytosis. Deposits in the subglottis and skin may also be observed.

The natural history of extranodal sinus histiocytosis is very variable. Most patients experience an indolent course, but in a few there may be dissemination of a histologically benign disease, resulting in death,[10] and in others death may occur from immunological deficiency.[11] In cases of nasal extranodal sinus histiocytosis, endoscopic resection appears to be effective treatment.[12] Although the aetiology still remains unclear, it has recently been proposed that a main mechanism for its pathogenesis is a process leading to immune-suppressive macrophages. This is suggested to occur due to stim-

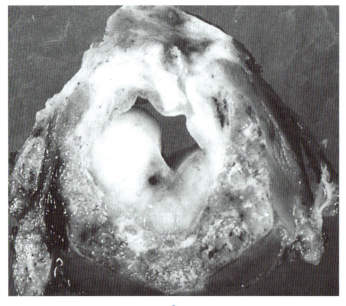

c

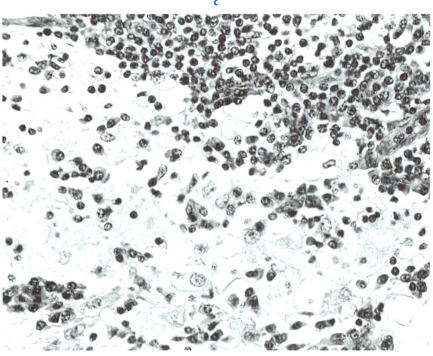

d

Figure 22.2 c,d

ulation of monocytes/macrophages by macrophage colony-stimulating factor M-CSF.[13]

Dermoid Cyst

Dermoid cysts are formed of tissue derivatives of one or more germinal layers. Unlike teratomas, they are not neoplasms. The nasal dermal cyst is one of many midline nasal masses and the differential diagnosis includes both congenital and aquired processes.

Nasal dermoid cysts are manifested soon after birth in 50% of cases. In the other cases the cyst develops later in childhood. The external appearance of the cyst is usually that of a sinus tract opening onto the bridge of the nose with sprouting hairs. Secondary infection usually takes place.

Microscopically the walls of the cyst are thick and fibrotic, being lined by epithelium which resembles skin in showing hair follicles and sebaceous glands. The cavity is filled with greasy material – the product of the sebaceous glands.

Nasolabial Cyst

The nasolabial cyst is a rare, often mucous-secreting, nonodontogenic developmental cyst. In a series of 16 patients with nasolabial cysts, the cyst was usually situated behind the ala nasi, extending backward beneath the nasal floor into the inferior meatus and forward into the labio-gingival sulcus behind the upper lip.[14] Most patients are female and in their fourth or fifth decade. The cyst is manifested as a painless lump beneath one ala. Histologically it is lined by ciliated columnar or cuboidal epithelium with some underlying mucous glands. An origin from cells trapped in the line of fusion between lateral nasal, medial nasal and maxillary processes is the usual explanation, but cell rests derived from the lower end of the nasolacrimal duct have also been suggested as the source.[15]

Teratoma and Teratocarcinoma

Teratomas of the nasal passages appear mainly in the nasopharynx and the subject is dealt with in that section (see Chapter 23). A particularly malignant form of teratoma has been described in the sinonasal tract by Heffner and Hyams.[16] Twenty cases of this neoplasm were reported. The ages of the patients ranged from 18 to 79 years, with a median of 60. The neoplasm combined the histological features of carcinosarcoma and malignant teratoma, components of the latter being malignant skeletal muscle and neuroblasts (Fig. 22.3). The average survival after treatment of such neoplasms was only 1.7 years. Since the report by Heffner and Hyams[16] it has been widely recognised that benign teratomas, with extremely rare exceptions, do not arise in the sinonasal tract. However, in total some 40 cases of sinonasal teratocarcinomas are now reported in the world literature. This is an aggressive tumour. It is still questionable whether this tumour is of germ cell origin and its histogenesis is not yet settled. Teratocarcinomas express a wide panel of antigens, for example CD99 (MIC-2), neurone-specific enolase, vimentin, epithelial membrane antigen and cytokeratins, but are usually negative for beta-human chorionic gonadotrophin, neurofilament and leukocyte common antigen.[17,18,19]

Mucocele

Mucoceles are common lesions of the frontal and ethmoid sinuses, but are unusual in the maxillary sinus. Most mucoceles are produced by obstruction of the ostium of the sinus, as a result of which the sinus itself becomes distended by the retained mucous secretion. The expanding sinus frequently erodes through the surrounding bone and in the case of the frontal sinus mucocele may also involve the contralateral frontal sinus or the orbit. Mucoceles present important clinical and radiological signs, but histopathological examination of their lining is only confirmatory and not diagnostic. Usually there is a fibrous tissue stroma bearing a

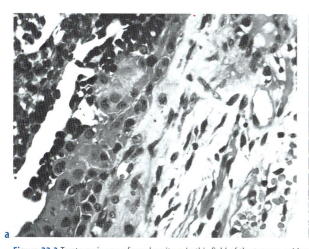
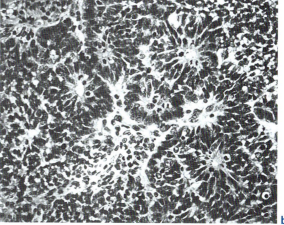

Figure 22.3 Teratocarcinoma of nasal cavity. **a** In this field of the tumour epidermoid tissue, undifferentiated and skeletal muscle fibres, some showing cross-striations, are present. **b** In another tumour of the same type there are neural rosettes

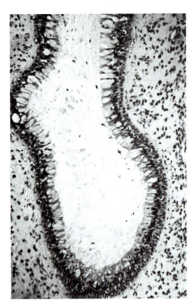

Figure 22.4 Mucocele of frontal sinus. There is goblet cell hyperplasia of the epithelium. The lamina propria shows an allergic type of inflammation with many eosinophils and plasma cells

columnar epithelial lining. The latter often shows many goblet cells. There may be numerous eosinophils in the mucosa and a thickened epithelial basement membrane, indicating a possible allergic type of inflammatory change (Fig. 22.4). During the last 10 years an increasing number of mucoceles has been seen in rhinological practice. There seems to be a correlation between the now widely used functional endoscopic sinus surgery and the increasing

number of mucocele cases, suggesting that some mucoceles today may be iatrogenic.[20]

Extragnathic Sinonasal Ameloblastoma

Neoplasms arising in the tooth germ may present in the nose and maxillary antrum. The most frequent, because of its invasiveness, is the ameloblastoma. The neoplasm may appear as a polypoid mass in the nasal cavity or maxillary sinus. Histologically the trabeculae of the neoplasm are embedded in fibrous stroma. They resemble the enamel organ of the developing tooth. The cells lining the periphery of the epithelial trabeculae resemble the ameloblastic layer (inner enamel epithelium), being columnar with nuclei polarised away from the basement membrane. The central component is made up of a loose stellate reticulum (Fig. 22.5). Squamous metaplasia is common. Cystic change within the stellate epithelium may result in an appearance mimicking that of adenoid cystic carcinoma.

The majority of sinonasal ameloblastomas are extensions from ameloblastomas arising in the maxilla or remnants of odontogenic epithelium in the oral cavity. There are, however, extragnathic ameloblastomas that arise in the sinonasal mucosa and thus are of primary sinonasal tract origin. In a recent series of 24 primary sinonasal ameloblastomas, these tumours showed a similar clinical behaviour to their gnathic counterparts, but had a predilection for men of older age.[21]

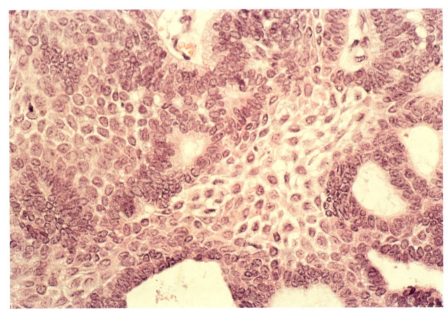

Figure 22.5 Ameloblastoma presenting in nasal cavity, showing islands of cells resembling stellate reticulum of enamel organ surrounded by a cubical epithelium

Ameloblastoma is, as mentioned, locally invasive and has a tendency to recur if not completely excised.

Metastatic Carcinoma

Metastasis via the bloodstream to the nose and sinuses is sometimes observed. It should be suspected by the pathologist in biopsies of neoplasms that do not resemble the usual pattern of primary growths in the sinonasal tract. The most frequent source of metastatic carcinoma to the nose and sinuses is renal cell carcinoma.[22] Carcinomas of the lung and breast, the thyroid, the gastrointestinal tract (even the stomach), prostate, pancreas, adrenal glands and malignant melanoma, have also been sources of metastatic neoplasm.

Metastatic Renal Carcinoma

Metastatic renal carcinoma usually causes epistaxis as a prominent symptom. Local swelling and nasal obstruction may also be present. Radiologically a destructive tumour is observed.

Grossly metastatic renal carcinoma is pale yellow in colour. Microscopically, the large, clearly defined, pale, vacuolated cells with a vascular stroma are characteristic. Useful histochemical aids in making the diagnosis are stains for the presence of lipid and glycogen in the tumour cells. These substances are also well seen as cytoplasmic inclusions with the electron microscope, and the presence of fine microvilli emanating from tumour cells is also helpful in identifying the renal origin of the tumour cells (Fig. 22.6). Metastatic carcinoma in the nose and paranasal sinuses is sometimes the first sign of the renal growth, which is confirmed on radiological investigation of the kidneys. On occasion the nasal metastasis is the only one that can be found and in such circumstances surgical removal of both the primary and the metastasis may result in cure.[23]

References

1. Wiltshaw E. The natural history of extramedullary plasmacytoma and its relation to solitary myeloma of bone and myelomatosis. Medicine 1976;55:217–238
2. Kapadia SB, Desai U, Chen VS. Extramedullary plasmacytoma of the head and neck. A clinicopathologic study of 26 cases. Medicine 1982;61:317–329
3. Haraguchi H, Ebihara S, Saikawa M et al. Malignant tumours of the nasal cavity: review of a 60-case series. Jpn J Clin Oncol 1995;25:188–194
4. Michaels L. Pathology of the larynx. Springer, Berlin, Heidelberg, New York, Tokyo, 1984
5. Soo G, Chan A, Lam D et al. Extramedullary nasal plasmacytoma – an unusual clinical entity. Ear Nose Throat J 1996;75:171–173
6. Leenen PJ, Egeler RM. Langerhans' cell histiocytosis is caused by dysregulation of the E-cadherin-beta-catenin cascade: a hypothesis. Immunol Cell Biol 1999; 77:460–467
7. Rosai J, Dorfman RF. Sinus histiocytosis with massive lymphadenopathy: a newly recognized benign clinicopathological entity. Arch Pathol 1969;87:63–70
8. Perry BP, Gregg CM, Myers S et al. Rosai-Dorfman disease (extranodal sinus histiocytosis) in a patient with HIV. Ear Nose Throat J 1998;77:855–858
9. Foucar E, Rosai J, Dorfman RF. Sinus histiocytosis with massive lymphadenopathy. An analysis of 14 deaths in a patient registry. Cancer 1984;54:1834–1840
10. Wright DH, Richards DB. Sinus histiocytosis with massive lympadenopathy (Rosai-Dorfman disease): report of a case with widespread nodal and extranodal dissemination. Histopathology 1981;5:697–709
11. Foucar E, Rosai J, Dorfman RF. Sinus histiocytosis with massive lymphadenopathy. Ear, nose and throat manifestations. Arch Otolaryngol 1978;104:687–693
12. Ku PK, Tong MC, Leung CY et al. Nasal manifestation of extranodal Rosai-Dorfman disease – diagnosis and management. J Laryngol Otol 1999;113:275–280
13. Middel P, Hemmerlein B, Fayyazi A et al. Sinus histiocytosis with massive lymphadenopathy: evidence for its relationship to macrophages and for a cytokine-related disorder. Histopathology 1999;35:525–533
14. Su CY, Chien CY, Hwang CF. A new transnasal approach to endoscopic marsupialization of the nasolabial cyst. Laryngoscope 1999;109:1116–1118.
15. David VC, O'Connell JE. Nasolabial cyst. Clin Otolaryngol 1986;11:5–8
16. Heffner DK, Hyams VJ. Teratocarcinoma (malignant teratoma?) of the nasal cavity and paranasal sinuses: a clinicopathologic study of 20 cases. Cancer 1984;53: 2140–2154
17. Fernández PL, Cardesa A, Alós L et al. Sinonasal teratocarcinosarcoma: an unusual neoplasm. Path Res Pract 1995;191:166–171
18. Luna MA. Critical commentary to "Sinonasal teratocarcinoma". Path Res Pract 1995;191:172
19. Pai SA, Naresh KN, Masih K et al. Teratocarcinosarcoma of the paranasal sinuses: a clinicopathologic and immunohistochemical study. Hum Pathol 1998;29: 718–722
20. Raynal M, Peynegre R, Beautru R et al. Sinus mucoceles and surgery in iatrogenic diseases. [In French] Ann Otolaryngol Chir Cervicofac 1999;116:85–91
21. Schafer DR, Thompson LDR, Smith BC et al. Primary ameloblastoma of the sinonasal tract. A clinicopathologic study of 24 cases. Cancer 1998;82:667–674
22. Miyamoto R, Helmus C. Hypernephroma metastatic to the head and neck. Laryngoscope 1973;83:898–905
23. Bernstein JM, Montgomery WW, Balogh K. Metastatic tumours to the maxilla, nose and paranasal sinus. Laryngoscope 1966;76:621–650

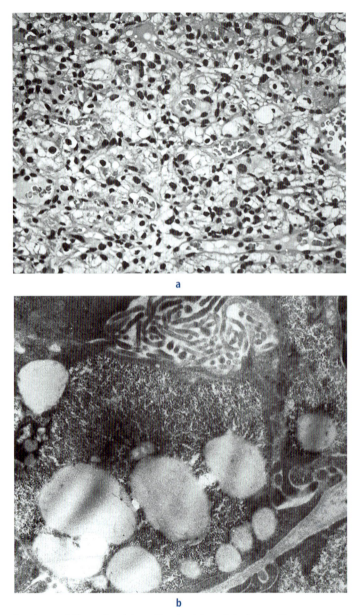

a

b

Figure 22.6 Metastasis of clear cell carcinoma of kidney to frontal sinus. **a** Vacuolated clear cells in clusters with numerous blood vessels. **b** Electron micrograph of the tumour shown in **a**. There are deposits of glycogen granules and large lipid-containing globules. A tangle of microvilli emanates from the upper part of the cell. Original magnification × 25 000

C

The
Nasopharynx

23 Normal Anatomy and Histology; Adenoids; Infections; Developmental Lesions

Anatomy

The nasopharynx (nasal part of the pharynx, epipharynx, post-nasal space) lies behind the nose, with which its lining and cavities are continuous. It has an arbitrary lower level at the posterior edge of the soft palate. The bony superior and posterior walls make a concavity composed of the body of the sphenoid above and the atlas and axis cervical vertebrae below. The mucosa and submucosa of the nasopharynx are separated from these bony structures by the retropharyngeal space, a layer of very loose connective tissue.

The Eustachian tube on each side opens into the nasopharynx, where it is bounded by an elevation that is produced by the medial end of the cartilage of the tube. The latter is shaped like a shepherd's crook (or an inverted J) so that the tubal elevation (torus) has a similar shape, the long limb being posterior (see Chapter 12). This appears even more elongated because the salpingopharyngeal muscle is attached to its lower end. The mucosa of the posterior wall of the nasopharynx shows an irregular bulging caused by the presence of lymphoid tissue in the mucosa, which is known as the pharyngeal tonsil. This is often excessive in children, when the bulges are commonly referred to as adenoids.

Examination at Autopsy

The nasopharynx may be examined by removing a wedge of sphenoid and adjacent occipital bone at the base of the skull. An alternative method is given in Chapter 12.

Histology

At birth the nasopharynx is lined by respiratory epithelium similar to that of the nose. However, later in childhood and in the adult most of the surface epithelium has become replaced by stratified squamous.[1] In the anterior wall 60% of the surface is lined by squamous epithelium except for the part adjacent to the posterior nares. On the posterior wall 80–90% is stratified squamous. Epithelium covering the pharyngeal tonsil and both lateral walls shows a pattern of alternating patches of respiratory and squamous epithelium, which are usually separated by islets of intermediate epithelium. Crypts lined by modified squamous epithelium of identical appearance to those found in the palatine tonsil (see Chapter 26) may also be seen in the nasopharynx.[1]

Seromucinous glands are also present in the submucosa of the nasopharynx. These are not as abundant as in the nose or oropharynx and are concentrated particularly in the region of the orifices of the Eustachian tube. Histologically they are both serous and mucous in type. Oncocytic alteration is frequently seen in these glands, particularly in older people. The lymphoid tissue of the nasopharyngeal tonsil is subepithelial and composed of diffusely scattered lymphocytes and secondary lymphoid follicles with germinal centres. Lymphoid cells have a particularly close relationship with the epithelium. Among the lymphocytes beneath the epithelium, both of the surface and of the crypts and gland ducts, plasma cells are found in abundance and this is their main location in the nasopharyngeal lymphoid tissue. Deep to the plasma cells, abundant reticulum cells with marked folding of cell membranes may be identified by the electron microscope. These relationships are relevant to the immunologic activity of the tissue, which is similar to that of the palatine tonsil (see Chapter 26).

The lymphoid tissue of the nasopharynx diminishes steadily throughout life. On its deep aspect is a well-marked connective tissue layer containing numerous blood vessels and infrequent lymphatic vessels.

Adenoids

The term "adenoids" is applied to an enlargement of the nasopharyngeal tonsil, which occurs in the majority of children between the ages of 3 and 7 years. The mass so formed may produce nasal obstruction by blocking the posterior choanae. Chronic sinusitis may also result from stasis of nasal secretions. Blockage of the nasopharyngeal opening of the Eustachian tube in children may lead to otitis media, adenoids being a frequent concomitant of the serous form, i.e. with an intact non-perforated tympanic membrane. Serous otitis media occurring in adults may similarly be the result of obstruction of the Eustachian tube, but when this is the case, a neoplasm of the nasopharynx such as undifferentiated carcinoma may be the cause of the obstruction (see Chapter 3). Examination of the nasopharynx including biopsy is, therefore, an important step in the investigation of an adult patient with secretory otitis media. The "adenoid facies" comprises an open mouth with prominent incisors and short upper lip, together with a thin nose, a hypoplastic narrow maxilla and a high vaulted palate. There is some doubt as to whether this is the result of severe nasal obstruction by adenoids or of a congenital malformation of the skull, which is associated with nasal obstruction.[2]

Pathological Appearances

Grossly adenoids show corrugated surfaces and pale grey fleshy cut surfaces. Microscopically the surface epithelium is of both stratified squamous and respiratory columnar varieties. The lymphoid follicles of the pharyngeal tonsil are enlarged and more numerous than normal. Their germinal centres are swollen and contain many tingible body macrophages (Fig. 23.1). Mitotic figures are numerous. Rarely acute inflammatory abscesses may contribute to the adenoidal enlargement.

Infections

Adenoidal enlargement may be frequently enhanced or even induced by local infection with bacteria or

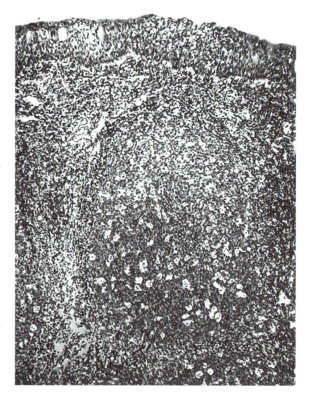

Figure 23.1 Adenoid. The epithelial covering is of respiratory type. There is a large lymphoid follicle, in which a cap of lymphocytes can be discerned on its epithelial side and, in its interior, a swollen germinal centre containing many tingible body macrophages

viruses. The whole of Waldeyer's ring is usually involved by the infective process. The subject will be discussed with inflammation of the palatine tonsil (see Chapter 26). Occasional cases of tuberculous infection are seen, which involve the nasopharynx solely, the palatine tonsil and oropharynx being unaffected. Grossly the nasopharyngeal tonsil appears to be swollen. Histologically well-demarcated tuberculoid granulomas are present in the lymphoid tissue of the nasopharynx, with caseation in some of the granulomas (Fig. 23.2).

Nasopharyngeal Lymphoid Tissue in HIV Infection

Hypertrophy of nasopharyngeal lymphoid tissue is common in HIV-1 infection.[3] This is likely to produce otitis media and it is possible that the clinically inapparent serous otitis media that is frequently revealed at autopsy temporal bone study of cases of AIDS[4] is produced by this change. Microscopic examination shows marked reactive follicular hyperplasia. Small lymphocytes, some with irregular nuclear profiles and a moderate infiltrate of plasma cells and immunoblasts, are present in the

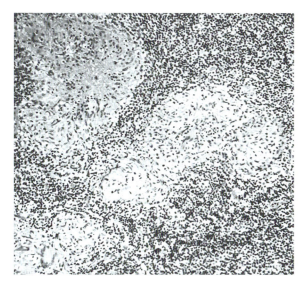

Figure 23.2 Tuberculoid granulomas in lymphoid tissue of nasopharynx. In one focus at the *top left* there is a central area of degeneration suggesting early caseation

interfollicular tissues and arterioles are prominent.[5] With the progression of the HIV infection into AIDS, follicles are reduced in number and size, with a background of moderate to marked lymphocytic infiltration or vascular fibrotic tissue.

Patients with HIV infection may present with a tumour-like nasopharyngeal mass, which is the result of the lesion described above, rather than a lymphoma.

Nodules and Cysts of Embryological Origin

The Pharyngeal Pituitary

Rathke's pouch is an ingrowth of the oral ectoderm, which can be detected as early as the fourth week of fetal life, when the embryo is about 3 mm in length. The subsequent deep penetration of the pouch is sited behind the future nasal septum, and cells at the tip of the pouch develop into the anterior lobe of the pituitary. Persistence of Rathke's pouch as tumour-like formations (craniopharyngomas) is encountered in the pituitary region, but is very rare in the nasopharynx. A residuum of Rathke's pouch that is found in virtually all nasopharynges is the pharyngeal pituitary. Melchionna and Moore discovered a pharyngeal pituitary in 51 of 54 cases at autopsy, in which they took a block for histological examination in the region of the vomerosphenoidal articulation.[6] In most cases it was located in the midline deep in the mucosa or in the periosteum and was from 0.22 to 6.62 mm in length and 0.21 to 1.15 mm in width.

A minority of the pharyngeal pituitaries showed small numbers of pituitary eosinophilic or basophilic cells, but in most cases the epithelial cells were undifferentiated. The pharyngeal pituitary rarely contributes to any physiological function or pathological change. A comparative statistical evaluation of seven hormone-producing cell types in the sellar and in the pharyngeal pituitary has indicated that, in most cases, the percentage of immunoreactive cells is significantly higher in the sellar pituitary.[7] Pituitary adenomas found in the nasopharynx are usually extensions from a primary tumour in the sella turcica (see Chapter 24). Extracranial pituitary tumours and pharyngeal hypopharyngeal cysts may rarely arise from the pharyngeal pituitary.[8]

Cysts

A deeply situated cyst in the midline of the nasopharynx may be found at any age. Its origin is said to be the median embryonal pharyngeal recess, an invagination of ectoderm found in relation to the tip of the primitive notochord and posterior to Rathke's pouch in about half of fetuses over 15 cm in length. Such a cyst is too deeply situated to be removed at adenoidectomy.

A shallow depression – the midline pharyngeal recess – is formed in the nasopharynx during development of the nasopharyngeal tonsil. This is thought to be the origin of a superficially occurring midline nasopharyngeal cyst, which could be removed during adenoidectomy and form part of the specimen.

Both cysts derived from the embryonal pharyngeal bursa and those from the midline pharyngeal recess probably fall into the classical designation of "Thornwaldt's bursa". An even more likely source of a midline nasopharyngeal cyst is obstruction of the duct of a seromucinous gland. The lining of all these cysts may be of squamous or columnar epithelium, or both.[9]

A cyst showing much lymphoid tissue in its wall and a lining of columnar or squamous epithelium may on rare occasions be found on the lateral wall of the nasopharynx. Although the designation "branchial cleft" cyst has usually been applied to such a structure, it seems more likely that the first branchial pouch is the source of this lesion.

Salivary Gland Anlage Tumour ("Congenital Pleomorphic Adenoma")

Salivary gland anlage tumour is a hamartomatous lesion of the nasopharynx that presents mainly in male infants with respiratory distress at birth or within the first few days or weeks of life. The tumours are in the midline and attached to the posterior pharyngeal wall by a pedicle. Microscopically a pattern of squamous nests and ducts at the periphery blends into predominantly mesenchymal-appearing nodules centrally. Ultrastructurally, the stromal-like cells show features of myoepithelial cells.[10]

Hairy Polyp (Teratoid Tumour)

A striking lesion of the nasopharynx arising during development is the hairy polyp or teratoid tumour. This lesion would seem to come under the designation of a choristoma, i.e. a formation of non-neoplastic tissue, which does not normally arise in that situation. It is possible that it may arise from the first branchial cleft area, representing an accessory auricle.[11] The epidermoid formation is a nodule of epidermis on the first branchial pouch and its derivatives and is also probably of first branchial cleft origin. It seems possible that it may give rise to the hairy polyp (see Chapters 1 and 5).

Sex and Age Incidence

Hairy polyps occur predominantly in females. They are frequently found at birth, but in some cases present later in childhood or even in young adults.

Site and Gross Appearance

Hairy polyps arise from the lateral wall of the nasopharynx or from the nasopharyngeal surface

of the soft palate. They are frequently pedunculated and may be up to 6 cm in diameter. They are grey or white structures, usually elongated to a sausage or pear shape with a hairy surface resembling skin.

Microscopic Appearances

The polyp is covered by skin with both hair follicles and sebaceous glands. More deeply adipose tissue, smooth and striated muscle, cartilage and bone may be found[12] (Fig. 23.3).

Neoplastic tissue is never seen and the lesion does not recur after removal.

Teratoma

A neoplasm composed of several tissues with predominance of neuroectodermal and neural tissue may occur in the nasopharynx (Fig. 23.4). Most of these lesions are benign even in the presence of primitive neural cells. Occasional teratocarcinomas have been seen in the nasopharynx. In these malignant lesions rapid intracranial invasion leads to the patient's demise; lymphatic and bloodstream metastases do not occur (see Chapter 22).

Congenital Choanal Atresia

Lack of communication between the nasal passages and the nasopharynx is occasionally present in the newborn. It is a life-threatening anomaly because mouth breathing is an acquired habit and the infant may die of asphyxia before this can be learned. At post-mortem the obstruction is detected by attempting to pass a probe through the nares into the pharynx. Unilateral atresia is also of importance because the normal side is easily obstructed during feeding or sleep, leading to a total occlusion of the airway. In about 90% of cases the obstruction to the choanae is of bone with some cartilage and in the remaining cases it is membranous. The embryological basis of the lesion is disputed.[13] The defect is rather more frequent in females than in males and has been reported in families. There may be other associated congenital defects, including Treacher Collins syndrome and abnormalities of the eye and external ear.

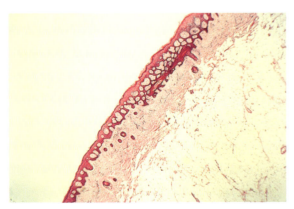

Figure 23.3 Hairy polyp (teratoid) of the nasopharynx showing hair follicles, one of which is aligned horizontally

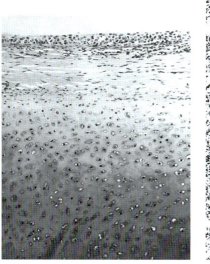
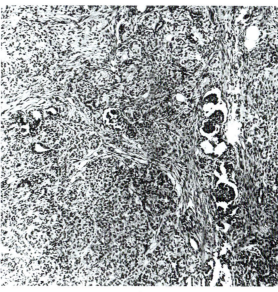

a b

Figure 23.4 Teratoma of maxilla from boy of 11 years. **a** Tissue resembling bronchial wall is shown with a surface of respiratory epithelium, beneath which is a layer of cartilage. **b** Another area of the tumour showing tissue of renal appearance with glomeruli and tubules (Courtesy of Dr. K. Lee, London)

References

1. Ali MY. Histology of the human nasopharyngeal mucosa. J Anat 1965;99:657–672
2. Klein JC. Nasal respiratory function and craniofacial growth. Arch Otolaryngol Head Neck Surg 1986;112: 843–849
3. Stern JC, Pi-Tang L, Lucente FE. Benign nasopharyngeal mass and human immunodeficiency virus infection. Arch Otolaryngol Head Neck Surg 1990;116:206–208
4. Michaels L, Soucek S, Liang J. The ear in the acquired immunodeficiency syndrome: I. Temporal bone histopathologic study. Am J Otol 1994;15:515–522
5. Shahab I, Osborne BM, Butler JJ. Nasopharyngeal lymphoid tissue masses in patients with human immunodeficiency virus-1. Histologic findings and clinical correlation. Cancer 1994;74:3083–3088
6. Melchionna RH, Moore RA. Pharyngeal pituitary gland. Am J Pathol 1938;14:763–772
7. Puy LA, Ciocca DR. Human pharyngeal and sellar pituitary glands: differences and similarities revealed by an immunocytochemical study. J Endocrinol 1986; 108:231–238
8. Fuller GN, Batsakis JG. Pharyngeal hypophysis. Ann Otol Rhinol Laryngol 1996;105:671–672
9. Guggenheim P. Cysts of the nasopharynx. Laryngoscope 1967;77:2147–2168
10. Dehner LP, Valbuena L, Perez-Atayde A et al. Salivary gland anlage tumour ("congenital pleomorphic adenoma"). A clinicopathologic, immunohistochemical and ultrastructural study of nine cases. Am J Surg Pathol 1994;18:25–36
11. Heffner DK, Thompson LD, Schall DG et al. Pharyngeal dermoids ("hairy polyps") as accessory auricles. Ann Otol Rhinol Laryngol 1996;105:819–824
12. Chaudry AP, Loré JM Jr, Fisher JE et al. So-called hairy polyps or teratoid tumours of the nasopharynx. Arch Otolaryngol 1978;104:517–525
13. Flake CG, Ferguson CF. Congenital choanal atresia in infants and children. Ann Otol Rhinol Laryngol 1964;73:458–473

24 Epithelial Neoplasms

Epidermoid Neoplasms

Papilloma

Benign epidermoid neoplasms of the nasopharynx, i.e. everted and inverted papillomas, are rare. There has been an occasional report of inverted papilloma arising in that situation, but, since the boundary between nose proper and nasopharynx is not clear-cut, it seems possible that these may be posteriorly situated nasal lesions.

Nasopharyngeal Carcinoma

Classification

There are three histological types of nasopharyngeal carcinoma in a classification formulated by the World Health Organization (WHO):[1]

1. Keratinising squamous-cell carcinoma.
2. Non-keratinising squamous-cell carcinoma.
3. Undifferentiated carcinoma.

Light and electron microscopic studies of surgical biopsies[2] and autopsy material[3] indicate that these three forms are each a variety of epidermoid carcinoma with greater or lesser degrees of stratified squamous differentiation. The 5-year survival rate of patients with WHO types 2 and 3 (65%) is, however, much higher than that of patients with type 1 (37%), presumably due to the greater radiosensitivity of the less differentiated types 2 and 3.[4]

Age and Sex Incidence

While the peak incidence of this cancer seems to be in the sixth decade, patients quite often present between 10 and 20 years of age and even younger. There is a male preponderance in the incidence of this disease of approximately 2:1.

Epidemiology and Aetiology

Nasopharyngeal carcinoma is infrequent in Europe and North America, but much more frequent among Mongoloid populations living in or derived from Southern China; groups with an intermediate incidence occur in the North African littoral and in East Africa. Convincing evidence has emerged from studies carried out in Hong Kong and Singapore that high-risk people in those areas, i.e. individuals of Southern Chinese origin, have a distinctive HLA profile.[5] Nasopharyngeal carcinoma is associated with an increased incidence of HLA-A2 and B sin 2, an association which holds for both initial susceptibility and for survival after diagnosis. Increased risk also seems to be associated with BW17, and a decreased risk with A11. The significance of altered HLA patterns in the aetiology of nasopharyngeal carcinoma among high-risk populations is unclear. The question of hypothetical disease susceptibility genes has been postulated, which may be linked with other genes that influence antibody responses.

Relationship to Epstein-Barr Virus

A close relationship between nasopharyngeal carcinoma and infection with Epstein-Barr virus is now extensively documented. Data based mainly on sero-epidemiological studies indicate an association that appears to operate in all groups investigated, broadly irrespective of ethnic origin or degree of risk. Nasopharyngeal carcinoma cells contain Epstein-Barr virus DNA and the characteristic nuclear antigen (EBNA), indicating the presence of Epstein-Barr provirus in the nuclei of the tumour cells. In situ hybridisation for EBV-encoded RNA (ISH EBER) is positive in almost all nasopharyngeal carcinomas and may be useful as a marker for the neoplasm.[6] EBV has also been detected by in situ hybridisation in the lymph node metastases of patients with nasopharyngeal carcinoma.[7]

Exogenous Carcinogens

Despite the obvious importance of genetic predisposition and exposure to Epstein-Barr virus, several other aetiologic features have been identified in carcinoma of the nasopharynx. There is a high risk associated with ingestion of salted fish in the southern Chinese population. In patients with WHO type 1 (i.e. keratinising type) nasopharyngeal carcinoma in the USA, a strong connection with cigarette smoking was found and an increased risk was also observed in heavy alcohol consumers.[8]

Bush Flying

An association between long exposure to the occupation of bush flying in Northern Canada and the development of nasopharyngeal carcinoma has been reported,[9] a possible explanation being the frequent opening and closing of the Eustachian tube with the passage of carcinogenic gasoline fumes across the nasopharynx many times a day during ascents and descents. So far there has been no confirmation of the occupational relationship.

Clinical Features

The most common presenting symptom of nasopharyngeal carcinoma is hearing loss, which is caused by otitis media, the result of blockage of the Eustachian tube by the tumour. Nearly as frequent is the initial complaint of a neck mass produced by cervical lymph node enlargement. Cranial nerve involvement – most often the fifth cranial nerve – is frequent. Other symptoms are nasal obstruction, epistaxis, nerve pains and headache.

Nasopharyngeal Biopsy

In some cases in which the patients present with cervical lymph node enlargement, the nasopharynx may appear normal, yet biopsy of the lymph node shows undifferentiated carcinoma of a type that is highly suggestive of an origin from the nasopharynx (see below). Random biopsies or even curettage of the nasopharynx would now be indicated to detect the small primary growth.

Site

The commonest site of origin for carcinoma of the nasopharynx is the lateral wall. The depression behind the inverted J-shaped prominence of the outlet of the Eustachian tube (see Chapter 23), known as the fossa of Rosenmüller, has been claimed as the commonest site of origin; the next most common site has been stated to be the posterior superior wall. Teoh[3] in an autopsy study was able to identify the site of origin from the posterior and lateral walls with certainty in only two cases, however, and origin specifically from the fossa of Rosenmüller could not be verified in any. Nevertheless, there is a strong clinical impression among surgeons with much experience of this form of cancer that the fossa of Rosenmüller is the source of this tumour, so a careful examination of this region is mandatory in the clinical examination of a suspected case of early carcinoma of the nasopharynx.

Gross Appearances

A full description of the pathological appearances of nasopharyngeal carcinoma has been derived only from observations in centres with large populations of southern Chinese. Work carried out elsewhere has had to depend on nasopharyngeal biopsies amplified by only an occasional autopsy. Biopsy specimens are small and often traumatised because of the difficulty in surgical access to the nasopharynx. The clasical autopsy study on 31 cases dying of this disease, conducted by Teoh in Hong Kong in 1957,[3] provides an authoritative basis for the following account.

The neoplasm had been irradiated in only one of them, so the appearances could usually be ascribed to the neoplasm itself rather than to a radiation reaction. In four of the 31 cases only did the tumour fill the nasopharynx. In the others it was of moderate size and showed superficial ulceration. In two cases it was very small, betrayed only by an indefinite granular patch in the nasopharyngeal mucosa.

Microscopic Appearance

Undifferentiated Form

Of the three WHO histological types of nasopharyngeal carcinoma[1] (see above), the undifferentiated one is the most frequently encountered and has given rise to the most confusion in terminology. It has been frequently described in the past as "lymphoepithelioma" because of the close association of the cells of the neoplasm with large numbers of lymphocytes and plasma cells, which surround clumps of, or infiltrate between, individual tumour cells. The mononuclear cells do not, however, form part of the tumour, since they are not present in metastases of the growth unassociated with normal lymphoid tissue.[3] Undifferentiated carcinoma cells often adopt a pattern of branching trabeculae or seemingly isolated masses. In some biopsies the tumour is composed of cells that lie loosely in connective tissue without any tendency to form groups. In others the tumour cells adopt a spindle shape similar to spindle cell carcinoma (a well-defined variant of squamous cell carcinoma – see Chapters 16 and 36). Between the tumour cells the stroma may be fibrous or show numerous lymphocytes and plasma cells. Occasionally a fibrous stroma may contain abundant fibroblasts.

Downgrowths of undifferentiated carcinoma from overlying squamous cell epithelium are frequently present. The epithelium may be either atypical or show actual in situ carcinoma.[2,3]

The cytology of undifferentiated carcinoma presents distinct features, no matter how the tumour cells are grouped. Nuclei have distinct membranes, but nuclear chromatin is very scanty. One or two nucleoli of eosinophilic appearance are prominent in most nuclei. The cytoplasm, on the other hand, is poorly defined, often presenting a syncytial appearance where a number of cells appear to merge together. The foregoing pattern is so characteristic of carcinoma of the nasopharynx that when it is seen in a biopsy of a cervical lymph node, as is fre-

quently the case, even without symptoms or signs of nasopharyngeal disease, an occult nasopharyngeal primary should be suspected (Fig. 24.1).

Keratinising and Non-keratinising Forms

Another form of squamous carcinoma in addition to the three WHO types described above is one composed of large glycogen-containing clear cells. Careful autopsy study[3] has shown that even in neoplasms that are predominantly undifferentiated, areas of definite keratinisation, non-keratinising and clear cell forms of squamous carcinoma are often intermixed in the same tumour. Thus there is a single entity only: squamous carcinoma of the nasopharynx comprising both undifferentiated and differentiated forms of carcinoma. The WHO types of nasopharyngeal carcinoma refer to the predominant pattern in any particular neoplasm.

Nasopharyngeal Carcinoma in Situ

In situ malignant change is common both in the overlying and in the adjacent tissue of nasopharyngeal carcinoma. It has now been shown that nasopharyngeal carcinoma in situ may exist without invasive carcinoma. The tumour cells are positive by in situ hybridisation for EBV-encoded RNA.[10] It would seem that radiotherapy for patients with nasopharyngeal carcinoma in situ is justified in view of the risk of cancer progression and the possibility of a coexisting invasive carcinoma.

Amyloid Deposits

Amyloid, which was potassium permanganate resistant, was found in 12% of 434 consecutive primary nasopharyngeal carcinomas, usually in the non-keratinising forms.[11] The amyloid was present both in tumour cells and in the stroma, often forming spherical structures similar to those seen in amyloid deposits of the larynx (see Chapter 31).

Electron Microscopic Appearances

On electron microscopic examination of undifferentiated carcinoma of the nasopharynx, little chromatin is detected in the nucleoplasm but the nuclear membrane is dense. Nucleoli are prominent in the nuclei. These features are indicative of the increased metabolic activity of the cells concomitant

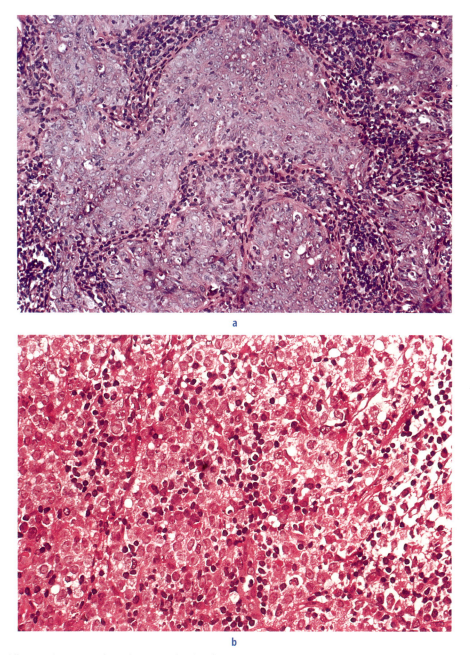

Figure 24.1 Undifferentiated carcinoma of nasopharynx. **a** Trabeculae of cells with vesicular nuclei and prominent nucleoli in a syncytial-like arrangement. A dense lymphocytic stroma surrounds the cell groups. **b** In this example lymphocytes and plasma cells infiltrate between tumour cells

with their reduced differentiation. Cytoplasmic processes characteristic of mature squamous cells are not present. The intimate contact of cytoplasm between neighbouring tumour cells gives rise to the indefinite cytoplasmic outline and syncytial appearances seen by the light microscope. All cases show desmosomes along the zones of cytoplasmic contact and, although scanty in some cases, there is often evidence of a little tonofilamentous material emanating from the desmosomes into the cytoplasm[2] (Fig. 24.2). These changes are more pronounced in tumours showing some degree of squamous differentiation. Numerous glycogen granules may also be present in the cytoplasm of tumour cells.

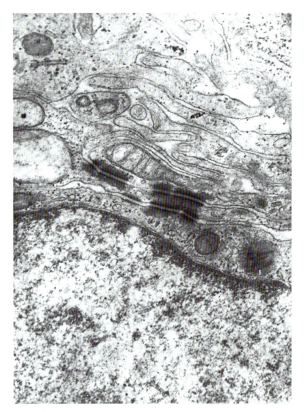

Figure 24.2 Electron micrograph of undifferentiated carcinoma cells. Three desmosomes are seen at the points of cytoplasmic contact between adjacent cells. A small wisp of tonofibrillary material is given off by the desmosomes. The nucleus shows a concentration of chromatin on the membrane and a deficiency of this material in the nucleoplasm. Original magnification × 25 000

Immunohistochemical Findings

A frequent source of difficulty in the diagnosis of undifferentiated nasopharyngeal carcinoma is its distinction from lymphoma. Immunochemical markers have served to increase the accuracy of histological diagnosis of this tumour by providing an objective means of its differentiation from lymphoma. To do this, two types of marker are used: one for keratin, such as CAM 5.2, and a general marker for leucocytes, such as PD7. Undifferentiated carcinoma cells give a positive result for keratin antigen but a negative result for the leucocyte common antigen. Lymphoma reacts to these two markers in the converse fashion.

Recent experimental evidence indicates that angiogenesis affects tumour growth and metastasis in general. Vascular endothelial growth factor (VEGF) is considered to be an important regulator of tumour angiogenesis. Increased expression of VGEF in nasopharyngeal carcinoma as shown by immunohistochemistry has been related to the degree of lymph node metastasis.[12] It is possible that this marker might be useful in the assessment of the prognosis of nasopharyngeal carcinoma by histological methods.

Spread

Direct Extension

At post-mortem in most cases, invasion of the basi-occiput and posterior part of the body of the sphenoid with erosion of the bone is revealed. In a few cases, there may also be new bone formation. Invasion as far as the intracranial cavity may occur, sometimes with superficial invasion of the brain. The sphenoid sinus and pituitary fossa are also often breached. It is possible for intracranial extension to take place without bone involvement by passage of tumour via the foramen lacerum and foramen ovale.[3]

Lymphatic

Cervical lymph node involvement in nasopharyngeal carcinoma is common. In Teoh's autopsy series,[3] 27 of 31 cases showed metastasis, sometimes massive. Cervical lymph nodes in several anatomical positions have been singled out as being specially prone to the reception of metastases from nasopharyngeal carcinoma:

1. The retropharyngeal node of Rouvière, which lies in the retropharyngeal compartment on each side.
2. Lymph nodes situated under the upper attachment of the sternomastoid muscle, just below the tip of the mastoid process at the apex of the posterior triangle.
3. Jugulodigastric lymph nodes, which lie above the point at which the omohyoid muscle crosses the carotid sheath.

With advance of the disease, inferior cervical lymph nodes also become affected. In two of the cases of Teoh[3] showing cervical lymph node metastasis, the primary nasopharyngeal carcinoma was inconspicuous. Neck veins are frequently invaded from cervical lymph node metastatic tumour.[13] In Teoh's series[3] there was invasion of the lumen of the internal jugular vein in some and compression of the vein wall from without, with associated proliferative phlebitis, in others.

Bloodstream

Metastases to remote organs, mainly liver, lungs and bones, in that order of frequency, were found in most cases at autopsy in Teoh's material.[3] Kidney and adrenal metastases were also found, each in one case. In each of the 11 cases in which cervical veins were invaded, there were also remote metastases.

Non-epidermoid Neoplasms

Adenocarcinoma, adenoid cystic carcinoma[14] and mucoepidermoid carcinoma are occasionally primarily located in the nasopharynx. The histopathological features of these tumours are identical to those in the nose and paranasal sinuses (see Chapter 17).

Pituitary Adenoma

Extension of pituitary tumours through the base of skull into the nasopharynx is a rare occurrence. The histological appearance of regular epithelial cells often forming acini may be confused with other epithelial tumours and immunohistochemical study for pituitary hormones, together with electron microscopy for the characteristic granules, is of diagnostic importance (Fig. 24.3). The pharyngeal pituitary (see Chapter 23) has only very rarely been associated with the development of neoplasia.

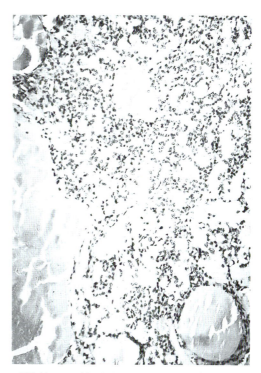

Figure 24.3 Adenoma of the pituitary presenting in the nasopharynx. It is composed of regular small epithelial cells. There is abundant amyloid between groups of cells, forming large, round masses in some places

References

1. Shanmugaratnam K, Sobin LH. Histological typing of tumours of the upper respiratory tract and ear. WHO international histological classification of tumours, 2nd edn. Springer-Verlag, Berlin, Heidelberg, New York, 1991
2. Michaels L, Hyams VJ. Undifferentiated carcinoma of the nasopharynx. A light and electron microscopical study. Clin Otolaryngol 1977;2:105–114
3. Teoh TB. Epidermoid carcinoma of the nasopharynx among Chinese: a study of 31 necropsies. J Pathol Bact 1957;73:451–465
4. Marks JE, Phillips JL, Menck HR. The National Cancer Data Base report on the relationship of race and national origin to the histology of nasopharyngeal carcinoma. Cancer 1998;83:582–588
5. Chan SH, Day NE, Kunaratnam N et al. HLA and nasopharyngeal carcinoma in Chinese – a further study. Int J Cancer 1983;15:171–176
6. Tsai ST, Jin YT, Mann RB et al. Epstein-Barr virus detection in nasopharyngeal tissues of patients with suspected nasopharyngeal carcinoma. Cancer 1998;82:1449–1453
7. Akao I, Sato Y, Mukai K et al. Localization of Epstein-Barr virus in lymph node metastasis with nasopharyngeal carcinoma. Acta Otolaryngol (Stockh) 1996;522(suppl):86–88
8. Vaughan TL, Shapiro JA, Burt RD et al. Nasopharyngeal cancer in a low-risk population: defining risk factors by histological type. Cancer Epidemiol Biomarkers Prev 1996:587–593
9. Andrews PAJ, Michaels L. Nasopharyngeal carcinoma in Canadian bush pilots. Lancet 1968;II:85–87
10. Cheung F, Pang SW, Hioe F et al. Nasopharyngeal carcinoma in situ: two cases of an emerging diagnostic entity. Cancer 1998;83:1069–1073
11. Prathap K, Looi LM, Prasad U. Localized amyloidosis in nasopharyngeal carcinoma. Histopathology 1984;8:27–34
12. Wakisaka N, Wen QH, Yoshizaki T et al. Association of vascular endothelial growth factor expression with angiogenesis and lymph node metastasis in nasopharyngeal carcinoma. Laryngoscope 1999;109:810–814
13. Willis RA. Spread of tumours in the human body, 2nd edn. Butterworth, London, 1952
14. Wang CC, See LC, Hong JH et al. Nasopharyngeal adenoid cystic carcinoma: five new cases and a literature review. J Otolaryngol 1996;25:399–403

25 Non-epithelial Neoplasms

Angiofibroma (Juvenile Nasopharyngeal Angiofibroma)

Angiofibroma, or juvenile nasopharyngeal angiofibroma, is a fibrous and vascular tumour-like swelling of the nasopharynx, which occurs only in young males.

Age and Sex Incidence

This is a lesion only of males. A few supposed cases have been described in women, but in each of these the histological diagnosis of the condition as angiofibroma has been equivocal, often suggesting an antrochoanal polyp with a particularly fibrovascular stroma. All patients with angiofibroma are boys or young men. In a large series of 52 patients, the average age of the patients at the onset of first symptoms was 15.3 years, the youngest being 10 and the oldest 25. The average age of this group at treatment was 16.4 years, the youngest being 11 and the oldest 26 years.[1]

Clinical and Imaging Features

The swelling is a large vascular mass in the region of the choana causing nasal obstruction and epistaxis in almost all cases. The larger tumours may enter the orbit and produce proptosis and diplopia and even become subcutaneous, forming a swelling of the sub- or infratemporal regions (see below). Imaging studies have detected the early growth in the region of the sphenopalatine foramen just in front of the choana. It is always unilateral in the early stages, but when it grows and fills the nasopharynx, both sides of the nose are obstructed. There is early involvement of the upper part of the medial pterygoid lamina. Bowing of the posterior wall of the maxillary antrum takes place later as the tumour presses against the bone in this region.

Site of Attachment and Extent

Very few detailed post-mortem studies are available and in most of these the tumour had already been completely eradicated. In one patient who died of postoperative meningitis, extensive tumour was still present. It was attached on a broad base to the lateral parts of the choana and nasal meatus.[1] At surgery determination of the exact site of attachment of the neoplasm is obscured by the bleeding, which frequently complicates the removal. The majority seem to involve the vault of the nasopharynx and also the choana. The sites and modes of involvement by angiofibroma modified in one description[2] are as follows:

1. Filling nasopharynx and posterior nasal cavity. May enter mouth from behind.
2. Filling sphenoid sinus and eroding sella turcica.
3. Eroding medial wall of antrum, which it then enters.
4. Spreading behind maxillary antrum, eroding pterygomaxillary fossa and entering middle cranial fossa.
5. Entering infratemporal fossa and also passing behind the zygoma, bulging in the supratemporal fossa.
6. Entering inferior orbital fissure and orbit.

Gross Appearances

When received in the laboratory the resected tumour shows a lobular surface and is grey or pinkish-grey depending on the degree of its vascularity. If the vascularity is marked, the cut surface will have a spongy appearance. In some cases the vessels near the surface of the tumour are so dilated that they appear as cysts with a smooth lining (Fig. 25.1).

In a maxillectomy specimen removed surgically in 1841 (before the anaesthetic era), the angiofibroma was seen to enter the infratemporal fossa, pass behind the zygoma and bulge into the supratemporal fossa[3] (Fig. 25.2).

Microscopic Appearances

Angiofibroma has a characteristic structure of blood vessels set in a stroma of mesenchymal cells and collagen. Blood vessels are thick walled in the deeper parts of the tumour. Here some vessels show gaps in their muscle and elastic layers. More superficially all vessels are thin walled with few or no muscle fibres. The capillary vessels are often extremely thin and elongated. In many angiofibromas the calibre of the vessels decreases towards the mucosal surface and the endothelial cells become plumper so that the pattern resembles a sclerosing haemangioma. The endothelial cells have been found to express CD34 antigen using two different antibodies (HPCA-1 and QBEND-10), indicating that they are of blood, not lymphatic vessel origin.[4] The stromal cells are stellate, show scanty cytoplasm with no tendency to be aligned in a particular direction and have vesicular nuclei, which may be atypical in appearance. The stromal cells may occasionally be multinucleate. They strongly express vimentin, but not CD34, indicating that they are of fibroblastic rather than endothelial origin and electron microscopy confirms the fibroblastic nature of the cells. Mitotic figures are

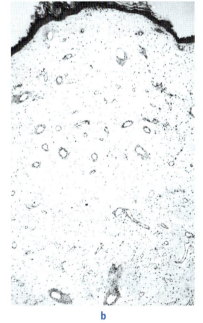

a

b

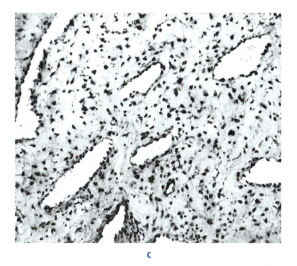

c

Figure 25.1 Nasopharyngeal angiofibroma. **a** Gross specimen: cut surface on *left* and outer surface on *right*. Cysts with smooth linings are the walls of blood vessels, some of which contain blood. **b** The surface is covered by keratotic squamous epithelium. Note small and large blood vessels, some with thickened walls distributed through the tumour. **c** Prominent blood vessels, between which are stromal cells. **d** Vessel with fibrin thrombus surrounded by stromal cells

(Figure 25.1 d, see overleaf)

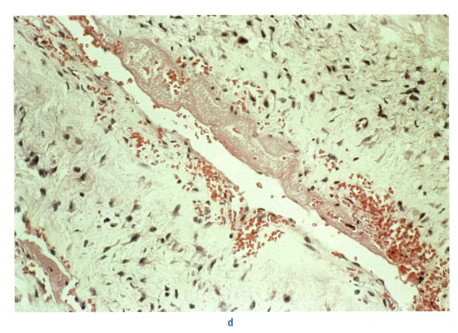

d

Figure 25.1 d

absent among these cells, however, the sole mitotic activity in angiofibromas occurring among the heaped-up vascular endothelial cells. Myofibroblasts occur only focally as both vimentin and actin positive, elongated cells, in the vicinity of collagenous areas and have been held to result from regressive changes.[5] Mast cells and lymphocytes may be quite frequent in angiofibromas.

Organised thrombi of various ages are seen in the lumina of some vessels. In some parts of angiofibroma pink-staining deposit is found around the periphery of the vessel walls.

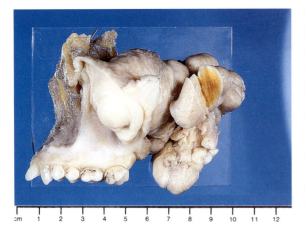

Figure 25.2 Advanced nasopharyngeal angiofibroma showing extension of nasopharyngeal growth lateral to maxilla. From a specimen of maxillectomy performed by Liston in 1841 at University College Hospital, London, and preserved as a museum specimen

The overlying epithelium of the tumour is most frequently of respiratory, occasionally of stratified squamous type.

Histogenesis

If the attribute of a benign neoplasm is its tendency to grow until satisfactorily treated, then the nasopharyngeal angiofibroma is such a condition. Its occurrence only in young males has not yet been explained, nor has the source of the fibrovascular tissue that constitutes the angiofibroma. Brunner[6] identified a fascial layer, the fascia basalis, in the posterior wall and roof of the nasopharynx resulting from the fusion of the pharyngeal aponeurosis, the upper tendon of the constrictor muscles of the pharynx, with the buccopharyngeal fascia, which is the outer layer of fascia of the constrictor muscles. The fascia basalis is distinct from the periosteum and contains many blood vessels. Brunner found in serial sections of a male and a female full-term infant that the fascia basalis was very extensive but he was convinced that it must undergo retrogression after birth. He suggested that it forms the matrix of angiofibroma, however. At an earlier stage in development we have found that the whole region of the sphenopalatine foramen and choana as well as the fascia basalis are occupied by a large amount of primitive mesenchyme. This is similar to that of the Eustachian tube and middle ear (see Chapter 1), with which it is contiguous in fetal life but from which it differs in being more vascular. The primitive mesenchyme of the sphenopalatine foramen may be the source of angiofibroma since it is from this region that radiological origin of the growth may be detected (see above). Further study is required of the development of the connective tissues of the nasopharynx in relation to the histogenesis of angiofibroma. In surgical specimens of angiofibroma the tumour may be seen to be continuous with the submucous vascular tissue of the nose. The latter is distinct from the neoplasm in having larger vessels of thicker calibre and a less cellular stroma. The two tissues appear to merge – an appearance suggesting that the neoplasm may be derived from the same anlage as the submucous vascular tissue.

Androgen receptors have been identified in both the endothelial and stromal cells of 75% of cases of juvenile angiofibromas[7] and there have been numerous reports showing indirect evidence for the presence of androgen, oestrogen, and progesterone receptors in these tumours, but the relevance of these findings to the histogenesis of this tumour in young males only is not yet clear.

Natural History

There is no solid evidence for the spontaneous involution of nasopharyngeal angiofibromas. The lesion seems to maintain its growth unless treated vigorously. However, malignant change does not occur. In the single acceptable case in the world literature[8] – a sarcoma which occurred after radiotherapy – it is most likely that the malignancy had been induced by irradiation.

Rhabdomyosarcoma

Malignant tumours of skeletal muscle are the commonest sarcoma in the head and neck. Most cases are of the embryonal type. The nasopharynx is the second most frequent situation within the head and neck, the orbit being the most frequent. (For a discussion of rhabdomyosarcoma of ear, see Chapter 4.)

Age and Sex Incidence

The average age at presentation is about 7 years. In 16 cases of rhabdomyosarcoma involving the nasal cavity or nasopharynx, the age range was from 10 months to 28 years; 12 patients were in the first decade and the average age was 7 years.[9] Most series of head and neck rhabdomyosarcomas show a slight preponderance of males.

Clinical Features

In rhabdomyosarcoma of the nasopharynx nasal bleeding is a prominent symptom and it is often accompanied by nasal obstruction. Otitis media due to Eustachian tube blockage may occur. Spread of the tumour to the orbit leads to proptosis.

Gross Appearances

Five of the 16 cases of Fu and Perzin[9] were composed of multiple grape-like polypoid masses. This gross feature gives rise to the designation of sarcoma botryoides. Apart from the presence of a cambial layer in some cases (see below), its histological appearance is identical with that of embryonal rhabdomyosarcoma. It is said to be less invasive than other forms. The surface of rhabdomyosarcomas is smooth and may be lobulated. There are frequently areas of haemorrhage and necrosis on the cut surface, which is otherwise pink or grey.

Microscopic Appearances

Rhabdomyosarcomas are classified into three histological forms. Pleomorphic rhabdomyosarcoma, which affects adults, is composed of differentiated rhabdomyoblasts, some of which show an eosinophilic cytoplasm with cross-striations. This form is uncommon in the head and neck and is very rare in the nasopharynx. Alveolar rhabdomyosarcoma is composed of non-cohesive cells arranged in an alveolar pattern (Fig. 25.3). This type of rhabdomyosarcoma is also unusual in the head and neck, although occasional examples are seen in the nasopharynx. Embryonal rhabdomyosarcoma has a primitive cellular structure corresponding to the early stages of the development of the skeletal muscle cell. It is this type that is the common form of rhabdomyosarcoma in the head and neck.

Embryonal Rhabdomyosarcoma

Most of the neoplasms in this category consist of loosely arranged primitive cells situated beneath the epithelium of the nasopharynx. Some cases of the polypoid form – sarcoma botryoides – show a condensation of tumour cells beneath the epithelium, the deeper cells being more loosely arranged. The

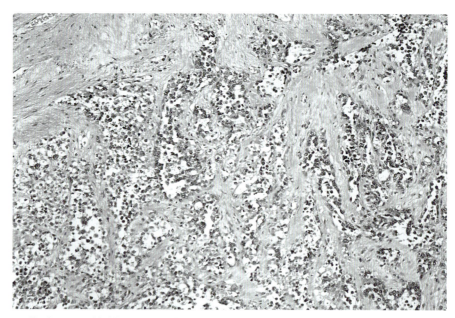

Figure 25.3 Alveolar pattern of rhabdomyosarcoma of nasopharynx. The cells are undifferentiated and arranged in a loose alveolar pattern

superficially condensed cell layer is often referred to as the cambial layer by analogy with plant tissue. The histological appearances of the botryoides form are in all other respects similar to those of other embryonal rhabdomyosarcomas.

The cells of embryonal rhabdomyosarcoma are round or somewhat elongated and the nuclei are usually hyperchromatic, irregularly shaped and showing numerous mitotic figures (Fig. 25.4). The cytoplasm in many areas shows vacuolation which, on special staining with periodic acid–Schiff reagent (with and without prior treatment by diastase), is revealed to be glycogen. This evidently reproduces the glycogen-containing phase present in the early development of normal skeletal muscle. Cross-striations are not usually observed, although they are sometimes found in a few tumour cells that are thin and elongated. Detection of cross-striations when they are present is usually easy in routinely stained sections; the examination of such sections in polarised light for the alternating light and dark stripes is sometimes useful, as is the staining of sections with phosphotungstic acid haematoxylin. Large round cells with abundant eosinophilic cytoplasm containing pink-staining masses but without cross-striations are much more frequent, however.

Immunohistochemistry

The presence of desmin is a valuable immunohistochemical marker for this neoplasm. Tumour cells are also vimentin-positive, and most of them also stain with antibodies to muscle-specific actin and show a co-expression of alpha-sarcomeric actin and myoglobin, but are negative with antibodies to alpha-smooth muscle actin.

Electron microscopy

Transmission electron microscopy is also of value in diagnosis, when the specific feature revealed is the presence of alternating thick (myosin) and thin (actin) filaments in the cytoplasm of tumour cells.

Spread

The neoplasm spreads deeply into the skull and often reaches the meninges. Lymph node metastases are seen in as many as 30% of cases.[10] Distant metastasis is also common, particularly to the lungs and bones.

Prognosis

Age at diagnosis is an independent predictor of outcome, it being more favourable in children and adolescents compared with adults. Additional factors contributing to the prognosis in patients with rhabdomyosarcoma are tumour invasiveness, presence of metastases, regional lymph node involvement and histopathologic subtype.[11] The common *PAX3-FKHR* and the variant *PAX7-FKHR* gene fusions have been observed in rhabdomyosarcoma

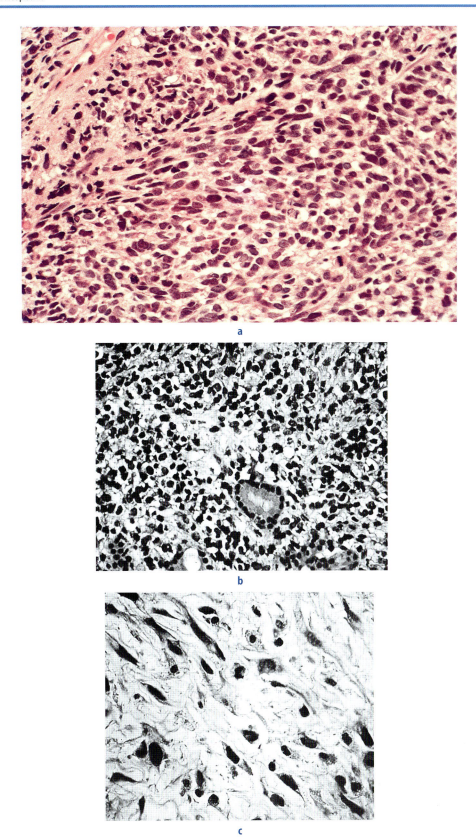

Figure 25.4 Embryonal rhabdomyosarcoma. **a** Spindle-shaped form showing cytoplasmic vacuolation. **b** Round cell variety with marked vacuolation due to accumulation of glycogen in the cytoplasm. **c** Another example of the spindle cell variety with looser cellular arrangement. Some of the cells show cytoplasm, which is eosinophilic in the original, and cross-striations

using reverse transcriptase polymerase chain reaction and a trend toward improved overall survival in the *PAX7-FKHR* group has been noted. These molecular changes may be of use both in diagnosis and prognosis of rhabdomyosarcoma.[12]

Chordoma

Chordoma is a neoplasm that is derived from the primitive notochord. The largest proportion of chordomas grow in the sacrococcygeal region, with rather smaller numbers in the cranio-occipital region, and it is members of this latter group that involve the nasopharynx. A third small group of chordomas occur along the vertebral column, most frequently in the cervical region.

Origin

The notochord is found within the bodies of the primitive vertebrae by the fifth week of life. Rathke's pouch seems to serve as an obstacle to the cranial extension of this structure, which thus terminates caudal to the pituitary fossa. Tumours arising from the cranial part of the notochord will in consequence lie posterior to the pituitary fossa and nasopharynx. Ectopic masses of notochordal tissue have been found in adults in the region of the clivus and in the submucosa of the nasopharynx.

Clinical Features

Although far fewer numbers of base of skull chordomas had been previously reported in the nasopharynx, Richter et al. stated that 11 of their 12 cases of base of skull chordoma had an important clinical extension to that region.[13] Cranial nerve involvement is frequent in this condition. Most of the cranial nerves may be affected. A mass in the nasopharyx is a frequent finding. In most cases this emanates from bone in the spheno-occipital source. In a few cases the tumour is confined to the nasopharynx. Imaging findings are those of destruction of the clivus and sphenoid and intracranial and nasopharyngeal masses.

Gross Appearances

At post-mortem chordoma has been described as producing a mass in the spheno-occipital region posterior to the pituitary, optic nerves and carotid vessels. There is infiltration through the body of the sphenoid into the nasopharynx.[14] The tumour shows a well-demarcated edge, often with a fibrous capsule. It may be lobulated. The cut surface is usually pale grey and mucoid with a rather softer, more mucoid texture than that presented by cartilage.

Microscopic Appearances

The histology of this tumour is very variable. However, three constant features may be recognised: (1) the formation of large lobules or alveoli of tumour; (2) strands of tumour cells; (3) "physaliferous" (bubble) cells. The lobules of growth may be enveloped by a fibrous capsule. In many places this is absent, however, and growth is seen in direct contact with surrounding normal tissue. The capsule may also intersect the tumour to produce fibrous septa. Within the tumour a characteristic growth pattern is the formation of strands of tumour cells within a mucoid ground substance. The cells in these strands frequently show indistinct boundaries. Physaliferous cells possess fine bubbles in their cytoplasm produced by droplets. They can usually be found in some parts of every chordoma. The fusion of the fine droplets to a single large vacuole gives the cell a "signet-ring" appearance and this may also be found in some chordomas. The droplets and vacuoles are empty spaces, unlike the mucous droplets of epithelial neoplasms such as adenocarcinoma.[15] Nuclei of chordoma cells show a variable degree of pleomorphism and mitoses are few. Sometimes there is much nuclear atypia, but this does not seem to be related to prognosis (Fig. 25.5). Stains for mucus are usually positive in the ground substance and the cytoplasm often contains glycogen.[15]

Immunohistochemistry

Immunohistochemical markers for cytokeratins are usually positive in chordoma, a finding that is of value in diagnosis. Forty-five per cent of chordomas exhibit S-100 protein.

Chondroid Chordoma

Chordomas seen in the base of skull (but not in the sacrococcygeal variety) have been observed in about one-third of cases to possess a chondroid appearance. In these areas the cellularity may be high, the nuclei large and many of the cells multinucleate. The ground substance surrounding these cells takes on a bluish staining (Fig. 25.5) so that the appearances may be closely similar to those of chondrosarcoma,

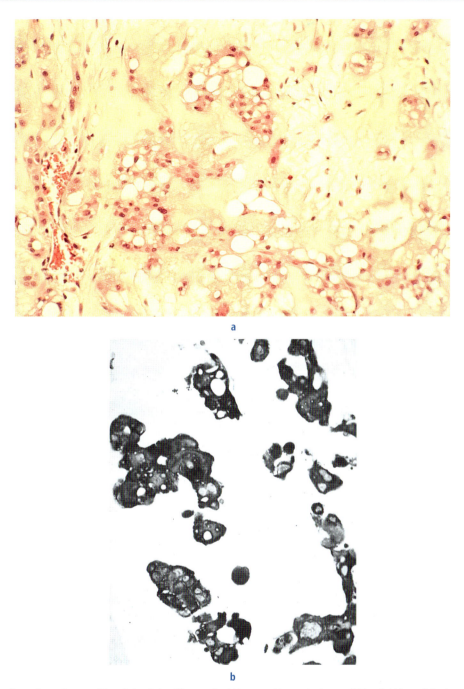

a

b

Figure 25.5 Chordoma of nasopharynx. **a** Distended and physaliferous cells within a mucoid ground substance. **b** Chondroid form of chordoma with extensive cartilage matrix-like ground substance. Note "soap-bubble" remnants of physaliferous cytoplasm within spaces in the ground substance. **c** Strongly positive cytoplasmic colouration (brown in original) after immunohistochemical staining for keratin. Immunoperoxidase after Cam 5.2 antibody

(Figure 25.5 c, see overleaf)

although more typical chordoma may be identified in adjacent parts of the section. Unlike the "classical" chordoma, only 32% of chondroid chordomas react for keratins, but 85% are positive for S-100 protein.

The separation of such a chondroid from the "classical" group has been thought to be important because patients with chondroid chordoma were thought to have a longer survival time than those with typical chordoma. It has been found, however, that regardless of tumour subtype, age is the single most important variable in determining survival; patients younger than 40 years of age do better than

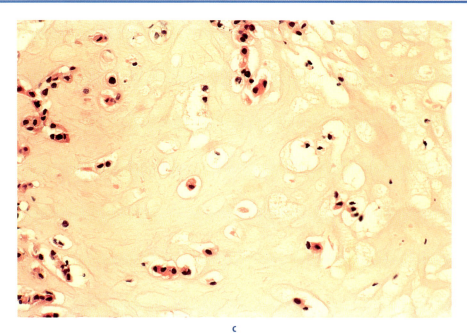

c

Figure 25.5 c

older patients. At 5 years, all patients younger than 40 years of age were found to be alive in both the classic and chondroid groups. In contrast, of patients older than 40 years of age, only 22% with classic chordomas and 38% with chondroid chordomas were found to be alive at 5 years.[16]

Spread

In most cases the spread of the tumour is into the bony tissue of the base of skull, outwards to the nasopharynx and inwards to the brain. Metastasis is rare.

Lymphoma

Lymphoma of the nasopharynx has similar pathologic features to that of other parts of Waldeyer's ring and is dealt with in detail in Chapter 27.

References

1. Härmä RA. Nasopharyngeal angiofibroma. A clinical and histopathological study. Acta Otolaryngol (Stockh) 1958;146(suppl):1–74
2. Neel HB 3d, Whicker JH, Devine KD et al. Juvenile angiofibroma – review of 120 cases. Am J Surg 1973;126:547–556
3. Myrhe M, Michaels L. Nasopharyngeal carcinoma treated in 1841 by maxillectomy. J Otolaryngol 1987;16:390–392
4. Beham A, Regauer S, Beham-Schmid C et al. Expression of CD34-antigen in nasopharyngeal angiofibromas. Int J Pediatr Otorhinolaryngol 1998;44:245–250
5. Beham A, Kainz J, Stammberger H et al. Immunohistochemical and electron microscopical characterisation of stromal cells in nasopharyngeal angiofibromas. Eur Arch Otorhinolaryngol 1997;254:196–199
6. Brunner H. Nasopharyngeal fibroma. Ann Otol Rhinol Laryngol 1942;51:29–65
7. Hwang HC, Mills SE, Patterson K et al. Expression of androgen receptors in nasopharyngeal angiofibroma: an immunohistochemical study of 24 cases. Mod Pathol 1998;11:1122–1126
8. Batsakis JG, Klopp C, Newman W. Fibrosarcoma arising in a "juvenile" angiofibroma following extensive radiation therapy. Am Surg 1955;21:786–793
9. Fu YS, Perzin KH. Nonepithelial tumours of the nasal cavity, paranasal sinuses and nasopharynx. A clinicopathologic study. V. Skeletal muscle tumours (rhabdomyoma and rhabdomyosarcoma). Cancer 1976;37:364–376
10. Holborow CA, White LL. Embryonic sarcoma (rhabdomyosarcoma) of the nasopharynx presenting with facial palsy. J Laryngol Otol 1958;72:157–165
11. La Quaglia MP, Heller G, Ghavimi F et al. The effect of age at diagnosis on outcome in rhabdomyosarcoma. Cancer 1994;73:109–117
12. Kelly KM, Womer RB, Sorensen PH et al. Common and variant gene fusions predict distinct clinical phenotypes in rhabdomyosarcoma. J Clin Oncol 1997;15:1831–1836
13. Richter HJ Jr, Batsakis JG, Boles R. Chordomas: nasopharyngeal presentation and atypical long survival. Ann Otol Rhinol Laryngol 1975;84:327–332
14. Unni KK, Dahlin DC. Bone tumours. General aspects and data on 11,087 cases, 5th edn. Lippincott Williams & Wilkins, Philadelphia, 1996
15. Perzin KH, Pushparaj N. Nonepithelial tumours of the nasal cavity, paranasal sinuses, and nasopharynx. A clinicopathologic study. XIV: Chordomas. Cancer 1986;57:784–796
16. Mitchell A, Scheithauer BW, Unni KK et al. Chordoma and chondroid neoplasms of the spheno-occiput. An immunohistochemical study of 41 cases with prognostic and nosologic implications. Cancer 1993;72:2943–2949

D

The Palatine Tonsil

26 Development; Normal Anatomy; Histology; Inflammatory Diseases

Development

The palatine tonsil is derived from the second pharyngeal pouch endoderm, which, like that of all the pharyngeal grooves, except the first, disappears early in development. A small recess, the tonsillar fossa, develops and the endodermal cells at its fundus proliferate. They are soon invaded by mesodermal cells and the closely associated cells of the two origins form the primordium of the palatine tonsil. A similar aggregation of mesodermal and endodermal cells is found on the first pharyngeal pouch, becoming the tubal tonsil, on the dorsum of the tongue, the lingual tonsil and on the dorsal pharyngeal wall, the adenoids. Thus the lymphoid/ epithelial conjunctions of Waldeyer's ring are not specifically related to pharyngeal pouches alone, but surround the whole inlet of the foregut.

In the later fetus, respiratory (essentially CK 18 positive, but CK 14 negative), multilayered and stratified squamous (essentially CK 14 positive, but CK 18 negative) epithelia are found.[1] In postnatal development there is progressive reduction of respiratory epithelium and although the multilayered epithelium is prominent in children (see below), it becomes less so in adult life. The lymphoid tissue in the 16th gestational week is composed of T cells, but later development of the primary follicles is characterised by increasing numbers of B cells.[2] Later development in childhood appears to be the result of immunological stimulation with secondary follicles and increasing numbers of intraepithelial lymphocytes and Langerhans cells.

Normal Anatomy

The palatine tonsil is composed of lymphoid tissue within which are channels lined by squamous epithelium – crypts – that open onto the surface. It is part of a ring of lymphoid tissue in the oral cavity and nasopharynx – Waldeyer's ring – which includes also the lingual tonsil at the base of the tongue and the pharyngeal tonsil or adenoid in the nasopharynx (see Chapter 23). The normal adult tonsil measures up to 2.5 cm in length, 2.0 cm in width and 1.2 cm in thickness. Its average weight is 1.5 g. There are about 20 crypts reaching the deepest part of the structure. Submucosal glands lie in the peripheral part.

The palatine tonsil adjoins laterally the superior constrictor muscle of the pharynx, from which it is separated by the fibrous capsule overlying that muscle. The tonsil is embedded between two mucosa-covered bands – the anterior and posterior pillars of the fauces. The former is produced by the palatoglossus muscle and the latter by the palatopharyngeus. The last-named gives rise to a muscle bundle, the tonsillopharyngeus muscle, which is inserted into the fibrous septae of the tonsil and may function by compressing it and so helping to cleanse the crypts of cellular debris. The lingual branch of the glossopharyngeal nerve passes below the lower pole of the tonsil into the oral region. It conveys the sense of taste and general sensation to the posterior one-third of the tongue.

Parapharyngeal Space

The parapharyngeal space is a potential recess, which lies deep to the tonsil and superior constrictor muscle. It is pyramidal in shape, with the skull as a base and the greater cornu of the hyoid bone as an apex. Medially are the superior constrictor muscle and the tonsil and laterally the medial pterygoid lamina, the inner surface of the mandibular ramus and the deep lobe of the parotid gland. Anteriorly it is bordered by the pterygomandibular ligament and posteriorly by the vertebral column and paravertebral muscles. The parapharyngeal space contains important vessels and nerves. Among these are: the internal carotid artery, internal jugular vein, the ninth, tenth, eleventh and twelfth cranial nerves, the cervical sympathetic chain, the vagal and carotid bodies and lymph nodes.

Tumours arising in the parapharyngeal space may grow inwards, causing medial displacement of the tonsillar fossa, soft palate and lateral pharyngeal wall. Alternatively they may grow downwards between the tail of the parotid and submandibular gland or behind the mandible.

Histology

Epithelium

The epithelium of the tonsillar surface is non-keratinising stratified squamous, similar to that covering the mucosa of the rest of the oral cavity. In the crypts, however, although continuous with the surface, the squamous epithelium has a more prominent component of basal cells and is infiltrated by lymphocytes and plasma cells. Particularly in children, the crypt epithelium conveys such an impression of activity that neoplasia may be suggested by those unfamiliar with this normal feature (Fig. 26.1). By scanning and transmission electron microscopy the crypt epithelium has been shown to be occupied by an extensive system of channels containing lymphocytes, plasma cells and mononuclear phagocytic cells. The last-named are probably identical with Langerhans cells (CD1-positive, dendritic cells). The overlying epithelium contains numerous so-called M cells (membrane cells). These cells transport antigenic matter across the mucosal membrane to initiate immune responses.[3] The cells in the lumina of the tonsillar crypts are desquamated squamous epithelial cells, lymphocytes, mononuclear phagocytes and plasma cells. Many are degenerate.

Lymphoid Tissue

Beneath the epithelium the tonsil is formed mainly by lymphoid follicles, which are surrounded by loosely distributed lymphoid tissue. Each follicle consists of a germinal centre and a lymphocytic cap, which becomes thicker towards the crypt. The germinal centre is composed of precursors of lymphocytes: centrocytes (cleaved cells), which have indented nuclei and indistinct cytoplasm, and centroblasts (large non-cleaved cells), which show nucleoli near the nuclear membrane and a thin rim of basophilic cytoplasm. There are also macrophages often containing numerous particles of phagocytosed material (tingible-body macrophages) and dendritic reticulum cells. The lymphocytic cap is composed entirely of B-lymphocytes. T-lymphocytes – mainly helper cells – are located in the perifollicular tissue.

During the last two decades it has become evident that the palatine tonsils, together with the other structures of Waldeyer's ring, have a regionalised immune function. In the human, muco-associated lymphoid tissue (MALT) structures of this region are mainly the palatine tonsils. However, it still unclear whether Waldeyer's lymphoid ring is functionally exactly comparable with nasal-associated lymphoid tissue in rodents and gut-associated lymphoid tissue in humans. Beneath the epithelium the tonsil is formed mainly by lymphoid follicles, which are surrounded by loosely distributed cells, mainly T lymphocytes and antigen presenting cells (APC). M cells are particularly present in the reticular areas of the tonsillar crypt epithelium. Antigens are transported from the mucosal surface through the M cells, or similar cells, to the immune cells and to APC. Antigens that thus have reached the MALT are then processed. Antigens are presented as immunogenic peptides to T cells, after having been processed by extrafollicular APC. Native antigens, on the other hand, are presented in immune complexes to B lymphocytes within the germinal centres, giving rise to memory B cells with a high receptor affinity for a specific antigen. These are subsequently distributed via lymph and peripheral blood to effector sites. Also the microenvironment, mainly cytokines and different adhesion molecules, plays an important role in the homing of lymphoid cells. In vivo production of as many as 19 different cytokines has been shown to occur in tonsillar tissue.[4] The cytokines and often pairs of adhesion molecules operate together to direct memory cells to their "home", i.e. the relevant effector site, where they may differentiate terminally to immunoglobulin-producing plasma cells. Although the composition of the mucosa of the gut and the upper respiratory tract varies with regard to such factors as exact location and numbers of CD4+, CD8+ T cells and numbers of APC, it appears very likely that homing of lymphoid cells also occurs in the MALT structures of the upper respiratory tract. Also, apparently only B cells with a potential for J-chain expression

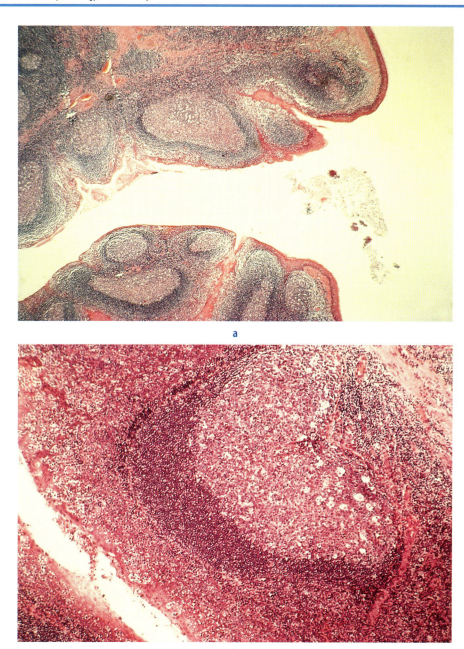

Figure 26.1 Normal histology of palatine tonsil. **a** Lining of crypt formed by squamous epithelium. Deep to this are lymphoid follicles, each composed of a germinal centre, and a lymphocytic cap, which is thickest towards the crypt. **b** Lymphoid follicle near lining of crypt. Note lymphocytic cap of follicle, which is thickest towards the crypt. **c** Deeper part of crypt. A shower of stratified squamous epithelial cells extend from keratinised epithelium towards underlying lymphoid follicles. **d** Lining of crypt showing loosening of basal epithelial cells and their close approximation to adjacent lymphoid cells. Note that many of the latter are plasma cells

(Figure 26.1 c and d, see overleaf)

are initially stimulated in MALT. Locally produced immunoglobulins (mainly dimers and large polymers of IgA) are pumped out by an epithelial receptor protein called transmembrane secretory component.[5]

Cartilage and Bone

Islands of bone and cartilage are found in about a fifth of all tonsils (Fig. 26.2). Bone is said to occur only in the presence of cartilage, but the latter may occur

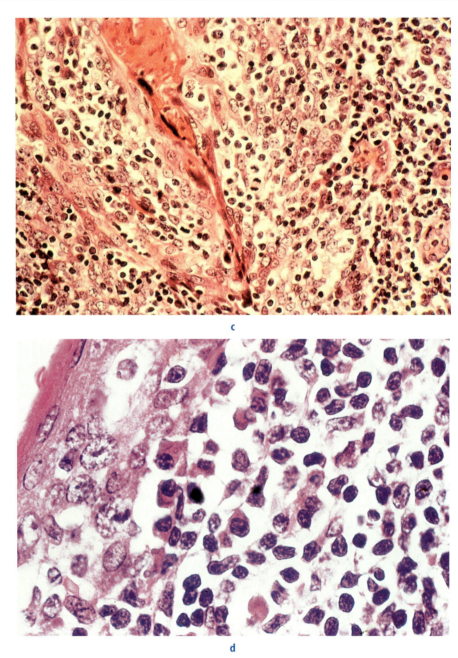

c

d

Figure 26.1 c,d

without bone. These tissues are present in older individuals, with an average age of about 24 years.[6]

Inflammatory Diseases

Tonsillitis

Attacks of tonsillitis are among the commonest of all infections. Children are the most frequent sufferers, but adults are not spared.

Clinical Features

Two forms are recognised depending on the appearances of the tonsils: acute parenchymatous, in which the surface of the tonsil and surrounding pharynx is red and swollen, but yellow spots are not present, and acute follicular, in which the tonsils are covered by yellow pus exuding from the tonsillar crypts. There would appear to be no essential difference between these forms in their microbiology or clinical symptomatology. Three symptoms are nearly always present in older children and adults: sore

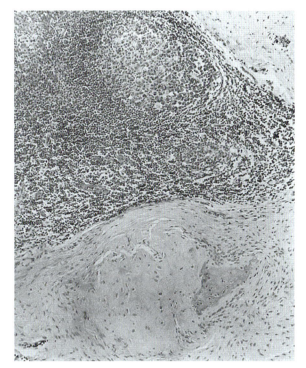

Figure 26.2 Normal cartilage and a small piece of bone, which have been deposited in the tonsil near lymphoid follicles

throat, pain on swallowing and pyrexia. Earache is frequent. On examination, apart from the tonsillar appearances mentioned above, swelling of the jugulodigastric lymph nodes in the neck is always found. Some patients have frequent recurrences and in a few of these autoimmune diseases, such as rheumatic fever or acute glomerulonephritis, may arise as complications. Scarlet fever is an acute tonsillitis caused by haemolytic streptococci type A, in which there is also an erythematous rash produced by an exotoxin of the streptococcus. Enlargement of the adenoids (see Chapter 23) frequently, but not invariably accompanies longstanding tonsillitis. Tonsillitis with negative throat cultures has been reported to be part of the so-called "periodic fever, aphthous stomatitis, pharyngitis and adenopathy syndrome". The children present with tonsillitis, episodes of fever, malaise, aphthous stomatitis, pharyngitis and cervical adenopathy. In some children also a mild hepatosplenomegaly is present. The disease appears to be self-limiting.[7]

Microbiology

The relationship of bacteria to tonsillitis is complex. Many organisms have been isolated from inflamed tonsils from time to time and these include: *Streptococcus pyogenes, Staphylococcus aureus, Haemophilus influenzae, Streptococcus pneumoniae, Candida albi-*

cans, enteric aerobes and anaerobes. More often the flora grown is a mixture of some of the above organisms. Latent virus infection of the tonsil by Epstein-Barr virus (EBV), adenovirus and herpes simplex virus is frequent and may last for long periods, in the case of the EBV even a lifetime. Activation of the virus may take place as a result of many local and general factors. The relationship of the viruses to the bacterial infections is still not clear.

Gross Appearances

The pathological changes characteristic of tonsillitis are difficult to define. The tonsils are rarely removed at the time of an acute attack and there is some uncertainty about the significance of the changes found between attacks.

The tonsils may be of equal or unequal size. The relative sizes are no reflection of the degree of pathological change in one or the other. The external (crypt orifice) surface may show crypts distended by white foci, greyish casts or even calcified casts of the crypt (tonsilloliths). Cut surface may show cysts filled with white debris or grey cast material. Fibrosis is rare.

We have found that the majority of surgically removed tonsils show no gross abnormalities.

Microscopic Appearances

The specific feature of inflammatory change in the tonsil is the presence of neutrophils under the crypt epithelium, which may form small abscesses and may extend through the epithelium to the lumen. The overlying squamous epithelium may be thinned or even ulcerated. In areas of resolved inflammation the crypt epithelium may show a papillary arrangement, in which numerous small swellings of squamous epithelium associated with plasma cells and lymphocytes project into the lumen (Fig. 26.3). Lymph follicles are swollen by enlargement of germinal centres, which contain many tingible body macrophages.

As a result of focal compression of the lumen of crypts by abscess formation or enlarged lymph follicles there may be a damming up of crypt products, leading to swelling of the crypt proximal to the obstruction with, eventually, the formation of a cyst lined by squamous epithelium and filled with squamous debris. In a few cases the stagnant material becomes calcified, resulting in a tonsillolith.

Another feature of crypt lumina in surgically excised tonsils is the presence of colonies of *Actinomyces* organisms. These may be found in up

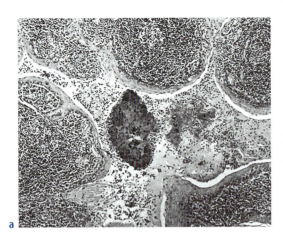 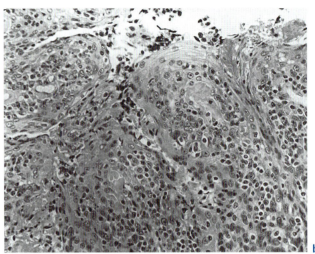

a   b

Figure 26.3 Inflammatory changes in tonsil. **a** Crypt containing *Actinomyces* and numerous pus cells. There is also papillary formation of the crypt mucosa. **b.** Higher power view of crypt papilla showing lymphoid cells and normal squamous epithelial covering

to 90% of surgically excised tonsils examined by step sections,[8] but are, of course, less frequently seen when the tonsils are examined by single sections only. The organisms are probably *Actinomyces israelii*, which are microaerophilic and, therefore, flourish well under the conditions existing in the crypt. It is doubtful how much they contribute to the inflammation of the tonsil. Actinomyces, acute inflammation and papillary change may be found in post-mortem tonsils from young people, apparently healthy individuals, who have died as a result of suicide or road traffic accidents. Actual actinomycosis of the tonsils may occasionally present a clinical picture mimicking a tonsillar tumour.[9]

Fibrosis is sometimes seen in tonsils. Although usually ascribed to previous inflammation, it is likely that it may also be the result of previous partial tonsillectomy.

Retrotonsillar Abscess (Quinsy)

If pus accumulates in the tonsil but is prevented from draining to the surface by blockage of affected crypts, it will tend to penetrate inwards. The path of least resistance is towards the loose areolar tissue situated behind the upper pole of the tonsil. There the abscess produces a quinsy with bulging of the overlying tonsil and contralateral deviation of the uvula and soft palate. If the quinsy is allowed to extend further, pus may enter the parapharyngeal space (see above), and spread upwards and downwards in that space to reach vital structures.

Infectious Mononucleosis

Infectious mononucleosis is an infection caused by the EBV. Changes are mainly in the mononuclear cells of the blood and in the lymph nodes and an antibody against sheep red cells is present in the blood. Complete recovery from the infection is the rule.

In a few cases the tonsils become markedly enlarged during the course of the infection and even impede swallowing and breathing.[10]

On examination of three pairs of tonsils removed surgically from cases of infectious mononucleosis to relieve serious throat obstruction, we have found massive replacement of crypt epithelium and follicles by lymphoid cells of blast cell appearance in each. In a few places the remains of keratinous cysts formed from crypt epithelium are present. An occasional surviving follicle is also seen. Areas of necrosis are frequent (Fig. 26.4). Some lymphoid cells may invade the walls of small arteries. In each case the patient recovered completely after tonsillectomy. The histological pattern would be highly suggestive of a lymphoma, but for the proven condition of infectious mononucleosis. Similar changes are described in the lymph nodes and spleen in this infection.[11] In the three cases mentioned above, immunohistochemical studies on the paraffin sections of tonsillar tissue were not possible. Immunoglobulin polyclonality, i.e. the presence of κ and λ light chains, has been constantly found in the proliferated cells of infectious mononucleosis. This immunohistochemical investigation is strongly recommended in doubtful cases to exclude the monoclonal immunoglobulin secretion of malignant lymphoma (see Chapter 27).

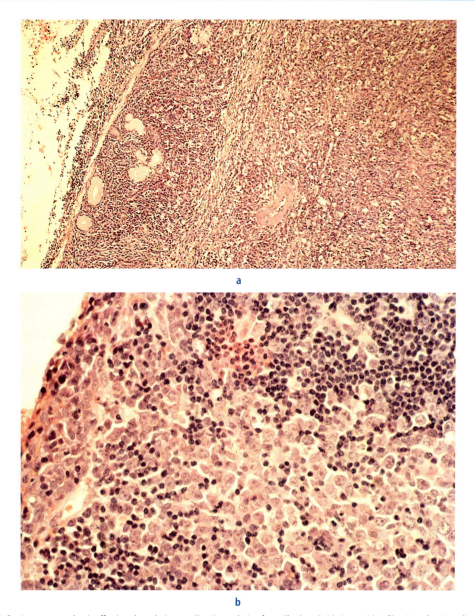

Figure 26.4 Infectious mononucleosis affecting the palatine tonsil. **a** Hyperplasia of tonsillar lymphoid tissue with infiltration of region of mucous glands. **b** Infiltration of atypical lymphoid cells with involvement of crypt epithelium on *left*

In situ hybridisation has demonstrated EBV in tonsillar tissue in cases of infectious mononucleosis. It appears that a limited number of cells only carry the EBV. These are both B and T cells. Using detection of small transcripts, a preferential accumulation in lymphocytes seems to be around crypts, within the surface squamous epithelium, and also within surrounding necrotic zones. Thus infected lymphocytes, and not epithelial cells, are the reservoir for EBV infection.[12,13] Interestingly, the tonsillar crypt squamous epithelial cells have been suggested to be possible progenitors of Hodgkin and Reed-Sternberg (HRS) cells in Hodgkin's disease. HRS cells express latent membrane protein (LMP), and it has been shown that adjacent to tonsillar crypts there are numerous HRS-like cells with strong LMP expression.[14]

Diphtheria

Diphtheria is an acute mucosal inflammation of the tonsils and adjacent soft palate produced by *Corynebacterium diphtheriae*. The organism is present in large numbers in the surface inflammatory exudate, and exotoxin produced by it enters the bloodstream and has a specific damaging effect on the myocardium. This is rare after active immunisation.

The gross appearance of the tonsillar inflammation is that of a dull greyish-yellow layer – the false membrane – which covers the surface of the tonsil and a variable amount of surrounding tissue. This membrane separates off with difficulty. The membrane may extend or may, indeed, be confined to the laryngeal or the nasopharyngeal mucosae. Microscopically the false membrane contains fibrin and neutrophils with, in the early stages, large numbers of diphtheria bacilli. The squamous epithelium of the tonsil forms part of the membrane.

Granulomas

Tuberculosis of the tonsil was once a common disease but has now been almost entirely eradicated by pasteurisation of milk or tuberculin testing of cows, as the lesion was always the result of infection by *Mycobacterium bovis* from infected cows' milk. Caseating granulomas within the lymphoid tissue of the tonsil constituted the main pathological feature of the condition. This was usually the primary focus of the bovine tuberculous disease; it was often overshadowed by the tuberculous lymphadenitis in the cervical region.

Non-caseating tuberculoid granulomas are occasionally seen in the tonsils. These are usually small and scattered evenly in the tonsillar lymphoid tissue. A few of these cases may show evidence of sarcoidosis on further investigation and also on very rare occasions the granuloma may be an extraintestinal manifestation of Crohn's disease.[15] The other cases remain unexplained.

Tangier Disease

Tangier disease is a familial disorder characterised by orange tonsils, cholesterol deposition in reticuloendothelial cells, abnormal chylomicron remnants, and a marked reduction in high-density lipoproteins. Recent sequence analysis of the human *ABC1* gene (containing 49 exons; a member of the ATP-binding cassette family) revealed that the proband for Tangier disease was homozygous for a deletion of nucleotides 3283 and 3284 in exon 22.[16] In the tonsils, as in the paranasal sinuses and middle ear, cholesterol ester crystals with foreign body giant cell reaction may result from a focal haemorrhage (see Chapters 3 and 14). In Tangier disease, which was first described among a group of families living on Tangier Island in Chesapeake Bay, Virginia, macrophages laden with cholesterol ester may accumulate also in the tonsil, plasma cholesterol levels are low, while a1-lipoproteins in plasma are absent.[17] The tonsils are enlarged by bright yellow streaks, which are composed of collections of macrophages containing fine lipid globules. These cells are present mainly between the lymphoid follicles. They are not accompanied by an inflammatory exudate of neutrophils and plasma cells. In Gaucher's disease the cytoplasmic granules stain green with Masson's trichrome. In the latter and most other reticuloendothelial storage diseases, the macrophages contain granules which stain red by the periodic acid–Schiff method. In Tangier disease the cytoplasmic granules do not stain by these methods. The affected cells may also be found in cases of Tangier disease in the nasopharyngeal adenoidal tissue (Fig. 26.5) and in lymph nodes, thymus, colon, pyelonephritic scars of the kidney and in the ureter.[18]

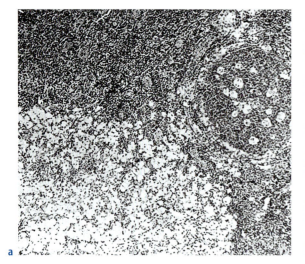
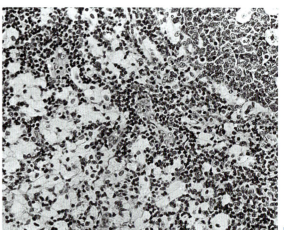

Figure 26.5 Tangier disease in nasopharyngeal biopsy. **a** Large numbers of pale-staining macrophages are present between lymphoid follicles. **b** Higher power of part of **a** showing macrophages with finely granular pale-staining cytoplasm at edge of lymphoid follicle

HIV Infection

Primary infection with the human immuno-deficiency virus (HIV) is generally followed by a burst of viraemia with or without clinical symptoms. Head and neck manifestations of HIV infection are common and include tonsillar and diffuse cervical lymphadenopathy, upper aerodigestive tract candidiasis, cutaneous and mucosal Kaposi's sarcoma, parotid lymphadenopathy and cysts. Histologic evaluation of the tonsils may show a spectrum of changes including florid follicular hyperplasia, follicle lysis, attenuated mantle zone, and presence of multinucleated giant cells. Similar changes may affect the nasopharyngeal lymphoid tissue in HIV infection (see Chapter 23). In most cases, immunohistochemical evaluation for the HIV p24 core proteins and in situ hybridisation for viral RNA have demonstrated localisation to follicular dendritic network, the multinucleated giant cells, scattered interfollicular cells, and cells within the surface or crypt epithelium.[19] Although cysts may be a feature of HIV and AIDS, their location in tonsils is not common. Most cystic lesions in tonsils represent dilated crypts with formation of cysts and are commonly seen in recurrent tonsillitis. In cases of developed AIDS, Kaposi's sarcoma may occur in the tonsils[20] (see also Chapters 11, 27 and 38).

References

1. Regauer S, Gogg-Kamerer M, Braun H et al. Lateral neck cysts – the branchial theory revisited. A critical review and clinicopathological study of 97 cases with special emphasis on cytokeratin expression. APMIS 1997;105:623–630
2. von Gaudecker B. Development and functional anatomy of the human tonsilla palatina. Acta Otolaryngol 1988;454 (suppl):28–32
3. Gebert A, Pabst R. M cells at locations outside the gut. Semin Immunol 1999;11:165–170
4. Andersson J, Abrams J, Björk L et al. Concomitant in vivo production of 19 different cytokines in human tonsils. Immunology 1994;83:16–24
5. Brandtzaeg P. The B-cell development in tonsillar lymphoid follicles. Acta Otolaryngol (Stockh) 1996;523(suppl):55–59
6. Eggston AE, Wolff D. Histopathology of the ear, nose and throat. Williams and Wilkins, Baltimore, 1947
7. Padeh S, Brezniak N, Zemer D et al. Periodic fever, aphthous stomatitis, pharyngitis, and adenopathy syndrome: clinical characteristics and outcome. J Pediatr 1999;135:98–101
8. Osborn GR, Roydhouse N. The tonsillitis habit. WP Roydhouse, Auckland, New Zealand, 1976
9. Valles Fontanet J, Oliva Izquierdo T. Actinomycosis of the tonsils with a pseudotumoral presentation: a clinical case [In Spanish]. Acta Otorrhinolaringol Esp 1995;46:444–446
10. Buchanan G. Infectious mononucleosis. Ear Nose Throat J 1982;61:557–561
11. Wright DH, Isaacson PG. Biopsy pathology of the lymphoreticular system. Chapman and Hall, London, 1983
12. Prange E, Trautmann JC, Kreipe H et al. Detection of Epstein-Barr virus in lymphoid tissue of patients with infectious mononucleosis by in situ hybridization. J Pathol 1992;166:113–119.
13. Anagnostopoulos I, Hummel M, Kreschel C et al. Morphology, immunophenotype, and distribution of latently and/or productively Epstein-Barr virus-infected cells in acute infectious mononucleosis: implications for the interindividual infection route of Epstein-Barr virus. Blood 1995;85:744–750
14. Isaacson PG, Schmid C, Pan L et al. Epstein-Barr virus latent membrane protein expression by Hodgkin and Reed-Sternberg-like cells in acute infectious mononucleosis. J Pathol 1992;167:267–271
15. Bozkurt T, Langer M, Fendel K et al. Granulomatous tonsillitis. A rare extraintestinal manifestation of Crohn's disease. Dig Dis Sci 1992;37:1127–1130
16. Remaley AT, Rust S, Rosier M et al. Human ATP-binding cassette transporter (ABC1): genomic organization and identification of the genetic defect in the original Tangier disease kindred. Proc Natl Acad Sci USA 1999;96: 12685–12690
17. Fredrickson DS. The inheritance of high density lipoprotein deficiency (Tangier disease). J Clin Invest 1964;43:228–236
18. Bale PM, Clifton-Bligh P, Benjamin BN et al. Pathology of Tangier disease. J Clin Pathol 1971;24:609–616
19. Wenig BM, Thompson LD, Frankel SS et al. Lymphoid changes of the nasopharyngeal and palatine tonsils that are indicative of human immunodeficiency virus infection. A clinicopathologic study of 12 cases. Am J Surg Pathol 1996;20:572–587
20. Chetty R, Batitang S. Kaposi's sarcoma of the tonsil. ORL J Otorhinolaryngol Relat Spec 1998;60:48–50

27 Neoplasms

Neoplasms of Squamous Cell Epithelium

The lymphoid tissue of the entire Waldeyer's ring, the tonsils included, has no afferent lymphatic channels leading to it. This anatomical feature explains the rarity of metastatic carcinoma in the tonsils (see below). Any carcinoma in the tonsils should be considered primary until proven otherwise. Before the age of immunohistochemistry it was frequently difficult for the pathologist to distinguish histologically between poorly differentiated carcinoma of the tonsil and "large cell" lymphoma.

Squamous Cell Papilloma

Squamous cell papilloma commonly arises on the surface of the palatine tonsil and adjacent oral epithelium. It has the appearance typical of an everted squamous papilloma seen elsewhere in the upper air and food passages, showing branching fronds and microscopically first, second and third order branching of the papillae from a central stalk. The papillary processes show a connective core and a covering of squamous epithelium. Malignant change does not occur.

In contrast to laryngeal papillomas, which frequently contain human papillomavirus (HPV) 6 and 11 (see Chapter 33), tonsillar squamous papillomas are rarely associated with HPV. HPV is, however, associated both with distinct morphological patterns of tonsillar squamous cell carcinomas, and with tonsillar squamous cell carcinomas lacking retinoblastoma protein (see below).

Squamous Cell Carcinoma

This neoplasm is said to be second in frequency to laryngeal carcinoma among malignant neoplasms of the upper air and food passages, although in some geographical regions squamous carcinoma of the tongue, lips and floor of mouth are probably more common. All series disclose a male predominance among patients with squamous carcinoma of the tonsil, and the average age is about 60 years. Both heavy smoking and excessive alcohol intake are important aetiological factors.

Common clinical features are sore throat, a throat lump, haemoptysis and deafness. Several tonsillar carcinomas are small and arise in crypts; metastatic deposits in ipsilateral neck lymph nodes will then constitute the first clinical sign.

Gross appearances are those of a tumour usually situated in the upper pole of one tonsil. In advanced cases there is involvement of the retromolar trigone, fauces, tongue and soft palate. The more highly keratinising growths are exophytic. The less differentiated ones are often ulcerated.

The microscopic structure of most cases of tonsillar primary carcinoma is of epidermoid malignancy with moderate degrees of keratinous differentiation. Dysplasia and carcinoma in situ are common in the adjacent squamous epithelium and may extend as far as the epithelium of the tongue and soft palate. In a small proportion of tonsillar carcinomas the neoplasm is completely undifferentiated and closely resembles undifferentiated carcinoma (lymphoepithelioma) of the nasopharynx (Fig. 27.1) (see Chapter 24). Such neoplasms grow rapidly. They metastasise more readily and are more sensitive to radiotherapy than the better differentiated squamous carcinomas. Extrapulmonary small cell carci-

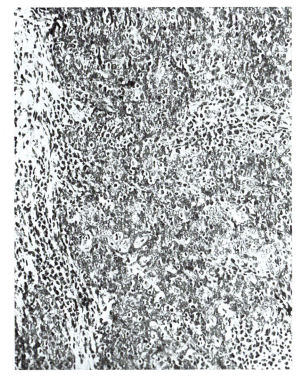

Figure 27.1 Undifferentiated carcinoma of the tonsil, showing large empty nuclei and syncytium-like associations of cytoplasm, with intimate relationship of lymphocytes and plasma cells

functional inactivation of the retinoblastoma protein by the viral E7 gene product.[3]

Lymph node involvement is present in about 65% of patients at the time of diagnosis. The commonest lymph node group to be affected is the jugulodigastric in the upper deep cervical chain.[4] Bloodstream metastasis is quite common. The cervical lymph node metastases frequently precede the clinical presentation of the primary in the tonsil. Cervical lymph node metastases are often cystic.[4] the cysts being covered by a rather bland, non-keratinising neoplastic epithelium (see Chapter 45). Treatment for squamous carcinoma of the tonsil is as a rule by radiotherapy. Surgery is carried out for persistent or recurrent disease and usually comprises a combined excision of the tonsil and adjacent involved tissues and radical neck resection of involved lymph nodes.

Salivary Gland Neoplasms

Salivary gland tumours may arise from the seromucinous glands situated near the palatine tonsil, or from the purely mucous supratonsillar salivary glands – Weber's glands. These include pleomorphic and basal cell adenoma, mucoepidermoid carcinoma and adenoid cystic carcinoma.

Lymphangiomatous Polyp

An uncommon benign tonsillar neoplasm is the lymphangiomatous polyp. It is covered by surface epithelium, although not a papilloma, and composed of abundant lymphatic channels. These polyps can be rather large, and sometimes have a prominent fibrous component.

Metastatic Tumours

Metastatic tumours are not frequent in the tonsils and only some 70 cases have been reported in the literature. Malignant melanoma, breast and lung carcinoma are the commonest sources.[5] Metastases of other adenocarcinomas, particularly from gastric and colorectal carcinomas, but also from renal cell carcinoma, are reported, as well as metastatic lung small cell carcinoma.

Malignant Lymphoma

The tonsils belong to the Waldeyer's ring that constitutes part of the human mucosa-associated

nomas of the amine precursor uptake and decarboxylation system are exceptionally rare, and less than ten cases of primary small cell carcinoma of the tonsil are reported.[1]

HPV DNA has been detected in as many as 60% of tonsillar squamous cell carcinomas, compared with 15% of all head and neck squamous cell carcinomas. A recent study has shown that HPV 16 is almost exclusively associated with a poorly differentiated tumour histology, whereas well-differentiated tonsillar squamous cell carcinomas lack HPV DNA. The well-differentiated carcinomas also show overexpression of cyclin D1 and/or p53, while the poorly differentiated tumours have a decreased expression of cyclin D1, p53 and retinoblastoma tumour suppressor protein, pRb. These findings suggest that HPV has a predilection for non-keratinising squamous cells, or alternatively that the virally transformed cells inhibit the process of keratinisation.[2] Another study, moreover, has demonstrated that tonsillar carcinomas show absence or pronounced reduction of the retinoblastoma tumour suppressor protein, pRb. Human HPV DNA was detected in tonsillar carcinomas defective of pRb, but not in pRb-positive tonsillar tumours. This is strongly in favour of a human HPV-associated aetiology of these tumours, and suggests also that there may be a

lymphoid tissue (MALT) structures of the upper respiratory tract. As discussed in Chapter 26, the tonsils have a regionalised immune function, and are formed mainly of lymphoid follicles, which are surrounded by loosely distributed cells, mainly T lymphocytes and antigen presenting cells. They have no afferent lymphatic channels leading to them, and it is still not entirely clear whether they are functionally exactly comparable with gut-associated lymphoid tissue. The majority of malignant lymphomas of the upper respiratory tract are found in Waldeyer's ring and the general opinion has been that lymphomas arising here should be considered as "nodal".[6] The new World Health Organization (WHO) Classification, which is based upon the Revised European–American Lymphoma (REAL) classification, is recommended for the classification of Waldeyer's ring lymphoma. MALT lymphomas occur also in the tonsils, however, and other parts of the Waldeyer's ring, and of particular interest may be the MALT lymphomas in children with AIDS (see below).

Gross Appearances

In the tonsil malignant lymphoma usually appears as a diffuse enlargement. The surface is smooth; ulceration or papilla formation as seen in carcinomas is not a feature of lymphomas. The cut surface is pink or grey and homogeneous with no surviving crypts. Occasional small cysts produced by obstruction of a crypt may be present. The lymphomatous process may extend to other parts of Waldeyer's ring, particularly the lingual tonsil and vallecula.

Site and Incidence

The tonsil is the commonest site of primary malignant lymphoma in the upper air and food passages. In a survey of non-Hodgkin's lymphoma referred to the Armed Forces Institute of Pathology, Washington, D.C. (L. Michaels, V.J. Hyams), there was involvement of the palatine tonsil in 34 cases (56%) (Table 27.1). In a study of 68 cases of lymphoma growing as a primary in Waldeyer's ring, Saul and

Table 27.1. Sites of origin of 60 cases of non-Hodgkin's lymphoma of upper air and food passages (Armed Forces Institute of Pathology, 1966–1977)

Site	No. of cases
Palatine tonsil and vallecula	34 (56%)
Nose and paranasal sinus	16 (27%)
Nasopharynx	10 (17%)

Table 27.2. Sites of origin of 116 cases of head and neck non-Hodgkin's lymphoma (after Economopoulos et al.[8])

Site	No. of cases
Tonsils	56 (48.3%)
Nasopharynx	15 (12.9%)
Mandible/gingiva	9 (7.8%)
Hard palate	7 (6%)
Parotid glands	6 (5.2%)
Nasal cavity	6 (5.2%)
Hypopharynx/larynx	6 (5.2%)
Thyroid	5 (4.3%)
Ocular adnexa	4 (3.5%)
Paranasal sinuses	2 (1.7%)

Kapadia found that 35 cases (51%) involved the tonsils.[7] In a large series of 116 non-Hodgkin's lymphoma, almost 50% of cases were located in the tonsils (Table 27.2).[8]

Microscopic Appearances

Lymphoma of the tonsil is always associated with the alteration or destruction of the architecture of that organ. The normal follicular arrangement is effaced by cells of the neoplasm. In some cases a nodular arrangement of the tumour cells may be present, but germinal centres of normal follicles are absent within tumour nodules. Crypts are obliterated and involvement of surviving crypts by tumour tissue is seen as compression into thin clefts or invasion of the crypt squamous epithelium. Plasma cells, although still identifiable in some places, particularly beneath the surface squamous epithelium, are less numerous.

At other sites of the upper air and food passages malignant lymphoma grows in the mucosa and may infiltrate deeply into adjacent bone, cartilage or skeletal muscle. Lymphoma cells infiltrate between the acini of seromucinous glands. The walls of small blood vessels often contain lymphoma cells without thrombosis or invasion of their lumina (Fig. 27.2). Necrosis and inflammation may be so severe as to destroy all tumour tissue in a particular biopsy, so that a histological diagnosis may not be possible. Lesions of this type occurring in the nose and paranasal sinuses have given rise to the erroneous conception of "midline granuloma" (see Chapter 22).

Non-Hodgkin's Lymphoma

Classification

Commencing in 1995 more than 50 leading pathologists worldwide were involved in a project aiming

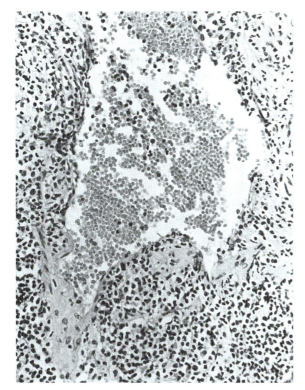

Figure 27.2 Small blood vessel of tonsil invaded by lymphoma. There is no thrombosis of blood in the lumen

Table 27.3. Proposed WHO classification of lymphoid neoplasms (after Harris et al.[10])

B-cell neoplasms
Precursor B-cell neoplasms
    Precursor B-lymphoblastic leukaemia/lymphoma
Mature (peripheral) B-cell neoplasms
    B-cell chronic lymphocytic leukaemia/small lymphocytic lymphoma
    Plasma cell myeloma/plasmacytoma
    Lymphoplasmacytic lymphoma
    Extranodal marginal zone B-cell lymphoma of MALT type
    Nodal mariginal zone B-cell lymphoma (+/– monocytoid B cells)
    Follicular lymphoma
    Mantle-cell lymphoma
    Diffuse large B-cell lymphoma
    Burkitt's lymphoma/Burkitt's cell leukaemia

T-cell and NK-cell neoplasms
Precursor T-cell neoplasms
    Precursor T-lymphoblastic lymphoma/leukaemia
Mature (peripheral) T-cell neoplasms
    Extranodal NK/T-cell lymphoma, nasal type
    Mycosis fungoides/Sezary syndrome
    Peripheral T-cell lymphoma, not otherwise characterized
    Angioimmunoblastic T-cell lymphoma
    Anaplastic large-cell lymphoma, T/null cell, primary systemic type

Hodgkin's lymphoma (Hodgkin's disease)
Nodular lymphocyte-predominant Hodgkin's lymphoma
Classic Hodgkin's lymphoma
    Nodular sclerosis Hodgkin's lymphoma (Grades 1 and 2)
    Lymphocyte-rich classic Hodgkin's lymphoma
    Mixed cellularity Hodgkin's lymphoma
    Lymphocyte depletion Hodgkin's lymphoma

for a consensus list of myeloid, lymphoid and histiocytic neoplasms. A new WHO classification, which applies and extends the REAL classification, has emerged from this.[9] Neoplasms are stratified primarily according to their lineage, e.g. myeloid neoplasms, lymphoid neoplasms, mast cell disorders and histiocytic neoplasms. A useful "Commentary" on the WHO classification has recently been published by the Steering Committee.[10] Within each category, distinct diseases are defined according to a combination of morphology, immunophenotype, genetic features and clinical syndromes. The Commentary emphasises that there is no gold standard, and the importance of various criteria for both definition and diagnosis differs among different diseases.[10] Below will follow a brief account only of the most common lymphoid neoplasms relevant to the tonsils and Waldeyer's ring. Readers interested in a more detailed description are referred to the WHO classification of lymphoma.

In regard to lymphoid neoplasms, the proposed WHO classification recognises B-cell neoplasms, T-cell/natural-killer (NK)-cell neoplasms and Hodgkin's disease. The B- and T-cell neoplasms are classified into precursor neoplasms (lymphoblastic) and mature (peripheral) B- and T-cell neoplasms. The mature B- and T-cell neoplasms are further grouped according to clinical presentation, thus predominantly disseminated/leukaemic, primary extranodal and predominantly nodal diseases (Table 27.3).

B-cell Neoplasms

Most tonsillar malignant lymphomas, like those of all of the Waldeyer's ring, are B-cell lymphomas.

B-cell small lymphocytic lymphoma (Fig. 27.3)

Synonyms are B-CLL (Kiel), well-differentiated lymphocytic, diffuse (Rappaport) and small lymphocytic, consistent with CLL (Working Formulation). The tumour consists of small lymphocytes, slightly larger than normal lymphocytes, and with clumped chromatin. The cells have faint SIgM, B-cell-associated antigen+, CD5+, CD23+, CD43+ and CD10−. The disease is one of elderly people and develops often very slowly, so that the patient eventually may die from an intercurrent illness rather than the lymphoma. Waldeyer's ring, particularly the tonsils, is affected in some cases.

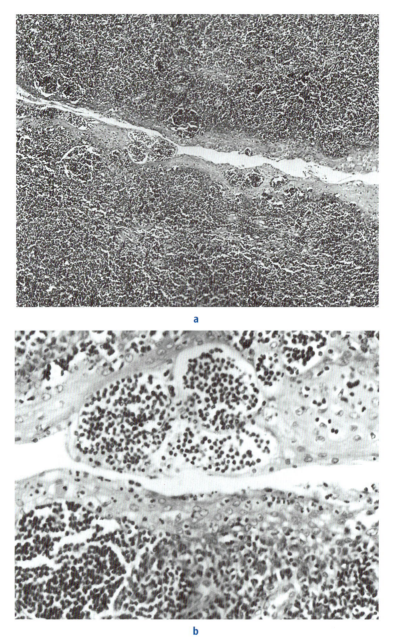

a

b

Figure 27.3 B-cell small lymphocytic lymphoma of the tonsil. **a** A deposit consisting solely of small lymphocytic cells has replaced a large part of the normal structure of the tonsil, but the crypt shown in the centre survives. It is infiltrated by clusters of small lymphocytes. **b** Higher power of crypt in **a**. Small lymphocytes in groups infiltrate the squamous epithelial lining

Plasmacytoma

Synonyms are plasmacytic malignant lymphoma (Kiel) and extramedullary plasmacytoma (Working Formulation). The tumour consists of mature and immature plasma cells, and most are B-cell-associated negative (CD19⁻, CD20⁻ and CD22⁻) but CD38⁺, CD79a$^{+/-}$, CD56$^{+/-}$, CD43$^{+/-}$ and epithelial membrane antigen (EMA)$^{-/+}$. There are in fact suggestions that

plasmacytomas may represent marginal zone B-cell zone lymphomas of MALT type that have undergone an extensive degree of plasmacytic differentiation. Plasmacytoma rarely affects the tonsils and the sites of its occurrence in the upper air and food passages are listed in Table 27.4. The nose and paranasal sinuses are the commonest sites for plasmacytoma in this region and a full account of it is given in Chapter 22.

Table 27.4. Site of initial presentation in 53 cases of extramedullary plasmacytoma of the upper air and food passages. Armed Forces Institute of Pathology Registry 1940–1980 (Courtesy of Dr. V.J. Hyams)

Site	No. of cases
Nose and paranasal sinuses	28 (52%)
Nasopharynx	10 (19%)
Pharynx (oropharynx and hypopharynx)	3 (6%)
Tonsil	3 (6%)
Larynx	9 (17%)

Extranodal Marginal Zone B-cell Lymphoma of MALT type

Synonyms are monocytoid B-cell lymphoma, immunocytoma (Kiel) and small lymphocyte B, lymphocytic-plasmacytic (Lukes-Collins). These lymphomas, often termed MALT lymphomas, are of special interest in head and neck pathology. Typically "MALT lymphomas" arise from sites normally devoid of lymphoid tissue, such as the mucosa of the nose and paranasal sinuses and the salivary glands. They also often arise in association with chronic, autoimmune inflammation, commonly seen for instance in the salivary glands. In the 1980s two tumours were described that were seemingly related (morphologically, immunophenotypically and clinically), and the use of the term monocytoid B-cell lymphoma for both nodal and extranodal disease was accordingly confusing. These tumours were the low-grade B-cell lymphoma of MALT type[11,12] and monocytoid B-cell lymphoma.[13] The term marginal zone B-cell lymphoma was proposed by the International Lymphoma Study Group[9] and the current nomenclature is thus extranodal marginal zone B-cell lymphoma of MALT type, and nodal marginal zone B-cell lymphoma (+/– monocytoid cells) (Table 27.2). The criteria for distinguishing MALT from non-MALT lymphoma at extranodal sites have recently been enlightened by Harris and Isaacson.[14] The tumour cells are the centrocyte-like marginal zone cells, which are small and atypical and with more cytoplasm than "proper" centrocytes. There are also plasma cells (often neoplastic), small lymphocytes and monocytoid B cells. Centroblast- and immunoblast-like cells are present. Around remaining reactive follicles neoplastic marginal zone or monocytoid B cells will occupy the marginal zone and the interfollicular region. In certain epithelial tissues, particularly the salivary glands, the marginal zone cells infiltrate the epithelium giving rise to the so-called lymphoepithelial lesions.

The tumour cells are SIg+ but lack IgD, B-cell-associated antigens+, CD19+, CD20+, CD22+, CD79a+, CD11c+/−, CD43−/+, CD5−, CD10− and CD23−. There is no rearrangement of bcl-2. Trisomy 3 has been reported in 60% of MALT lymphomas.[15] These tumours have a slight female predominance and are tumours of adults. Extranodal marginal zone B-cell lymphoma of MALT type develops not infrequently in patients with autoimmune disease, e.g. Sjögren's syndrome or Hashimoto's thyroiditis.

For a long time it has been noticed that extranodal marginal zone B-cell lymphoma of MALT type often arise from a background of chronic inflammatory lesions and can transform into high-grade tumours. It also has been observed that chronic inflammation is associated with genetic instability and thus theoretically genetic instability may play a role in the pathogenesis of MALT lymphomas. To this extent it was recently shown that the replication error phenotype (RER+; a manifestation of genetic instability) apparently is a common genetic feature of extranodal marginal zone B-cell lymphoma of MALT type. Furthermore, this study demonstrated homogeneous and heterogeneous microsatellite alterations between so-called low- and high-grade components, which likely indicate their clonal lineage and genetic diversity.[16] Also, it appears that most gastric extranodal marginal zone B-cell lymphomas of MALT type arise in response to *Helicobacter pylori* infection and that the growth of the lymphoma is driven by contact between neoplastic B cells and *H. pylori*-specific intra-tumoural T cells (antigen-driven). Moreover, "high-grade MALT lymphomas" have been associated with p53 inactivation, for example, deletions of p16 and t(8;14).[17] Nevertheless, the new WHO classification recommends that the term high-grade MALT lymphoma should not be used.[10] Very recently a novel gene, *MALT1*, located at 18q21, has been identified and is thought to play an important role in the pathogenesis of extranodal marginal zone B-cell lymphoma of MALT type.[18]

Follicular Lymphoma (Fig. 27.4)

Synonyms are centroblastic/centrocytic follicular lymphoma (Kiel) and follicle centre lymphoma (REAL). The tumour is composed of follicle centre cells, usually a mixture of cleaved follicle cells (centrocytes) and large non-cleaved follicle centre cells (centroblasts). For the rare case of purely diffuse lymphoma that seems to be of follicle centre origin (predominance of centrocytes, rare centroblasts, bcl-2 rearranged), the term follicle centre lymphoma, diffuse, will be retained as a separate category.[10] In Waldeyer's ring, including the tonsils, there is a higher incidence of the diffuse type compared with the lymph nodes, perhaps due to the more disseminated nature of the disease when presenting in this anatomical location. Follicular lymphoma is recommended to be graded by the

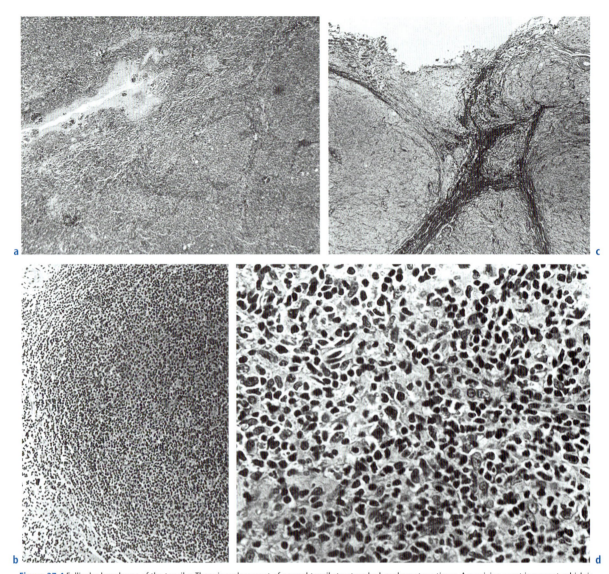

Figure 27.4 Follicular lymphoma of the tonsil. **a** There is replacement of normal tonsil structure by lymphomatous tissue. A surviving crypt is present, which is invaded by groups of lymphoma cells. The tumour shows a follicular structure. **b** A tumour follicle from another tonsillar neoplasm. **c** Follicular structure is outlined by reticulin fibres in tumour shown in **b**. Reticulin stain. **d** Higher power of tumour shown in **b** and **c**. The smaller cells are centrocytes. The larger ones with vesicular nuclei, often showing nucleoli near the nuclear membrane, are centroblasts

number of large cells. Thus Grade 1: zero to five centroblasts/high power field (HPF); Grade 2: six to 15 centroblasts/HPF; and Grade 3: >15 centroblasts/HPF. The presence of diffuse areas will also be reported (predominantly follicular: >75% follicular; follicular and diffuse: 25–75% follicular; and predominantly diffuse: <25% follicular). At the Royal National Throat, Nose and Ear Hospital, six cases of Grade 3 follicular lymphoma were identified over a period of 15 years. Four were located in the tonsils, one in the nasopharynx and one in the nose (Fig. 27.5).

The immunophenotype is characterised by the tumour cells being usually SIg+, B-cell-associated antigen+, CD10+/−, CD23−/+, CD43−, etc. The BCL-2 protein is present in most follicular lymphomas while absent in reactive follicles. In 70–95% of cases the translocation t(14;18) is present, involving rearrangement of the *bcl-2* gene. Follicular lymphoma has an equal sex incidence, occurs predominantly in adults, and generally has an indolent clinical course and is usually not curable with available treatment.[9]

Mantle-Cell Lymphoma

This tumour is defined according to the Kiel classification criteria for centrocytic lymphoma. Synonyms are centrocytic lymphoma (Kiel), small

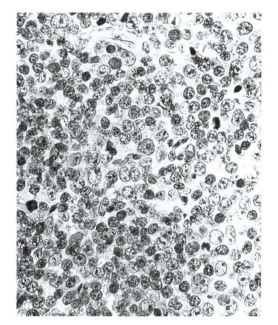

Figure 27.5 Centroblastic lymphoma of tonsil. The tumour consists of large cells with pale-staining nuclei showing peripheral nucleoli

cleaved follicular centre cell lymphoma (Lukes-Collins) and small cleaved cell, diffuse or nodular (Working Formulation). This lymphoma does not arise from true follicle centre centrocytes, but rather from a subset of follicle mantle B cells. The tumour cells are small to medium-sized with scant cytoplasm. The nuclei are irregular or cleaved. The growth pattern is diffuse or vaguely nodular, but rarely follicular. Some cases may contain scattered epithelioid histiocytes, thus creating a "starry-sky" appearance. There are no large cells. Retrospective examination of lymphomas seen at The Royal National Throat, Nose and Ear Hospital over some 15 years revealed five patients with mantle-cell lymphoma in the upper air and food passages. In two, the palatine tonsils were affected; in a further two, the nasopharynx, and in one patient the tumour grew in the nasal passages.

The tumour cells are SigM+, usually IgD+, B-cell-associated antigen+, CD5+, CD10-/+, CD23-, CD43+. CD5 can thus be an useful marker to distinguish between follicular and mantle-cell lymphoma, and the absence of CD23 in distinguishing mantle cell lymphoma from B-cell small lymphocytic lymphoma (B-CLL). In the majority of cases there is a chromosomal translocation t(11;14) that results in an overexpression of the *PRAD1* gene, which encodes cyclin D1. Cyclin D1 is not normally expressed in lymphoid cells. Mantle-cell lymphoma has a strong male predominance and has a moderately aggressive clinical behaviour. At present it appears to be incurable, with median survival ranging from 3 to 5 years.[9] The new WHO classification recommends that mantle-cell lymphoma should not be subclassified/graded for clinical purposes.[10]

Diffuse large B-cell lymphoma (Fig. 27.6)

Synonyms are centroblastic, B-immunoblastic, large cell anaplastic (Kiel) and diffuse large cell cleaved, non-cleaved or immunoblastic (Working Formulation). The tumour cells are large, i.e. at least twice the size of a small lymphocyte. The cells have vesicular nuclei and prominent nucleoli, and a basophil cytoplasm. The cells resemble a large non-cleaved cell (centroblast) or an immunoblast, or a mixture thereof. Diffuse large B-cell lymphoma is rare in the tonsil.

The tumour cells are SIg+/-, B-cell-associated antigens+, CD19+, CD20+, CD22+, CD79a+, CD45+/-, CD5-/+, CD10-/+. In about 30% of cases the *bcl-2* gene is rearranged, and the *c-myc* gene occasionally. Diffuse large B-cell lymphomas have a broad age range with a median age in the sixth decade, although they can be seen in children. This tumour is aggressive with a rapidly enlarging mass at a single node, or extranodal site (almost 40% are

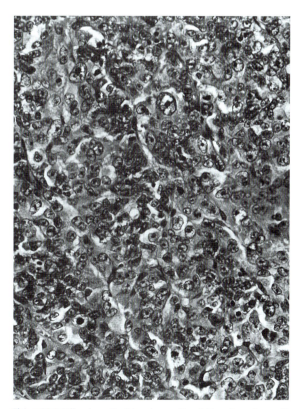

Figure 27.6 Diffuse large B-cell lymphoma of tonsil. The cells are large with prominent central nucleoli and abundant cytoplasm

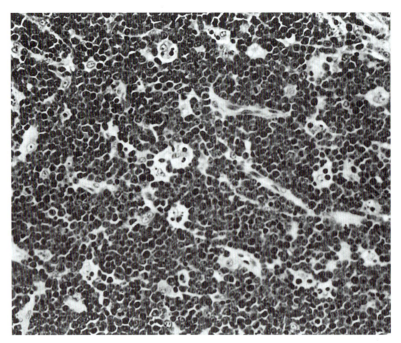

Figure 27.7 Burkitt's lymphoma of the larynx in a 9-year-old English boy. Note "starry sky" formation of blast cells in which there are scattered larger histiocytic cells with phagocytosed cytoplasmic debris

extranodal), but potentially curable with aggressive therapy.

Burkitt's lymphoma (Fig. 27.7)

Synonyms are Burkitt's lymphoma (Kiel), undifferentiated lymphoma, Burkitt's type (Rappaport) and small non-cleaved cell lymphoma, Burkitt's type (Working Formulation). The tumour cells are medium-sized and rather monomorphic. They have round nuclei and multiple nucleoli and abundant basophil cytoplasm.

The tumour cells are SIgM[+], B-cell-associated antigens[+], CD19[+], CD20[+], CD22[+], CD79a[+] and CD10[+] but CD5[-] and CD23[-]. Epstein-Barr virus can be demonstrated in most African cases, and in up to 40% of cases with AIDS, but less frequently in non-African, non-immune-deficient cases.[9] Translocation t(8;14) is found in most cases (c-myc on chromosome 8 to Ig heavy chain region on chromosome 14), but also t(2;8) and t(8;22) are reported. The tumour is most common in children and there is a male predominance. In the head and neck area, the jaws are often involved followed in incidence by the salivary glands. Burkitt's lymphoma is highly aggressive but potentially curable.

T-cell and NK-cell neoplasms

Many T-cell and NK-cell lymphomas show variation in the size of the cells and immunophenotypic variation exists within disease entities. The location, i.e. nodal versus extranodal, is more important in determining the biological behaviour than is the case of B-cell lymphomas. Therefore, it has been recommended that clinical syndromes are integral to the definition of peripheral T/NK-cell lymphomas.[9] The extranodal NK/T-cell lymphoma, nasal type (Table 27.3) is described in Chapter 14.

Peripheral T-cell lymphoma, not otherwise characterised (Fig. 27.8)

Synonyms are T-zone lymphoma, lymphoepithelioid cell lymphoma. Lennert's lymphoma (Kiel), T-immunoblastic lymphoma (Lukes-Collins) and diffuse small cleaved cell, diffuse mixed small and large cell, large cell immunoblastic (Working Formulation). The tumours consist of a mixture of small and large atypical cells admixed with rather numerous eosinophils and epithelioid histiocytes. The tumour cells have irregular nuclei and show great variation in shape and size, with occasional large hyperchromatic cells that resemble Reed-

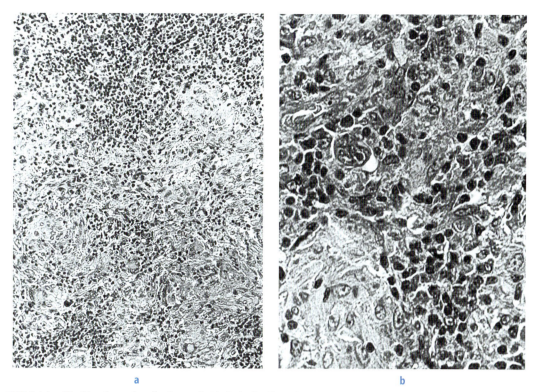

Figure 27.8 Peripheral T-cell lymphoma of tonsil. **a** Groups of epithelioid cells infiltrate the tonsil and there are some multinucleate giant cells. **b** High-power view of tumour showing epithelioid cells, blast cells and a giant cell, which bears a resemblance to a Reed-Sternberg cell

Sternberg cells. These latter cells were probably the cause of confusion with Hodgkin's lymphoma in the past and in fact Hodgkin's lymphoma is very rare in the tonsil and elsewhere in Waldeyer's ring. Lymph nodes are mainly affected, but tonsillar involvement at the outset in a substantial number of cases.

The tumour cells have variable T-cell-associated antigens, CD3$^{+/-}$, CD2$^{+/-}$, CD5$^{+/-}$, CD7$^{-/+}$, and may be CD4$^-$CD8$^-$. B-cell-associated antigens are lacking but occasionally the tumour cells may express CD45RA and CD20. *TCR* genes are usually but not always rearranged.[9] Peripheral T-cell lymphoma, not otherwise characterised, affects adults, usually with generalised disease. They comprise less than 15% of all lymphomas in Europe and the USA but are more common in other parts of the world. A recent study from Korea reported as many as 30% of cases in a series of 501 non-Hodgkin's lymphomas to be T- and NK-cell lymphomas.[19] The clinical course is often rather aggressive and relapses are more common than in B-cell lymphomas. However, the tumours are potentially curable.

Lymphoma in HIV-positive patients

An increased incidence of non-Hodgkin's lymphoma is seen in patients with immunodeficiency from any cause. In children with HIV infection, non-Hodgkin's lymphoma is the most frequent malignancy, followed in frequency by leiomyosarcoma.[20] Extranodal marginal zone B-cell lymphoma of MALT type appears to be one of the most frequent types of lymphoma associated with HIV infection, particularly in children.[21,22,23] Also Hodgkin's lymphoma is associated with HIV infection. Rubio[24] reported that in 43 of 46 patients, Hodgkin's lymphoma was the manifestation of HIV infection. In 16 of these 46 patients, AIDS developed after the diagnosis of Hodgkin's lymphoma.

Hodgkin's lymphoma

Although no consensus was reached concerning the nomenclature – Hodgkin's disease or Hodgkin's lymphoma – it was proposed that both names could be used.[10] In the upper air and food passages, Hodgkin's lymphoma is very rare or may exist only as an extension from lymph nodes. Cases previously identified in this region as Hodgkin's lymphoma were probably peripheral T-cell lymphoma, not otherwise characterised (see above). Below will be given only a brief account of the different immunophenotypes.[9]

Nodular lymphocyte-predominant Hodgkin's lymphoma has atypical cells, which are CD45$^+$, B-cell-associated antigens$^+$ (CD19, 20, 22, 79a), CDw75$^+$, EMA$^{+/-}$, CD15$^-$ and CD30$^{-/+}$. Of the classic Hodgkin's lymphoma, the nodular sclerosis type has cells that are CD30$^+$, CD15$^{+/-}$, CD45$^-$ and EMA$^-$. Tumour cells of mixed cellularity Hodgkin's lymphoma are CD30$^+$, CD15$^{+/-}$, CD45$^-$ and EMA$^-$. Lymphocyte depletion Hodgkin's lymphoma has cells that are CD30$^+$, CD15$^{+/-}$, CD45$^-$, B-cell-associated antigens$^-$, T-cell-associated antigens$^-$ and EMA$^-$. The lymphocyte-rich classical Hodgkin's lymphoma has atypical cells with immunophenotypes similar to nodular sclerosis and mixed cellularity. Recently it was reported that the malignant cells of Hodgkin's lymphoma (NOS) express an abundance of heat shock proteins (particularly hsp89 and hsp60). This expression of heat shock proteins was not seen in other lymphomas, and may imply a pathogenic role of Hodgkin's lymphoma.[25]

References

1. Bawa R, Wax MK. Small cell carcinoma of the tonsil. Otolaryngol Head Neck Surg 1995;113:328–333
2. Wilczynski SP, Lin BT, Xie Y et al. Detection of human papillomavirus DNA and oncoprotein overexpression are associated with distinct morphological patterns of tonsillar squamous cell carcinoma. Am J Pathol 1998;152:145–156
3. Andl T, Kahn T, Pfuhl A et al. Etiological involvement of oncogenic human papillomavirus in tonsillar squamous cell carcinomas lacking retinoblastoma cell cycle control. Cancer Res 1998;58:5–13
4. Thompson LD, Heffner DK. The clinical importance of cystic squamous cell carcinomas in the neck: a study of 136 cases. Cancer 1998;82:944–956
5. Fernandez Acenero MJ, Pascual Martin A, Martin Rodilla C et al. Tonsillar metastases: report on two cases and review of literature. Gen Diagn Pathol 1996;141:269–272
6. Isaacson PG, Norton AJ. General features of extranodal lymphomas. In: Extranodal lymphomas. Churchill Livingstone, London, 1994, pp 1–4,
7. Saul SH, Kapadia SB. Primary lymphoma in Waldeyer's ring. Clinicopathologic study of 68 cases. Cancer 1985;56:157–166
8. Economopoulos E, Fountzilas G, Kostourou A et al. Primary extranodal non Hodgkin's lymphoma of the head and neck in adults: a clinicopathological comparison between tonsillar and non tonsillar lymphomas. (Hellenic Cooperative Oncology Group). Anticancer Res 1998;18:4655–4660
9. Harris NL, Jaffe ES, Stein H et al. A revised European–American classification of lymphoid neoplasms: a proposal from the International Lymphoma Study Group. Blood 1994;84:1361–1392
10. Harris NL, Jaffe ES, Diebold J et al. World Health Organization classification of neoplastic diseases of the hematopoietic and lymphoid tissues: report of the Clinical Advisory Committee Meeting – Airlie House, Virginia, November 1997. J Clin Oncol 1999;17:3835–3849
11. Isaacson P, Wright D. Malignant lymphoma of mucosa associated lymphoid tissue. A distinctive B cell lymphoma. Cancer 1983;52:1410–1416
12. Isaacson P, Spencer J. Malignant lymphoma of mucosa-associated lymphoid tissue. Histopathology 1987;11:445–462
13. Cousar J, McGinn D, Glick A et al. Report of an unusual lymphoma arising from parafollicular B lymphocytes or so-called "monocytoid" lymphocytes. Am J Clin Pathol 1987;87:121–128
14. Harris NL, Isaacson PG. What are the criteria for distinguishing MALT from non-MALT lymphoma at extranodal sites? Am J Clin Pathol 1999;111(1 suppl 1):S126–132
15. Wotherspoon AC, Finn TM, Isaacson PG. Trisomy 3 in low-grade B-cell lymphomas of mucosa-associated lymphoid tissue. Blood 1995;85:2000–2004
16. Peng H, Chen G, Du M et al. Replication error phenotype and p53 gene mutation in lymphomas of mucosa-associated lymphoid tissue. Am J Pathol 1996;148:643–648
17. Isaacson PG. Gastric MALT lymphoma: from concept to cure. Ann Oncol 1999;10:637–645
18. Akagi T, Motegi M, Tamura A et al. A novel gene, MALT1 at 18q21, is involved in t(11;18)(q21;q21) found in low-grade B-cell lymphoma of mucosa-associated lymphoid tissue. Oncogene 1999;18:5785–5794
19. Lee SS, Cho KJ, Kim CW et al. Clinicopathological analysis of 501 non-Hodgkin's lymphomas in Korea according to the revised European-American classification of lymphoid neoplasms. Histopathology 1999;35:345–354
20. McClain KL, Joshi VV, Murphy SB. Cancers in children with HIV infection. Hematol Oncol Clin North Am 1996;10:1189–1201
21. Wotherspoon AC, Diss TC, Pan L et al. Low grade gastric B-cell lymphoma of mucosa associated lymphoid tissue in immunocompromised patients. Histopathology 1996;28:129–134
22. Joshi VV, Gagnon GA, Chadwick EG et al. The spectrum of mucosa-associated lymphoid tissue lesions in pediatric patients infected with HIV: a clinicopathologic study of six cases. Am J Clin Pathol 1997;107:592–600
23. Corr P, Vaithilingum M, Thejpal R et al. Parotid MALT lymphoma in HIV infected children. J Ultrasound Med 1997;16:615–617
24. Rubio R. Hodgkin's disease associated with human immunodeficiency virus infection. A clinical study of 46 cases. Cooperative Study Group of malignancies associated with HIV infection of Madrid. Cancer 1994;73:2400–2407
25. Hsu PL, Hsu SM. Abundance of heat shock proteins (hsp89, hsp60 and hsp27) in malignant cells of Hodgkin's disease. Cancer Res 1998;58:5507–5513

The Larynx and Hypopharynx

28 Normal Anatomy and Histology

Development

The basic outlines of development of the larynx are clear and uncontroversial. It is accepted that the epithelium of the larynx arises from the upper end of an outgrowth from the endoderm of the ventral wall of the pharynx. In growing caudally this outgrowth eventually produces the trachea, and bifurcates to produce the bronchi and lungs.

The subsequent fate of the epithelium of the larynx has been subjected to detailed analyses, but there is little evidence for the idea (see Chapter 35) of segregation of the larynx into three regions – supraglottic, glottic and subglottic – with sharply separated epithelial fields producing tumours that usually retain their positions within those regions. This concept has formed the basis of the TMN system of classification of laryngeal squamous carcinoma. The further development of the larynx, particularly the cartilages and muscles, takes place from a condensation of mesenchyme around the epithelium of the early larynx.

The epithelial bud arises in the 12 mm (6 weeks) embryo and is surrounded by a median ventral bud – the epiglottic swelling – and a right and left lateral bulge – the arytenoid swellings. By 8 weeks (30 mm) the outlines of the larynx are well-delineated with all the main cartilages and the thyroarytenoid, interarytenoid and posterior cricoarytenoid muscle precursors established. The thyroid and cricoid develop as cartilaginous masses on each side and subsequently the thyroid fuses in the midline anteriorly and the cricoid fuses both anteriorly and posteriorly. The origin of the laryngeal epithelium from the foregut epithelium is still evident. Figure 28.1 shows transverse sections of the larynx of an embryo of about this stage. Figure 28.1a shows the upper end of the primitive larynx. The pharynx is U-shaped ventrally and a cartilaginous styloid process can be seen behind one limb of the U. From the centre of the U, the median central epithelial groove is given off and joins the horizontal portion of the laryngeal epithelium. Ventral to this epithelial layer, a condensation of mesenchyme is seen, which is the future epiglottic cartilage. Figure 28.1b shows a transverse section of the same embryo larynx taken more caudally. The arytenoid cartilages and vocal processes are well-delineated and the thyroarytenoid and interarytenoid muscles are established already. The saccule arises as an outpouching of the laryngeal cavity at about this stage and is prominent in the late fetal and infant larynx.

Anatomy

The larynx is basically a hollow tube with a flap at its upper end (the epiglottis), which serves to protect the airway from inspiration of food material, and highly mobile vocal cords lower down, which function in phonation.

Regions

Mainly for purposes of classification of neoplasms, the larynx has been divided into three regions: supraglottis, glottis and subglottis. The supraglottis is that region above the true vocal cords, including the epiglottis, the false cords, the ventricles and the saccules. The glottis comprises the vocal cords, the vocal processes of the arytenoids, and the anterior and posterior commissures. The subglottis is that region of the larynx below the true vocal cords

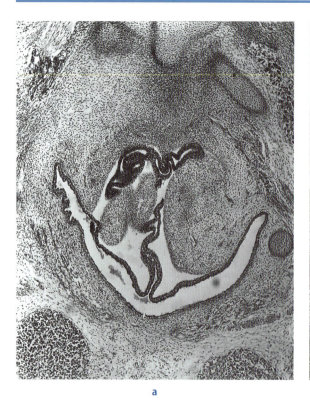

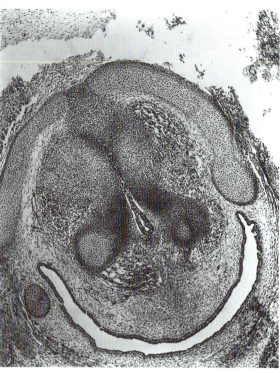

a   **b**

Figure 28.1 Transverse sections of larynx of 33 mm fetus at 9 weeks' gestation. **a** Cranial end. **b** More caudal part than that shown in **a** (Courtesy of Armed Forces Institute of Pathology, Washington, D.C., Dr. P.I. Yakovlev)

down to the level of the lower border of the cricoid cartilage, below which the trachea commences.

Cartilages and Elastic Membranes

The complexity of laryngeal anatomy is the result of the curious relationships that exist among the five laryngeal cartilages. A useful approach to depicting these relationships has been made by Paff,[1] and is reproduced in Figure 28.2. In this figure, the cartilages of the larynx are built up in their final relationship to each other.

Intrinsic Muscles

The intrinsic muscles of the larynx stretch between the cartilages. A knowledge of their anatomy is of importance in understanding laryngeal pathology.

Cricothyroid

The two cricothyroid muscles arise from the arch of the cricoid cartilage and are inserted on the inferior border of the lamina and the anterior border of the inferior cornu of the thyroid cartilage.

Posterior Cricoarytenoid

Each of the two posterior cricoarytenoid muscles arises from a shallow depression on the posterior aspect of the lamina of the cricoid cartilage (shown as two series of parallel short lines in Fig. 28.2) and is inserted into the muscular process of the arytenoid cartilage. These muscles have been described as the most important in the body, since they are the sole abductors of the vocal cords, i.e. the only muscles opening the glottic valve for entry of air into the lungs (Fig. 28.3).

Lateral Cricoarytenoid

These two muscles arise from the arch of the cricoid cartilage and the superior surface of the conus elasticus. Fibres pass posteriorly and upwards to be inserted into the anterior surface of the muscular process of the arytenoid.

Thyroarytenoid and Vocalis Portion

The two thyroarytenoid muscles arise from the internal surface of the inferior half of the thyroid cartilage close to the angle formed by the thyroid

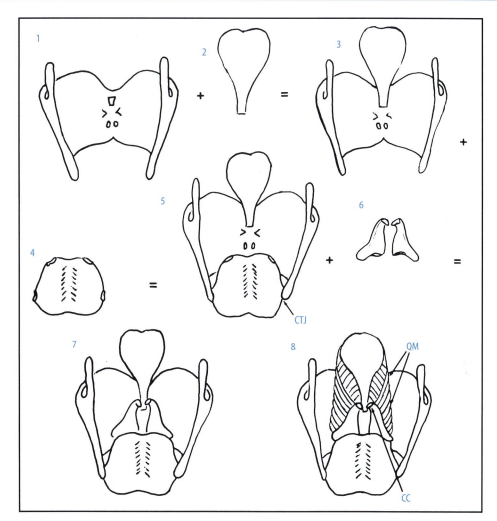

Figure 28.2 The cartilaginous framework of the larynx. In this series of diagrams the cartilages of the larynx are built up into their actual relationships with each other: 1 shows the shape of the thyroid cartilage from behind; 2 shows the epiglottic cartilage, placed in position in 3; 4 shows the cricoid lamina from behind; the ring of the cricoid is not seen; 5 shows the position of the lamina in relation to the thyroid cartilage, forming a joint with it, the cricothyroid joint, *CTJ*. The arytenoids are seen in 6 and are placed in position in 7, the inferior thyroid cornu forming a joint with the cricoid lamina – the cricoarytenoid joint – on each side. In 8 the elastic quadrangular membrane (*QM*) is in place. This is the elastic frame of the laryngeal cavity. The *vertically hatched* part of this represents the aryepiglottic folds; *cc*, position of insertion of cuneiform cartilage at apex of arytenoid[1]

lamina and the superior surface of the conus elasticus. The muscle fibres extend posteriorly in a horizontal plane to be inserted into the body of the arytenoid cartilage. Slips of muscle leave the thyroarytenoid to be inserted along the length of the vocal ligaments, and it is these that constitute the vocalis portions of the thyroarytenoid muscles.

Transverse Arytenoid

The transverse arytenoid is not a paired muscle, but extends from the lateral surfaces of the bodies (the apices) of each arytenoid to the other.

Thus there are four paired intrinsic muscles and an unpaired muscle. The posterior cricoarytenoid is the sole abductor. All the other intrinsic muscles function in adduction of the vocal cords.

Nerve Supply

All the intrinsic laryngeal muscles except the cricothyroid muscle are supplied by the recurrent laryngeal branch of the vagus nerve. The cricothyroid muscle is supplied by the superior laryngeal branch of the vagus nerve.

The Cords; the Ventricle and Saccule

The false and true cords of the larynx are two pairs of mucous folds situated above and below (respec-

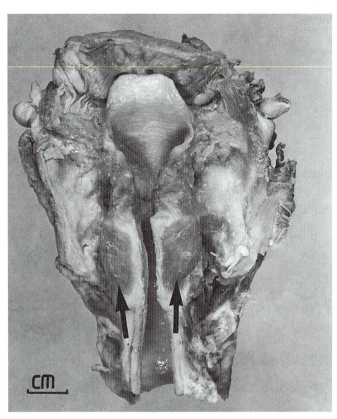

Figure 28.3 Post-mortem larynx seen from behind and opened by a vertical cut through the cricoid lamina. The *arrows* point to the two posterior cricoarytenoid muscles. Note the prominent bellies of these muscles. They pass upwards and laterally from an origin on the posterior surface of the cricoid lamina to be inserted into the muscular process of the arytenoid

tively) an invagination of the laryngeal mucosa known as the ventricle. The false cords enclose fibrous and adipose tissue and many seromucinous glands. The lower border of the false cords forms a free crescentic margin, which constitutes the upper boundary of the laryngeal ventricle.

The true cords are composed of elastic tissue covered by mucosa, and extend from the angle of the thyroid cartilage anteriorly to the vocal process of the arytenoid cartilage posteriorly. The ventricle is an oblong fossa between the two cords on each side and extends for most of their lengths. The anterior part of the ventricle leads upwards into a blind pouch of variable length – the saccule.

Examination of Specimens of Larynx

Laryngeal Biopsy Specimens

Following the successful use of the colposcope for observation of diseases of the cervix uteri, a microscopic procedure was introduced for direct laryngoscopy. Not only can the mucosa of the larynx be observed under magnification, but also operative manipulations, especially biopsy, can be carried out with precision. This is now part of the standard technique for the investigation of laryngeal diseases. In some cases frozen section for the rapid diagnosis of laryngoscopy biopsy specimens may be useful, as in cases that have been repeatedly subjected to biopsy, but no definite result obtained or where the surgeon would need to initiate surgical therapy under the same general anaesthetic.

The Partial Laryngectomy Specimen

Partial laryngectomy procedures were devised to resect malignant laryngeal lesions, but at the same time to allow breathing to take place through the remaining laryngeal lumen without a permanent tracheostomy and also to conserve phonation by retaining the vocal cords and their essential musculature. There are broadly three types of partial laryngectomy, devised to resect completely carcinomas of different sites and extent in the larynx: partial vertical laryngectomy, supraglottic horizontal laryngectomy and subtotal laryngectomy.

Partial Vertical Laryngectomy

This procedure is used to remove carcinoma confined to or with little spread from the true vocal cord. The structures removed are: the whole vocal cord on the affected side, including the carcinoma, the ipsilateral arytenoid cartilage, an adjacent part of the ipsilateral thyroid cartilage and, if there is some subglottic spread, part of the adjacent cricoid cartilage.

Supraglottic Horizontal Laryngectomy

This procedure is used for supraglottic neoplasms. The structures removed are: the epiglottis, the hyoid bone, the thyrohyoid membrane and the upper half of the thyroid cartilage. Resection margins are through the ventricles, the aryepiglottic folds and the valleculae.

Subtotal Laryngectomy

This procedure is used for an extensive laryngeal neoplasm involving both glottis on one side only and supraglottis. The structures removed are: the supraglottic larynx as for supraglottic laryngectomy together with the vertical half of the affected glottis and subglottis with the neoplasm, leaving one vocal cord intact for phonation.

When examining the partial laryngectomy specimen it is essential first to identify grossly the normal structures and the neoplasm within the resected specimen. The resection margins may be painted with India ink to assist in their identification in the histological specimen. It is most useful in these specimens to slice the specimen vertically using a scalpel with a large disposable blade, which is usually heavy enough to cut through the cartilage and overlying mucosa. In each vertical slice the same side is presented for sectioning in the embedded specimen, conveniently the lateral side. This is ensured by marking the opposite surface with a daub of India ink before embedding.

Sections are assessed, as in the whole laryngectomy specimen (see below), for origin of squamous carcinoma and extent of invasion, particular care being paid to the inspection of surgical resection margins for extension of neoplasm.

Laryngectomy Specimens

To obtain an adequate picture of the extent of spread of tumour in the laryngectomy specimen, multiple sections of the whole specimen are required. One means of achieving this has been the whole-organ serial sectioning method. By this method the whole larynx is cut serially after decalcification and embedding in celloidin or in paraffin wax. The coronal plane is favoured for the serial sectioning of most laryngeal tumours. By contrast, serial sectioning of epiglottic tumours is performed in the sagittal plane.

A variation of this method using horizontal whole organ serial sections has recently been employed for the study of non-neoplastic lesions of the larynx in autopsied infant larynges.[2,3]

Serial sectioning of the larynx is, however, far too time consuming for use in most histopathology laboratories. The method necessitates prior decalcification of the whole organ, a process that requires longer exposure to acid than is necessary for smaller blocks of tissue, and therefore leads to inferior histological appearances. In addition, with this method the opportunity for gross study of special areas is lost, and the application of modern histological methods, such as frozen sections, plastic embedding, immunocytochemistry and electron microscopy, is not possible. Whole-organ serial sectioning requires long periods of embedding, which do not suit the clinical need for a reasonable quick laboratory assessment of the degree of tumour spread.

The introduction of computerised tomography allowed a series of horizontal radiographs of the larynx to be taken at 5-mm intervals. To correlate the appearances of such radiographs with pathological changes, horizontal slicing of surgically resected larynges at similar intervals, using a slicing machine, were prepared. The blade of the slicing machine cutting smoothly through the ossified cartilages allowed a complete gross picture of the tumour in situ in the larynx to be obtained, following which satisfactory histological studies could be carried out in the material so sliced. The method has proved over many years to be suitable for the routine examination of whole laryngectomy specimens in the histopathology laboratory.[4]

Preparation Technique

The larynx is fixed in 10% buffered formol-saline for at least 48 h. It is then opened by a vertical cut along the midline of the posterior surface, and the lesion is photographed. After the gross appearances of the interior of the larynx have been described, the hyoid bone is carefully dissected off the larynx. If tumour is seen in the pre-epiglottic space, either grossly at this stage or microscopically at a later stage, the hyoid is sectioned transversely by sawing, and sampled for histological examination.

The larynx is then sliced transversely in a slicing machine of the ordinary meat-slicing motorised type used by delicatessen shops. The machine is always supplied with special grindstone equipment for sharpening the circular blade. It is very important to do this before cutting each larynx so that the slicing of ossified areas will take place easily. Slicing is carried out transversely. It is advantageous to slice the epiglottis vertically using a stout scalpel before the transverse slicing of the rest of the larynx with the slicing machine.[5] The machine is set for cutting slices of 4 mm thickness. Four millimetres is the maximum thickness of a block of tissue that can be inserted into a tissue capsule for embedding.

Appearances of Transverse Slices

By slicing the fixed larynx with a slicing machine, material for an accurate gross study is provided quickly and easily. The following normal structures may be identified in the tissue slices: epiglottis, laminae of the thyroid and cricoid cartilages, corniculate and cuneiform cartilages, false vocal cords, ventricles and saccules, true vocal cords, arytenoid cartilages, inferior cornua of the thyroid cartilage, intrinsic muscles, cricoarytenoid joints, cricothyroid membrane and arch of the cricoid cartilage (Fig. 28.4). Any small structure that is not displayed on the surface of a block for microscopy may be included within a paraffin block and can be subsequently displayed in histological section by cutting down on to the required area during microtomy.

Portions of hypopharynx that are removed with the larynx can be studied in the horizontal sections, and the method described is also suitable for studying hypopharyngeal carcinoma that has been treated by pharyngolaryngectomy (see Chapter 39).

In addition to the normal structures mentioned above, the intrinsic laryngeal muscles may be conveniently displayed and sampled for histological examination by this method.

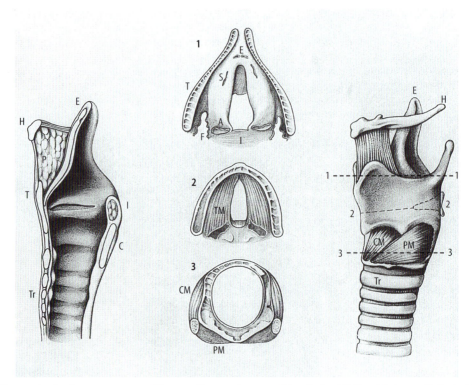

Figure 28.4 Diagrams showing the gross appearance of the normal larynx on transverse slicing. *On the right*, the whole larynx with the hyoid bone (*H*) and epiglottis (*E*) is viewed from the left side. The *broken line (2)* shows the position of the glottic transverse slice, passing through the true vocal cords and arytenoid. The *broken lines (1) and (3)* indicate the positions of the supraglottic and subglottic slices. *On the left*, the larynx has been bisected in a vertical plane and the right half is viewed from the left side. Note the hyoid bone (*H*) and the epiglottic (*E*), thyroid (*T*), cricoid (*C*) and tracheal (*Tr*) cartilages in the vertical section. Note also the fatty pre-epiglottic space (*P*) and the interarytenoid muscle (*I*) (the latter above the cricoid lamina (*C*)). Transverse slices are taken from the supraglottis (*1*), glottis (*2*) and subglottis (*3*). The supraglottic slice (*1*) is bounded by the thyroid cartilages (*T*) at the sides. The gap anteriorly represents the thyroid notch. Note the epiglottic cartilage (*E*) in transverse section. Behind it on each side is a slit-shaped saccule (*S*). The apical portions of the arytenoids (*A*) are seen posteriorly. Behind them and joining them is the interarytenoid muscle (*I*). At its two sides are the piriform fossae (*F*) of the hypopharynx. The transverse slice through the vocal cords (*2*) shows the prominent thyroarytenoid muscles (*TM*) at this level. The lower slice (*3*) is taken at the level of the cricoid ring. Note the cricothyroid muscles (*CM*) laterally and the posterior cricoarytenoid muscles (*PM*) posteriorly[4]

Histology

Epiglottis

The pear-shaped epiglottic cartilage contains elastic tissue and does not undergo ossification (Fig. 28.5). The elastic cartilage is perforated in the lower two-thirds by numerous foramina, which are produced by seromucinous glands that open through the posterior epithelial surface (Fig. 28.6). The mucosa lining the anterior epiglottic surface is stratified squamous epithelium in continuity with that of the posterior surface of the tongue (vallecula) and surrounding hypopharynx. The posterior (or laryngeal) epiglottis is covered by a similar stratified squamous epithelium in its upper half, but lower down this changes into the ciliated pseudostratified columnar type characteristic of most of the internal laryngeal lining. The submucosa of the lingual epiglottic surface is comparatively loose areolar tissue, compared with the dense compact connective tissue of the posterior epiglottic surface.

False Cords

The epithelium of the false cords is of the respiratory type. However, squamous metaplasia is common. The submucosa is characterised by a large

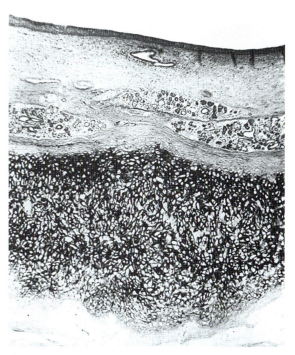

Figure 28.5 Posterior (laryngeal) surface of epiglottis with cartilage. The network of elastic fibres of the epiglottic cartilage is outlined in black. Weigert's elastic stain

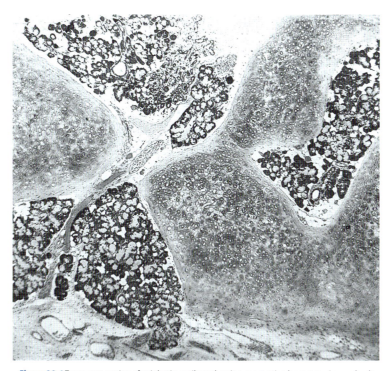

Figure 28.6 Transverse section of epiglottic cartilage showing penetration by seromucinous glands

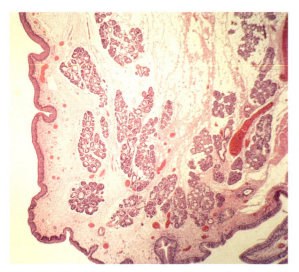

Figure 28.7 False cord. The commencement of the ventricle is seen at the bottom right. The laryngeal lumen is at the bottom. Note the large amount of seromucinous glands and adipose tissue between them

number of seromucinous glands embedded in a fibro-areolar stroma, which is admixed with strands of striated muscle fibres extending superiorly from the thyroarytenoid (vocalis) muscle. These glands are also found within the loose fibres of the quandrangular membrane (Fig. 28.7). In some larynges from elderly people, a considerable amount of adipose tissue is seen in the false cord, which imparts a yellowish colour to it when seen in cross-section. Metaplasia of the connective tissue of the false cord to elastic cartilage is seen frequently. This new formation of cartilage may encroach on the laryngeal lumen, but should not be mistaken for a neoplasm.

True Vocal Cords

The epithelium of the true vocal cord is of stratified squamous variety from early in develop-
ment. This epithelium continues for a variable distance on to the floor of the ventricle and downwards towards the subglottis. The deep margin of the epithelium lining the ventricular floor (horizontal portion) is smooth, but the airway part of the vocal cord shows rete ridges. Melanocytes may be found among the squamous epithelial cells regardless of the race of the individual[6] (see Chapter 37). The lamina propria of the true vocal cord is bounded on its deep aspect by the vocal ligament, and at its upper and lower extents by respiratory mucosa. It contains no seromucinous glands. This vocal cord lamina propria is said to be deficient in lymphatic drainage and forms a space (Reinke's space). The vocal ligament (which is continuous below with the conus elasticus) is a nodular thickening composed of elastic tissue to which the vocalis portion of the thyroarytenoid muscle is tethered (Figs 28.8, 28.9 and 28.10). The region of the vocal ligament may contain nodules of elastic cartilage (Figs 28.11 and 28.12).

Anterior and Posterior Commissures

A poorly demarcated area at the junction of the vocal cords anteriorly – the anterior commissure – is a region where the mucosa is not folded into vocal cords, but where it is in close proximity to the thyroid cartilage at the angle region. The core of the anterior commissure is fibrous tissue containing blood vessels and lymphatics. The epithelium in this region is repiratory in type, and there is an extensive tubo-alveolar system of glands, which drains into the lower part of the anterior commissure region and the adjacent subglottis. The interarytenoid area of the glottis is sometimes known as the posterior commissure. The epithelium here is also respiratory in type. Abundant seromucinous glands are present in this area and may extend deeply, even into the interarytenoid muscle.

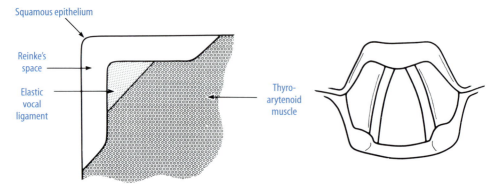

Squamous epithelium

Reinke's space

Elastic vocal ligament

Thyro-arytenoid muscle

Figure 28.8 Diagrams of true vocal cord seen from above (*right*) and in vertical section with component structures (*left*)

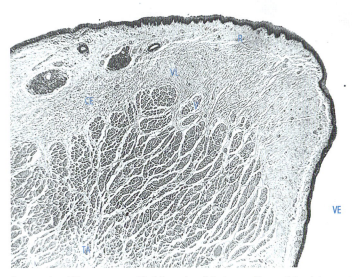

Figure 28.9 Vertical sections of true vocal cord. The squamous epithelial covering of the laryngeal lumen (*above*) shows rete ridges, but that of the vestibule (*right*) does not. *CE*, conus elasticus; *R*, Reinke's space; *TA*, thyroarytenoid muscle; *V*, vocalis fibres of thyroarytenoid muscle; *VE*, space of ventricle; *VL*, vocal ligament

Ventricle and Saccule

The ventricle and saccule are the proximal and distal parts (respectively) of an out-pouching of the laryngeal mucosa between the true and false cords. The saccule, which is of variable length, is an upward extension of the ventricle, derived from its anterior part. A similar lining consisting of respiratory epithelium with numerous glands is present in both the ventricle and the saccule. Squamous metaplasia is unusual. The saccule often shows villiform-like projections and these are always prominent in the infant saccule. A chronic inflammatory exudate is commonly found in the mucosa of the saccule, sometimes concentrated into lymphoid aggregates (Fig. 28.13).

Laryngeal Joints

Both the cricoarytenoid and the cricothyroid joints are diarthrodial – that is, they contain a joint cavity.

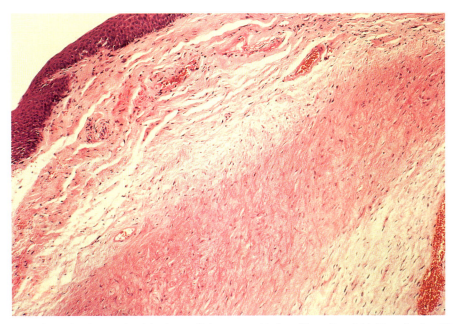

Figure 28.10 Surface region of true vocal cord showing stratified squamous epithelium with rete ridges, Reinke's "space" and vocal ligament

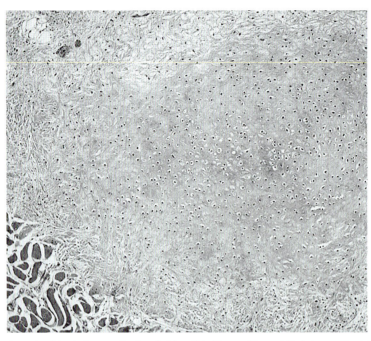

Figure 28.11 Elastic cartilage has replaced the elastic connective tissue in this section of the vocal ligament. The lesion was biopsied as a nodule of the vocal cord

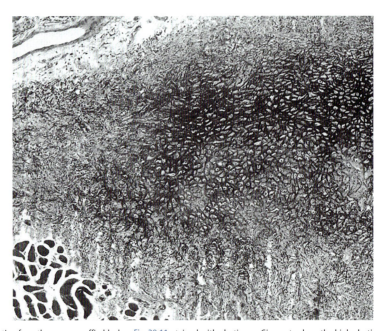

Figure 28.12 Another section from the same paraffin block as Fig. 28.11, stained with elastic-van Gieson, to show the high elastin content of the cartilaginous nodule

The articular surfaces are smooth and composed of a layer of cartilage, the thickness of which depends on the degree of ossification of the underlying arytenoid, cricoid and thyroid cartilages. The synovial membranes are lined by flattened synovial cells, beneath which there is a connective tissue layer. Synovial membrane is confined to a recess which surrounds the articular cartilaginous surface but does not cover it. A tongue of synovium is regularly seen springing from the lateral recess of the cricoarytenoid joint (Fig. 28.14).

Subglottis

Histological sections of the larynx in the subglottic region are characterised by the solid cartilaginous

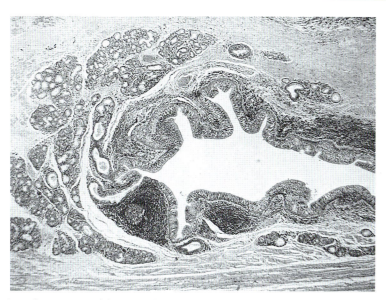

Figure 28.13 Saccule showing surface projections of the mucosa. There are collections of lymphocytes under the epithelium gathered (in some places) into lymphoid follicles, one of which shows a germinal centre

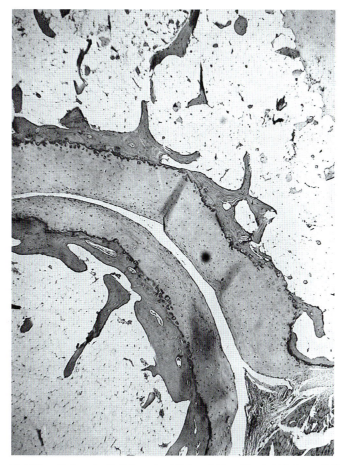

Figure 28.14 Normal cricoarytenoid joint. The articular ends of both the arytenoid (*above right*) and the cricoid (*below and left*) are covered by hyaline cartilage. A tongue of synovium is arising from the lateral recess of the joint (*bottom right*)

lamina of the cricoid behind, and in the lower part of the subglottis the ring is completed by the cricoid arch anteriorly. In the upper part of the subglottis, between the lower border of the thyroid cartilage and the cricoid arch, the cricothyroid membrane is seen – a thick elastic lamina that is perforated by blood vessels and lymphatic channels. At least one lymph node is usually found near the outer surface of the cricothyroid membrane.

Laryngeal Cartilage

The thyroid, cricoid and arytenoid cartilages are hyaline in nature. The apex (body) of the arytenoid has been stated to be elastic cartilage; the epiglottis, corniculate and cuneiform cartilages are definitely so. Hyaline cartilage undergoes ossification with developing age; elastic cartilage does not.

In hyaline cartilage of the larynx and trachea that has been stored for at least 5 years in dilute buffered formaldehyde solution before processing for histology, large numbers of petal-like birefringent crystals are found, which are insoluble in water and in the organic solvents used in histological processing, but soluble in dilute acids. These crystals appear to contain calcium, and special staining by the silver rubeanate test indicates that they are calcium oxalate. Electron probe analysis confirms the presence of calcium. The crystals are not found in cartilages that have been stored for less than 5 years, nor in elastic cartilage or any other tissue. These crystals of calcium oxalate have an identical appearance to those found in the kidney in ethylene glycol poisoning and oxalosis, but the significance of these storage artefacts of laryngeal cartilage is unknown.

Ossification of hyaline cartilage is always present to a variable degree in adult larynges, and the degree of ossification increases with age. This process begins later and advances more slowly in women than in men. It starts in the thyroid cartilage, involves the cricoid next, and occurs last in the arytenoid cartilage. It is frequently found in the cartilage near the cricothyroid and cricoarytenoid joints, near the zones of the cartilage where muscles are inserted, and in the vicinity of squamous carcinoma. There does not appear to be a regular arrangement of ossifying areas similar to that of ossification of bones. Woven bone is formed in the early stages of active ossification. Later, lamellar bone is deposited. Bone marrow with haemopoietic cells and adipose tissue is frequently present in the regions of ossification. Ossified laryngeal cartilage is vascular, like bone elsewhere; but unossified cartilage contains no vessels. A perichondrium (a fibrovascular layer from which cartilage cells grow and are nourished) completely envelops each laryngeal cartilage (see Chapter 31).

Laryngeal Muscles

The laryngeal muscles show the features of normal skeletal muscles. On routine staining, we have found, however, that the posterior cricoarytenoid muscles constantly show abnormal features; the transverse arytenoid, thyroarytenoid, cricoarytenoid and lateral cricoarytenoid muscles show lesser degrees of such changes or none at all.[7] The changes in the posterior cricoarytenoid muscles are the presence of focal deposits of coarse brown pigment granules (lipofuscin) situated in the sarcoplasm near the sarcolemma, rows of up to 30 small, deeply staining nuclei near the sarcolemma, a segmented eosinophilic change in a short length of the fibre, leaving the rest of the fibre normal and a loss of transverse striation. In many areas histiocytic cells accompany and infiltrate the necrotic areas and in a few cases there was fibrous tissue replacing muscle in some areas. Some fibres are shrunken to atrophic bands less than a quarter the width of normal fibres (Figs 28.15 and 28.16). It is likely that these changes in some way reflect the intense activity that these muscles undergo throughout life. The posterior cricoarytenoid muscles are the sole abductors of the vocal cords. They function with every inspiration and are active in phonation. They have a higher proportion of type 1 fibres than the other laryngeal muscles, a greater aerobic metabolic activity, and a more abundant capillary blood supply. Similar changes, but with more fibrosis, may be found in the cricopharyngeus muscle in association with symptoms of dysphagia (see Chapter 34).

Recurrent Laryngeal Nerve

The recurrent laryngeal nerve (containing the motor nerve supply for the larynx and lower pharynx) comes off the vagus. On the right side it passes in front of the right subclavian artery, and on the left side in front of the arch of the aorta. On both sides the nerve ascends between the trachea and oesophagus, and passes under the inferior constrictor muscle, which it supplies. Above this muscle an important relationship is maintained to the cricothyroid joint, which lies anterior to the recurrent laryngeal nerve. It first gives off a branch to the posterior cricoarytenoid muscle and then enters the larynx to supply all the intrinsic muscles except the cricothyroid, which is supplied from the superior laryngeal nerve (Fig. 28.17).

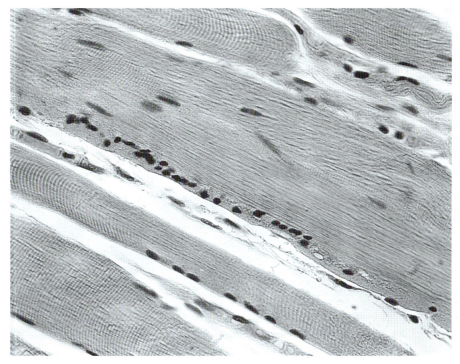

Figure 28.15 Muscle fibres from posterior cricoarytenoid muscle showing strings of sarcolemmal nuclei and central muscle nuclei[7]

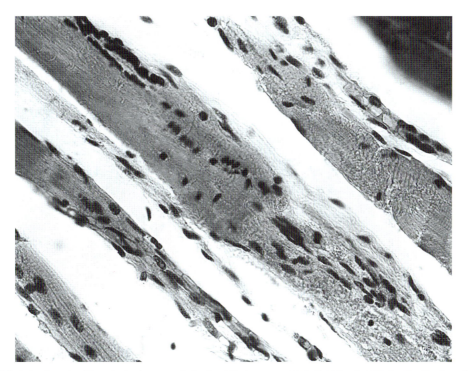

Figure 28.16 Posterior cricoarytenoid muscle showing segment of eosinophilic change associated with histiocytic infiltration. One fibre is greatly shrunken[7]

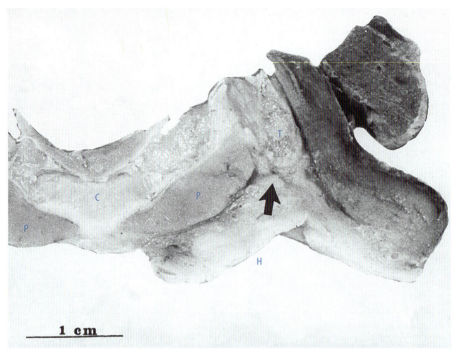

Figure 28.17 Transverse slice of larynx at level of cricoid lamina (*C*) showing position of right recurrent laryngeal nerve (*arrow*) posterior to inferior cornu of thyroid cartilage (*T*) in region of cricothyroid joint. The nerve is also near the posterior cricoarytenoid muscle (*P*). *H*, hypopharyngeal mucosa

In plastic-embedded transverse sections of the recurrent laryngeal nerve, large and small transverse, myelinated fibres may be seen (Fig. 28.18).

Laryngeal Paraganglia

Paraganglia have been discovered in the larynx, and are said to be the source of the tumours resembling paraganglioma that are occasionally seen in the larynx (see Chapter 37).

Paraganglia occur at two principal sites in the larynx. The upper one – named the superior laryngeal glomus by Kleinsasser[8] – is up to 3 mm in diameter and is situated on each side in the upper and anterior one-third of the false cord, adjacent to the superior margin of the thyroid cartilage and in relation to the internal branch of the superior laryn-

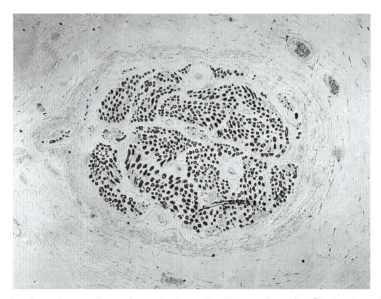

Figure 28.18 Transverse section of normal recurrent laryngeal nerve, showing small and large myelinated fibres[9] Methacrylate embedded 1 μ section, Sudan black stain

geal nerve and artery. The inferior laryngeal glomus is situated between the cricoid cartilage and first tracheal ring on each side and measures about 0.4 mm in diameter.[8] Other inconstantly placed glomus bodies have been found in the larynx. The paraganglia are often situated near small autonomic ganglia in the larynx. The histological structure of the laryngeal paraganglia is similar to that of the normal carotid body and paraganglia of the temporal bone (see Chapter 5).

References

1. Paff SGE. Anatomy of the head and neck. Saunders, Philadelphia, 1973
2. Holinger LD. Histopathology of congenital subglottic stenosis. Ann Otol Rhinol Laryngol 1999;108:101–111
3. Liu H, Chen JC, Holinger LD et al. Histopathologic fundamentals of acquired laryngeal stenosis. Pediatr Pathol Lab Med 1995;15:655–677
4. Michaels L. Examination of specimens of larynx. J Clin Path 1990;43:792–795
5. Slootweg P, de Groot GA. Surgical pathological anatomy of head and neck specimens. A manual for the dissection of surgical specimens from the upper aerodigestive tract. Springer, London, 1999
6. Goldman JL, Lawson W, Zak FG et al. The presence of melanocytes in the human larynx. Laryngoscope 1972;82:824–835
7. Guindi GM, Michaels L, Bannister R et al. Pathology of the intrinsic muscles of the larynx. Clin Otolaryngol 1981;6:101–109
8. Kleinsasser O. Das Glomus laryngicum inferior. Ein bisher unbekanntes, nichtchromaffines Paraganglion vom Bau der sog. Carotisdrüse im menschlichen Kehlkopf. Arch Ohr Nas Kehlkopfheilk [In German] 1964;184:214–224
9. Bannister R, Gibson W, Michaels L et al. Laryngeal abductor paralysis in multiple system atrophy. A report on three necropsied cases, with observations on the laryngeal muscles and the nuclei ambigui. Brain 1981;104:351–368

29 Congenital Anomalies, Laryngocele and Other Developmental Anomalies

Congenital Anomalies

Congenital anomalies of the larynx are uncommon. The reason for this may in part be that the patency of the laryngeal airway is necessary for life. This is not the whole explanation, because serious laryngeal anomalies are rare in autopsies performed on neonatal deaths and stillborn infants.

The three most common congenital disorders, in descending order of frequency, are:[1]

1. Laryngomalacia.
2. Vocal cord paralysis.
3. Congenital subglottic stenosis.

Laryngomalacia

The term "laryngomalacia" is applied to a common anomaly of the newborn in which the infant produces an inspiratory stridor. This may be produced by the bulky folds, which are softer and less rigid than normal, projecting from the laryngeal wall into the lumen.[1] The infant usually grows out of the symptoms in the second year and no therapy is required. The cause is not known.

Vocal Cord Paralysis

Like laryngomalacia, this is a functional, not structural, anomaly and has many possible aetiologic bases. Unilateral vocal cord paralysis is usually left-sided because the recurrent laryngeal nerve has a longer course on that side. Stretching of the neck at birth may be a factor in many cases. This form of paralysis is usually also temporary, lasting up to 4 weeks after birth.

Bilateral vocal cord paralysis is more usually the result of central nervous system damage such as intracerebral bleeding, encephalocele, hydrocephalus and dysgenesis of the nucleus ambiguus, and so is more likely to be permanent.

Congenital Subglottic Stenosis

Congenital subglottic stenosis is the commonest serious cause of stridor in the newborn. The pathologist faced with the identification of the pathological changes in these small larynxes has difficulty in studying the gross and histological changes that may be present. In order to observe the changes in the infantile larynx a special processing technique is required.

Techniques for Examination

In the method of horizontal serial sectioning of the whole infantile larynx, the larynx, including the hyoid bone and hypopharynx, is fixed in 10% formalin solution, decalcified and embedded in Parlodion.[2] It is then serially sectioned and every 20th section is mounted and stained with haematoxylin and eosin. A less time-consuming method, which we have found useful, is to slice the larynx, with the hypopharynx but without the hyoid bone, horizontally after fixation into three parts, approximately representing the supraglottic, glottic and subglottic portions. These are then embedded in paraffin wax and step-sectioned horizontally at about 300-μm intervals.[3]

Pathological Changes

The pathological bases for subglottic stenosis in the newborn are classified into two groups:

1. Cricoid cartilage deformity. This is the result of a developmental anomaly of the cricoid cartilage, which may have grown in an abnormal shape, be abnormally thick or distorted by a cleft in the cartilage. The lesions in this group account for almost all cases of congenital subglottic stenosis.[2]
2. "Soft" tissue obstruction. Here there is a swelling which is maximal 2–3 cm below the true vocal cords. This swelling is composed of hypertrophied mucous glands, ductal cysts, granulation or fibrous tissue. These lesions are usually acquired (see Chapter 31).

Cricoid Cartilage Deformities

Holinger has provided a useful analysis of cricoid cartilage deformities.[2] The shape of the cricoid lumen may be normal, but the diameter abnormally small. The minimum accepted diameter of the cricoid in the newborn is 3.5 mm. The commonest abnormal shape causing congenital subglottic stenosis is the elliptical one. The flattened cricoid has a transverse diameter greater than its anteroposterior one. Anterior laminar thickening and flattened cricoid may each be associated with a trapped first tracheal ring, which rides up inside the cricoid in a telescopic fashion, further reducing the anteroposterior diameter. Generalised thickening of the whole cricoid may also be a cause of congenital subglottic stenosis.

Laryngeal clefts are usually posterior. Variable degrees of cleft formation may be present. A posterior laryngeal cleft is the result of failure of fusion of the tracheoesophageal septum and may penetrate the cricoid lamina and communicate with the hypopharynx. The posterior submucous (occult) cleft does not communicate with the hypopharynx.

Acquired subglottic stenosis

Acquired subglottic stenosis is a lesion that is found in some premature infants. Histopathological observations indicate that the lesion is a surface necrosis with an acute inflammatory perichondritis involving the arytenoid and cricoid cartilages. These changes are almost certainly the result of intubation, which is required in all these infants to maintain adequate respiration (see Chapter 31). It is likely that the congenitally narrowed larynx has a greater chance of being traumatised by an endotracheal tube than does the normal airway.

Less Common Anomalies

Laryngeal Webs

Laryngeal webs would seem to have their origin in the stage of development of the larynx at which the lumen does not yet exist, but at which epithelium has formed a solid lamina. It is subsequent to this that the hollowing out of this epithelial lamina leads to formation of the laryngeal lumen. Incomplete development at this stage will result in a laryngeal lumen that is partially obstructed – a condition that is known as a web. In rare cases there may be complete obstruction – a condition known as laryngeal atresia, which is incompatible with life. Most webs are seen as thin transparent sheets covering the anterior part of the glottis between the true vocal cords to varying degrees. The upper surface is flat, with a sharp concave posterior border. Occasionally a supraglottic web may be present. The upper surface is composed of squamous epithelium, often hyperplastic and keratinised, below which is a connective tissue layer. The lower surface is said to show normal respiratory mucosa.

Bifid Epiglottis

The existence of the rare anomaly of bifid epiglottis would seem to support a bilateral embryological origin of this structure. The patients have the symptoms of persistent respiratory stridor and dyspnoea due to the inspiration of the halves of the epiglottis into the glottis.[4] Aspiration of ingested food may also take place. The appearance of this condition is of an epiglottis that is split in the midline down to its base.

Congenital Laryngoptosis

A few cases have been described in which the larynx has been found to be in an unusually low position. In these cases the trachea cannot be palpated and is short. No serious symptoms result from this abnormality, but it gives rise to difficulty in intubating the patient.

The larynx is high up behind the mandible in fetal life. It begins to descend later in fetal life and this descent continues during infancy. It would seem likely that this lesion results from an excessive degree of descent.

Laryngocele

Definition and Classification

A laryngocele is a dilatation of the laryngeal saccule, which is filled with air. Three forms are recognised: (1) external, in which the swelling appears in the neck above the thyrohyoid membrane; (2) internal, in which the dilatation of the saccule is confined to the larynx, inferior to the thyrohyoid membrane; and (3) mixed, comprising the features of both (1) and (2).

Incidence

Laryngocele is a rare condition. However, by studying case reports in the literature of 130 patients and adding nine of their own, Stell and Maran were able to come to some useful conclusions regarding the incidence of laryngoceles.[5] They saw nine laryngoceles in 8 years and 500 laryngeal carcinomas in the same time. On the basis of the known incidence of carcinoma, they calculated that laryngoceles occur about once per 2 500 000 population per annum in the UK. From the published literature, laryngoceles appear to be commonest in the white race, and far commoner in men – the ratio of men to women with this lesion being about 7:1. The commonest age incidence is in the fifties. Most laryngoceles are unilateral. About one-half of all laryngoceles are represented by the mixed type.

Clinical Features

The patient with an internal laryngocele usually complains of hoarseness, dyspnoea and cough. At laryngoscopy the lesion is seen as a submucosal swelling in one side of the supraglottis. External laryngocele usually presents as a bulge in the side of the neck, which varies in size, swelling up when intralaryngeal pressure is increased, and may be compressed from outside. Laryngoceles are easily confirmed by straight X-rays of the neck, which show the air-filled sac in the characteristic lateral position.

On rare occasions, laryngoceles may undergo secondary infection and become filled with pus. Such "laryngoceles" are very dangerous since they carry a risk of causing death from asphyxia or mediastinitis.

Pathological Appearances

The pathological anatomy of laryngocele was first described by Virchow. A laryngocele may be observed on gross examination of the larynx before dissection as a bulge of the lateral supraglottic mucosa or lateral to the aryepiglottic fold. On dissection or transverse slicing, it will be seen that the bulge represents a dilatation of the saccule filled with air, which communicates with the mucosal surface of the larynx via the ventricle. An internal laryngocele is confined to the interior of the larynx and extends posterosuperiorly towards the false cord into the aryepiglottic fold. An external laryngocele extends superiorly by bulging out above the thyrohyoid membrane, the "internal" portion of the saccule remaining of normal size. The protrusion of the dilated saccule through the thyrohyoid membrane takes place where the superior laryngeal nerve, artery and vein penetrate that membrane. The mixed type of laryngocele shows features of both external and internal types. Histological examination of the laryngocele wall shows the lining to be composed of respiratory epithelium in all cases. Like the normal saccular lining from which it is derived, this epithelial surface may be somewhat papillated, although many laryngoceles have lost this feature of the saccular epithelium, presumably because of distension and stretching. There is a variable degree of chronic inflammation beneath the epithelium and a fibrous lamina propria.

A laryngocele contains air. A structure with identical appearance but filled with mucus as a result of obstruction in the ventricle is known as a mucocele (Fig. 29.1).

Laryngocele and Neoplasia of the Larynx

There is an association between neoplasia of the larynx and laryngocele. Stell and Maran, reviewing the literature and in their own cases, found 7 of 139 laryngoceles to be associated with squamous carcinoma, and two to be associated with papilloma.[5] Large saccules, which extended beyond the thyroid cartilage, have been found in 17% of larynxes from larygneal carcinoma cases.[6]

Carcinoma may be related to a laryngocele in three possible ways:

1. Carcinoma of the contralateral glottis may grow towards the lumen and produce a valvular-type obstruction of the homolateral ventricle. The saccule above this then becomes distended with air to produce a laryngocele.

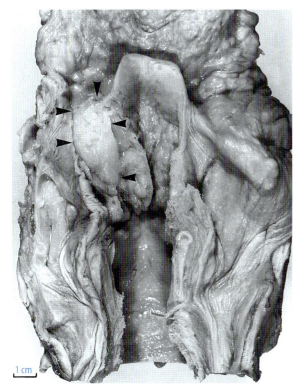

Figure 29.1 Mucocele of larynx (*arrowheads*). The lesion has the same structure as a mixed type of laryngocele (internal *and* external swelling of saccule), but is filled with mucus, not air. The mucocele has been opened lateral to the left aryepiglottic fold to reveal the mucous content

2. The tumour may involve the ventricle or the saccule on the same side with a one-way valvular effect producing a laryngocele on the same side.

3. Carcinoma may grow in the wall of a preformed laryngocele. This was observed in one of the larynxes of a series of cases of ventriculo-saccular carcinoma[7] as a multifocal squamous carcinoma arising from the epithelium of the laryngocele at a number of sites (see Chapter 35).

In many cases, however, the carcinoma may be found to be associated with a mucus-containing cyst of the saccule produced by complete obstruction proximally, with retention of mucus beyond the obstruction, rather than a laryngocele (see below).

Pathogenesis

Stell and Maran[5] dismiss out of hand the concept that laryngoceles are acquired by repeated blowing, as in glass blowers or trumpeters. They give the following reasons for their view:

1. There is hardly ever a history of much blowing before the onset of the laryngocele.
2. Most laryngoceles are unilateral.
3. They are rare, whereas people frequently blow as part of their occupation or leisure activity.
4. The recurrence of laryngoceles after simple removal has not been observed.

Stell and Maran conclude that laryngoceles are an atavistic remnant corresponding to the lateral laryngeal air sacs of the higher anthropoid apes. In the presence of such a congenitally large saccule, the clinical appearance of a laryngocele may become manifest in response to a sudden increase of intralaryngeal pressure caused by coughing, straining at stool or trumpet playing. Mention should be made here of the remarkable results of a study in Canada in which radiographs of the necks of 94 wind-instrument bandsmen were carried out during raised intrathoracic pressure.[8] The study revealed that 56% of the bandsmen had laryngoceles!

The relative importance of congenital enlargement and increased intralaryngeal pressure in the pathogenesis of laryngocele is not yet completely settled. Both factors do, in fact, seem to play a part.

Cysts of the Saccule

Saccular cysts, unlike laryngoceles, are associated with stenosis of the saccular lumen at one point and so do not communicate with the laryngeal airway. Distal to the obstruction, the cyst becomes dilated with mucus. Saccular cysts may be present on a congenital or an acquired basis.

Congenital saccular cysts are usually related to a congenital atresia at the proximal (ventricular) end of the saccule. If the saccule is short, the cyst derived from it will present as a bulge in the anterior part of the ventricle, i.e. between the false cord and the true cord. If the saccule is longer, the cyst derived from it will present as a smooth swelling of the lateral laryngeal wall. Thus congenital saccular cysts are customarily divided into anterior and lateral varieties.[9]

Acquired saccular cysts are the result of occlusion of the saccule at any point along its course. A frequent cause of the occlusion is squamous carcinoma (see above). Saccular cysts resulting from supraglottic carcinoma are seen projecting through the thyrohyoid membrane.

Saccular cysts may, like laryngoceles, be complicated by infection and acute inflammation to produce a laryngopyocele – a very dangerous complication because it will produce acute airway obstruction.[10]

Prolapse and Eversion of the Ventricle

A process of bulging of the mucosa of the laryngeal ventricle has been variously described as prolapse and eversion:[11]

1. Prolapse is polypoid formation of the ventricle caused by adipose tissue formation in the submucosa.
2. Eversion, on the other hand, is a protrusion of tissue into the laryngeal lumen from between the true and false vocal cords, secondary to pulsion or traction by an associated laryngeal lesion. Examples of pulsion eversion of the ventricle are chondroma or lymphoid hyperplasia, which "pushes" the ventricular mucosa, and ductal cyst, which "pulls" the ventricular mucosa into the airway.

Other Cysts

Cysts of the larynx are of the squamous or columnar variety. Both types are produced by obstruction of the ducts of laryngeal glands. The majority of cysts are lined by columnar epithelium (Fig. 29.2) and are situated most commonly in the ventricle or false cord. A large proportion of these columnar cysts are lined by oncocytic cells, and a similar oncocytic change is very common in the adjacent seromucinous glands (Fig. 29.3). Since these glands are normally very abundant in the false cords, the change of oncocytosis produces a large amount of pink-staining glandular epithelium; this has given rise to the erroneous concept that these lesions are neoplasms – "cystadenomas" of oncocytes. The electron microscopic appearance of oncocytes is one of cytoplasm packed with mitochondria to the exclusion of other organelles. Thus the oncocyte may be a less active and more degenerated cell than its normal precursor in the laryngeal glands. Such cells are seen more frequently with advancing age. Therefore, the presence of oncocytes in the lining and in nearby glands of a cyst is most likely to be a degenerative change due to the pressure of the cyst. These columnar cysts rarely attain a large size in adults, although in children they may attain sufficient size to narrow the airway to a significant degree.

Squamous-cell-lined cysts are usually seen in the upper part of the larynx, on the posterior surface of the epiglottis or aryepiglottic fold.

In columnar and squamous cell cysts, the cause of the duct obstruction is only occasionally visible in the biopsy specimen, since most cysts are removed surgically with little adjacent tissue. When the whole

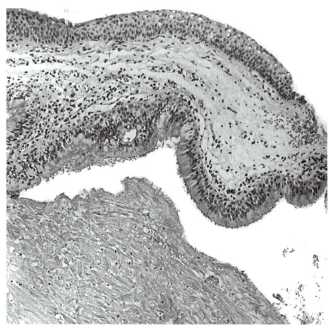

Figure 29.2 Retention cyst of false cord. The cyst is lined by ciliated columnar epithelium and contains fibrillar threads of mucus. The lining of the false cord is seen *above*

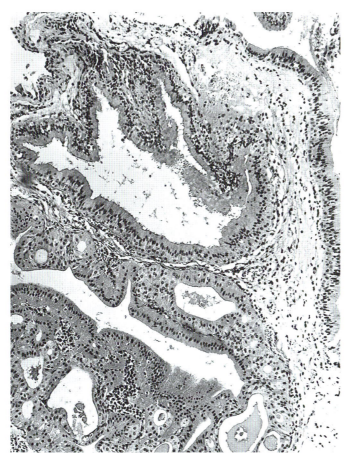

Figure 29.3 Cyst of false cord with oncocytic change. The cyst lining near the *right edge* of the figure and adjacent seromucinous glands consists of oncocytic (pink-staining in the original) epithelium

area of larynx is available for study (as at autopsy), the obstruction of the duct will often be found to be due to squamous metaplasia of the duct epithelium, the new epithelium either causing sufficient thickening to narrow the lumen of the duct or producing keratinised squames, which, by blocking the lumen, achieve the same effect. In the case of oncocytic-lined cysts, the oncocytes, which are swollen columnar cells, may themselves by their presence produce obstruction of a duct leading to cyst formation.

Thyroid Tissue Within the Larynx

It is well known that thyroid gland tissue may be found along the pathway of embryological descent of the thyroid gland from the tongue downwards. Thyroid tissue may also be found within the subglottic larynx and upper trachea. The usual position for such aberrant thyroid gland is between the lower border of the cricoid cartilage and the upper rings of the trachea just beneath the mucosa.[12] In laryngectomy specimens removed from carcinoma,

it is common to find islands of thyroid gland tissue within the fibrous capsule of the larynx and trachea, just outside the cricothyroid membrane. Occasionally thyroid tissue is internal to the cartilage of the larynx and trachea, often extending over a broad area of the subglottis. The thyroid tissue in these cases is usually not recognised grossly, but is a chance finding on routine examination of the larynx specimen. The follicles of the thyroid are small and regular in such cases, with well-formed colloid, and are in proximity to seromucinous glands of the laryngeal mucosa (Fig. 29.4). Whether within the laryngeal connective tissue just outside the larynx, or within the laryngeal mucosa, the thyroid tissue does not usually show continuity with the main thyroid gland.[13]

On rare occasions an actual mass is present in the subglottic larynx or upper trachea, which produces symptoms of respiratory obstruction. This is usually seen in females, and is composed in most cases of benign thyroid tissue, which has increased in size presumably by physiological mechanisms or as part of a goitre in iodine-deficiency areas. The usual situ-

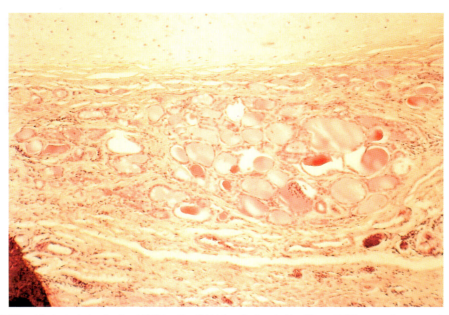

Figure 29.4 Thyroid heterotopia showing thyroid follicle with colloid *internal* to the cricoid cartilage, which lies across the upper part of the figure

ation for such swellings is posterolaterally in the subglottic region.[14] On even rarer occasions a primary malignant tumour may arise within the aberrant laryngotracheal thyroid tissue.[15]

It has been suggested that thyroid gland tissue that forms in the larynx is split off from the main thyroid gland during development by the formation of the thyroid cartilage anlage on each side.[16] It is difficult to understand why, if that were the mechanism, thyroid tissue is always seen in a subglottic and tracheal position within the airway mucosa and not higher. The thyroid gland is normally wrapped around the lower larynx and trachea, and aberrant thyroid is usually seen within the mucosa at the same horizontal levels as the normally situated gland. It seems more likely that ectopic thyroid tissue arises from the already descended gland by growth of thyroid follicles into the adjacent laryngotracheal wall during further development; this tissue subsequently loses connection with the main thyroid gland. This would explain the presence of isolated areas of thyroid tissue both inside and outside the laryngotracheal wall.

Tracheopathia Osteochondroplastica

In tracheopathia osteochondroplastica, multiple ingrowths of cartilage derived from the cartilages of tracheal rings are present. Ossification of these cartilaginous ingrowths frequently takes place. It is usually symptom free and not discovered until bronchoscopy for another condition or autopsy, when the lesion may present as irregular protuberances under the mucosa of the trachea and bronchi. The cricoid cartilage may also be involved.

On histological examination, cartilage or lamellar bone is seen under the epithelium within and beneath the mucosa. Depending on the plane of the section, the aberrant cartilage or bone may be seen as a protrusion of the main cartilage towards the lumen (Fig. 29.5) or an isolated mass of mucosal tissue. The condition would seem to produce no harmful effects. Bone morphogenetic protein-2, a factor in ectopic bone and cartilage formation by the induction of differentiation of mesenchymal cells to osteoprogenitor cells, has been detected in mesenchymal cells and chondroblasts lining the nodules in the tracheal submucosa. Transforming growth factor beta-1 (TGF-beta 1), a factor that stimulates the production of extracellular matrix protein by chondrocytes, appeared in this study in chondrocytes and osteocytes of the nodules. It has been suggested that the two substances act synergistically with each other to promote an inductive cascade resulting in cartilage and bone formation in the tracheal submucosa.[17]

References

1. Cotton RT, Richardson MA. Congenital laryngeal anomalies. In: Symposium on congenital disorders in otolaryngology. Otolaryngol Clin North Am 1981;14:203–218
2. Holinger LD. Histopathology of congenital subglottic stenosis. Ann Otol Rhinol Laryngol 1999;108:101–111
3. Gould SJ, Howard S. The histopathology of the larynx in the neonate following endotracheal intubation. J Pathol 1985;146:301–311

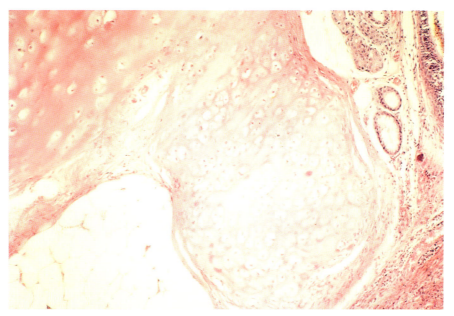

Figure 29.5 Tracheopathia osteochondroplastica. There is an ingrowth of cartilage from the tracheal ring into the tracheal mucosa

4. Montreuil F. Bifid epiglottis; report of a case. Laryngoscope 1949;59:194–199

5. Stell PM, Maran AGD. Laryngocoele. J Laryngol Otol 1975;89:915–924

6. Birt D. Observations on the size of the saccule in laryngectomy specimens. Laryngoscope 1987;97:190–200

7. Michaels L, Hassmann E. Ventriculosaccular carcinoma of the larynx. Clin Otolaryngol 1982;7:165–173

8. MacFie DA. Asymptomatic laryngoceles in wind instrument bandsmen. Arch Otolaryngol 1966;83:270–275

9. Holinger LD, Barnes DR, Smid LJ et al. Laryngocele and saccular cysts. Ann Otol Rhinol Laryngol 1978;87:675–685

10. De Santo LW. Laryngocele, laryngeal mucocele, large saccules and laryngeal saccular cysts; a developmental spectrum. Laryngoscope 1974;84:1291–1296

11. Barnes DR, Holinger LD, Pelletiere EV. Prolapse of the laryngeal ventricle. Otolaryngol Head Neck Surg 1980;88:165–171

12. Willis RA. The borderland of embryology and pathology, 2nd edn. Butterworth, London, 1962

13. Richardson GM, Assor D. Thyroid tissue within the larynx. Case report. Laryngoscope 1971;81:120–125

14. Bone RC, Biller HF, Irwin TM. Intralaryngotracheal thyroid. Ann Otol Rhinol Laryngol 1972;81:424–428

15. Prisel A. Primäres Karzinom einer intratrachealen Struma. Monatschr Ohren [In German] 1921;55:593–599

16. Randolph J, Grunt J, Vawter GF. The medical and surgical aspects of intratracheal goiter. N Engl J Med 1963;268: 457–465

17. Tajima K, Yamakawa M, Katagiri T et al. Immunohistochemical detection of bone morphogenetic protein-2 and transforming growth factor beta-1 in tracheopathia osteochondroplastica. Virchows Arch 1997;431:359–363

30 Infections

The larynx is subject to infections caused by a wide variety of organisms. Table 30.1 lists the bacterial, viral and fungal infections that a review of the literature shows the larynx to have endured from time to time. Those infections that are represented by only a very small number of case reports in the literature have not been listed. In spite of this omission, it will be seen that none of the laryngeal infections on the list is represented in clinical practice with any frequency. The reason for this is partly that infection in general is now less common, with improved hygienic practices and much better methods of treatment. Other important reasons for the paucity of laryngeal infections are that few infecting organisms settle in the larynx, and those that do are efficiently eliminated.

Origin

Upper Respiratory

The most important pathway for the exposure of organisms to the larynx is via the upper respiratory tract airway. The nose acts as a highly efficient filter of all large particles; only those smaller than 1 μm reach and settle in the lungs. Thus the great majority of dust particles or droplet nuclei containing bacteria, viruses or fungi that enter the respiratory tract either remain in the nose or pass directly into the terminal part of the respiratory tree. Those organisms that do drop off at the level of the larynx are probably efficiently dealt with by the local mucous stream and by the standard immunological mechanisms. The slight tendency that the true vocal cords may have to act as a net for microorganisms by virtue of their projection into the air flow is, no doubt, counteracted by the greater resistance to

Table 30.1. Infections of the larynx

Infection	Causative agent	Principal site
Bacterial (and related)		
Epiglottis	*Haemophilus influenzae*	Lung
Tuberculosis	*Mycobacterium tuberculosis*	Lung
Leprosy	*Mycobacterium leprae*	Nose
Other mycobacterial infections	*Mycobacterium avium intracellulare* and *Mycobacterium scrofulaceum*	Buccal mucosa and draining lymph nodes
Diphtheria	*Corynebacterium diphtheriae*	Nose and pharynx
Glanders	*Pfeiferella mallei*	Nose
Typhoid fever	*Salmonella typhi*	Blood-borne
Anthrax	*Bacillus anthracis*	? Pharynx
Scleroma	*Klebsiella rhinoscleromatis*	Nose
Actinomycosis	*Actinomycosis israelii*	Tonsil and neck
Typhus	*Rickettsia prowazekii*	Blood-borne
Fungal		
Histoplasmosis	*Histoplasma capsulatum*	Lung
Coccidioidomycosis	*Coccidioides immitis*	Lung
N. American blastomycosis	*Blastomyces dermatidis*	Lung
Candidosis	*Candida albicans*	Lung or pharynx
Rhinosporidiosis	*Rhinosporidium seeberi*	Nose
Viral		
Variola	Virus	Skin
Herpes simplex	Virus	Skin
Influenza	Virus	Lung
HIV and AIDS	Wide variety of viral, bacterial, fungal and protozoal agents	Cells of immune system leading to immunosuppression
Protozoal		
Leishmaniasis	*Leishmania braziliensis*	Mouth and pharynx
Parasitic		
Trichinosis	*Trichinella spiralis*	Skeletal muscle

infection of the stratified squamous epithelium covering those structures.

In fact, in each of the infections listed in Table 30.1, the larynx suffers disability of secondary importance only. The sites of primary importance for each of these infections are listed in the third column of the table.

In leprosy, diphtheria, glanders, scleroma and rhinosporidiosis, the major site of the infection is usually in the nasal passages. The laryngeal infection in these cases is probably the result of an overspill of organisms from the nose into the larynx.

Pharyngeal

In acute epiglottitis, actinomycosis, the mucocutaneous forms of candidosis, leishmaniasis and perhaps anthrax, the infection attacks the larynx from the adjacent pharynx, the organisms and their attendant inflammatory reaction entering either from above between the thyroid cartilage and quadrangular (elastic) ligament, as in acute epiglottitis, or by penetrating the thyroid cartilage directly, as in some cases of actinomycosis and candidosis.

Pulmonary

In tuberculosis and the fungus infections histoplasmosis, coccidioidomycosis, North American blastomycosis and some cases of systemic candidosis, the major infection is in the lungs. Thus it would seem possible that the laryngeal infection in these cases is the result of organisms being coughed up and infecting the larynx en route to the mouth. However, there is a possibility in at least some of those illnesses that the organisms may be conveyed to the larynx from the lung via the bloodstream (see below).

Bloodstream

It is certain that some infections do reach the larynx only via the bloodstream. This is the case with typhoid fever, typhus and syphilis. Laryngeal infections by these organisms are now so rare as to be of historical importance only.

Virus Infections

Influenza

The position of the larynx with regard to virus infections is perplexing. It is part of clinical lore that the larynx is involved in serious respiratory virus infections such as influenza. Yet the symptom complex described for influenza does not emphasize laryngeal symptoms. Those cases who have severe infection suffer mainly pulmonary changes, laryngeal symptoms in both children and adults being unusual. A careful pathological study of the respiratory tract in fatal cases of influenza by Hers[1] included the examination of histological sections taken from the larynx as well as the tracheobronchial tree and the lungs soon after death. A specific histological finding in the respiratory epithelium of the trachea and bronchi in influenza was "necrobiosis", in which the superficial epithelial cells became swollen and degenerated, and eventually the whole thickness of the epithelium became necrotic. The larynx was not affected by those specific changes in the nine cases in which it was examined, although in those same cases and in eight others, necrobiosis was present lower in the respiratory tract. Lymphocytic infiltration, sometimes heavy and with the formation of lymphoid follicles, was present in many of the larynges, possibly representing a non-specific reaction to the serious inflammation lower down the respiratory tract. A similar change is seen under the posterior epithelial covering of the epiglottis in acute epiglottitis (see below).

Herpes Zoster and Simplex

It is difficult to find any reference to specific pathological changes in other virus diseases possibly affecting the larynx. Laryngeal changes are mentioned as part of the syndrome of the skin virus affection of herpes – both zoster and simplex – in the older German literature.[2] This was before the laboratory identification of viruses, and modern histological studies are not available.

HIV Infection and AIDS – the Immunocompromised Larynx

The larynx is subject to infection when in the immunocompromised state. The latter may occur as a result of the use of glucorticoid inhalants in asthma or in cases of AIDS. Once again serious infections are unusual in either of these situations.

It is difficult to escape the conclusion that, apart from the induction of papillomas of the larynx by human papillomavirus type 6/11 (see Chapter 33), the larynx is singularly free from damaging viral infection.

Acute Inflammation

Acute inflammation may take a variety of forms in the larynx. There are four groups, each with a characteristic aetiological basis and pathological appearance, into which most cases would seem to fit:

1. Acute epiglottitis. This is usually caused by bacteria, in the majority of cases *Haemophilus influenzae*.
2. Acute laryngotracheobronchitis. This inflammatory lesion is probably caused by viruses, and the glottis and subglottic regions are particularly affected.
3. Allergic laryngitis.
4. Diphtheritic laryngitis.

The majority of cases are children in whom, because of the narrowness of the airway, the obstruction is serious and sometimes fatal.

Acute Epiglottitis

Acute epiglottitis was not recognised as a pathological entity until the early 1940s, when the association with *H. influenzae* type B was noted in many cases.

Clinical Features

Vague prodromata of upper respiratory infection are followed by sore throat and pain on swallowing. The voice is relatively unaffected and there is little cough. The condition progresses rapidly with shock, leading to severe respiratory obstruction in from 1 to 24 h. The child's dyspnoea is exacerbated in the supine position. The clinical diagnosis is confirmed by observation of the fiery red, swollen epiglottis above the tongue.

Incidence

Acute epiglottitis was an unusual condition, affecting males more commonly than females, with a peak age incidence of about 3 years, but was being detected more frequently in adults. The situation has now changed with the introduction of *H. influenzae* type B vaccination in a general childhood programme, which has had a dramatic effect in reducing the incidence of acute epiglottitis. In Sweden, for instance, it has achieved not only a greater than 90% reduction in the incidence of the disease in the youngest age group, but also a reduction in the inci-

dence in the older age groups and among adults.[3] A few cases may present as sudden unexpected natural deaths.[4]

Bacteriology

H. influenzae type B is the causative agent of acute epiglottitis in children. There is a high yield of the organism on culture of the blood. In adults a broader spectrum of organisms, especially pyogenic cocci, have been associated with acute epiglottitis.

Pathological Appearances

At autopsy, not only does the epiglottis show signs of acute inflammation, but the adjacent tongue and pharyngeal structures are also swollen. An accentuation of the normal posterior concavity of the epiglottis is seen in some cases. The aryepiglottic folds are swollen, and the laryngeal inlet is greatly narrowed (Figs 30.1 and 30.2).

In an unpublished study of microscopic sections from 15 fatal cases, taken across the whole thickness of the epiglottis, we saw in all cases that an acute inflammatory exudate with neutrophils, red cells and fibrin infiltrated the anterior part of the epiglottis deep to the squamous epithelium (Figs 30.3 and 30.4). The latter was sometimes itself infiltrated by pus cells, and was occasionally ulcerated. The inflammatory exudate extended widely in the pre-epiglottic space, but never penetrated the epiglottic cartilage posteriorly. In all cases there was a lymphocytic exudate in the posterior epiglottic mucosa. This varied from moderate to severe in amount, and in five of the 11 children there were germinal centres in the posterior mucosal exudate (Fig. 30.5).

In some of the cases, sections were taken from the posterior part of the larynx, hypopharynx, supraglottic larynx, including aryepiglottic folds, and vocal cord region. They all showed acute inflammatory exudate similar in intensity to the anterior epiglottic region affecting the vallecula, hypopharynx and aryepiglottic fold region. The exudate was also present in the deep tissues of the larynx, extending downwards deep to the thyrohyoid, thyroarytenoid and interarytenoid muscles, but the false and true cord mucosae did not show this change, exhibiting only a lymphocytic exudate similar in degree to that seen in the posterior epiglottis. Organisms were not seen, even on special staining, in the acute inflammatory exudate.

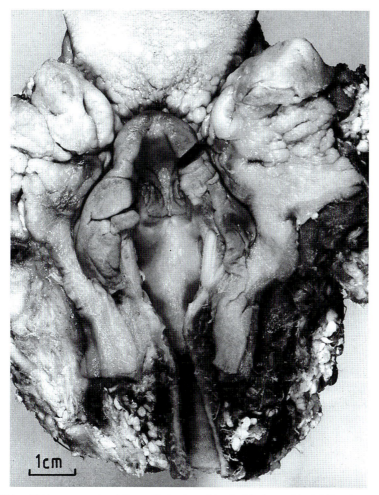

Figure 30.1 Acute epiglottitis in a child (necropsy specimen). Note marked oedema of rim of epiglottis, aryepiglottic folds and posterior pharyngeal wall. A wedge of tissue has been removed from the right side of the epiglottis for histological section

Pathogenesis

It is clear from the above description that acute epiglottitis does not originate as a laryngeal disorder, but as an acute inflammatory condition affecting the oropharynx and hypopharynx. The anterior mucosa of the epiglottis, the pre-epiglottic space and the aryepiglottic folds are involved as part of this inflammatory process, and the inflammation tracks downwards through the deep muscular tissues of the larynx, but does not involve the mucosal surface of the larynx because the latter is on the airway side of the quadrangular membrane (Figs 30.3 and 30.6). Therefore, obstruction of the laryngeal airway takes place by pressure from outside. The clinical features of acute epiglottitis are in keeping with this distribution of the inflammatory process. Pain in the throat and difficulty in swallowing are important symptoms; hoarseness is not. Difficulty in breathing is a late symptom of acute epiglottitis, related to airway obstruction.

Haemophilus influenzae is a common organism in the normal upper respiratory tract flora. The B antigen seems to convey especial pathogenicity. It is likely that this organism gains entry to the submucous tissues through the pharyngeal epithelium, perhaps through a crypt of the lingual tonsil, and, on finding a suitable soil in a particular case, induces a severe pharyngitis, which eventually occludes the laryngeal inlet tissues in the way described. The reason why the condition has been given the designation acute epiglottitis, rather than pharyngitis, is that the epiglottic component is the most conspicuous one clinically and at autopsy. The

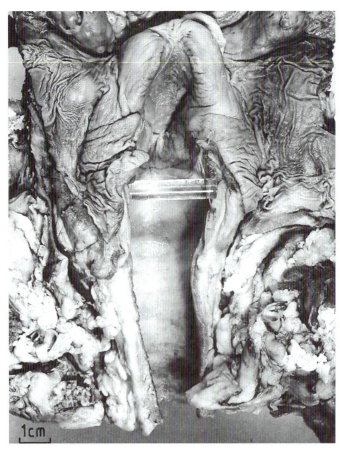

Figure 30.2 Acute epiglottitis in an adult (necropsy specimen). The aryepiglottic folds are markedly oedematous, as is the rim of the epiglottis

actual airway obstruction is related to the deep extension of the acute inflammation in the larynx and not to the swelling of the epiglottis itself.

In Adults

Although primarily a disease of children, acute epiglottitis affects adults more frequently than has been generally realised. *Haemophilus influenzae* type B has also been incriminated in many adult infections, but pyogenic cocci play a greater role than in childhood acute epiglottitis.

Epiglottic Abscess

A complication of acute epiglottitis may be seen in adults in which an actual abscess develops in the epiglottis. The abscess most frequently comes to a point on or near the lingual surface of the epiglottis. From the above description of the pathology of acute epiglottitis, it would seem that epiglottic abscess is just a late manifestation of the acute condition.

Acute Laryngotracheobronchitis

The synonyms for acute laryngotracheobronchitis – subglottic laryngitis, non-diphtheritic croup, virus croup and fibrinous laryngotracheobronchitis – indicate the likely aetiologic and pathologic bases as well as the characteristic anatomical location of this inflammatory disease.

Incidence

Acute laryngotracheobronchitis affects a rather younger age group than acute epiglottitis. The majority of cases are less than 3 years of age, and some cases occur in the first year of life. A preponderance of the cases are male children.

Clinical Features

The onset of the condition is more gradual than that of acute epiglottitis. When fully developed, there is a croupy cough with inspiratory and expiratory

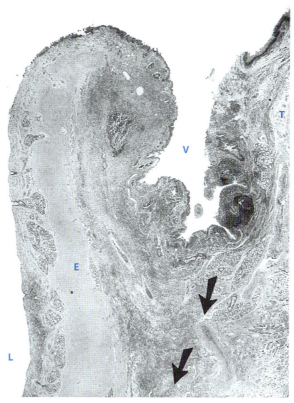

Figure 30.3 Sagittal section through the epiglottis, vallecula and posterior surface of tongue in a case of acute epiglottitis. Note severe accumulation of inflammatory exudate (neutrophilic – see Fig. 30.4) in mucosa of anterior epiglottis, under vallecula and in deeper tissue behind epiglottic cartilage. Posterior epiglottic mucosa is only mildly inflamed (lymphocytic – see Fig. 30.5). *Arrows* indicate direction of spread of inflammation from vallecula into larynx. *E*, epiglottic cartilage; *L*, laryngeal cavity; *T*, back of tongue; *V*, vallecula

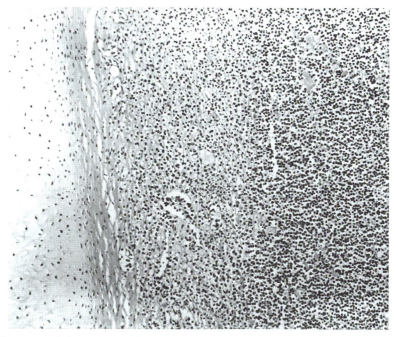

Figure 30.4 Deep part of squamous epithelium and mucosa of anterior surface of epiglottis in a case of acute epiglottitis. There is a dense accumulation of neutrophils beneath the epithelium

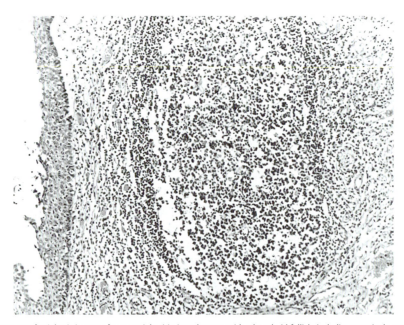

Figure 30.5 Posterior mucosa of epiglottis in case of acute epiglottitis. Lymphocytes with a lymphoid follicle including germinal centre are present under the epithelium

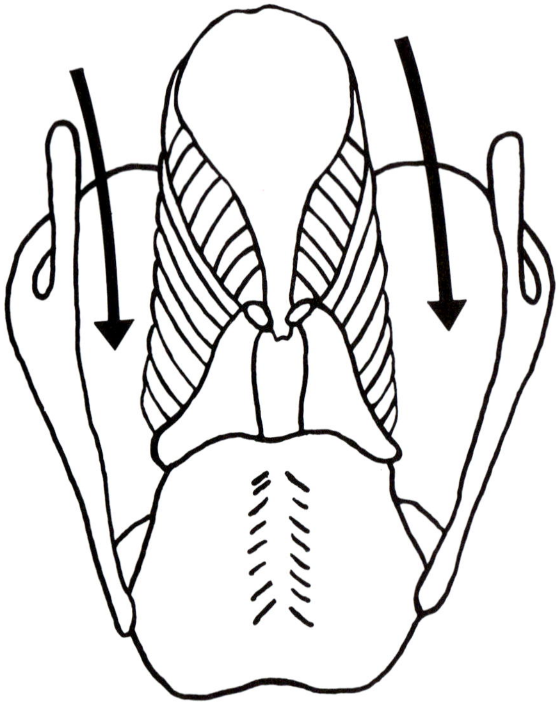

Figure 30.6 Pathway of spread of inflammation into larynx in acute epiglottitis. The inflammatory exudate tracks from the pharynx downwards in the direction of the *arrows* outside the quadrangular membrane, which is shown by parallel lines (Adapted from Paff[5])

stridor, features that are not characteristic of the latter (see above).

Microbiology

Acute laryngotracheobronchitis in children has been ascribed to a variety of viruses, including influenza A2, influenza B, parainfluenza 2 and respiratory syncytial viruses, the evidence being based on serological methods, but there have been few cases available in recent years for pathological study. It is likely that there is a superadded bacterial infection in some cases.

Pathological Appearances

The mortality from acute laryngotracheobronchitis has been very low for many years. Thus, to obtain a description of the pathological appearances, it is necessary to refer to accounts given before the antibiotic era. According to the study of Brennemann et al.,[6] they are characterised by neutrophil exudate in the subglottis, accompanied by mucus and fibrin, with degeneration of epithelial cells. A gummy, rope-like exudate and crusting of necrotic epithelium are observed grossly. These changes take place mainly at the subglottic level in the larynx. There is a sparing of the seromucinous glands until late in the disease (unlike diphtheritic laryngitis, in which a specific necrosis of glands takes place with sparing of the surrounding tissue). The process extends downwards as tracheitis, bronchitis and bronchiolitis associated with similar rope-like secretions and dried crusts. Interstitial pneumonia, atelectasis and pulmonary oedema may also be present following the changes in the tracheobronchial tree.

In contrast to this earlier study, Szpunar et al.[7] found "round cell infiltration" of the inflamed tracheobronchial tree, suggestive of a viral aetiology.

Allergic Laryngitis

Although clinical features of laryngeal involvement are common in hypersensitivity reactions, there has been little opportunity for study of the pathological basis of allergic conditions.

A large number of possible inhaled allergens have been cited as relevant to allergic laryngitis, including house dust, moulds, feathers, animal danders and volatile oils or emanations from plants. Food antigens have also been incriminated.

The pathological feature of allergic laryngitis takes the form of varying degrees of oedema involving the epiglottis, aryepiglottic fold and vocal cords, the most severe being "glottic oedema" related to anaphylactic reaction. In this condition the location of the oedema would seem to be similar to that of the acute inflammatory process of acute epiglottitis, i.e. the anterior surface of the epiglottis, aryepiglottic fold, base of tongue and hypopharynx, and it seems possible that the respiratory obstruction is produced in a similar way by allergic oedema rather than by acute inflammatory exudate. Miller[8] showed that the submucous areolar tissue extends from the base of the tongue continuously to the tip of the epiglottis, and the existence of a layer of such tissue could account for the spread of fluid in both allergic laryngitis and acute epiglottitis.

Angioneurotic Oedema (Angioedema)

In angioneurotic oedema, episodes of oedema take place in the larynx, principally in the epiglottis and supraglottis (for the anatomical reasons described above), and by prejudicing the airway, may endanger life. Two important forms may be recognised:

1. Angioneurotic oedema associated with urticaria. This is the already mentioned acute form of allergic laryngitis.
2. Hereditary angioneurotic oedema. In this form there is no urticaria, but attacks of colic as well as laryngeal oedema are common. The condition is inherited as an autosomal dominant so

that there is usually a strong family history. There is a deficiency of inhibitor of the serum complement factor C1 due to a mutation in the C1 inhibitor gene. Complement factors C1, C4 and C2 are used up and their serum levels are very low. CT inhibitor is also lacking in many of the relations of the patients. The condition is treated by administration of an androgenic drug such as the synthetic androgen danazol, which, surprisingly, raises the level of C1 inhibitor and prevents attacks of angioneurotic oedema.

Diphtheritic Laryngitis

Diphtheria is an acute mucosal inflammation of the fauces, soft palate and tonsils, produced by *Corynebacterium diphtheriae* (see Chapter 26). The mucosal inflammation of diphtheria may spread to, or may be confined to, the larynx. In these cases the epiglottis, false cords and true cords are covered by a false membrane, a dull greyish yellow thickened layer, which may extend down into the trachea.

Microscopically the false membrane is composed of fibrin and neutrophils with, in the early stages, large numbers of diphtheria bacilli. On the deeper aspects, the laryngeal epithelium is included with the membrane. Where this epithelium is respiratory columnar in type, the membrane peels easily off the basement membrane (it may indeed be coughed up), but in the squamous-epithelium-lined vocal cords the false membrane separates off with difficulty and airway obstruction may result. The submucosal seromucinous glands underlying the diphtheritic membrane often show necrosis; in other forms of acute laryngitis this is said not to happen.[6]

Chronic Bacterial Infections and Related Conditions

Tuberculosis

Tuberculosis of the larynx is a disease that is almost always associated with tuberculosis of the lungs.

Incidence

In common with pulmonary tuberculosis, laryngeal tuberculosis has become unusual in developed countries. In the early years of the 20th century, the great majority of tuberculous patients at post-mortem had tuberculous lesions of the larynx. By 1946, the autopsy incidence of laryngeal involvement in cases of pulmonary tuberculosis was down to 37.5%.[9] In the last quarter of the 20th century, both pulmonary and laryngeal tuberculosis became uncommon. In recent years, however, both seem to be on the increase again, but many cases of laryngeal tuberculosis now present without or with minimal pulmonary involvement.

The age incidence of laryngeal tuberculosis was mainly under 40 years in the pre-chemotherapy era. Now most of the patients are older.

Clinical Features

In the earlier era, the laryngeal tuberculosis was clinically overshadowed by the pulmonary tuberculosis that invariably accompanied it. In present-day practice, however, patients have little constitutional disturbance. Hoarseness and painful dysphagia are usually complained of. The laryngoscopic appearances are those of a localised lesion, usually mimicking laryngeal carcinoma, with no tendency to be sited in the posterior part of the larynx. The disease now responds well to chemotherapy.

Pathological Appearances

There is little opportunity nowadays for a gross examination to be made of advanced tuberculosis of the larynx. The older descriptions speak of nodule formation going on to ulceration of true vocal cords, false cords and epiglottis. Involvement of cartilage with extensive excavation of large areas was common. By contrast, recent experience indicates that most cases have a small area of involvement only affecting most often the true vocal cords, sometimes the false cords. The lesions are often nodular, sometimes ulcerated.

Microscopic examination may show the fully developed appearance of tuberculosis. The epithelium may be intact or ulcerated. Pseudo-epitheliomatous hyperplasia is common. Variable areas of mucosa are occupied by inflammatory tissue consisting of epithelioid cells, lymphocytes and Langhans' giant cells. Caseous necrosis is present to a variable degree. If the epithelium is ulcerated, acute inflammatory changes may be present (Fig. 30.7). Special stains may reveal acid-fast bacilli in some cases, but very often these are not seen.

The clinical diagnosis of tuberculous laryngitis is usually made as a result of the pathologist's suspicions from his examinations of the endoscopic biopsy material. Since the histological appearances may be indefinite, the pathologist should adopt a

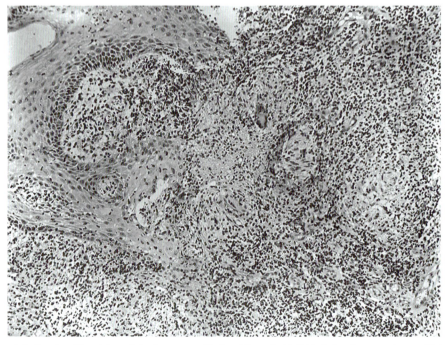

Figure 30.7 Tuberculosis of vocal cord. There is hyperplasia of squamous epithelium. A focus of epithelioid cells, lymphocytes and neutrophils is present with some caseation. There is a single Langhans-type giant cell adjacent to the caseous area

high index of suspicion with regard to tuberculosis, especially in the presence of giant cells of any type, granulomatous lesions or unusual necrotic changes.

Pathogenesis

In the older, more severe form of the disease, the spread of the tuberculous process from the lungs to the larynx was clearly the result of transmission of organisms along the tracheobronchial tree. In recent cases the evidence is often more in favour of blood-borne dissemination.[10]

Sarcoidosis

Definition

Sarcoidosis is seen in the upper respiratory tract, mainly in the nose (see Chapter 13). It is characterised histologically by the presence of epithelioid cell tubercles without caseation, which are converted into hyaline fibrous tissue.

Clinical Features

The symptoms are those of airway obstruction rather than disorders of phonation, because the supraglottic region rather than the vocal cords is usually affected.

Gross Appearances

In the reported cases, the disease process commences and develops near the mucosal surface of the posterior aspect and edges of the epiglottis, the aryepiglottic folds, the false cords and the arytenoid region. These tissues are symmetrically affected with a pale, diffusely swollen appearance.[11]

Microscopic Appearances

Microscopically the characteristic change is one of rather uniform tubercles composed of groups of epithelioid cells with no caseation (although a limited degree of central necrosis is often present). Foreign body or Langhans-type giant cells are usually present and may contain a variety of crystalline, calcified or other inclusions (see Chapter 13). Fibrosis of the tubercle takes place around the periphery and grows to involve the whole of it. Later

stages may be seen as a group of uniform round, hyaline fibrous masses.

Involvement of the Recurrent Laryngeal Nerve

Sarcoid deposits are known to involve nervous tissue of the central and peripheral nervous systems. The recurrent laryngeal nerves on one or other side may be involved by sarcoid leading to vocal cord palsy. It is possible that sarcoid tissue in cervical or mediastinal lymph nodes may spread in such cases to involve those nerves.[12]

Leprosy

Leprosy is an infective disease of the skin, mucosa of upper respiratory tract and peripheral nervous system, caused by *Mycobacterium leprae*. A spectrum of the disease exists between lepromatous leprosy, in which numerous mycobacteria are present, and tuberculoid leprosy, with few organisms. The difference between these forms is based on the immunological relationship of the host to the organism, the lepromatous form representing a state of low cell-mediated immunity and the tuberculoid a high one (see Chapter 13).

Leprosy frequently attacks the larynx as well as the nose. Laryngeal involvement is seen only in the lepromatous, not the tuberculoid, form of the disease. Thirty-six per cent of lepromatous leprosy patients in a study in India have been found to have laryngeal involvement.[13] In most of the cases there are lepromata of the epiglottis – nodules of inflammation terminating in destruction of tissue and scarring to produce a shrunken and incurved epiglottis – but not usually ulceration. The nodules also involved the aryepiglottic fold and arytenoids, and in a few cases the vocal cords. The deep infiltration by the lepromatous tissue may involve intrinsic laryngeal muscles and thereby diminish the mobility of the vocal cords (Fig. 30.8).[14]

Microscopic Appearances

The laryngeal lepromatous lesion consists in its active stage of a mucosal thickening containing macrophages, many of which appear as large foam cells (Virchow cells). The latter contain the acid-fast bacilli of *M. leprae* in large numbers (Figs 30.9, 30.10). The organisms also appear in round, basophilic structures known as globi, which represent degenerated macrophages.

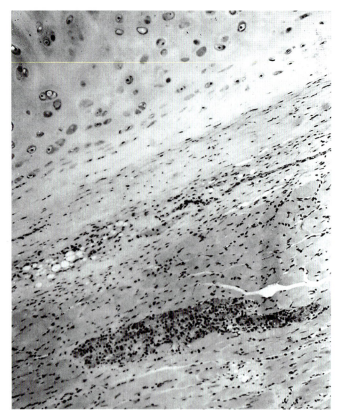

Figure 30.8 Lepromatous leprosy involving the thyroarytenoid muscle. The focus consists of foamy macrophages and lymphocytes. The thyroid cartilage is seen in the *upper part* of the photograph (Courtesy of Dr. S. Lucas)

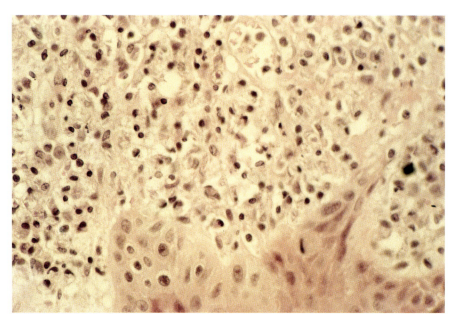

Figure 30.9 Lepromatous leprosy involving the supraglottic mucosa. Near the epithelium (below) there is an inflammatory exudate composed of foamy macrophages and lymphocytes

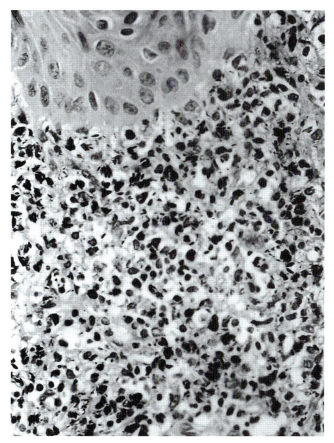

Figure 30.10 Lepromatous leprosy of supraglottic mucosa showing large numbers of short rod-shaped and beaded bacilli amid the foamy macrophages (Courtesy of Dr. S. Lucas) Wade-Fite stain

Scleroma

Definition

Scleroma (often termed "rhinoscleroma") is a chronic inflammatory condition usually affecting the mucosa of the nose, in which large, deforming masses of tissue distend the nasal cavity. For a detailed description see Chapter 13.

Laryngeal Involvement

Laryngeal lesions are common in scleroma, being present in as many as 40% of patients with the nasal lesions,[15] but are a relatively minor aspect of the condition. The lesions are usually found in the subglottic region.[16]

Syphilis

Syphilis is a venereally acquired infective condition caused by the spirochaete *Treponema pallidum*. Mackenzie found 308 cases of laryngeal syphilis in 10 000 consecutive cases of throat disease examined at the Throat Hospital, London.[17] One hundred and twenty years later in that hospital, now expanded to the Royal National Throat, Nose and Ear Hospital, London, cases of laryngeal syphilis are extremely rare. Mackenzie did not have the Wassermann reaction to help him with the diagnosis; it was not introduced until 1906. He made the diagnosis on the history of the patient, on the laryngoscopic appearances and on the course of the disease. The introduction of penicillin to treat syphilis has eliminated laryngeal syphilis in advanced countries. The following is a summary of the pathological lesions of laryngeal syphilis as they once were seen.

Primary Syphilis

Primary syphilis was excessively rare, even in the heyday of syphilis, since it is derived by primary contact with a diseased part.

Secondary Syphilis

Secondary syphilis was often manifested as congestion of the laryngeal mucosa. Mucous patches were seen in the epiglottis. Condyloma lata – polypoid lesions of epithelial hyperplasia – were common. They presented as smooth yellow projections up to 1 cm in diameter, situated on the epiglottis and interarytenoid region, and occasionally on the vocal cords. Microscopically the squamous epithelial proliferation was sometimes confused with carcinoma. There is a dense infiltrate of plasma cells and lymphocytes, often around blood vessels. These lesions contain large numbers of spirochaetes.

Tertiary Syphilis

Tertiary syphilis was usually manifested in the larynx by gummata, granulomatous foci that commenced as nodules, but which broke down eventually to form ulcers. These ulcers were scattered throughout the larynx, but were commonest on the epiglottis. They were often very deep, even penetrating the laryngeal cartilage. The ulcers eventually healed to produce scars, which underwent severe contraction, greatly distorting the structure of the larynx and sometimes producing severe stenosis. The distortion resulting from healed gummatous syphilis was occasionally so severe that it was "almost impossible to identify the various parts" of the larynx.[17] Microscopically the centre of the gumma shows coagulation necrosis. This is surrounded by an inflammatory exudate composed of plasma cells, lymphocytes, epithelioid cells and fibroblasts with variable numbers of giant cells. There is usually marked obliterative endarteritis.

Neurological Syphilis

The larynx was often involved secondarily by affection of the nervous system with syphilis. The vagus nerve was involved, leading to vocal cord paralysis. In tabes dorsalis there were sudden severe sensory disturbances and these were sometimes manifested by spasm of the vocal cords.

Syphilis is increasing in incidence and it is possible that laryngologists and pathologists will be renewing acquaintance with the laryngological aspects of tertiary syphilis.

Mycotic Infections

Mycotic infections of the larynx are unusual, and are all examples of deep mycoses. In contrast to superficial mycoses, in which the infecting fungi are present only in the epidermis and its surface appendages (hair and nails) or in the more "external" mucosae (mouth, vulva, vagina), the deep, or "systemic", mycoses relate to fungus infections of the dermis and deeper parts of the body. Many mycoses of the larynx are associated with bronchopulmonary infection by the same fungus, in the same way as tuberculosis of the larynx is related to pulmonary tuberculosis. A "primary complex" of the mycotic infection is set up by the formation of a lung lesion accompanied by metastatic infection by the fungus to the hilar lymph nodes. Transmission of the organism to the larynx takes place through the air passages or bloodstream. In some cases, as in candidosis, the lesion often spreads to the larynx via the upper air and food passages. In a very few cases of laryngeal mycosis, the lesion is primary and is found in no other organ.

Histoplasmosis

Histoplasmosis is caused by *Histoplasma capsulatum*. The fungus infection is endemic in many parts of the world and is particularly common in the Ohio River Valley of the USA. The disease, which is usually benign and self-limiting, takes the form in most cases of a primary pulmonary infection with secondary hilar lymph node spread. The histological appearance is that of chronic inflammatory infiltrate, often in the form of a tuberculoid granuloma. The organism is seen within histiocytic cells of the granulomas as budding yeast-like structures 1–3 μm in diameter. A mycelial phase of the organism is seen in culture on Sabouraud's medium, but never in the tissue lesion.

The disease is often confined to the larynx and the lesions resemble papillomas,[18] but in three patients reported by Calcaterra[19] the laryngeal lesions appeared to be part of a wider-spread condition affecting also the mouth and throat. Histological changes are mostly those of epithelioid granulomas showing variable numbers of the organisms (Figs 30.11, 30.12). There is often pseudo-epitheliomatous hyperplasia of squamous epithelium.

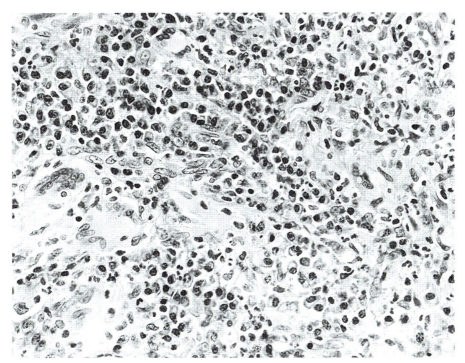

Figure 30.11 Histoplasmosis of the larynx. There is a granulomatous reaction with giant cells, macrophages and plasma cells. A few organisms are present, but are difficult to locate in this preparation (Courtesy of Dr. V. J. Hyams)

Coccidioidomycosis

This infection, caused by the fungus *Coccidioides immitis*, is endemic in the San Joaquin Valley of California. The usual form of the disease is a primary complex in the lung, but spread, particularly to the brain, may occur.

Lesions caused by this fungus have been described in the larynx. They are usually part of a generalised infection. Histologically the organisms are seen as thick-walled spherules, 30–60 μm in diameter, containing endospores. These give rise to a granulomatous reaction.

North American Blastomycosis

North American blastomycosis, which is produced by the fungus *Blastomyces dermatidis*, is usually associated with a suppurative pneumonia, which may lead to pyaemia with abscesses in prostate, brain, bone, skin and elsewhere. Cutaneous lesions may develop by blood-borne infection from the lungs.

Pathological Appearances

The disease has been seen in the larynx sufficiently often to permit its description as a sequence of gross

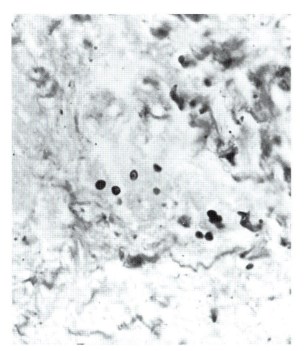

Figure 30.12 Yeast-like organisms of *Histoplasmosis capsulatum* from same tissue block as that of Fig. 30.11. Note budding. Gomori's methanamine silver stain

changes.[20] At first there is marked reddening and a granular appearance of the vocal cords and surrounding structures. This is followed by the appearance of minute pinhead-size greyish papules, with occasional yellowish nodules. Ulceration then takes place and a greyish membrane covers the ulcer, which, when removed, leaves a red patch. Healing by fibrosis slowly develops and results in scarring of the vocal cords. Abscesses may extend from the larynx into the neck.

Microscopically there is often hyperplasia of squamous epithelium of the vocal cords or metaplastic laryngeal epithelium. Abscesses may be present within the thickened epithelium. The inflammatory exudate is composed of neutrophils, plasma cells, lymphocytes and giant cells, often with areas of necrosis. The organisms are seen as double-contoured yeast-like bodies, 8–15 microns in diameter, within the inflammatory exudate, staining (like most fungi) strongly with periodic acid-Schiff and methenamine silver stains.

South American Blastomycosis (Paracoccidioidomycosis)

This fungus disease, caused by *Blastomyces brasiliensis*, is found mainly in Central and South America. The lesions are usually in the lungs as a primary complex, or in the buccal mucous membrane, where they may develop particularly after removal of a tooth.

Secondary laryngeal involvement is said to take place often.

Actinomycosis

Actinomycosis is caused by *Actinomyces israeli*, which is not a true fungus, but is (by general agreement among microbiologists) classed with the higher bacteria. There are clinical similarities between actinomycosis and fungal infection, so it is usually considered with the latter. The organism is found normally in the tonsillar crypts (see Chapter 26) and gum margins. Infection usually takes the form of a suppurating mass in the neck or jaw as a result of the *Actinomyces* entering the tissues, possibly through an abrasion. Spread to the skin surface and to the deep mucosal aspects of the lesion with the formation of sinuses is common.

Involvement of the larynx by actinomycosis is rare and it is usually secondary to cervical or pharyngeal actinomycosis.[21] The true vocal cord is involved. The cellular reaction in actinomycosis is an acute one with large numbers of neutrophils and some histiocytes (Fig. 30.13). The organisms can sometimes be identified grossly within the inflammatory exudate as minute yellow "sulphur granules".

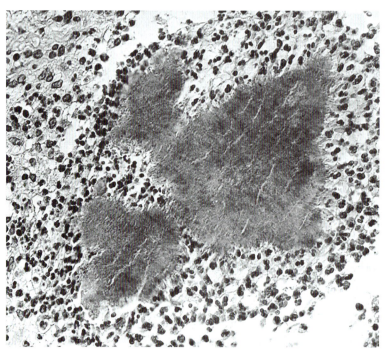

Figure 30.13 Colony of *Actinomyces* surrounded by neutrophil reaction. From a case of laryngeal actinomycosis described by Bennett[20] (Courtesy of Dr. G.A.K. Missen)

Microscopically *Actinomyces* are identified as long, slender, Gram-positive, branching filaments. There are generally also Gram-negative peripheral club-like processes. Culture of this organism requires anaerobic or microaerophilic conditions.

Candidosis (Candidiasis, Moniliasis)

Candida albicans, the causative agent of candidosis, is a saprophytic organism, which inhabits the throat under normal conditions. Candidosis may arise in the presence of host resistance lowered by disease, corticosteroid therapy, immunosuppression, drugs or radiation (see Chapter 36) or in the presence of altered normal flora by prolonged therapy with broad-spectrum antibiotics. It also occurs in the presence of debilitating general diseases such as diabetes mellitus. In most cases of laryngeal candidosis there is marked pulmonary involvement, while laryngeal involvement is secondary. In a few cases the *Candida* infection is primary in the larynx. The disease may spread directly to the laryngeal mucosa or cartilages from a hypopharyngeal, mouth and skin infection (mucocutaneous candidosis).

The lesions are found in the laryngeal mucosa or more deeply, depending on the site of entry of the organism. If in the laryngeal mucosa, there is frequently a marked hyperplastic reaction of squamous epithelium that may be confused grossly or microscopically with squamous cell carcinoma.

A variable inflammatory reaction of lymphocytes and plasma cells is present, and the organism is easily recognised by the presence of yeast forms together with pseudohyphae and hyphae.

Aspergillosis

Although *Aspergillus* spp. are commonly found in lesions of both the lower and the upper respiratory tract (maxillary sinuses) as well as the external ear (see Chapters 2 and 13), such lesions are rare in the larynx except in immunocompromised patients. In the few cases recorded the lesions had a proclivity for the vocal cord. There may be hyperplasia of the stratified squamous epithelium and an acute inflammatory reaction to the fungus.[22]

Rhinosporidiosis

In rhinosporidiosis there are intranasal or conjunctival polyps of chronic inflammatory tissue containing large and small cysts, some filled with endospores, which represent the causative organism, *Rhinosporidium seeberi* (see Chapter 13). A few cases have been noted with lesions of the epiglottis or vocal cords, as well as nose and conjunctiva.[23]

The Immunocompromised Larynx

The larynx is subject to infection when in the immunocompromised state. The latter may occur as a result of the use of glucorticoid inhalants in asthma or in cases of AIDS.

Occasional infections – viral, bacterial, protozoal – may be related to steroid inhalants that the patient was taking for bronchial asthma. We have seen cases of herpes simplex of the vocal cord (Fig. 30.14), *Mycobacterium avium intracellulare* (Fig. 30.15) and leishmanial infections of the larynx in such patients.

The main effect of AIDS on the larynx is one of wasting – a remarkable appearance in which the organ is reduced to its basic cartilaginous skeleton of cartilage and fibroelastic bands, covered by mucosa on its luminal surface. We have observed this appearance in the majority of cases of AIDS at autopsy. This is, of course, part of the HIV wasting syndrome, a condition not related to infection at all but probably the result of the poor nutrition in AIDS sufferers due to gastrointestinal disease.[24]

Infections caused by the viruses, bacteria including mycobacteria, fungi and protozoa in the list in Table 30.1 do occur in the larynx in AIDS, but are unusual. The larynx is occasionally the seat of an infection in patients immunocompromised by AIDS. The infecting organisms in reported cases are rather different from those seen in non-immunocompromised patients. Cases of epiglottitis are described but none have been associated with *H. influenzae*, staphylococci or streptococci being the causative bacteria.[25] Laryngeal tuberculosis without a pulmonary source has been reported in an occasional patient with HIV infection.[26] Primary laryngeal cryptococcosis is very rare in the non-immunocompromised patient, but several cases are described in patients with AIDS.[27] Primary infection of the larynx with *Aspergillus* spp. is rare even in AIDS. It is more commonly seen as part of a wider infection involving the respiratory system in AIDS. Cytomegalovirus is the most important viral opportunist in patients with AIDS and is commonly seen on microscopic examination of the larynx at autopsy of such patients. In the non-immunocompromised patient it is very rarely seen in this situation.[28] Visceral leishmaniasis is increasingly being associated with HIV infection so that, although rare, an occasional report of this protozoal infection in the larynx of a case with AIDS should not be surprising.[29] Thus infections of the larynx in AIDS,

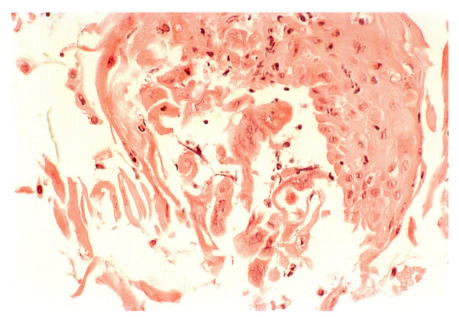

Figure 30.14 Herpes simplex infection of vocal cord in child of 2 years who was treated with prolonged steroid inhalant for severe bronchial asthma. Note necrosis of stratified squamous epithelium with some cells showing multiple nuclei, clear nuclei and nuclear moulding

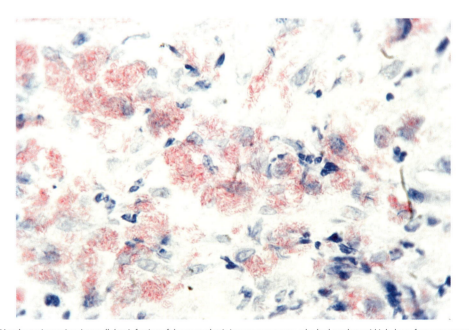

Figure 30.15 *Mycobacterium avium intracellulare* infection of the supraglottis in a young woman who had used steroid inhalants for many years. There are vast numbers of red-staining rod-shaped organisms in the cytoplasm of macrophages. Acid-fast stain

with the exception of the frequent incidence of sub-clinical cytomegalovirus infection, are unusual.

Parasitic Diseases

Leishmaniasis

Leishmaniasis is an infection caused by a protozoon of the genus *Leishmania*. Three distinct clinico-pathological entities exist:

1. Tropical sore.
2. Mucocutaneous leishmaniasis.
3. Disseminated anergic cutaneous leishmaniasis.

The larynx may be affected in the mucocutaneous form.

Histological examination of upper respiratory tissue shows hyperplasia of squamous epithelium in reaction to a granulomatous process in the affected tissue in which the organisms are found. The para-sites are ovoid or round structures 1.5–3.0 μm in diameter. They have a large nucleus and a rod-shaped kinetoplast. The organism is transmitted by blood-sucking flies.

Detailed case reports in which there was laryngeal leishmaniasis are rare.

Trichinosis

Trichinosis is a parasitic infestation caused by the roundworm *Trichinella spiralis*. The adult worms reach and inhabit the intestine as a result of inges-tion of insufficiently cooked pork infested with *Trichinella* larvae. Larvae enter the blood through the intestinal wall and settle particularly in skeletal muscles (including the intrinsic laryngeal muscles) throughout the body. The clinical features of trichinosis are systemic as well as those related to infestation of particular muscles, the brain or myocardium. The presence of *Trichinella* larvae in laryngeal muscles does not give rise to local symptoms.

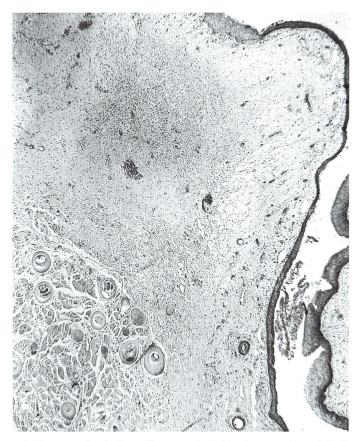

Figure 30.16 Trichinosis of larynx showing true vocal cord with vocal ligament and underlying thyroarytenoid muscle. The last-mentioned contains numerous larvae of *Trichinella spiralis* (Courtesy of Dr. V.J. Hyams)

Microscopic Appearances

The larvae of *Trichinella* are usually found by chance on histological examination of laryngeal muscle sampled after endoscopic biopsy, laryngectomy for carcinoma, or at autopsy. The larvae are most commonly seen in the thyroarytenoid muscle, probably because this is the muscle most commonly examined histologically with the vocal cord. Many muscle fibres contain encysted larvae, which are coiled up within the substance of the fibre. The sarcoplasm adjacent to the larva undergoes a basophilic granular change (Fig. 30.16). Adjacent fibres show hyaline degeneration, and the muscle tissue is infiltrated with eosinophils, neutrophils, lymphocytes and histiocytes.

References

1. Hers JFP. The histopathology of the respiratory tract in human influenza. HE Stenfert Kroese, Leiden, 1955
2. Hajek M. Pathologie und Therapie der Erkrankungen des Kehlkopfes, der Luftröhre und der Bronchien. Curt Kabitzsch, Leipzig, 1932
3. Garpenholt O, Hugosson S, Fredlund H et al. Epiglottitis in Sweden before and after introduction of vaccination against *Haemophilus influenzae* type b. Pediatr Infect Dis J 1999;18: 490–493
4. Siboni A, Simonsen J. Sudden unexpected natural death in young persons. Forensic Sci Int 1986;31:159–166
5. Paff SGE. Anatomy of the head and neck. Saunders, Philadelphia, 1973
6. Brennemann J, Clifton WM, Frank A et al. Acute laryngotracheobronchitis. Am J Dis Child 1938;55:667–695
7. Szpunar J, Glowacki J, Laskowski A et al. Fibrinous laryngotracheobronchitis in children. Arch Otolaryngol 1971;93: 173–178
8. Miller VM. Edema of the larynx. A study of the loose areolar tissues of the larynx. Arch Otolaryngol 1940; 31:256–274
9. Auerbach O. Laryngeal tuberculosis. Arch Otolaryngol 1946;44:191–201
10. Hunter AM, Millar JW, Wightman AJ et al. The changing pattern of laryngeal tuberculosis. J Laryngol Otol 1981;95: 393–398
11. Benjamin B, Dalton C, Croxson G. Laryngoscopic diagnosis of laryngeal sarcoid. Ann Otol Rhinol Laryngol 1995;104: 529–531
12. Colover J. Sarcoidosis with involvement of nervous system. Brain 1948;71:451–475
13. Soni NK. Leprosy of the larynx. J Laryngol Otol 1992;106: 518–520
14. Munor MacCormick CE. The larynx in leprosy. Arch Otolaryngol 1957;66:138–149
15. Fajardo-Dolci G, Chavolla R, Lamadrid-Bautista E et al. Laryngeal scleroma. J Otolaryngol 1999;28:229–231
16. Soni NK. Scleroma of the larynx. J Laryngol Otol 1997;111: 438–440
17. Mackenzie M. A manual of diseases of the throat and nose, vol 1. Diseases of the pharynx, larynx and trachea. Churchill, London, 1880
18. Sataloff RT, Wilborn A, Prestipino A et al. Histoplasmosis of the larynx. Am J Otolaryngol 1993;14:199–205
19. Calcaterra TC. Otolaryngeal histoplasmosis. Laryngoscope 1970;80: 111–120
20. Bennett M. Laryngeal blastomycosis. Laryngoscope 1964;74:498–512
21. Shaheen SO, Ellis FG. Actinomycosis of the larynx. J R Soc Med 1983;76:226–228
22. Nakahira M, Saito H, Miyagi T. Left vocal cord paralysis as a primary manifestation of invasive pulmonary aspergillosis in a nonimmunocompromised host. Arch Otolaryngol Head Neck Surg 1999;125:691–693
23. Pillai OS. Rhinosporidiosis of the larynx. J Laryngol Otol 1974;88:277–280
24. Macallan DC. Wasting in HIV infection and AIDS. J Nutr 1999;129(1S Suppl):238S-242S
25. Rothstein SG, Persky MS, Edelman BA et al. Epiglottitis in AIDS patients. Laryngoscope 1989;99:389–392
26. Singh B, Balwally AN, Har-El G et al. Isolated cervical tuberculosis in patients with HIV infection. Otolaryngol Head Neck Surg 1998;118:766–770
27. Browning DG, Schwartz DA, Jurado RL. Cryptococcosis of the larynx in a patient with AIDS: an unusual cause of fungal laryngitis. South Med J 1992;85:762–764
28. Marelli RA, Biddinger PW, Gluckman JL. Cytomegalovirus infection of the larynx in the acquired immunodeficiency syndrome. Otolaryngol Head Neck Surg 1992;106:296–301
29. Canovas DL, Carbonell J, Torres J et al. Laryngeal leishmaniasis as initial opportunistic disease in HIV infection. J Laryngol Otol 1994;108:1089–1092

31 Non-infective Inflammatory Conditions

The Vocal Cord Polyp and Other Exudative Processes of Reinke's Space

Reinke's space is a potential space of the true vocal cord bounded above and below by the junctions of squamous with respiratory epithelium, anteriorly by the anterior commissure, and posteriorly by the tip of the vocal process of the arytenoid. The squamous epithelium of the vocal cord and the elastic tissue of the vocal ligament represent the superficial and deep boundaries of Reinke's space, respectively. It is suggested that, because Reinke's space does not possess an adequate lymph drainage, blood products may accumulate in it without resolution and give rise to tissue reactions; together the blood products and their tissue reactions in Reinke's space constitute the vocal cord polyp and some other lesions of the true vocal cord.

Aetiology

A variety of aetiological factors have been described in the formation of exudates into Reinke's space. It is clear that any cause of inflammatory reaction stimulating the blood vessels supplying the epithelium of the vocal cord may lead to this process. The following are some of the factors that have been invoked to explain these lesions:

1. Trauma of vocal cord abuse, particularly overviolent adduction so that the cords flap against each other.
2. Cigarette smoking producing irritation of the vocal cords.
3. Other airborne irritants such as oil fumes, oil dusts, chemical vapours and steam

4. Nasal disease, particularly severe nasal obstruction, in which the air reaching the larynx is abnormally dry.

Hypothyroidism has been suggested as a possible factor, but a careful study has shown that it is not an aetiological factor in the development of Reinke's oedema.[1]

Clinical and Gross Appearances

The gross appearance of the upper surfaces of some of these lesions corresponds to that of coronal sections across the vocal cord, as shown in Figure 31.1.

Microscopic Appearances

The histological appearances of these lesions show combinations of the following features:

1. Blood products and tissue fluid.
2. Connective tissue cellular reaction.

These two features are present in all cases. In a small number of cases there may also be present:

3. Changes in the stratified squamous epithelial covering.

Fibrin is the main blood product, which has exuded into the space in most of these lesions. This is observed as hyaline pink-staining amorphous material, sometimes with threads, which is usually extravascular (Fig. 31.2). It often surrounds blood vessels and is frequently accompanied by a blue-staining amorphous mucoid material, probably formed by sulphated glycosaminoglycans. Lakes of

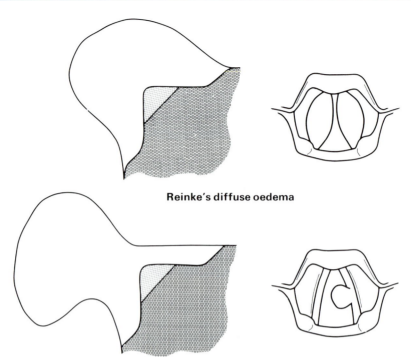

Reinke's diffuse oedema

Figure 31.1 Diagrams of coronal section (*left*) and direct laryngoscopic view to illustrate gross distinction between Reinke's diffuse oedema and vocal cord polyp. The coronal sections show (from *left* to *right*) Reinke's space, vocal ligament and thyroarytenoid muscle. In Reinke's oedema the full lengths of both Reinke's spaces are diffusely oedematous. In the vocal cord polyp there is a localised swelling of Reinke's space on one side.

oedema fluid are frequently seen. Occasionally fibrin may be present within blood vessels as part of thrombus (Fig. 31.3). Frank haemorrhage is also often present in these lesions. That this represents a real part of the tissue change and is not an artefact resulting from the surgery may be confirmed by the frequent presence of haemosiderin (Figs 31.4, 31.5).

Variable, often extensive, degrees of connective tissue proliferation always contribute to the subepithelial swelling of vocal cord polyp or the other related lesions. Fibroblasts are always abundant. Frequently they are small and stellate, and vocal cord polyps with a predominance of such cells have been described as "myxoid" (Fig. 31.6). Blood vessels – arteries, veins and capillaries – are often very prominent, particularly in the presence of fresh haemorrhage. Thrombosis may be seen within some of them. Cysts lined by flat cells sometimes develop among the connective tissue cells (Fig. 31.7).

Only a minority of Reinke's space exudative lesions show squamous epithelial changes of the following types:

1. Hyaline thickening of the basement membrane (Figs 31.2, 31.7).
2. Epithelial abnormalities of mild degree.
3. Keratosis, rarely severe, of the epithelial surface.

Clearly these changes are in reaction to the florid alterations taking place immediately below the epithelium and they rarely pose diagnostic problems. Vocal cord polyp and Reinke's oedema are so frequent that they may be associated with vocal cord carcinoma, another common condition and the two conditions may even be found within the same biopsy.

Three distinct clinical entities have each been associated with specific combinations of histological features:[2]

1. Polyp – grossly a sessile or pedunculated lesion on the anterior third of the true vocal cord, very mobile if pedunculated; microscopically there is evidence of recent haemorrhage, haemosiderin and fibrin and thrombosis.

2. Reinke's oedema – grossly a unilateral or bilateral white swelling of the vocal cord; microscopically there is swelling of the basement membrane of the squamous epithelium, lakes of oedema fluid, extravascular red cells and increased thickness of the walls of blood vessels in the submucosa.

3. Nodule – small bilateral lesions symmetrically placed on the border of the anterior and middle third of the cords and immobile during phonation; microscopically, like Reinke's oedema there is swelling of the basement membrane of the squamous epithelium, but no haemorrhage and no oedematous lakes.

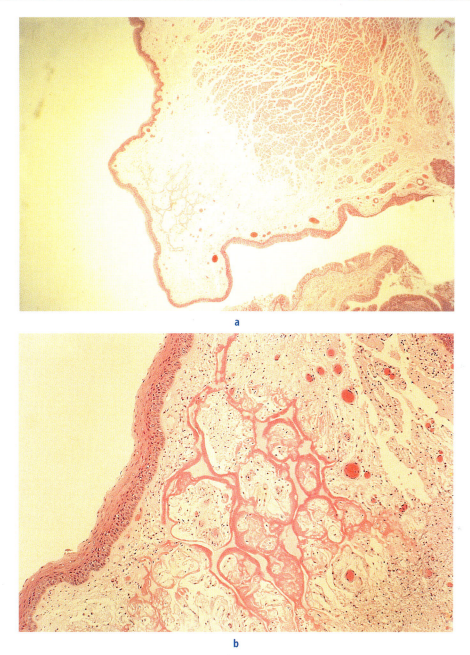

Figure 31.2 Fibrin exudation into Reinke's space. **a** Widening by exudation of fibrin threads. **b** Higher power view showing threads of fibrin in Reinke's space. Note slight hyalinisation of basement membrane

Laryngeal Joints

Ageing Changes

To attempt to ascertain whether degeneration of laryngeal joints may be responsible for senescent vocal quality, an autopsy histological study was carried out of cricoarytenoid joints at different ages.[3] No changes were found in the joints, but there was progressive cricoid and arytenoid ossification and periarticular muscular atrophy and fibrosis, suggesting that other laryngeal changes may play a greater role rather than changes within the cricoarytenoid joint itself.

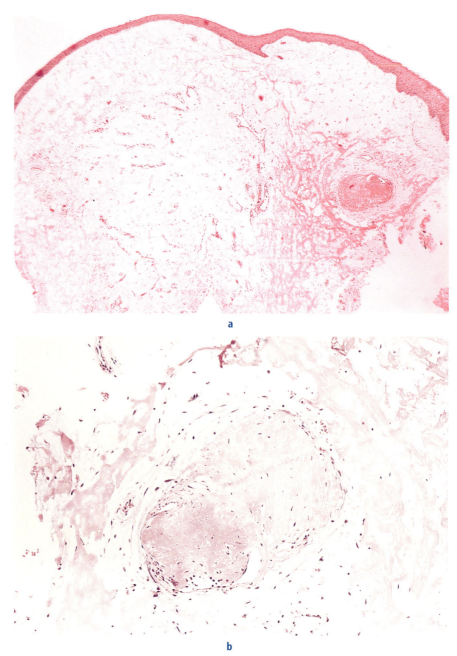

Figure 31.3 Thrombosed blood vessel in vocal cord nodule. **a** Note also abundant fibrin and small blood vessels in Reinke's space. **b** Higher power of a thrombosed blood vessel. Note fibrin in blood vessel and surrounding it

Arthritis of Laryngeal Joints

By far the commonest disease process producing inflammation of the laryngeal joints is rheumatoid arthritis. Other causes are rare. They include infections, trauma or following prolonged immobilization, as in longstanding paralysis caused by intrinsic laryngeal muscular paralysis.

Laryngeal Rheumatoid Arthritis

Rheumatoid arthritis is a chronic systemic disease manifested primarily by inflammatory arthritis of the peripheral joints, but also by systemic disorders including abnormalities of the blood, lungs, nervous system, heart and blood vessels, and the deposition of rheumatoid nodules.

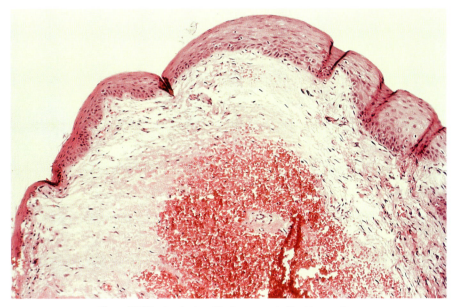

Figure 31.4 Vocal cord polyp with a large amount of fresh haemorrhage

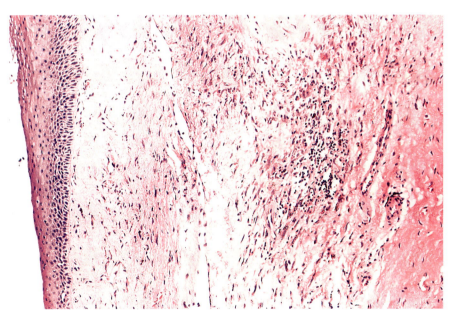

Figure 31.5 Fibrosis in vocal cord polyp. Note also brownish granules of haemosiderin remote from surface epithelium

The disease may show itself in the larynx in one or both of two ways:

1. By the development of an arthritis affecting the cricoarytenoid and cricothyroid joints.
2. By the formation of a granuloma – the rheumatoid nodule.

Joint Involvement

Rheumatoid arthritis affecting the cricoarytenoid and cricothyroid joints passes through two successive phases of development, and each stage has characteristic clinical features and pathological changes.

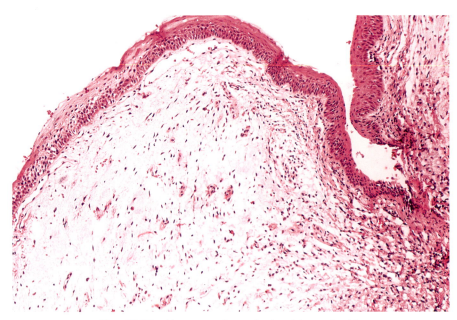

Figure 31.6 Myxoid appearance of connective tissue in laryngeal nodule

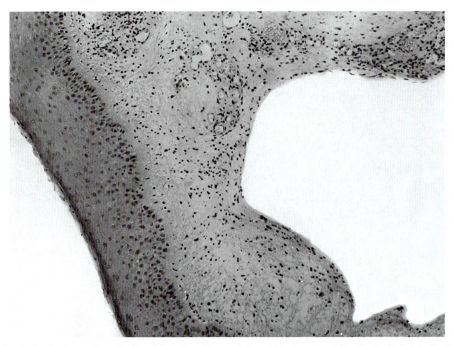

Figure 31.7 Vocal cord polyp showing cyst formation. There is fibrin deposition, newly formed blood vessels and fibroblastic cells. Note hyaline thickening of basement membrane of squamous epithelium

Acute Phase – Synovitis. Symptoms and signs at this early stage can be slight, or there may be acute pain, with swelling of the laryngeal mucosa over the joints, and voice disturbances.

The pathological changes at this stage are confined to the synovium, which becomes thickened and may be villous or papillary due to accumulation of plasma cells and lymphocytes. There may be a fibrinous exudate into the joint cavity, but the articular surfaces remain normal.

Chronic Phase – Joint Destruction and Ankylosis. The chronic stage is more dangerous clinically, for the ankylosed laryngeal joints leave the vocal cords in adduction. The patient may have stridor and respiratory obstruction requiring tracheostomy.

The pathological appearances are of the inflammatory tissue covering the joint surfaces. The two joint surfaces become welded together by a mass of fibrous tissue with the resolution of the inflammatory process (Fig. 31.8).

Rheumatoid Nodules (Granulomata)

Rheumatoid nodules may be found in the larynx in the subhyoid area (possibly in relation to the bursa occasionally found there), or in the postcricoid region, which is subject to recurrent trauma from deglutition.[4] Rheumatoid nodules may (as mentioned) coexist with arthritis in the larynx and so increase the tendency to respiratory obstruction.

The histological structure of the rheumatoid nodule is characterized by an eosinophilic zone of central necrosis. Around the necrotic centre of the nodule is a serpiginous margin of histiocytes, which are arranged radially with their long axes at right angles to the border of the nodule (Fig. 31.9). There is often also a surrounding fibroblastic reaction. The lumina of nearby blood vessels are reduced by intimal fibrosis.

Gout

Definition

Gout is usually manifested as an acute arthritis, most frequently in the big toe joint. The arthritis is related to deposition of sodium urate crystals in the joint capsule and as tophi, particularly in the ear cartilage (see Chapter 2) but also elsewhere. The larynx is a rare site for the deposition of tophi. Most of the gouty tophi of the larynx described in the literature have shown a similar appearance and position as white patches in or near the true vocal cord.

Gouty Cricoarytenoid Arthritis

In a post-mortem study of a gouty larynx, both cricoarytenoid joints showed massive deposits of urates, surrounded by macrophages and giant cells.

There was destruction of joint cartilage and, in some places, of underlying ossified cartilage.[5]

Hyaline Deposits: Amyloid and Lipoid Proteinosis

Amyloid Deposits

Amyloidosis, whether primary or secondary, usually involves more than one internal organ. Solitary lesions of amyloid deposition giving rise to symptoms and signs also occur in, for example, the upper respiratory tract, urinary bladder, skin and conjunctiva, but are most common in the false cord of the larynx.

Site

In the majority of patients the lesion is found in the false cord. In addition the subglottic area, the oropharynx, nasopharynx and nasal cavity may occasionally be involved by amyloid deposition.[6]

Natural History

The disease can usually be controlled by surgical procedures, sometimes repeated, to clear the airway. Occasionally spread to the bronchi may take place.

Clinical Features

The majority of patients complain of hoarseness related to a lesion of the false cord. No evidence of amyloidosis outside the respiratory tract need be expected.

Gross Appearances

The affected area, usually the false cord is swollen, even to the extent of being described as polypoid. The surface is smooth, sometimes "bosselated".

Microscopic Appearances

In haematoxylin- and eosin-stained sections, the amyloid is seen as pink, almost acellular material prominently infiltrating the lamina propria of the tissue, but always leaving intact the covering epithe-

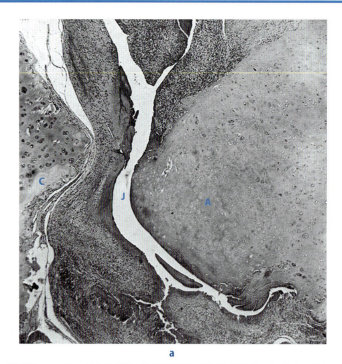

a

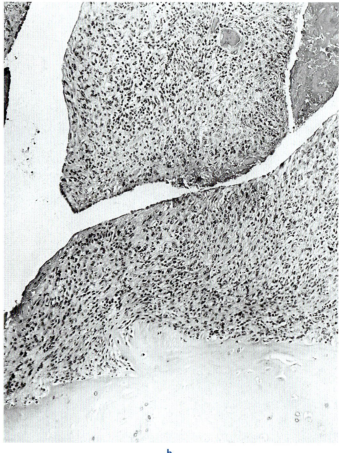

b

Figure 31.8 Chronic phase of rheumatoid arthritis of the cricoarytenoid joint. **a** The whole articular surface of the cricoid cartilage is covered by a layer of chronic inflammatory granulation tissue. The sides of the arytenoid cartilage are similarly eroded. A layer of fibrin is seen lining the joint space on the cricoid side. *A*, arytenoid cartilage; *C*, cricoid cartilage; *J*, joint space. **b** Higher power of part of Fig. 31.5 showing inflammatory tissue eroding arytenoid cartilage. Note the fibrin in the joint cavity at *top right*

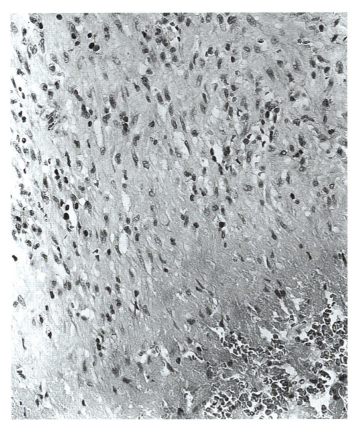

Figure 31.9 Rheumatoid nodule of the larynx. The centre of the nodule is seen at the *bottom right*. It is eosinophilic in the original and shows deposited red cells. Surrounding the necrotic area is a layer of histiocytes and fibroblasts, which are aligned at right angles to the circumference of the necrotic centre

lium – usually pseudostratified columnar epithelium or, in a few cases, stratified squamous epithelium. Sometimes large areas are distended by amyloid, with only the ducts of glands remaining of the surviving normal tissue. In most biopsies a striking feature is the disappearance of seromucinous glands – structures that normally constitute a large part of the tissues from which the biopsies were derived – and their replacement by amyloid (Fig. 31.10).

In all biopsies the amyloid is deposited as thin flecks and also as large rounded masses of variable size. It is frequently possible to observe that the latter are derived from replacement by amyloid of seromucinous glands, since all stages may be seen in this process, from partial involvement of individual acini to the loss of entire glands, the final result being a number of uniform regular "balls" of amyloid or a diffuse replacement of tissue (Figs 31.11, 31.12). Perivascular amyloid deposit is also frequent. Foreign body-type giant cell reaction to the amyloid is often present.

In all cases the amyloid stains positively with Congo red and gives a greenish birefringence. Laryngeal amyloid deposits retain their Congo red positivity after treatment by potassium perman-

ganate solution, suggesting that they are composed of immunoglobulin amyloid (AL) rather than AA amyloid. Immunostaining of laryngeal amyloid has confirmed this, showing it to be composed of lambda-light chains in 71% of cases and kappa-light chains in 29%, indicating that laryngeal amyloidosis is a form of localised amyloidosis characterised by monoclonal light-chain deposition.[7]

Trabeculae of woven bone are sometimes found in the amyloid material. A cartilage-like appearance is assumed by the amyloid in a few places (Fig. 31.13). Irregular, partly ossified, cartilaginous outgrowths derived from the tracheal rings are sometimes present, resembling tracheopathia osteoplastica (see Chapter 29).

Electron Microscopy

Electron microscopic studies on a case of primary amyloid deposit of the false cord, in which deposits of amyloid material were present around the acini and ducts of seromucinous glands, showed areas in which amyloid appeared to be replacing the basal lamina of a duct. In some areas, parallel fibres with

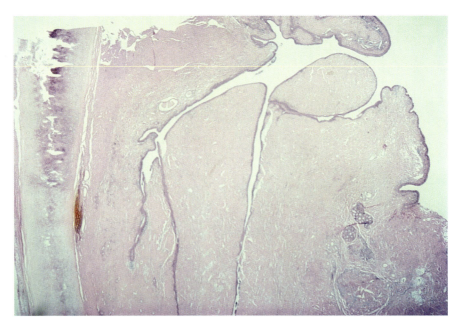

Figure 31.10 Amyloid deposit of false cord of larynx. Hyaline eosinophilic amorphous material has almost completely replaced the normally abundant seromucinous glands of this part

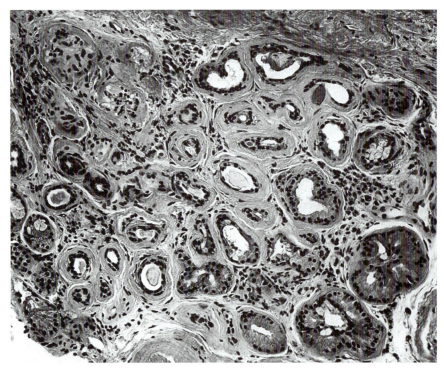

Figure 31.11 Amyloid deposit involving seromucinous glands of the larynx. The amyloid is at an early stage of deposition around the acini of seromucinous glands. The epithelium of the acini is still intact[6]

similar dimensions to amyloid were present within basal cells of the epithelium, and were situated between the more densely stained tonofibrils of the cell and the cytoplasmic membrane. There was a loss of definition of the latter, and the fibrils appeared to merge into the randomly orientated amyloid fibrils adjacent to the epithelium (Fig. 31.14). In the lumina of some ducts, amorphous material was present in which randomly arranged fibrils with a diameter of about 10 nm, indicating amyloid, were seen.[6]

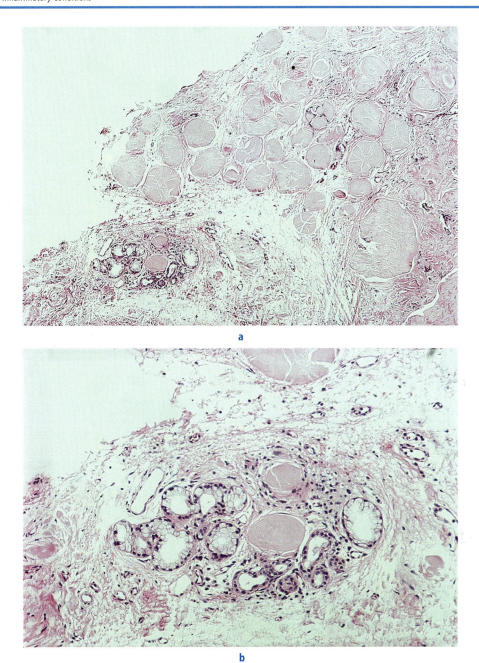

Figure 31.12 Later stage than Fig. 31.11 with complete amyloid replacement of some seromucinous glands. **a** Numerous large round masses of amyloid and origin of two such "balls" of amyloid in lower left hand corner. **b** Higher power view of seromucinous glands from **a** showing complete replacement of gland lumen and epithelium by amyloid. **c** Reddish staining of amyloid deposit by Congo red. **d** Same field of Congo red section as that depicted in **c**, viewed through crossed polaroids. The amyloid shows a greenish birefringence

(Figure 31.12 c and d, see overleaf)

Lipoid Proteinosis

Synonyms

The disease has several synonyms: Urbach-Wiethe disease, lipoidosis cutis et mucosae, hyalinosis cutis et mucosae and lipoglycoproteinosis.

Clinical Features

The features are those of papules, plaques and nodules, involving the skin widely and also the mucosae of the upper air and food passages. There is a particular predilection for involvement of the mucous membrane of the larynx and in approximately two-

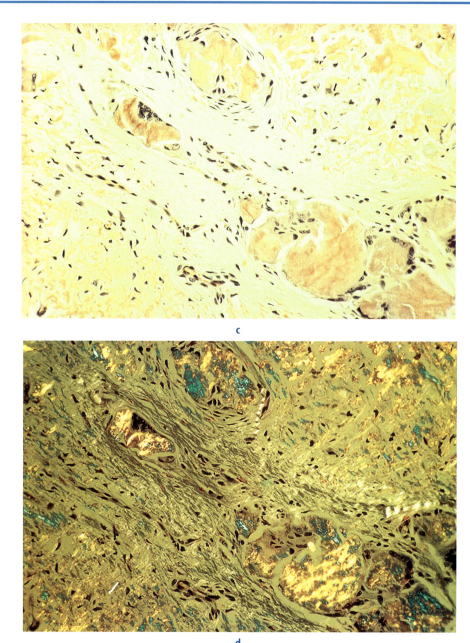

c

d

Figure 31.12 c, d

thirds of cases, voice change secondary to laryngeal involvement, occurring at birth or early in infancy, is the first manifestation of the disease. It has been thought to be inherited as an autosomal recessive.

Pathological Appearances

In the larynx, nodules are present most frequently in the mucosae of the epiglottis, aryepiglottic fold and vocal cords.

The essential microscopic abnormality is the presence of eosinophilic hyaline foci around the capillaries. An oil-soluble fat stain will disclose lipid in areas of hyalinisation. The overlying epithelium is frequently hyperplastic and may be hyperkeratotic. The hyaline deposits are composed of glycoprotein, which gives a strongly positive periodic acid–Schiff reaction in paraffin as well as frozen sections.

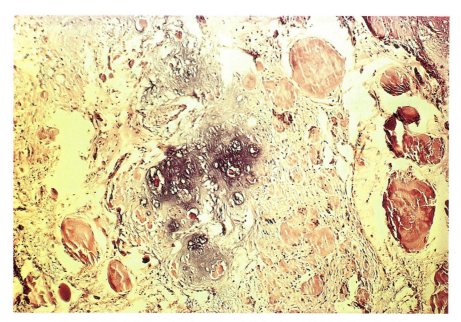

Figure 31.13 Metaplastic cartilage deposit in amyloid of trachea, which is in the form of "balls"

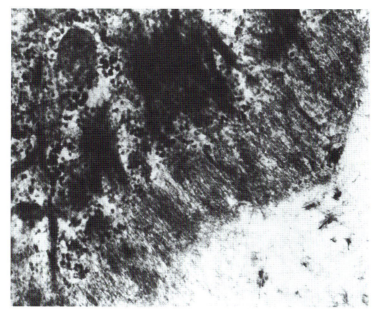

Figure 31.14 Electron micrograph of part of epithelial cell from seromucinous gland in case of amyloid deposit in false cord at a phase of amyloid deposition similar to that shown in Fig. 31.11. The darker tonofibrils of an epithelial cell appear to merge with the fibrils of amyloid in the vicinity of the cell membrane, and similar fibrils pass beyond the region of the cell membrane to the basal lamina. The latter is greatly thickened with amyloid in this area[6]

Relapsing Polychondritis

The cartilage of the ear is most frequently affected in relapsing polychondritis, but when the laryngeal cartilages are involved in this condition, the pathological processes become life-threatening. A full account of this condition is given in Chapter 2.

Wegener's Granulomatosis

Wegener's granulomatosis affects the nose, lung and kidney in almost all cases (see Chapter 14). There have been cases of Wegener's granulomatosis in the recent literature in which the larynx was involved also. In these the inflammatory process was usually in the subglottic region and trachea, and this has been so severe sometimes as to produce obstruction requiring tracheostomy. In all cases serological tests for circulating autoantibodies against both cytoplasmic and perinuclear constituents of neutrophils (ANCA test) were positive. In some cases the only clinical features were those of subglottic stenosis and a positive ANCA test. Such cases are thought to be a *forme fruste* of Wegener's granuloma.[8]

Strangulation

It might be thought that part or all of the fatal effects of strangulation are produced by traumatic damage to the larynx. This is not so. After fatal strangulation, the deep tissues of the neck show haemorrhage on either side of the larynx. No fracture, haemorrhage or oedema can usually be seen in any part of the laryngeal wall, hyoid bone or laryngeal mucosa. It seems death from strangulation may result from cerebral ischaemia caused by common carotid artery compression and from nervous shock transmitted by the vagus nerve.

Pathological Changes after Intratracheal Intubation

Acute Effects

A tube inserted through the mouth and larynx into the trachea is commonly used to provide an airway during anaesthesia, and also for prolonged respiratory care and artificial ventilation. The method is of immense value, but is not free from complications – which are brought about by the damaging effect of the tube on the mucosa and underlying tissues of the larynx. The endotracheal tube tends to lie in the larynx in a posterior position. This is so for two reasons. First, the glottis has a triangular shape, the apex of the triangle being anterior and the base posterior. A tube inserted into the larynx is more likely to come to lie against the flat base and sides of the triangle, i.e. the posterior laryngeal surface and the vocal process region. Second, the cervical vertebral column normally shows lordosis, which pushes the cricoid cartilage forward and so enhances the tendency of the posterior laryngeal wall to make contact with the tube. It is thus to be expected that pathological changes following prolonged intubation will be found principally on the posterolateral part of the larynx.

There are two groups of patients in whom intubation is especially frequently required, and so in whom the deleterious results of intubation represent a major problem:

1. Adults undergoing anaesthesia and resuscitation.
2. Neonates with respiratory distress. The pathological changes in the two groups are similar.

In Adults

Patients in whom intubation has been carried out for longer than 72 h are unable to swallow fluids for some days because of the frequent aspiration into the airway. Some are hoarse, a situation that may be persistent. On examination of the larynx, varying degrees of inflammation and oedema of the aryepiglottic folds, epiglottis and vocal cords are seen in those who have been intubated for less than 48 h. In those who have been intubated for longer, arytenoid and posterior vocal cord ulceration are usually seen.[9,10]

At autopsy it has been found that the brunt of the damage inflicted by the tube is over the vocal processes of the arytenoids and the subjacent mucosa of the subglottis, overlying the cricoid lamina. The degree of pathological change depends on the length of time of the intubation. In larynges intubated for less than 12 h, pale ovoid areas were present on the vocal processes and subjacent posterior cricoid laminae; these corresponding microscopically to loss of epithelium and empty capillaries. Intubation for between 12 and 48 h results in ulceration of those areas, with deep stromal necrosis. The non-ulcerated perichondrium of the arytenoid is inflamed in all cases with longer than 12 hours' intubation. After 48 hours' intubation, the ulcers on the vocal processes and subglottis are broader and deeper. Often the perichondrium of these cartilages was exposed, and after 96 h there was actual excavation of the cartilage. After 120 hours' intubation, at least one vocal process becomes loose and partly or completely separated from the rest of the vocal cord. After repeated intubation or in larynges that are relieved of the tube for more than 12 h, a pseudomembrane develops over the cartilages with a heavy inflammatory response, although there is no significant inflammatory exudate in cases with continuous intubation. The lesions inflicted by continuous intubation may thus be ischaemic; subsequent removal of the tube allows resumption of vascular flow and this leads to the inflammatory and pseudomembrane formation.[10]

In Neonates

Damage from intubation of neonates is common and results in some cases in the serious long-term complication of acquired laryngeal stenosis.

Pathological Appearances

A pioneering pathological study of this problem found post-intubation changes in the neonate with a similar reaction to those of the adult.[11] The earliest changes of loss of epithelium and ulceration take place at the outer angles of the glottic triangle over the vocal processes of the arytenoid within hours of intubation. The subglottic epithelium inferior to this area is also affected. Ulceration develops, and the perichondrium of the vocal process and cricoid lamina, and eventually the cartilages themselves, become eroded (Figs 31.15, 31.16, 31.17). The observation in adults of inflammatory involvement of the vocal process perichondrium in its antiluminal surface was confirmed in neonatal larynges to occur after 3 days of intubation. A similar acute inflammatory layer of the antiluminal cricoid lamina perichondrium was also constantly present (Fig. 31.18), and this was seen to be changing to fibrous granulation tissue in some cases. It is possible that the tube causes movement of these cartilages, with the cricoarytenoid joint as a fulcrum. The inner aspects of these cartilages are damaged by ischaemic necrosis caused by the direct pressure effect of the tube, but the outer surfaces might suffer from a tearing and abrasive action on the cartilage surface with acute inflammation resulting from this movement. In this study it was not felt that laryngeal stenosis could result from the changes described since the larynx usually healed despite the continued presence of the endotracheal tube.

A more recent study of neonatal intubation damage using horizontal whole-organ serial sections (see Chapter 29) has provided, however, an explanation for the laryngeal stenosis resulting from intubation through the larynx in infants.[12] While minor abrasions caused by the tube can heal by primary intention, more serious ulceration is followed by granulation tissue with exposure of cartilage. This often resolves, but sometimes produces considerable fibrosis, which can decrease the size of the laryngeal lumen or after contraction cause its distortion. The diameter of the laryngeal airway can also be compromised after intubation by the mucous gland hyperplasia that it stimulates or by mucus-containing ductal cysts, which are formed as a result of obstruction of gland ducts by the scarring.

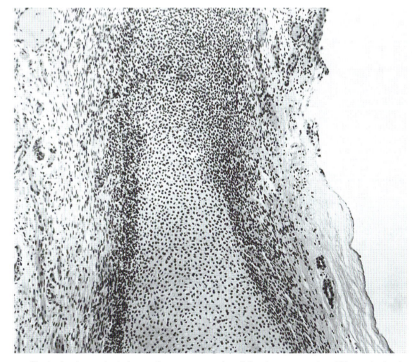

Figure 31.15 Early changes of intubation damage in the larynx of a premature newborn infant (necropsy specimen). The section is taken through the posterolateral angle of the glottic region. The epithelium has been almost entirely denuded in this area. The mucosa immediately beneath it is free from inflammatory change and shows a fibrillary alteration of connective tissue. There is an intense inflammatory reaction in the perichondrial region on both the luminal and the antiluminal surfaces (Courtesy of Dr. S. Gould)

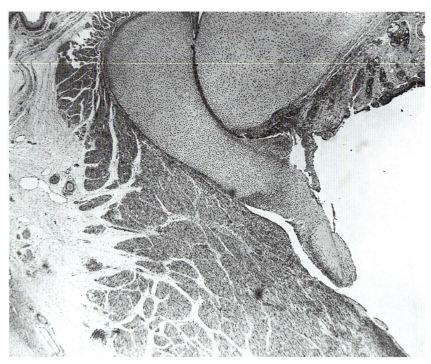

Figure 31.16 Intubation damage of posterolateral angle region of glottis of premature infant at a later stage than Fig. 31.15. The vocal process of the arytenoid is denuded of mucosa, is necrotic and is displaced into the laryngeal lumen (Courtesy of Dr. S. Gould)

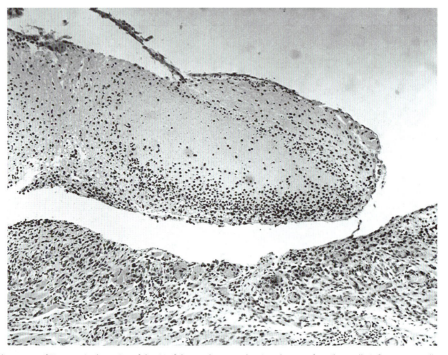

Figure 31.17 Higher power of Fig 31.16 in the region of the tip of the vocal process showing absence of cartilage cells. Inflammatory cells are mainly near the surface on the deeper aspect of the vocal process and within the underlying muscle

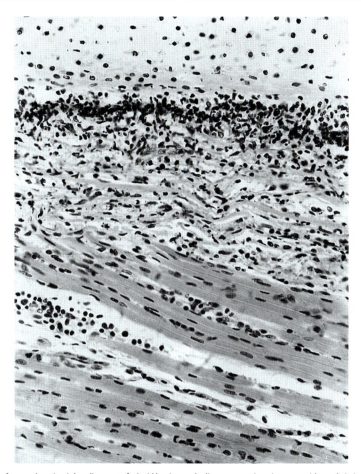

Figure 31.18 Perichondrial surface on deep (peripheral) aspect of cricoid lamina, and adjacent posterior cricoarytenoid muscle in intubation damage of premature newborn. There is a brisk chronic inflammatory reaction at the perichondrium, which extends into the muscle

Long-term Effects

Intubation Granuloma

An unusual complication of endotracheal anaesthesia is the slow development and persistence of a mass of granulation tissue over the vocal process of the arytenoid. The major symptom of this development is hoarseness, which usually does not commence until about 2 months after the operation; in some cases this symptom is delayed for up to 1 year. The lesion is found predominantly in adult females, perhaps because the smaller size of the female larynx renders it more susceptible to the damaging effect of the tube.

The gross appearances of these lesions are those of a reddish, spherical or oval swelling situated at the posterior end of the upper surface of a vocal cord. Microscopically the granuloma has a round outline. The surface is usually covered by a layer of fibrin. The main component of the lesion is a network of capillary blood vessels, between which

are plasma cells, lymphocytes, fibroblasts, neutrophils and eosinophils (Figs 31.19, 31.20). At the base, the origin of this tissue from the underlying lamina propria can be identified. Traces of arytenoid cartilage are never seen in biopsy specimens of intubation granuloma. In some cases a stalk can be identified, the sides of which show squamous epithelium, which gives way to the fibrin surface that covers most of the lesion.

The pathogenesis is clearly that of trauma by the intratracheal tube, the acute manifestations of which are described above. The persistence and recurrence of the lesion may be related to vocal abuse or to non-linguistic laryngeal trauma such as recurrent harsh coughing or persistent throat clearing. In some cases such habits may be associated with gastro-oesophageal reflux disease (see below). The histological appearances of intubation granuloma are indistinguishable from those of pyogenic granuloma. It should also be said that intubation granuloma cannot be easily distinguished from contact ulcer (see below).

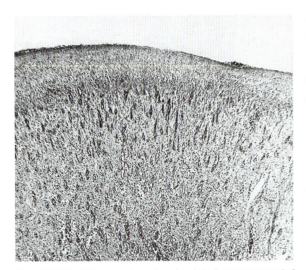

Figure 31.19 Intubation granuloma of vocal cord. The lesion is composed of granulation tissue with surface necrosis

Intubation granulomas are usually treated by surgical removal of the lesion endoscopically. There is, however, a marked tendency of the lesion to recur. In some cases four or five recurrences will take place after treatment before the lesion subsides. The material removed shows in each biopsy the presence only of inflammatory granulation tissue, and with such a histological basis the essentially benign nature of the process need not be in doubt, in spite of repeated recurrences.

Contact Ulcer (Vocal Process Granuloma)

Although contact ulcer is not due to intubation, it is considered in this section because the sites of occurrence and histological appearance are similar to those of intubation granuloma. Contact ulcer of the larynx has been ascribed to violent coughing at night due to aspiration of oral secretions.[13] Hyperacidity with aspiration of gastric acid from the patient's hiatus hernia is probably an important factor.

Contact ulcer is a lesion affecting both the vertical portion of the arytenoid and the vocal process. In some cases the edges of the ulcer are raised and the vocal process of the opposite arytenoid fits into the bowl-like lesion, giving rise to the term "contact" ulcer. In a few patients the surface of the other arytenoid may become similarly ulcerated.

Histological examination shows only non-specific granulation tissue and chronic inflammatory exudate. It is not possible to separate this lesion on a histological basis from intubation granuloma and there is a similar tendency to recur.

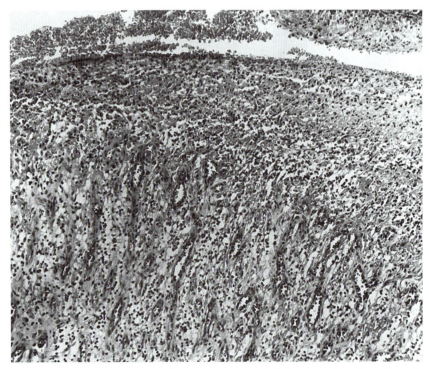

Figure 31.20 Surface of intubation granuloma shown in Fig. 31.19. The granuloma is composed of inflamed granulation tissue with a surface cap of fibrin, necrotic tissue and red cells

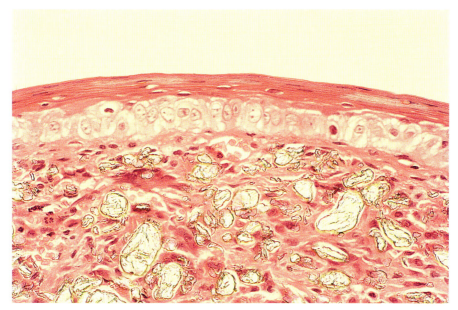

Figure 31.21 Teflon particles beneath true vocal cord epithelium. The inflammatory reaction at this stage is mainly one of macrophages

Reaction to Teflon Injection

Teflon is a polymer of tetrafluorethylene and is used to treat vocal cord disability, particularly that caused by hemiparesis. It is usually made up as a paste. The size of the particles of Teflon is uniform in a particular sample, and varies according to the method of manufacture from between 6 and 12 μm to between 50 and 100 μm. Studies of the larynx at post-mortem in patients who have had Teflon injected for the treatment of a paralysed vocal cord have shown a reaction to the Teflon particles by histiocytes, neutrophils and lymphocytes.[14] A large granuloma may be formed (Fig. 31.21). One of the complications associated with Teflon paste injection is migration of the paste into the surrounding tissues. In one case Teflon had migrated from the right vocal cord where it had been injected to the left vocal cord and some particles were found in a periarterial lymphatic vessel.

References

1. White A, Sim DW, Maran AG. Reinke's edema and thyroid function. J Laryngol Otol 1991;105:291–292
2. Dikkers FG, Nikkels PG. Benign lesions of the vocal folds: histopathology and phonotrauma. Ann Otol Rhinol Laryngol 1995;104:698–703
3. Casiano RR, Ruiz PJ, Goldstein W. Histopathologic changes in the aging human cricoarytenoid joint. Laryngoscope 1994;104:533–538
4. Bridger MWM, Jahn AF, van Nostrand AWP. Laryngeal rheumatoid arthritis. Laryngoscope 1980;90:296–303
5. Goodman M, Montgomery W, Minette L. Pathologic findings in gouty cricoarytenoid arthritis. Arch Otolaryngol 1976; 102:27–29
6. Michaels L, Hyams VJ. Amyloid in localised deposits and plasmacytomas of the respiratory tract. J Pathol 1979;128:29–38
7. Lewis JE, Olsen KD, Kurtin PJ et al. Laryngeal amyloidosis: a clinicopathologic and immunohistochemical review. Otolaryngol Head Neck Surg 1992;106:372–377
8. Gans R, de Vries N, Donker AJ et al. Circulating anti-neutrophil cytoplasmic autoantibodies in subglottic stenosis: a useful aid in diagnosing vasculitis in this condition? Q J Med 1991;80:565–574
9. Hedden M, Ersoz CJ, Donnelly WH et al. Laryngotracheal damage after prolonged use of orotracheal tubes in adults. JAMA 1969;207:703–708
10. Donnelly WH. Histopathology of endotracheal intubation. An autopsy study of 99 cases. Arch Pathol 1969;88: 511–520
11. Gould SJ, Howard S. The histopathology of the larynx in the neonate following endotracheal intubation. J Pathol 1985;146:301–311
12. Liu H, Chen JC, Holinger LD et al. Histopathologic fundamentals of acquired laryngeal stenosis. Pediatr Pathol Lab Med 1995;15:655–677
13. Jackson C. Contact ulcer of the larynx. Ann Otorhinolaryngol 1929;37:227–230
14. Boedts D, Roels H, Kluyskens P. Laryngeal tissue responses to Teflon. Arch Otolaryngol 1967;86:562–567

32 Neuromuscular Diseases

The important action of the larynx is that of opening and closing the vocal cords. Any disturbance of this process is observed clinically as a voice disorder and, on laryngoscopy, as a failure of movement of the vocal cord. Inability to abduct the vocal cord is a frequent manifestation of such paresis.

Vocal cord paralysis of the neurological type is always based on pathological changes in the lower motor neurone supplying vocal cord movement, which extends from the nuclei ambigui in the medulla to the intrinsic laryngeal muscles. A summary of such lesions is given in Table 32.1.

Investigation of the Histopathology of a Lower Motor Lesion of the Neuromuscular Pathway of Vocal Cord Movement

In the analysis of any lower motor disorder associated with vocal cord paralysis in which the cause is not known, a pathological study of the neuromuscular pathway of phonation is necessary (Table 32.2). This would involve investigation of the nucleus ambiguus, the vagus, recurrent and superior laryngeal nerves and the intrinsic laryngeal muscles.

Nucleus Ambiguus

The nucleus ambiguus extends throughout the whole length of the medulla on each side so that step or serial sections of the whole medulla would be required.

Table 32.1. Classification of lower motor neurone lesions of vocal cord movement (after Smith and Ramig[1])

Abnormalities of muscle	Myopathies, muscle dystrophies
Abnormalities of neuromuscular junctions	Myaesthenia gravis
Abnormalities of peripheral nerves: Recurrent laryngeal nerve Superior laryngeal nerve Upper vagus nerve	Trauma (e.g. overstretching of neck), neoplasia (usually carcinoma of the lung), iatrogenic (surgery e.g. thyroid surgery, drugs, radiation), Guillain-Barré, syndrome
Abnormalities of nuclei ambigui in brainstem	Wallenberg's syndrome (thrombosis of posterior inferior cerebellar artery), Arnold-Chiari malformation, syringobulbia, neoplasia, trauma

Vagus, Recurrent and Superior Laryngeal Nerves

The nerve fibre pathway of vocal cord movement includes the vagus nerve and its recurrent laryngeal and superior laryngeal nerve branches. A complete pathological study of this part of the pathway would require its gross dissection and observation with microscopic observations of transverse sections of parts of the nerves.

Intrinsic Laryngeal Muscles

In such a pathological study of the final, muscular part of the pathway, some or all of the intrinsic laryngeal muscles would be examined grossly and histologically. It happens that the intrinsic laryngeal

Table 32.2. Studies of pathological changes in the neuromuscular pathway of vocal cord movement

Reference	Disease Patient numbers Type of study	Nuclei ambigui	Vagus and recurrent laryngeal nerve	Intrinsic laryngeal muscles
Guindi et al.[2]	Normal 58 Autopsy	–	Normal	Myopathic changes
Bannister et al.[4]	Shy-Drager syndrome 3 cases Autopsy	No change	Loss of small axons	Neurogenic atrophy in each case
DeReuck and Van Landegem[5]	Shy-Drager syndrome 2 cases Surgical specimens compared with carcinomatous surgical larynges	–	–	Type 1 fibre atrophy in both c ases. Group atrophy ? neurogenic atrophy also in 1 case
Hayashi et al.[6]	Multiple system atrophy 6 cases, 4 with vocal cord palsy, 2 without Autopsy study	Gliosis in 1 case with vocal cord palsy	Small myelinated fibres reduced in all 6 cases. Large myelinated fibres reduced in 4 with vocal cord palsy	Neurogenic atrophy in cases with vocal cord palsy
Quiney and Michaels[7]	Carcinoma of left lung Paralysed left vocal cord 1 case Autopsy		Normal invaded by tumour	Atrophy of all muscles on left

– Not examined

muscle of the greatest pathological importance is easiest to investigate at autopsy. The posterior cricoarytenoid (PCA) muscle may be observed grossly on each side simply by dissecting away the hypopharynx over the posterior aspect of the cricoid lamina and then removing the fascia over the muscle (see Chapter 28). Adenosine triphosphatase and other enzyme studies for typing the muscle fibres can be carried out in surgical specimens if the larynx is obtained fresh after resection. In most cases information about disease states affecting vocal cord movements would only be obtained from autopsy larynges. If the lesion is in the nerve cells of the nucleus ambiguus or in the nerve itself, a neurogenic type of atrophy would be observed in affected muscles, i.e. shrinkage of groups of muscle fibres. Myopathic changes, i.e. conditions in which the presumed causes act directly on the muscle fibres and not via the nerve supply, might also be observed, in appropriate cases.

Changes in the Neuromuscular Pathway of Vocal Cord Movement in Some Vocal Cord Palsies

Little work has been done on the histopathological changes in the neuromuscular pathway of vocal cord movement in cases of vocal cord palsy where the cause is unknown. The results of investigations of the neuromuscular pathway that have been carried out in some of these conditions are listed in Table 32.2. The range of these few investigations is very small, in the light of the clinical frequency of vocal cord paralysis.

Myopathy in "Normal" Larynges

In a study of 54 post-mortem larynges by Guindi et al.,[2] the intrinsic laryngeal muscles were examined histologically in all cases and the recurrent laryngeal nerves in a few. These were all from patients without vocal cord defects. Myopathic changes were frequently found in these "normal" larynges, and the results are provided in Chapter 28. These findings should be considered as baseline controls in the histopathological investigation for pathological changes in intrinsic laryngeal muscles.

Multiple System Atrophy with Progressive Autonomic Failure (Shy-Drager Syndrome)

The Shy-Drager syndrome is a condition characterised by severe orthostatic hypotension with syncope or seizures when the patient stands up. This is associated with features of autonomic failure such as anhydrosis, loss of hair, decreased basal metabolic rate, reduced adrenaline production, deficient secretion of salivary and lacrimal glands, sexual impotence, bladder atony and absence of tachycardia on standing. The pathological changes in the central nervous system are those of multiple system atrophy, atrophy of the intermediolateral column cells of the spinal cord, and those usually found in parkinson-

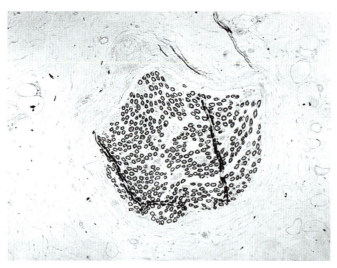

Figure 32.1 Transverse section of recurrent laryngeal nerve from a case of Shy-Drager syndrome. There is an absence of small myelinated fibres so that the fibres appear to be larger and their total number smaller than normal.[4] Compare Fig. 28.18. Methacrylate-embedded 1 μm section, Sudan black stain

ism.[3] Stridor due to abductor paralysis of the vocal cords is fairly common in the Shy-Drager syndrome and commences as excessive snoring and sometimes sleep apnoea. It is frequently necessary for tracheostomy to be carried out to relieve the respiratory obstruction caused by this abductor palsy of the vocal cords. Patients often die even after this measure, probably from cardiac or respiratory centre failure.

Pathological changes in the neuromuscular pathway of vocal cord movement in three cases of Shy-Drager syndrome were studied.[4] The nuclei ambigui were examined in two cases by cell counting; no quantitative or qualitative change could be found in the motor cells. One recurrent laryngeal nerve was examined in a position just inferior (proximal) to its branch to the PCA muscle. It showed fibres that were larger and less numerous than those in the normal control (Fig. 32.1; see also Chapter 28). In each case there was a marked gross atrophy of the PCA, but the other intrinsic laryngeal muscles were not atrophic (Figs 32.2, 32.3). Histologically there was clear evidence of denervation atrophy of the PCA muscles in two of the three cases, as shown by the presence of large groups of atrophic muscle fibres (Fig. 32.4). In the third case the changes were obscured by a severe degree of the myopathic alteration noted in "normal" larynges (see above). It seemed likely, however, that the atrophy (even in the third case) was the result of loss of nerve supply. Subtle undetected changes of a chemical nature were suggested to take place in the cells of the nucleus ambiguus, in keeping with a widespread attack on central nervous system cells that is prevalent in the Shy-Drager syndrome.[4] This then is presumed to give rise to atrophic changes in the recurrent laryngeal nerve. Although all muscles of vocal cord movement would be affected, the abductor muscles – the PCAs – are particularly vulnerable.

In a later study of two cases of Shy-Drager syndrome with stridor, one them showing a clear-cut

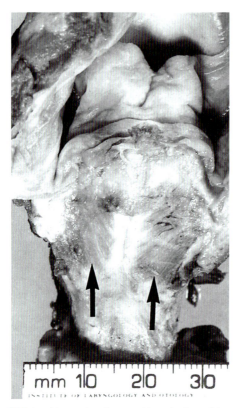

Figure 32.2 Atrophic posterior cricoarytenoid muscles (*arrows*) in a case of Shy-Drager syndrome seen from behind.[4] Compare Fig. 28.3

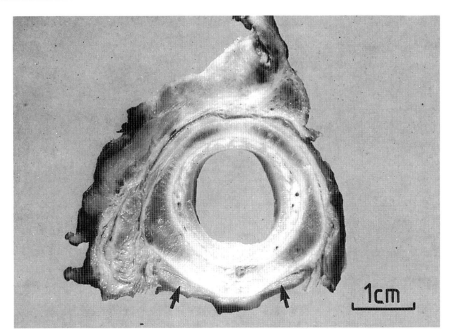

Figure 32.3 Transverse slice of larynx from a case of Shy-Drager syndrome showing atrophic state of both posterior cricoarytenoid muscles (*arrows*).[4] Compare Fig. 28.17

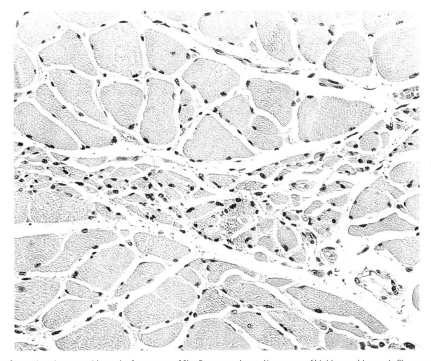

Figure 32.4 Section of posterior cricoarytenoid muscles from a case of Shy-Drager syndrome. Note group of highly atrophic muscle fibres contrasting with normal fibres on each side of it[4]

laryngeal abductor palsy,[5] the PCAs were examined at biopsy and the changes compared with those seen in similar studies on PCAs taken from laryngectomy specimens. In all of the larynges with carcinoma, well-marked neurogenic atrophy was present, but this could not be seen in one of the two Shy-Drager PCAs; the other case displayed some group atrophy of the PCA, but it was not certain whether or not this was due to denervation. Both cases displayed a pronounced type 1 muscle fibre atrophy (low adenosine triphosphatase activity). The gross appearance of the muscles in these two cases was not described. The muscle changes were, as in the earlier study,[4] ascribed to chemical changes in the brainstem.

Multiple System Atrophy Without Progressive Autonomic Failure

Patients with multiple system atrophy without autonomic failure also commonly show vocal cord palsy. An autopsy study providing more information on the basis of the palsy was carried out on six cases of multiple system atrophy without autonomic failure, four of whom had vocal cord palsy. In one of the patients with vocal cord palsy the nuclei ambigui showed gliosis. In all six cases nerve fibre counts identified a loss of small myelinated nerve fibres in the recurrent laryngeal nerve, but in the four with palsy counts showed also a loss of large myelinated fibres. All four with palsy showed thin PCA muscles, which histologically displayed neurogenic atrophy. This study demonstrates that small fibres in the recurrent laryngeal nerve are affected first without clinical signs of palsy. Later large fibres are lost and, these being the fibres that innervate the intrinsic laryngeal muscles, vocal cord palsy results.[6]

Carcinoma of the Left Lung with Left Recurrent Laryngeal Nerve Involvement

A left-sided vocal cord palsy is a well-known complication of carcinoma of the lung, resulting from involvement of the left recurrent laryngeal nerve by mediastinal tumour in the passage of the nerve below the aorta on the left side. The left vocal cord is often fixed in the "cadaveric" or laterally displaced postion. This has not been satisfactorily explained. An autopsy study was carried out on a patient who had had the complication of a left recurrent nerve palsy during his terminal course.[7] The paralysed left vocal cord was seen during life to be fixed in the cadaveric (abducted) position (Fig. 32.5). This was explained by the marked atrophy of all the intrinsic laryngeal muscles on the left that was found. The left vagus and recurrent laryngeal nerve were invaded by carcinoma below the level of the subclavian artery.

References

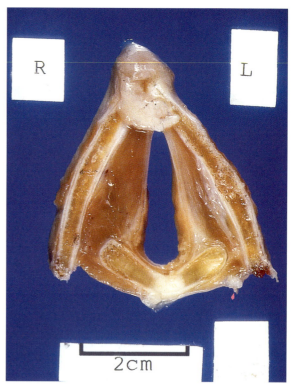

Figure 32.5 Transverse slice of larynx from a patient with carcinoma of the left lung who had a left recurrent nerve palsy during his terminal course. The slice is from the cricoid region and is viewed from below. Note marked atrophy of the intrinsic laryngeal muscles on the left side. This had caused an apparent fixation of the left vocal cord in the cadaveric (laterally displaced) position. *L*, left side. *R*, right side

1. Smith ME, Ramig L. Neurological disorders and the voice. In: Rubin JS, Sataloff RT, Korovin GS et al. (eds) Diagnosis and treatment of voice disorders. Igaku-Shoin, New York, 1995, pp 203–224

2. Guindi GM, Michaels L, Bannister R et al. Pathology of the intrinsic muscles of the larynx. Clin Otolaryngol 1981;6:101–109

3. Bannister R, Oppenheimer DR. Degenerative disease of the nervous system associated with autonomic failure. Brain 1972;95:457–474

4. Bannister R, Gibson W, Michaels L et al. Laryngeal abductor paralysis in multiple system atrophy. A report on three necropsied cases, with observations on the laryngeal muscles and the nuclei ambigui. Brain 1981; 104:351–368

5. DeReuck J, Van Landegem W. The posterior crico-arytenoid muscle in two cases of Shy-Drager syndrome with laryngeal stridor. Comparison of the histological, histochemical and biometric findings. J Neurol 1987;234:187–190

6. Hayashi M, Isozaki E, Oda M et al. Loss of large myelinated nerve fibres of the recurrent laryngeal nerve in patients with multiple system atrophy and vocal cord palsy. J Neurol Neurosurg Psychiatry 1997;62:234–238

7. Quiney RE, Michaels L. Histopathology of vocal cord palsy from recurrent laryngeal nerve damage. J Otolaryngol 1990;19:237–241

33 Squamous Cell Papilloma

Squamous cell papillomas are frequent in the larynx of adults. They also found in children where, because of the much narrower diameter of the airway, the more widespread involvement in the larynx and the greater tendency to recurrence, the symptoms are more serious, and treatment is more urgent and difficult. It is thus customary to divide the condition on the basis of the age of the patient into juvenile and adult types. In some juvenile cases the papillomas persist into adult life. The pathological changes are similar at all ages, and will be described first before a discussion of the natural history of the lesion.

Sites

By far the commonest site of occurrence of squamous papilloma of the larynx is the vocal cord. The anterior half of the cord is more frequently affected than the posterior. The false cord, the vestibule and the subglottis are sometimes affected, but rarely are squamous papillomas seen on the epiglottis and in the trachea and bronchi (Fig. 33.1). Multiple papillomas may exceptionally spread upwards to the pharynx and soft palate.

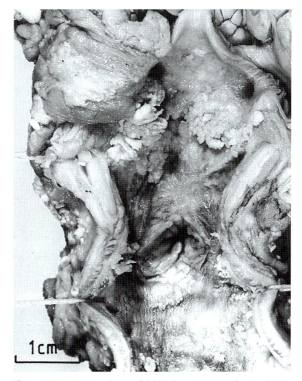

Figure 33.1 Post-mortem larynx of child with squamous papillomatosis. Note papillomas also in trachea, below tracheostomy opening

Gross Appearances

Squamous papillomas range from white to red, and are delicate, granular, polypoid structures, which vary from 1 to 10 mm in diameter, most being less than 5 mm. In florid cases that require laryngectomy, the papillomas form a solid field of mucosal thickening without invasion deep to mucosa. Under magnification, small individual papillae can be discerned as blunt finger-like processes with branches, which never become long and filiform (Fig. 33.2).

Microscopic Appearances

The papillary processes arise from the epithelium of the larynx as cylindrical projections. In sections of some papillomas, smaller cylinders of squamous-

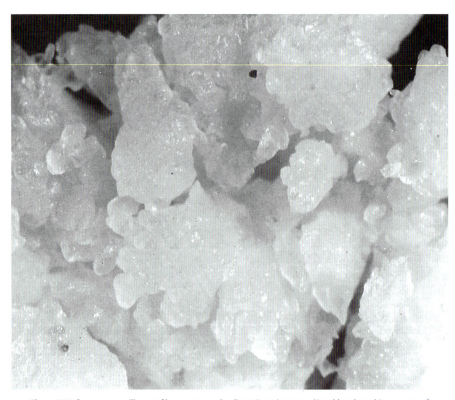

Figure 33.2 Squamous papillomas of larynx seen under dissecting microscope. Note blunt branching processes[8]

cell-covered epithelium are present in the vicinity of the larger papillae and are cut in various planes. These represent second- or even third-order branching of the papillary structures (Figs 33.3, 33.4).

The numbers of layers of squamous epithelial cells lining the papilloma depend on the thickness of the particular papilla examined, which is related to the order of branching that the papilla represents. First-order papillae show up to 15 layers of squamous epithelium; third-order ones show only five or six; second-order ones show intermediate numbers of layers.

In many papillomas nuclei are retained up to the keratinised surface, but in a minority of cases there

is keratosis in which layers of completely keratinised anucleate cells are seen on the surface of the papillae. This may be very extensive, and in these cases the papillae appear to be immersed in a large area of keratin. In these lesions the rete ridges of the squamous cell epithelium are always short and regular, unlike those in verrucous squamous carcinoma (see below and Chapter 37). In all cases with keratosis, a granular layer of keratohyaline is present beneath the keratinised layer, where it forms a zone of variable prominence (Figs 33.5, 33.6).

The basal two or three layers of squamous papillomas are composed of small cells, which are quite distinct from the more superficial "prickle" cells. The basal cells lie loosely on a well-defined basement membrane, which frequently shows hyalinisation.

"Abnormal" Changes

In some cases the epithelium of the papilloma may show changes that may be classified as "dysplastic" or "atypical". These terms have connotations of premalignant change. In our observation such changes are rare in laryngeal papilloma; when present, careful study of the specimens should be carried out to exclude a malignant process. We would prefer to use the terminology of the Ljubljana classification of

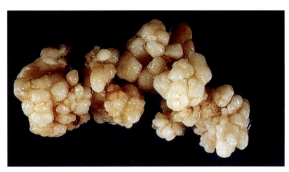

Figure 33.3 Papillomas removed from the vocal cord of an adult

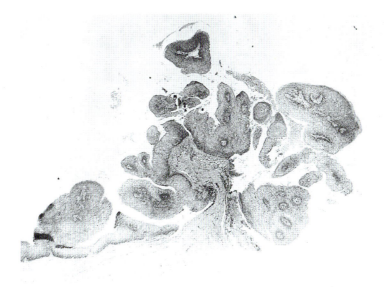

Figure 33.4 Squamous papilloma originating from squamous epithelium of larynx. Note branching of exophytic processes

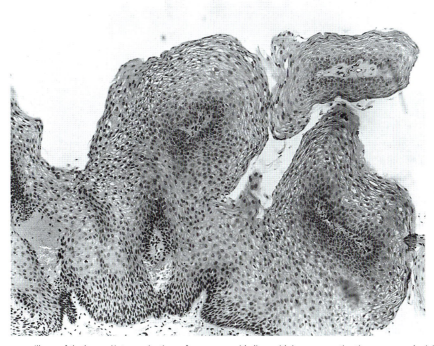

Figure 33.5 Squamous papilloma of the larynx. Note evaginations of squamous epithelium with inner connective tissue cores, and origin of second-degree papilla from primary squamous papilloma

laryngeal hyperplastic lesions,[1] referring to such changes as "abnormal" if there are no features suggesting premalignant change (see Chapter 34). Two types of such abnormality are commonly seen in laryngeal papillomas: basal cell hyperplasia and koilocytosis. In basal cell hyperplasia there is an increase in numbers of rows of basal cells from the normal two or three. The hyperplastic basal cells

may show some enlargement of nuclei and increased content of cytoplasm. Koilocytosis is a change that is frequently present in squamous papillomas at any site and has been studied particularly in condyloma acuminatum of the vulva and cervix, in which its relationship to infection of the squamous epithelium by human papillomavirus (HPV) has been stressed. Koilocytosis is very frequently seen in the upper

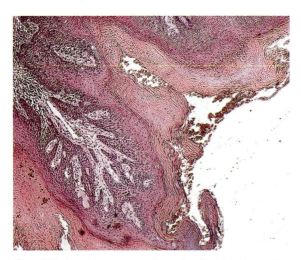

Figure 33.6 Keratotic squamous papilloma of vocal cord showing papillary processes embedded in acellular keratin

intermediate zone and superficial squamous epithelium of squamous papillomas of the larynx. It consists of a spherical enlargement of the cells of the lesion, accompanied by perinuclear vacuolation, so that no stained cytoplasm is seen in the cell or, if it is, it is present as a thin rim around the cell periphery. The nucleus is central and often enlarged, angular or wrinkled. It may exhibit moderate degrees of dysplasia. Since infection of the cells of squamous papillomas of the larynx by HPV is very

frequent, perhaps invariable (see below), it is not surprising that koilocytosis is so commonly seen in papillomas (Fig. 33.8).

In a few cases of papillomatosis, some of the material shows a papillary process not only of squamous cell epithelium, but also of respiratory epithelium. The latter comprises non-malignant respiratory epithelium featuring both ciliated cells and goblet cells. Areas of "stratification" of this respiratory columnar epithelium are seen where cells are heaped up. Papillomas showing such respiratory epithelial hyperplasia have a decided tendency to recur. The appearances of the columnar cell papillomas are similar to those of cylindric cell papilloma of the nose and paranasal sinuses (see Chapter 15). In some squamous papillomas, Alcian-blue stains for mucopolysaccharide show mucin-containing goblet cells and even cysts containing mucin amid the squamous cells of the papillary epithelium, indicating the participation of respiratory epithelium in the papillary process (Figs 33.9–33.12). Papillomas comprising cylindric cell areas should be treated with great care because they have a particularly strong tendency to recur.

Differential Diagnosis

Difficulty may be experienced in distinguishing two other types of neoplastic lesion, which occur par-

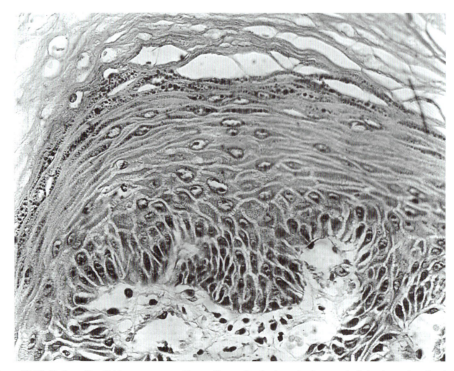

Figure 33.7 Epithelium of keratinising squamous papilloma of larynx showing keratohyaline granules below keratotic surface layers[8]

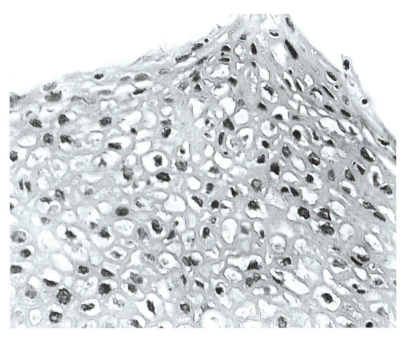

Figure 33.8 Koilocytosis of squamous epithelium on surface of squamous papilloma

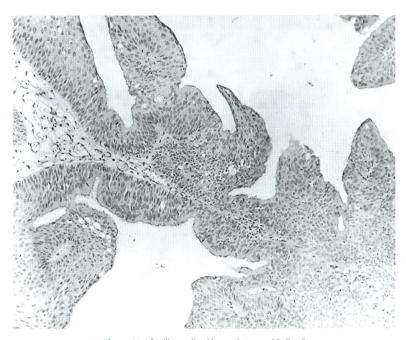

Figure 33.9 Papillomas lined by respiratory epithelium[8]

ticularly often on the vocal cords, from squamous papilloma: keratotic plaque and carcinoma of both verrucous squamous and regular types.

Raised plaques, which have been referred to as verrucous hyperplasia,[2] and are composed of thickened, often abnormal, squamous epithelium with keratinised surface, are seen quite frequently in biopsy. A careful examination of the whole biopsy material for evidence of cylinders of papilloma formation and the branching that is associated with them will usually suffice to distinguish this lesion from verrucous hyperplasia. The degree of abnormal or atypical change exhibited by the plaque is often more severe than would be expected in a papilloma. It has been suggested that some of these plaques may be precursors of verrucous squamous carcinoma.[2,3]

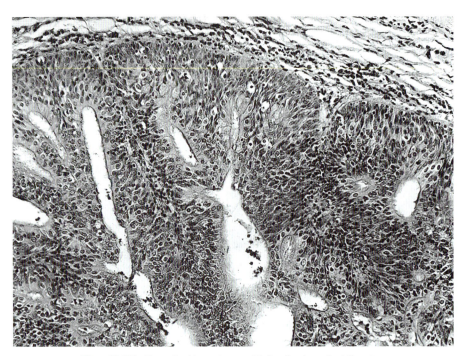

Figure 33.10 Papillomas lined by respiratory epithelium forming a gland-like pattern

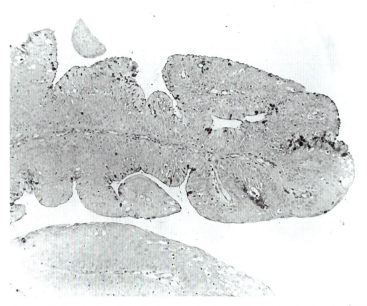

Figure 33.11 Goblet cells in respiratory epithelium-lined papilloma showing as small dark areas (blue in original) near surface.[8] Alcian blue–periodic acid–Schiff stain

Squamous carcinoma may exhibit true papilloma formation and be mistaken for benign squamous papilloma. The pattern is not, however, as symmetrical as in papillomas and second- or third-degree branching is not seen. Verrucous squamous carcinoma often displays very long papillae, without branching. The rete ridges are irregular and the basement membrane is never hyalinised. The latter is frequently seen in papillomas. Squamous cells of the intermediate layer in verrucous carcinomas are larger than those of the corresponding layer in squamous papillomas, showing a mean area of more than 300 μm^2 (see Chapter 36). Regular squamous carcinoma shows evidence of invasion into the lamina propria.

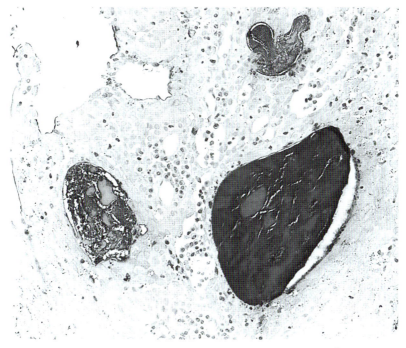

Figure 33.12 Cysts containing mucus (dark-staining areas, blue in original) in squamous papilloma of the larynx.[8] Alcian blue–periodic acid–Schiff stain

Natural History

Juvenile Papilloma

Squamous papillomas arising in childhood have been regarded as distinct from the adult form. Their incidence has a female preponderance,[4] unlike those occurring in adults, which have a male preponderance (see below). They may arise at any age of childhood and have been described as early as 18 months. It has been found that HPV DNA persists in adjacent, normal-appearing mucosa and it is likely that this serves as a reservoir for viral reseeding and regrowth of the papilloma after surgery.[5] Malignant alteration of juvenile papillomatosis has been described. A few cases are on record in which malignancy took place many years after treatment of juvenile papillomatosis by radiotherapy, in which it must be presumed that the carcinoma was the result of the radiation.[6] Cases are also on record in which carcinoma of the lung developed in adults after extensive laryngotracheal papillomatosis since childhood in the absence of radiation therapy.[7]

Adult Papilloma

Laryngeal papillomas arise in twice as many adult males as adult females.[8] The condition may start as juvenile papillomas and continue into adult life. The maximum incidence of onset is in the fourth decade. The condition may take one of three gross forms in the larynx:

1. A solitary mass of varied size. In these patients no recurrence need be expected after a single endoscopic operation to remove the papilloma.
2. Two or more distinct laryngeal lesions separated by clinically normal epithelium. Under these circumstances it is likely that several endoscopic operations will be required to remove recurrences.
3. Florid papillomatosis, where there is involvement of every part of the larynx with an aggressive growth. In these cases symptoms usually date from juvenile life. The condition will necessitate frequent removals over a lengthy period and tracheostomy, and rarely even laryngectomy, may be required.[8]

Rare cases of sudden death, usually from asphyxia due to airway occlusion by a single large papilloma, have been described.[9] In one case that we have encountered the patient complained of asthma-like symptoms and death was ascribed to status asthmaticus until the laryngeal papilloma was revealed at autopsy.

Are Juvenile and Adult Papillomas Different Entities?

The separation of juvenile and adult papillomas as two distinct entities is not realistic, in spite of the reported differences in sex incidence (see above). The two conditions show identical pathological appearances, and juvenile disease may persist into adult life, when it is still similar in appearance to the purely adult cases. An aggressive form may commence de novo in an adult and the mild form in children.[10] In children the condition is more serious because of a greater tendency to recur and the narrowness of the larynx. The outlook is poor for patients with juvenile-onset papillomas that persist after 16 years of age. The majority of patients with adult-onset papillomas have a fair eventual prognosis.

Viral Aetiology

Squamous papillomas of the larynx are caused by HPV, which is known to give rise also to the lesions of verruca vulgaris and condyloma acuminatum. HPV is a member of the PAPOVA group of viruses, which comprises *PA*pilloma-producing viruses and *PO*lyoma virus-producing tumours of mice. HPV has not been propagated in culture. Electron microscopic observations have only occasionally been successful in the search for virus particles in laryngeal papillomas. The localisation of HPV in laryngeal papillomas has been frequently carried out in recent years, however, using other techniques. The immunoperoxidase method for HPV antigen identifies the latter to be situated in the squamous cells of the papillomas, near the surface in most cases.[11] The position of antigen for virus is closely correlated with that of koilocytosis in routinely stained sections (see above). The technique of DNA in situ hybridisation detects HPV genome in laryngeal papillomas in the majority of cases (Fig. 33.13). Another molecular biological method that has been used to identify type 6/11 HPV in laryngeal papillomas is the polymerase chain reaction.

Using the in situ hybridisation technique, about 66% of both adult and juvenile cases are positive for HPV types 6/11, but groups 16/18 and 31/33/35, which have been reported in malignancies of the head and neck as well as in those of the uterine cervix, have not been found in the laryngeal lesions.[12] The proportion of cases giving positive signals for HPV is much higher in cases with multiple confluent lesions than in those with single isolated lesions. It seems possible that the detection of HPV 6/11 in biopsy specimens at initial endoscopy might be a useful prognostic indicator, because those patients whose biopsy tissue shows many nuclei positive for HPV type 6/11, especially on more than one occasion, are more likely to have a worse eventual outcome. The presence of HPV 6/11 may also be used to monitor interferon treatment.[13]

The tendency of papillomas of the larynx to recur and the frequent failure of thorough surgical removal to eradicate laryngeal papillomatosis may be

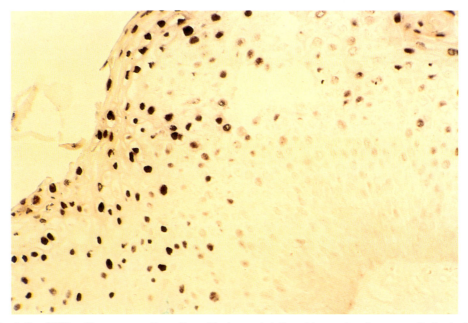

Figure 33.13 Localisation of HPV type 6 in squamous papilloma of larynx. Virus is concentrated in nuclei near surface of squamous epithelium. In situ hybridisation

explained by the presence of the HPV in adjacent normal tissues. In a study of 11 adults with recurrent papillomas of the larynx, it was found that eight had HPV in the contralateral (non-diseased) vocal cord or ventricular fold.[14] The polymerase chain reaction method used to detect the HPV in these areas is far more sensitive than that of immuno-histochemistry or in situ hybridisation, and it seems likely that the copy number of the virus in the non-diseased areas was lower than that in the papillomatous areas. Nevertheless, this study would indicate that laryngeal papillomas are a clinical manifestation of a widespread HPV infection of the laryngeal epithelium.

Transmission of HPV

Condyloma acuminatum is histologically similar to laryngeal papilloma and it has been similarly found to be related to infection with type 6/11 HPV. It is natural therefore to suspect that transmission of the virus from the mother's genital wart to the child's larynx may occur during pregnancy or parturition. Such an association has been confirmed in some series.[15,16] The question as to whether all infants of pregnant mothers with condyloma acuminatum should be delivered by Caesarian section has not yet been answered, however.

References

1. Hellquist H, Cardesa, Gale N et al. Criteria for grading in the Ljubljana classification of epithelial hyperplastic laryngeal lesions. A study by members of the Working Group on Epithelial Hyperplastic Laryngeal Lesions of the European Society of Pathology. Histopathology 1999;34:226–233

2. Murrah VA, Batsakis JG. Proliferative verrucous leukoplakia and verrucous hyperplasia. Ann Otol Rhinol Laryngol 1994;103:660–663

3. Michaels L. The Kambic-Gale method of assessment of epithelial hyperplastic lesions of the larynx in comparison with the dysplasia grade method. Acta Otolaryngol (Stockh) 1997;527(suppl):17–20

4. Lindberg H, Oster S, Oxland I et al. Laryngeal papillomatosis; classification and course. Clin Otolaryngol 1986;11:423–429

5. Bauman NM, Smith RJ. Recurrent respiratory papillomatosis. Pediatr Clin North Am 1996;43:1385–1401

6. Walsh TE, Beamer PR. Epidermoid carcinoma of the larynx occurring in two children with papilloma of larynx. Laryngoscope 1950;60:1110–1124

7. Bewtra C, Krishnan R, Lee SS. Malignant change in non-irradiated juvenile laryngotracheal papillomatosis. Arch Otolaryngol 1982;108:114–116

8. Capper JWR, Bailey CM, Michaels L. Squamous papillomas of the larynx in adults. A review of 63 cases. Clin Otolaryngol 1983;8:109–119

9. Balazic J, Masera A, Poljak M. Sudden death caused by laryngeal papillomatosis. Acta Otolaryngol (Stockh) 1997;527(suppl):111–113

10. Doyle DJ, Gianoli GJ, Espinola T et al. Recurrent respiratory papillomatosis: juvenile versus adult forms. Laryngoscope 1994;104:523–527

11. Lack EE, Jenson AB, Smith HG et al. Immunoperoxidase localization of human papillomavirus in laryngeal papillomas. Intervirology 1980;14:148–154

12. Rimell F, Maisel R, Dayton V. In situ hybridization and laryngeal papillomas. Ann Otol Rhinol Laryngol 1992;101:119–126

13. Steinberg BM, Gallagher T, Stoler M et al. Persistence and expression of human papillomavirus during interferon therapy. Arch Otolaryngol 1988;114:27–32

14. Rihkanen H, Aaltonen L-M, Syrjanen SM. Human papillomavirus and its adjacent normal epithelium. Clin Otolaryngol 1993;18:470–474

15. Quick CA, Watts SL, Krzyzek RA et al. Relationship between condylomata and laryngeal papillomata. Clinical and molecular virological evidence. Ann Otol Rhinol Laryngol 1980;89:467–471

16. Hallden C, Majmudar B. The relationship between juvenile laryngeal papillomatosis and maternal condylomata acuminata. J Reprod Med 1986;31:804–807

34 Squamous Cell Carcinoma: Epidemiology, Early Lesions, Biopsy Diagnosis

Squamous cell carcinoma is by far the commonest neoplasm of the larynx, arising directly in many cases from the squamous epithelium covering the vocal cords; it also frequently arises from the covering epithelium of other parts of the larynx. It is well established that precancerous states frequently precede squamous carcinoma. The fully developed tumour may show a large number of histological variations depending on, among other features, the appearances of its proliferating cells and the amount of keratin produced by them. In addition there are several special forms of squamous cell carcinoma, including verrucous squamous cell carcinoma, spindle cell carcinoma, adenoid squamous carcinoma and basaloid squamous carcinoma, which will be dealt with separately.

Incidence

Squamous carcinoma of the larynx may present as early as the second decade of life and as late as the ninth decade. The mean and median ages of presentation for a sample of 371 patients were found to be 60 years.[1] Laryngeal carcinoma occurs mainly in men. There is evidence that women are becoming increasingly involved by this cancer. In a study over two recent 15-year periods, the male-to-female ratio declined from 5.6:1 to 4.5:1, reflecting a greater incidence among women.[2]

Epidemiological Factors

Cigarette Smoking

There is very strong evidence of a relationship between squamous carcinoma of the larynx and cigarette smoking. The vocal cords are the most susceptible in this regard.[3] As further proof of this causative relationship, it has been found that precancerous lesions are also related to smoking. The degree of precancerous change in autopsy larynges was found to be significantly higher in smokers in proportion to the degree of smoking.[4] More recently, in 148 vocal cords at post-mortem, precancerous changes were found in only 4.2% of non-smokers, and in 12.5% of light smokers, 22.5% of moderate smokers and 47.2% of heavy smokers. In those who had smoked previously but given up, the precancerous changes were present to the same degree as in light smokers, i.e. 12.5%.[5]

Alcohol

Evidence is growing that alcohol may play a part in carcinoma of the larynx. Alcohol carcinogenesis is more difficult to explain than that due to cigarette smoking, in which known carcinogens are involved. The mechanism of carcinogenesis could involve alcohol-related nutritional deficiencies such as zinc or vitamin A.[6] Another possible mechanism could be a synergistic effect on a known carcinogen. Combined alcohol and tobacco consumption shows such an action. In some recent studies the risk ratio of excessive tobacco with excessive alcohol showed an increase that was more in a multiplicative than in an additive manner.[7]

Asbestos Exposure

The inhalation of asbestos fibres predisposes not only to neoplasia of the pleural mesothelium, but also to carcinoma of the lung. It seemed possible that asbestos might act as a carcinogen similarly in the upper part of the respiratory tract. A retrospective study in 1973[8] indicated that laryngeal carcinoma was related to asbestos inhalation. A number of prospective and retrospective studies have been carried out more recently and have shown no definite relationship between asbestos exposure and laryngeal cancer.[9–12] Asbestos bodies have been recovered from the post-mortem larynx after digestion in commercial bleach in two patients who were exposed to asbestos and had asbestos-related pulmonary pathology, but no asbestos bodies or dysplastic changes were seen on histological examination of the mucosa.[13] It is possible that the asbestos bodies in the larynx in these cases were coughed up from the heavily contaminated lungs, rather than having been inhaled and absorbed directly into the larynx.

Exposure to Other Extrinsic Agents

Besides the above extrinsic agents, several others have been considered to be related to carcinoma of the larynx. Mineral oils used in the automobile industry are associated with an almost two-fold excess in larynx cancer risk. Possible risk factors also in this industry are elemental sulphur and polycyclic aromatic hydrocarbons.[14]

Origin

Since the larynx is the commonest site for development of squamous cell carcinoma in the ear, nose and throat and the pathology of squamous carcinoma is similar in most sites, this neoplasm will be discussed in detail in this work only in relation to the larynx.

It is likely that many cases of squamous carcinoma pass through a stage in which malignant changes are present for a time in the epithelium of the larynx without actual deep invasion. Such changes are termed precancerous, and it is important to consider them because it is likely that they represent the earliest treatable form of the malignant process. A precancerous state can be identified at present only by the histological features that the epithelium displays. Active changes that do not usually arouse suspicions of a possible malignant outcome may be identified in the epithelia in which carcinoma frequently grows. Because such changes may sometimes be confused with precancerous changes, we believe that it is preferable to consider them together with the definite precancerous changes under the general designation of hyperplastic lesions.

Squamous carcinomas in the larynx develop not only from the epithelium of the vocal cord, which is normally lined by squamous epithelium, but also from other areas of epithelium, which are normally lined by respiratory epithelium.

Even in large squamous carcinomas of the larynx, histological features are present by which the position of surface origin of the growth may be detected. These features are: (1) hyperplastic changes in the stratified squamous epithelium adjacent to the invading neoplasm and (2) a smooth covering of epithelium from the deep surface of which tongues of carcinoma are emanating. This epithelial surface, which may be keratinised or non-keratinised, is usually carcinomatous itself (Fig. 34.1). Sometimes it is non-malignant epithelium with clearly precancerous features; occasionally squamous epithelium exhibiting a benign-appearing hyperplasia will be seen giving rise to carcinoma (Fig. 34.2). Sometimes even normal-appearing ciliated respiratory epithelium will be the direct source of neoplastic cells, although more usually ciliated epithelium first becomes metaplastic to epidermoid epithelium.

Although the growth of the cancer is at first in the form of a broad band emanating from the field of origin, at certain points tongues of tumour appear to grow more rapidly and penetrate more deeply than the main tumour mass. This may occur anywhere in the field of tumour, and invasion will take place into anatomical structures – muscle, cartilage, ligaments – that are contiguous with the tumour. Certain regions of the larynx, such as the connective tissue adjacent to the saccule or the anterior commissure, seem to be particularly favourable to the spread of squamous carcinoma, and tumour is often seen infiltrating these regions, where it sends out malignant tongues away from the main field.

Hyperplastic Lesions

Since the diagnosis, treatment, and, to some extent, prognosis of laryngeal lesions are related to the histological changes that may be present, it is important that pathologists have a common language among themselves by which they can communicate the histological changes that are present and their interpretation in terms of the expected clinical behaviour of the lesion. It is also essential that clinicians responsible for treating the patients should be familiar with this language. To achieve such communication it is necessary for the histological features of epithelial hyperplastic lesions of the larynx (EHLL) to be separated together into sub-groups, each sub-group having specific microscopic changes and clinical behaviour to be expected. Pathologists and clinicians with experience of working with

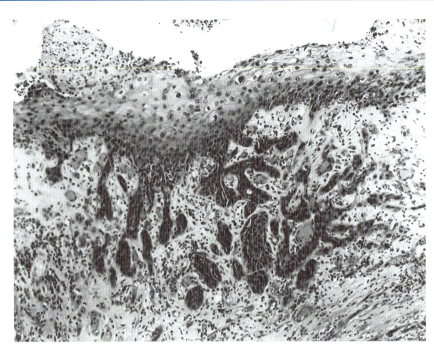

Figure 34.1 Origin of squamous carcinoma from malignant surface squamous epithelium

precancerous lesions will acknowledge the importance to their work of a classification of EHLL common to their colleagues.

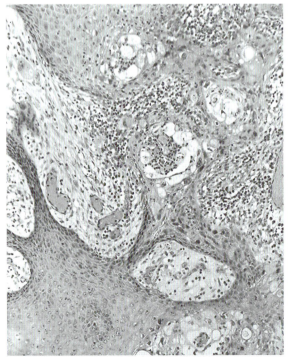

Figure 34.2 Origin of carcinoma from hyperplastic, but not dysplastic, squamous epithelium (*top*)

During the last three decades, however, many classifications of EHLL have been proposed, but comparisons between some of them have proved difficult or even impossible because of inconsistencies in the criteria used for evaluation of the histological features of the EHLL. The majority of such classifications have followed criteria similar to those in common use for the grading of stratified squamous epithelial lesions of the uterine cervix.[15] One of the most widely used of such classifications is that described by the World Health Organization (WHO).[16] In the formal description of EHLL we will first present the features of this one.

It must be admitted that systems of classification for precancerous cervical conditions are not entirely suitable models for laryngeal precancer, however. Recent findings in the epidemiology and molecular biology of laryngeal and cervical squamous epithelial lesions have indicated considerable differences in the aetiology of comparable lesions in the two regions. On the basis of the detection of papillomavirus DNA by molecular hybridisation techniques, a link between human papillomavirus (HPV) infection and cervical precancerous aberrations and carcinoma of the cervix has been well documented in at least 90% of the lesions.[17] Recent investigations, on the other hand, do not support HPV as an important factor in the pathogenesis of EHLL.[18,19] The aetiology of laryngeal carcinoma is more likely to be related to cigarette smoking, alcohol abuse and exposure to other extrinsic irritants, as described above. These factors probably trigger a different pathway of genetic events, not entirely identified, from those recently established in cervical cancer. It would thus be expected that the histological features of precancerous lesions of the larynx might be somewhat different from those seen in the cervix and this is, indeed, the experience of pathologists working in both fields. Classifications of cervical squamous intraepithelial lesions should not, in consequence, be uncritically applied to the laryngeal ones.

Moreover, in regard to laryngeal lesions, there is a pressing need to identify, in the one biopsy, conditions with the substantial hazard of becoming malignant; although still important, such a requirement is not quite so critical with cervical lesions. The laryngeal mucosa is less accessible than the uterine cervix for careful surveillance and biopsy. Furthermore, no operation has been devised on the laryngeal mucosa corresponding to the cone biopsy in the cervix, which removes the whole of the cancer-bearing area and thereby reduces the need for accurately distinguishing between potentially malignant and actual preinvasive carcinoma of the cervix. This distinction is, in contrast, very important in the larynx, where the two lesions are treated differently.

A classification of EHLL, proposed and tested in Ljubljana,[20] does not follow the criteria used for classifying cervical lesions, but was devised to cater to the special clinical and histological problems presented by laryngeal conditions. We will, therefore, first describe the WHO classification and then follow with a description of the the Ljubljana classification of EHLL.

WHO Classification

The WHO classification of EHLL[16] is based on the degree and topographic extent of "dysplasia". Dysplasia of squamous epithelium is defined in the WHO classification as a "precancerous lesion characterised by cellular atypia and loss of normal maturation and stratification short of carcinoma in situ". A benign lesion of "squamous cell hyperplasia" in which there is acanthosis without cellular atypia is also recorded.

Three degrees of dysplasia are recognised:

1. Mild dysplasia – slight nuclear abnormalities, most marked in the basal one-third of the epithelium. A few mitoses may be present in the parabasal layers.
2. Moderate dysplasia – more marked nuclear abnormalities than in mild dysplasia, with prominent nucleoli; changes present in the lower two-thirds of the epithelium. Cell matura-

tion and stratification still evident in the upper layers. Mitoses present in parabasal and intermediate layers.
3. Severe dysplasia – marked nuclear abnormalities and loss of maturation involving more than two-thirds of the epithelial thickness. Maturation and stratification still present in the most superficial layers. Mitoses may be present high up the epithelium and there may be some atypical mitoses.

A fourth precancerous grade of "carcinoma in situ (intraepithelial carcinoma)" is included in the WHO classification of EHLL. In this group the full thickness of the squamous epithelium shows the cellular features of carcinoma without stromal invasion.

The Ljubljana Classification

The main feature by which the Ljubljana classification of EHLL differs from that of the WHO and others is the distinction that is made between benign hyperplasia of basal and parabasal epithelial cells (abnormal hyperplasia) on the one hand and potentially malignant (atypical or risky hyperplasia) cells on the other. We have been involved in a study to examine the criteria for grading in this classification[21] and believe that the use of the Ljubljana classification will improve the accuracy of diagnosis, and, as a result, the efficacy of treatment of laryngeal hyperplastic and early neoplastic lesions.

The grades of the Ljubljana classification are as follows:

1. Simple hyperplasia – a benign hyperplastic process with retention of the normal pattern of the laryngeal epithelium. Epithelium is augmented because of an increased prickle cell layer, with no cellular atypia (Fig. 34.3).
2. Abnormal hyperplasia – a benign augmentation of the basal or parabasal layers. Stratification, a smooth transition from the epithelium of the more basal cells, which are aligned perpendicularly to the basement membrane, to that of the more superficial part, in which the cells are aligned horizontally to the basement membrane, is fully retained. Occasional typical mitoses may be found in or near the basal layer only (Fig. 34.4).
3. Atypical (risky) hyperplasia – a recognisable alteration of epithelial cells towards malignancy. Stratification is still preserved, but nuclei are enlarged and the nuclear contour may be irregular with marked variations in staining intensity. Nucleoli may be increased in number, prominent in size and with enhanced staining

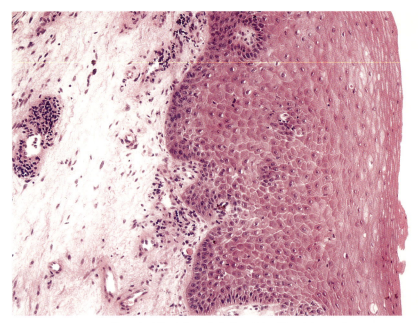

Figure 34.3 Simple hyperplasia. The prickle cell layer is increased

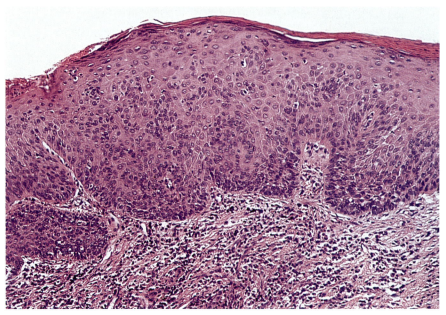

Figure 34.4 Abnormal hyperplasia. There is a marked, but benign augmentation of the basal and parabasal cells

intensity. The nuclear/cytoplasmic ratio is increased. Mitoses are increased, but not numerous and not abnormal. Dyskeratotic cells are frequent (Fig. 34.5). Civatte bodies with hyaline, eosinophilic cytoplasm and pyknotic nuclei may be present (Fig. 34.6). A basal cell type, with no intercellular "prickles" and no increased eosinophilia of cytoplasm or a spinous cell type, with intercellular prickles and

increased eosinophilia of cytoplasm, may be recognised.

4. Carcinoma in situ, in which the features of carcinoma without invasion are present. This can be diagnosed if there are: (1) loss of stratification of epithelium as a whole apart from some superficial compressed and sometimes cornified cells; (2) marked cellular alterations of the type found in invasive carcinoma; and

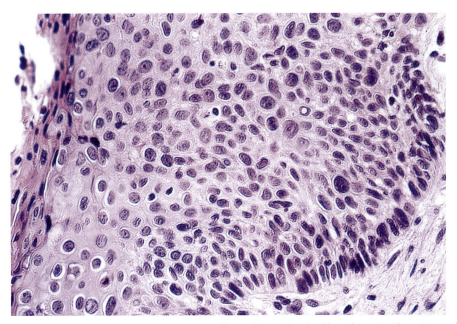

Figure 34.5 Atypical (risky) hyperplasia. Stratification is preserved, but nuclei are enlarged and hyperchromatic with prominent nucleoli

(3) many mitotic figures with some abnormal mitoses (Fig. 34.7). Civatte bodies (see above) may also be present. As in the atypical (risky) hyperplasia grade, the lesion may be designated in some cases as falling within a basal cell type or a spinous cell type. It should be noted that these criteria are advanced and that carcinoma in situ, as diagnosed by these criteria, is rare. It is possible that some EHLL lesions that appear to be earlier forms of precancer may in fact be intraepithelial carcinoma,[22] but this is a defect of all current systems of grading, which do not yet refer to *molecular* rather than morphologic distinctions.

The value of the distinctions made in the Ljubljana classification between the benign, the potentially and the actually malignant forms of epithelial hyperplasias in the larynx has been corroborated not only by many years of experience of its use in Ljubljana, but also by quantitative morphometric analyses and by following up patients with these conditions. In addition studies have been carried out with several supplementary techniques, which reduce reliance on subjective evaluation of epithelial changes. These include numbers of silver-staining nucleolar organiser regions, use of the the proliferative marker, Ki-67 antigen and the demonstration of p53 protein immunoreactivity in greater concentration and more widespread appearance. For each technique an increase in the parameter measured was seen in potentially malignant (atypical) lesions and a further increase in actually malignant (carcinoma in situ) lesions.[21]

Pitfalls in the Diagnosis of EHLL

The diagnosis of EHLL is usually made after examination of small punch biopsies removed at endoscopy. The first requisite for an accurate histological assessment is the correct selection of tissue for biopsy by the surgeon. Failure to remove a representative area for biopsy, or the removal of insufficient tissue, may result in a mistaken histological interpretation of the lesion, which may not be recognised until the patient returns with more advanced

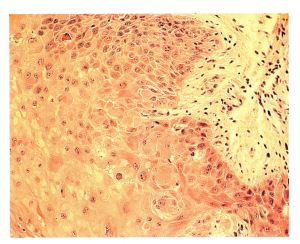

Figure 34.6 Atypical (risky) hyperplasia with Civatte bodies

disease. Some regions are difficult or impossible to

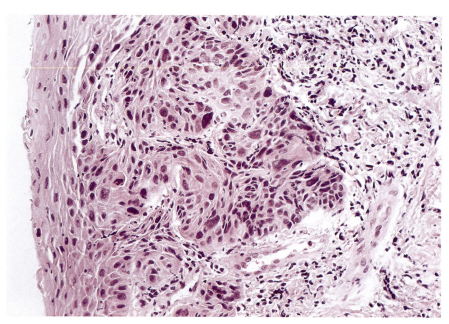

Figure 34.7 Carcinoma in situ. There is loss of stratification, except for a flattening of the superficial part of the epidermis. There is marked nuclear abnormality and numerous mitoses

inspect with the laryngoscope – the subglottis for example, because of the overhanging vocal cords, and the vestibule because of the overhanging false cord or the deep and narrow saccule. The presence of severe inflammatory change and oedema may make it impossible to obtain an adequate biopsy, although it must be admitted that such severe changes are usually to be found in the presence of invasive carcinoma rather than EHHL alone. There is an impression among clinicians that precancerous histological alterations will always provide some gross surface appearances, which, at most sites, will be detected by careful microlaryngoscopy. There is no doubt, however, that some areas of atypical hyperplasia (severe dysplasia) carcinoma in situ, or even invasive carcinoma may be associated with an unremarkable surface appearance. These areas would not be detected and so would not biopsied at laryngoscopy. The clinician may hinder the pathological assessment by tearing the biopsy fragments in the course of removal so that severe artefacts are seen in the final histological preparation.

In the laboratory, correct handling by technologists is very important. Endoscopic punch biopsies are small, and experience in their correct embedding is required to avoid the production of tangential sections of epithelium; with such sections, the diagnosis of EHLL versus invasive carcinoma is difficult since a decision about the presence or absence of invasion requires observation of the relationship of surface epithelium to lamina propria.

Differential Diagnosis

Inflammatory and other non-malignant lesions may be associated with simple hyperplasia and even dysplasia (WHO) of the overlying squamous epithelium, often because of possible confusion with invasive squamous carcinoma, called "pseudo-epitheliomatous hyperplasia". Such changes are well known in relation to tuberculosis (see Chapter 30) and granular cell tumour (see Chapter 37). The specific histological features of tuberculosis in the larynx may, in particular, be slight, and the amount of material available is often very small. The site of a previous biopsy and the surface of a laryngeal nodule may be associated with changes that cause concern with regard to the possibility of a precancerous lesion. One of the commonest causes of such change in laryngeal biopsies, which is unrelated to malignancy, is previous irradiation. The pathologist should always be aware of the clinical history, particularly with regard to previous lesions of the larynx and their treatment.

Carcinomatous tissue identified below the surface of the covering epithelium does not always mean that invasive carcinoma is present. Dysplasia (WHO), (i.e. atypical change, Ljubljana) often develops deep to the columnar cells of the ducts of seromucinous glands of the larynx (Fig. 34.8). The columnar cells may degenerate and disappear or they may not be visible at that site of the particular lesion, and the appearances may be misinterpreted as a focus of invasive squamous cell carcinoma.

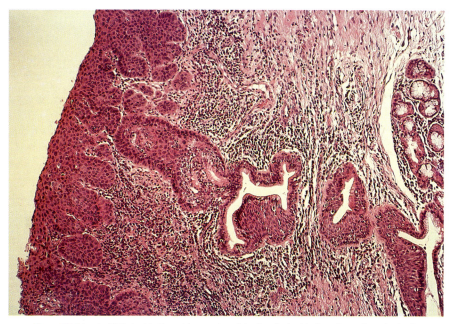

Figure 34.8 Atypical (risky) epithelium with extension of the disturbed epithelium along a duct of a gland

Laryngeal Biopsy

Laryngoscopy

The larynx is a relatively inaccessible organ, and the difficulties of reaching its inner surface during life, of inspecting it and of sampling it for histological examination have hampered the understanding of its disease processes. In the 19th century, examination with a mirror – indirect laryngoscopy – was carried out with very great skill by the master laryngologists such as Sir Morell Mackenzie. Even biopsy was carried out by this means – a remarkable feat when it is recalled that topical anaesthesia by the use of cocaine was not introduced until 1884.

Observation and biopsy using a mirror were later replaced by direct observation and biopsy through a laryngoscope tube. This latter procedure, which can be carried out either under local or, more usually, general anaesthesia, has led to an intimate knowledge of the changes in the larynx with disease.

Following the use of the colposcope for diseases of the cervix uteri, a microscopic procedure was introduced for direct laryngoscopy. With such an instrument, not only could the mucosa of the larynx be observed under magnification, but also operative manipulations, especially biopsy, could be carried out with the greatest precision. Microlaryngoscopy under general anaesthesia is now the standard method in most ear, nose and throat clinics for the investigation of the pathology of laryngeal diseases.

At microlaryngoscopy the surgeon clearly observes the superior surfaces of the vocal cords, and even the subepithelial capillary plexus of the cords is seen. Some of the subglottis can be seen and a better view is obtained by gently displacing the vocal cords laterally. The respiratory epithelium covering the posterior surface of the epiglottis, the false cords and the rest of the supraglottis is dull red in colour, in contrast to the whiteness of the true vocal cords. The lower part of the laryngeal ventricle can be observed by some gentle displacement of the false cords. The appearances of the interior of the larynx can be photographed in still photography, moving picture and television camera for recording on videotape. Remarkably vivid magnified photographs have been produced by these means.

Biopsy Procedure

An important factor in the success of laryngoscopic biopsy as a diagnostic procedure is the rapid and efficient handling of the specimen as soon as it is removed. The great majority of biopsies will be fixed in 10% formaldehyde solution, and subsequently processed and embedded in paraffin wax prior to histological sectioning. The biopsy fragment is conveniently fixed immediately by washing the tip of the biopsy forceps in formaldehyde fixative as soon as they are removed from the patient. Specimens may also be required in a fresh unfixed state for frozen section, microbiological culture, or other laboratory studies. Under these circumstances they should be handled in the necessary way immediately in the operating room; if this is not possible, great speed is required in transporting them to the laboratory because drying is very rapid. If the laboratory is more than 3 min away, the specimen should be wrapped in gauze moistened with saline and placed in a closed bottle.

Range of Pathological Conditions that may be Diagnosed by Laryngoscopic Biopsy

A wide range of pathological conditions of the larynx may be diagnosed by endoscopic laryngeal biopsy. A list would cover almost the whole spectrum of laryngeal pathology.

A large proportion of laryngeal biopsies are from vocal cord nodules or polyps. Tissue is removed in these cases primarily as treatment for the lesion, but the opportunity is usually taken to submit the material removed to the pathologist for confirmation of the diagnosis. Other inflammatory lesions with a non-specific histological appearance that may be submitted are intubation and pyogenic granulomas. These are composed of granulation tissue and situated in the posterior part of the glottis so that it is important for the pathologist to know the site of the lesion on the vocal cord.

Post-irradiation biopsies are frequently carried out to detect persistence or regrowth of the neoplasm in the larynx. A problem that frequently causes difficulty is when should an irradiated cancer be biopsied so as to be sure that any carcinomatous tissue present is "viable", i.e. truly composed of actively growing malignant tissue? There may be cancer cells present that have been inactivated by the irradiation so that they will not grow, and will eventually disappear. These cells may show no morphological difference from growing cancer cells. A categorical answer to this question thus cannot be given. There is probably a marked variation in the reaction to irradiation of neoplasms of different patients and of different parts of a single neoplasm in the same patient. There is a period of time after irradiation when the tumour cells that are about to die appear normal; this period is subject to those very variations. In most clinics a period of 6 weeks is allowed to elapse after irradiation before a biopsy procedure is carried out, but it must be admitted that this is a purely arbitrary period. In the interpretation of biopsy material taken after radiation therapy, a policy that we would recommend is as follows:

1. If overt cancer tissue is found it should be reported as such. The decision as to whether it

is "viable" or "non-viable" must rest with the clinician who has been observing the area where tumour has been present. Growth in the area would suggest active tumour. Increased ulceration may be entirely an irradiation effect.

2. Histological features that are less definite for malignancy are reported on conservatively. In these cases the Ljubljana classification is particularly useful since it allows a clear separation between non-malignant (abnormal) and potentially malignant (atypical).

Frequently the only hope for successful treatment after failed irradiation is drastic surgery such as laryngectomy. A report of malignancy must, therefore, be given only with confidence. Thus if there is any doubt, an equivocal diagnosis should be rendered and rebiopsy requested.

Frozen Section

Frozen sections for rapid diagnosis of laryngoscopy biopsy specimens should be used only rarely. Modern methods of producing frozen sections with a cryostat microtomy for sectioning of the frozen tissue often produce excellent results and the technique is useful in making surgical decisions when fairly large biopsies of tissue can be provided. However, laryngoscopic biopsies are usually small. Frozen section of such specimens is technically more difficult and, because of the small size of the specimen, is more likely to lead to artefacts resulting from the freezing procedure. The appearances of a block of tissue that has once been frozen and then thawed and subjected to routine paraffin procedures are somewhat impaired for purposes of diagnostic pathology. Such deterioration is of little import when large specimens are available for histological sampling, for other slices can be subjected to the more usual fixation and embedding procedures while the frozen section is being carried out. Thus conventionally processed sections will be available afterwards as well as the somewhat distorted tissue obtained from thawed frozen section blocks. Such a procedure is not usually possible with the very limited biopsy material obtained at laryngoscopy. If these specimens are frozen, the pathologist will obtain permanent sections only of the tissue fragments that have suffered from freezing and then thawing.

There are, however, indications for the occasional frozen section to be carried out on laryngoscopy specimens:

1. In some cases no histological diagnosis can be obtained after repeated direct laryngoscopies (each requiring a general anaesthetic) with

biopsy have been carried out. Such cases include those of carcinoma with overhanging areas of inflammation or oedema so that diagnostic tumour tissue cannot be obtained. Under these circumstances a frozen section may be of help in guaranteeing that the biopsy has yielded some diagnostic material.

2. Special procedures may be required in a particular case, such as electron microscopy, microbiological culture or immunological assay. Frozen sections may be obtained so that an immediate decision can be made as to whether such special laboratory procedures should be carried out and what they should be.

References

1. Huygen PLM, Van den Broek P, Kazem I. Age and mortality in laryngeal cancer. Clin Otolaryngol 1980;5:129–137
2. DeRienzo DP, Greenberg SD, Fraire AE. Carcinoma of the larynx. Changing incidence in women. Arch Otolaryngol Head Neck Surg 1991;117:681–684
3. Stell PM. Smoking and laryngeal cancer. Lancet 1972;I:617–618
4. Auerbach O, Hammond EC, Garfinkel L. Histologic changes in the larynx in relation to smoking habits. Cancer 1970;25:92–104
5. Müller KM, Krohn BR. Smoking habits and their relationship to precancerous lesions of the larynx. J Cancer Res Clin Oncol 1980;96:211–217
6. McCoy GD, Hecht SS, Wynder EL. The roles of tobacco, alcohol and diet in the etiology of upper alimentary respiratory tract cancers. Prev Med 1980;9:622–629
7. Maier H, Dietz A, Gewelke U et al. Tobacco and alcohol and the risk of head and neck cancer. Clin Investig 1992;70:320–327
8. Stell PM, McGill T. Asbestos and laryngeal carcinoma. Lancet 1973;II:416–417
9. Hinds MW, Thomas DB, O'Reilly HP. Asbestos, dental X-rays, tobacco and alcohol in the epidemiology of laryngeal cancer. Cancer 1979;44:1114–1120
10. Newhouse ML, Gregory MM, Shannon H. Etiology of carcinoma of the larynx. In: Lyon JC (ed) Biological effects of mineral fibres, vol. 2. IARC Scientific Publications, no. 30, 1980, pp 687–695
11. Ahrens W, Jockel, KH, Patzak W et al. Alcohol, smoking, and occupational factors in cancer of the larynx: a case-control study. Am J Ind Med 1991;20:477–493
12. Muscat JE, Wynder EL. Tobacco, alcohol, asbestos, and occupational risk factors for laryngeal cancer. Cancer 1992;69:2244–2251
13. Roggli VL, Greenberg SD, McLarty JL et al. Asbestos body content of the larynx in asbestos workers. A study of five cases. Arch Otolaryngol 1980;106:533–535
14. Eisen EA, Tolbert PE, Hallock MF et al. Mortality studies of machining fluid exposure in the automobile industry. III: A case-control study of larynx cancer. Am J Ind Med 1994;26:185–202
15. Scully RE. Histological typing of female genital tract tumours, 2nd edn. Springer, Berlin, 1994
16. Shanmugaratnam K, Sobin LH. Histological typing of tumours of the upper respiratory tract and ear. WHO international histological classification of tumours, 2nd edn. Springer-Verlag, Berlin, Heidelberg, New York, 1991
17. zur Hausen H. Papilloma virus infections – a major cause of human cancers. Biochim Biophys Acta 1996;1288:F55-F78
18. Gallo O, Bianchi S, Giannini A et al. Lack of detection of human papillomavirus (HPV) in transformed laryngeal keratoses by in situ hybridisation (ISH) technique. Acta Otolaryngol (Stockh) 1994;114:213–217
19. Rihkanen H, Peltomaa J, Syrjanen S. Prevalence of human papillomavirus (HPV) DNA in vocal cords without laryngeal papillomas. Acta Otolaryngol (Stockh) 1994;114:348–351
20. Kambic V, Gale N. Epithelial hyperplastic lesions of the larynx. Elsevier, Amsterdam, 1995
21. Hellquist H, Cardesa A, Gale N et al. Criteria for grading in the Ljubljana classification of epithelial hyperplastic laryngeal lesions. A study by members of the Working Group on Epithelial Hyperplastic Lesions of the European Society of Pathology. Histopathology 1999;34:226–233
22. Hellquist H, Cardesa A, Gale N et al. (Letter) Histopathology 1999;35:181

35 Pathology of Invasive Squamous Cell Carcinoma

The TNM system of staging of laryngeal carcinoma divides laryngeal tumours into supraglottic, glottic and subglottic.[1] The terms are not used purely as anatomical descriptions, but, more than this, to designate three embryologically distinct regions, each of which gives rise to its own type of neoplasm. Origin of a carcinoma from two adjacent regions is held to indicate "invasion" or "extension" from one of these regions to the other and hence to necessitate a higher, i.e. more serious, grading. The concept of the separate embryological development of the three parts of the larynx is unproven, however. The most frequent site for the localisation of carcinoma is the anterior part of the vocal cords and the diameter of the tumour is usually small. It may be that a similarly small neoplasm happens to arise across the arbitrarily designated boundary of glottis and supraglottis or glottis and subglottis. The behaviour of such a neoplasm is not necessarily more aggressive. Laryngeal neoplasms, however, do possess different innate biological properties of growth activity and aggressiveness, which may be related to original size but cannot be predicted from involvement of more than one region.

Gross Appearances

The commonest site for squamous carcinoma of the larynx is at the anterior part of the true cord. However, the lesion may be seen anywhere in the larynx. It is least frequent in a posterior situation. Whatever its size and situation, by far the most usual gross appearance is that of a flat plaque with a well-defined, somewhat raised, edge and a surface that ranges from occasional furrows to marked corrugation. Cut surface reveals this structure to consist of a pale-grey band of variable thickness (Figs 35.1–35.6).

Ulceration is sometimes present. Transverse slices of the larynx through the neoplasm reveal that the ulcerated areas represent merely superficial losses of tumour. They rarely extend to the depths of the neoplasm, and do not involve normal laryngeal tissues. Tumours, particularly in the supraglottic region, frequently show one or more sinuses, which extend deeply into the growth. Sometimes these are very narrow and slit-like (Fig. 35.1). Histological examination always shows a malignant squamous epithelial surface lining the whole sinus or slit, often with areas of necrosis and fibrin exudation. These deficiencies of the tumour may be related to ischaemia in parts furthest away from the blood supply.

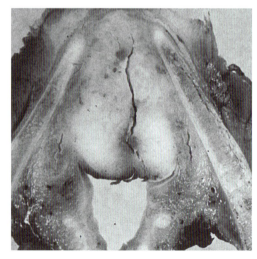

Figure 35.1 Transverse slice of supraglottic carcinoma showing deep slit in substance of tumour

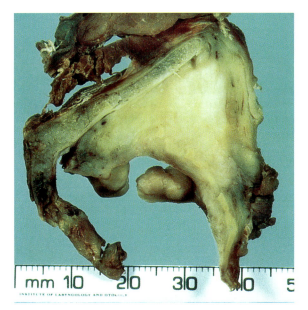

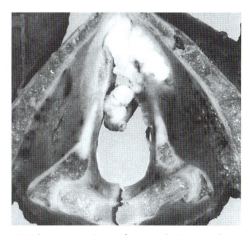

Figure 35.4 Squamous carcinoma of anterior glottic region. The neoplasm shows a papillary aspect as well as that of a flat plaque

Figure 35.2 Supraglottic carcinoma with deep invasion of pre-epiglottic space. Note pale yellow bars of epiglottic cartilage through which tumour has invaded

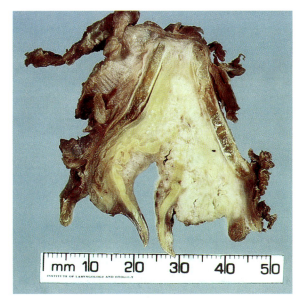

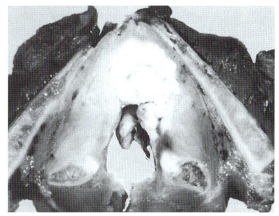

Figure 35.5 Anterior right squamous carcinoma of glottic region. Note the papillary part of the neoplasm. The fits into the anterior part of the left laryngeal ventricle. There was a saccular mucocele above this on the left side

Figure 35.3 Supraglottic portion of origin of extensive carcinoma. There is penetration of the epiglottic cartilage by growth, and the tumour has reached the piriform sinus on the right side

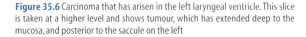

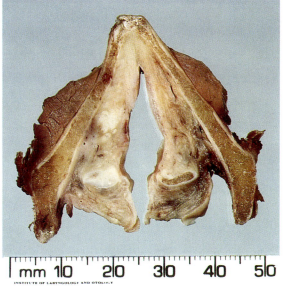

Figure 35.6 Carcinoma that has arisen in the left laryngeal ventricle. This slice is taken at a higher level and shows tumour, which has extended deep to the mucosa, and posterior to the saccule on the left

In a small proportion of cases the tumours may show one or more papillary elements (Figs 35.4, 35.5). These are most common in the glottic and subglottic regions, but are occasionally found in the supraglottic portion of a laryngeal neoplasm. When arising from the vocal cord they may grow into the contralateral ventricle and, by occluding it, give rise to a mucocele of the saccule on that side (Fig. 35.5) (see Chapter 29). Papillary areas of squamous cell carcinoma usually coexist with the flat type of neoplasm; they rarely exist as a single gross entity.

Microscopic Appearances

The histological features of squamous carcinoma are extremely variable, and in a particular neoplasm result from the proportions of the different epidermoid components that are present (Fig. 35.7). Like normal squamous cell epithelium, these include undifferentiated basal cells, intermediate "prickle" cells, cells containing keratohyaline granules and acellular keratinous material. Glycogen is also found in varying amounts, sometimes large, within the epithelial cells of a squamous carcinoma. So squamous carcinoma of the larynx may display trabeculae formed largely of proliferated malignant basal cells, prominent groups of large pale cells with intercellular bridges ("prickles"), large areas of fully keratinised cells, often anucleate, or many cells vacuolated from the presence of cytoplasmic glycogen. Malignant basal type cells, sometimes including a few "prickle" cells, in other instances composed of rows of single cell width, may give an irregular

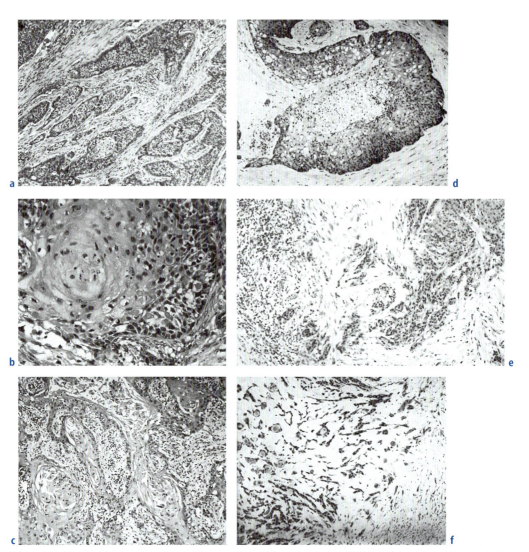

Figure 35.7 Histological features of squamous carcinoma of larynx. **a** Basal cell form of carcinoma. **b** "Prickle" cell hyperplasia with keratohyaline granules. **c** Abundant keratin formation. **d** Numerous glycogen-filled (clear) cells. **e** Irregular jagged margin. **f** Invading cells rows of but one cell thick

jagged margin to the tumour. Tumour edges composed of "prickle" cells and keratinised cells tend to form large round masses sometimes referred to as "pushing" margins, suggesting that they invade by pressure rather than by cell infiltration. Some squamous carcinomas show a constant "mix" of the squamous elements throughout the whole tumour. The majority, however, show considerable variation from one part of the neoplasm to another.

Relation of Differentiation to Prognosis

Assessment of the degree of differentiation is often carried out by pathologists to obtain an impression of the aggressiveness of the neoplasm. An overall impression of the degree of differentiation of the worst differentiated area is the method commonly used, using the categories of well, moderately and poorly differentiated. The validity of this method is open to serious doubt because of its subjective nature and the variations in differentiation which may be frequently observed in different parts of the same neoplasm.

To address these problems attempts have been made to quantitate the assessment of differentiation. These range from simply counting the proportion of differentiated cells in the neoplasm[2] (the Broders method) to quantifying the features of differentiation at the growing edge of the cancer.[3,4] None of these quantitative methods have become widely used by pathologists probably because of their time-consuming nature and doubts about reproducibility and interpretation.

A method of assessing biopsies that is simple, reproducible and highly predictive for the outcome of the cancer growth in laryngeal and hypopharyngeal squamous carcinomas has been put forward, but is not yet widely used in diagnostic histopathology. In the method the histopathologist need assess only whether the tumour is "well-differentiated", i.e. contains keratin, or "anaplastic", i.e. is without keratin.[5] Using this system there was an over 98% agreement between the initial report and that given by a reviewer. In an analysis of 1315 patients there was a highly significant difference between the observed survival and tumour-free rates for patients with well-differentiated and anaplastic lesions over a 10-year period, the well-differentiated group having the better outlook.

Spread from Laryngeal Airway Origin

The anatomical routes of invasion of squamous carcinoma arising from the epithelium of the laryngeal airway depend on the site of origin of the neoplasm within the larynx. The tumour usually invades outwards at right angles to the surface of origin. In some places the spread of the carcinoma is favoured in a different plane, e.g. adjacent to the saccule.

Supraglottic Region

Epiglottic Region

In the supraglottis, tumours that arise from the laryngeal surface of the epiglottis invade towards and then through the epiglottic cartilage. The perforating seromucinous glands of that cartilage often provide pathways for its penetration, but penetration of the elastic cartilage itself by the tumour is sometimes seen. Anterior to the fixed portion of the epiglottis lies a zone of adipose connective tissue – the pre-epiglottic space – and entry of carcinoma therein is frequent after its passage through the epiglottic cartilage (Figs 35.2, 35.3). In some cases the full thickness of the pre-epiglottic space is traversed by the neoplasm as far as the anterior boundary, which is the hyoid bone; sometimes even that structure may be entered. Thus the hyoid bone should be examined for tumour grossly and microscopically at least whenever the pre-epiglottic space has been found to be deeply invaded by neoplasm.

A special form of carcinoma in the epiglottic region has been separated by German authors and designated "Winkelkarzinom" or "corner carcinoma".[6] This arises laterally in the region of the edge of the epiglottic cartilage. It invades into the pre-epiglottic space by passing around the edge of the epiglottic cartilage and only at a late stage of the tumour is the lateral edge of the epiglottic cartilage destroyed.

Aryepiglottic Fold Region

Lower down the supraglottis and more laterally, the aryepiglottic fold epithelium may be the source of tumour, which may invade that thin fold from medial to lateral side to attain and even invade the mucosa of the piriform fossa.

False Cord Region

Tumours originating on the false cords and glottis may also reach this surface, since the piriform fossa extends downwards from a level behind the upper supraglottis to the upper subglottis. In its path of invasion, lower supraglottic tumour first encounters the thyroarytenoid muscle. The thyroid cartilage laterally and the arytenoid cartilage posteriorly may then be invaded by tumour arising at this level. Carcinoma arising from the laryngeal ventricular epithelium in continuity with higher supraglottic or lower vocal cord epithelium seems to have a special tendency to invade laryngeal connective tissue in an upward direction in relation to the laryngeal saccule, the presence of which seems to facilitate local growth of that tumour to its medial, lateral or posterior aspects (Fig. 35.6). (Carcinoma arising from ventricle alone with or without saccular origin seems to spread only outward, and slowly – see Chapter 36.)

Posterior Supraglottic Region

Rarely squamous carcinoma arises from the posterior supraglottic epithelium. Invasion then is into the apical portion of the arytenoid cartilage, interarytenoid muscle and hyopharyngeal submucosa.

Glottic Region

The field of carcinoma that includes the glottic area often shows origin of carcinoma in the region of the anterior commissure. Here the neoplasm is separated from the angle of the thyroid cartilage by only a very small band of connective tissue (Fig. 35.8); as a result, invasion of the thyroid cartilage in this region is very common. More posteriorly, neoplasm arising on the vocal cord passes into the thyroary-

tenoid muscle and then on to the thyroid cartilage. Invading posterolaterally, it can reach the piriform fossa and posteriorly the arytenoid cartilage.

Posterior origin of glottic carcinoma is rare. It is especially noteworthy because, unlike the region of vocal cord where the lymph supply of Reinke's space is poor, the lymphatics of this region are similarly abundant to those in the supra- and subglottis. Lymph node metastases from tumours in the posterior glottis thus should be expected early.

Subglottic Region

Anterior Superior

That portion of the neoplasm that arises in the subglottic region, if anterior, will come against the cricothyroid membrane. This sometimes, but not always, is penetrated by subglottic carcinoma (Figs 35.9, 35.10). Frequently, tumour that has penetrated the cricothyroid membrane has arisen from above, where it is derived from neoplasm that has entered the thyroid cartilage in the supraglottic and/or glottic region, and then expanding ("ballooning" out, see below) that cartilage as it spreads within it as far as its inferior end. It then enters the cricothyroid ligament and may grow out of the larynx easily from that situation.

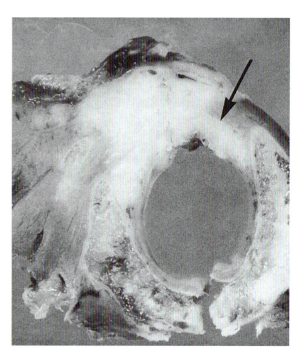

Figure 35.9 Invasion of the cricothyroid membrane by carcinoma. The intact membrane on the right not yet invaded is shown by an *arrow*

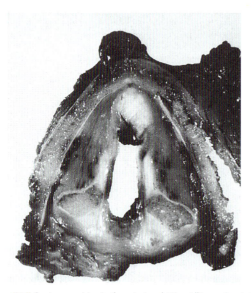

Figure 35.8 Carcinoma arising in the anterior glottic midline region. In the midline the tumour has penetrated the narrow anterior commissure connective tissue almost as far as the thyroid cartilage

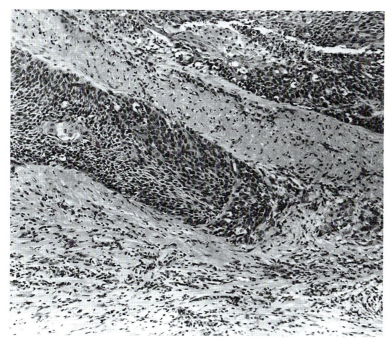

Figure 35.10 Histological section of cricothyroid membrane from Fig. 35.9. Columns of carcinoma are seen infiltrating the elastic fibres of the membrane

One or two lymph nodes are inconstantly found anterior to the cricothyroid membrane. These are termed the Delphian nodes and may be the seat of metastases from tumours invading in this region.[7]

Posterior and Lateral

In other parts of the subglottis, tumour will tend to invade the local muscles and cartilages in which it finds itself; the cricoarytenoid joint and cricoid lamina are sometimes invaded by posteriorly located neoplasm (Fig. 35.11). On rare occasions the tumour will penetrate the lamina of the cricoid and reach the posterior cricoarytenoid muscle. The lateral cricoarytenoid muscle, on the other hand, is frequently invaded by subglottic neoplasm, and the lower thyroid lamina above and the cricoid ring below are potential cartilage targets for invasion by such tumours.

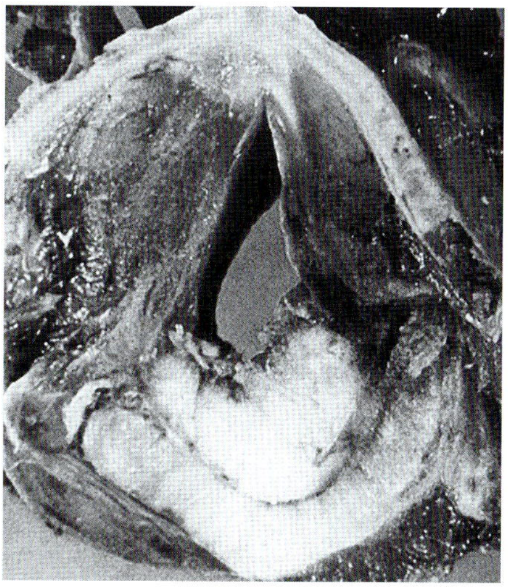

Figure 35.11 Posterior origin and growth of squamous carcinoma in subglottic region in vicinity of cricoid lamina, which lies immediately behind the tumour

Invasion of the Cartilaginous Framework

It has been accepted for many years that hyaline cartilage in areas such as the epiphyseal plate, bronchus, intervertebral disc and larynx is highly resistant to invasion by carcinoma or sarcoma. This has been studied particularly with regard to osteosarcoma, a malignant tumour that usually arises in the metaphyseal region of a long bone. As it grows it fills the marrow space in the bone and replaces the cancellous bone, but when it reaches the epiphyseal plate further penetration appears to be halted until a very late stage of the disease. With regard to the larynx, it has been repeatedly stressed in the literature that invasion takes place preferentially into ossified areas, and that invasion of non-ossified areas is rare. These statements are not in keeping with our observations on the invasion of the laryn-

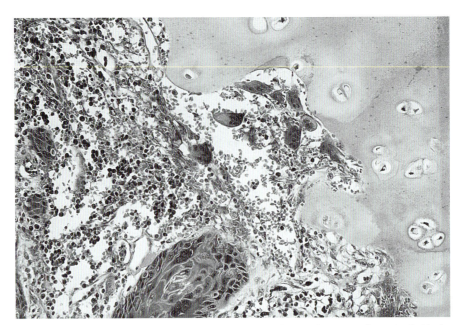

Figure 35.12 Invasion of non-ossified thyroid cartilage by squamous carcinoma. Note layer of multinucleate giant cells associated with a lacuna at the interface between tumour and cartilage

geal framework by squamous carcinoma. Gross and microscopic study of laryngeal squamous carcinoma that is invading the cartilage frequently shows extensive invasion in non-ossified cricoid and thyroid cartilages. At the interface of squamous carcinoma with cartilage, multinucleated giant cells are present in most cases, and the giant cells are frequently lodged in lacunae, indicating that they are producing resorption of cartilage (Fig. 35.12).

The thyroid cartilage is much more ossified in the presence of non-invading carcinoma than when the carcinoma actively invades the cartilage.[8] The most probable explanation for this is that the thyroid cartilage frequently ossifies near squamous carcinoma, especially where there is no invasion. Histological examination of the cartilage near the tumour in these larynges shows that it has formed woven bone; this may be seen in the cricoid and arytenoid in the vicinity of carcinoma as well as in the thyroid. It is thus possible that where a neoplasm is insufficiently aggressive to invade cartilage, its continued presence near the cartilage may induce ossification. This observation may be of diagnostic value in the radiological demonstration of carcinoma by computerised tomography usually in the vicinity of the arytenoid.[9] The arytenoid was most often affected by sclerotic bony change in these cases, and showed increased density on the side affected by tumour in comparison with its fellow on the normal side. The pathological changes shown at the sites of involvement were proximity of tumour to cartilage, often with perichondritis apparently provoked by adjacent tumour and associated with woven bone formation.

A striking mode of spread of squamous carcinoma through the thyroid cartilage – "ballooning" – is seen in some cases. Tumour enters the thyroid cartilage, often in the anterior commissure region (see above), and then burrows through the cartilage and appears to blow out the outer shell of cartilage from within (Figs 35.13, 35.14). Most of the ballooned thyroid cartilage is unossified. In this way tumour frequently reaches the lower border of the thyroid cartilage, enters the cricothyroid membrane, and may leave the larynx.

Spread Outside the Larynx

Stomal Recurrence

In approximately 10% of cases the operation of laryngectomy for squamous carcinoma is followed by recurrence in the tracheostomy stoma. Risk factors for this are particularly an advanced primary tumour in the larynx (stage T4), subglottic involvement of the primary carcinoma, and the necessity for a preoperative tracheostomy having to be done.[10] The deposits of carcinoma grow not in the main skin scar, but in the mucocutaneous junction of the tracheostomy that is produced at the laryngectomy.

The mechanism for tracheostomal recurrence is still not known. It has been suggested that it may result from deposition of cancer cells in the wound from the main specimen at the time of operation. Other suggestions that have been made are exten-

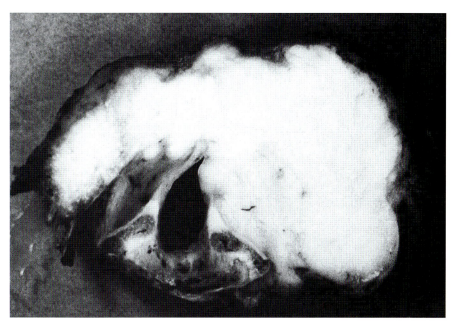

Figure 35.13 Invasion of thyroid cartilage by carcinoma in glottic region with ballooning effect. A thin rim of surviving cartilage can be seen around the neoplasm in some places

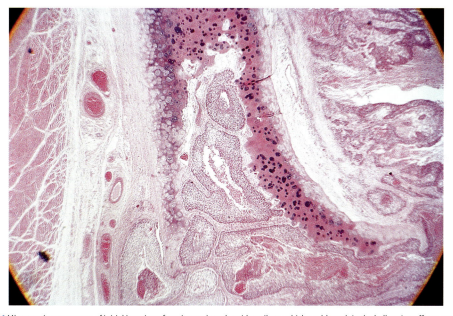

Figure 35.14 Microscopic appearance of initial invasion of carcinoma into thyroid cartilage, which could result in the ballooning effect seen in Fig. 35.13

sion from nearby lymph nodes involved by metastasis, development of an additional primary and extension of neoplasm from the margin of resection. Recurrences nearly always take place in the presence of extensive inoperable neoplasm, although the latter is often occult. Histological observations on specimens of stomal recurrences would favour the concept of a new primary derived from the tracheal mucosa near the mouth of the stoma. In two biopsy specimens of stomal recurrence, the squamous carcinoma was clearly arising from the mucosal epithelial covering of the tracheostomy in the manner described in Chapter 34. In one of these two cases, no nodule had been detected in the tracheostomy stoma clinically. The primary growth was a hypopharyngeal one, with extension of tumour into the larynx, and tracheostomy had been required before the operation to relieve airway obstruction.

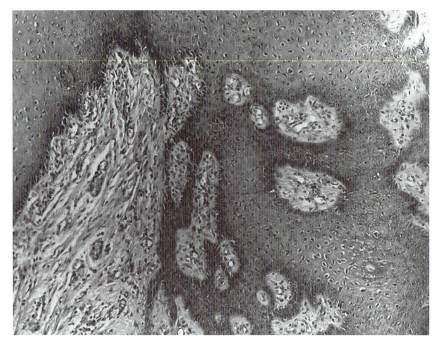

Figure 35.15 New primary squamous carcinoma in tracheostomy opening, which had been made before resection of larynx

Resection of the pharynx, larynx and tracheostomy stoma was carried out. There was no gross abnormality of the stoma, but on examination of a routine section of the tracheostomy opening, an early invasive carcinoma arising from the local mucosa was found (Fig. 35.15). These observations would suggest that the presence of extensive local squamous carcinoma induces the epithelium of the tracheostomy to become malignant.

Lymph Node Metastasis

Squamous cell carcinoma of the larynx has a high tendency to metastasise to cervical lymph nodes. This is particularly prominent in larger invasive tumour; in such cases a careful study of the histological sections of the primary growth will often reveal evidence of invasion along lymphatic vessels. In smaller localised tumours, particularly of the glottis, lymph node metastasis is unusual. In larger tumours, particularly of the supra- and subglottis, metastases in lymph nodes are frequent (see Chapter 44).

Bloodstream Metastasis

In any post-mortem study on patients dying of carcinoma of the larynx, it is found that the majority have bloodstream metastases.[11,12] Bloodstream metastases from squamous carcinoma of the larynx are most common in the lungs. They are also frequently seen in the liver, bones and mediastinal lymph nodes. In all cases showing bloodstream metastases, cervical lymph node metastases are present or have become manifest and have been treated.

Radiation Perichondritis

Synonyms for radiation perichondritis are radiation necrosis and chondroradionecrosis. Clinical features suggestive of perichondritis of laryngeal cartilage are sometimes encountered at a later stage in patients who have been irradiated for malignant disease of the larynx. The incidence of this complication varies greatly between centres. In one, it was stated to be "extremely rare";[13] in another, it occurred in nine out of 123 patients (7%).[14] The use of hyperbaric oxygen as a concomitant to radiotherapy for carcinoma of the larynx appears to increase markedly the risk of radiation perichondritis.[15] Pathological examination of larynges removed after radiation therapy for carcinoma in yet another centre showed radiation necrosis in 26%.[16] In that paper, necrosis of cartilage was equated with acute inflammation, and the necrotic changes as so defined were ascribed in many of the cases to the presence of tumour. Using criteria only of gross and microscopic damage to cartilage following irradia-

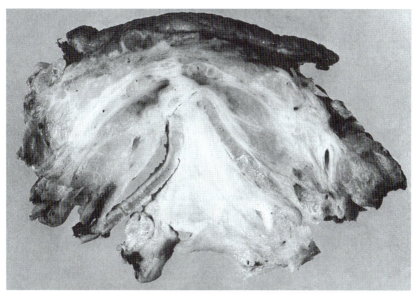

Figure 35.16 Transverse slice of larynx from aryepiglottic fold region. Radiation perichondritis of left thyroid ala. There is cavitation along both medial and lateral surfaces of the left thyroid ala. The edges of the cavities are lined by pale-grey material (yellow in original), which corresponds to purulent deposit, and there is fine irregular erosion of the edges of the adjacent cartilage. The mucosa, lamina propria and surrounding strap muscles are markedly thickened by fibrosis

tion, we have examined larynges with such damage (unpublished observations). In most of these cases laryngectomy was carried out because conservative treatment for the radiation perichondritis was not successful. In some there was a clinical impression, uncorroborated by biopsy, that the larynx contained an advancing carcinoma.

Gross Appearances

Gross examination of the larynx usually shows fibrous thickening of the mucosa with narrowing of the airway. Cartilaginous change is present at the perichondrial surface as a pale-yellow, opaque area. In some places the yellowed cartilage is fragmented. There are always gaps in the substance of the cartilage in this region. These gaps are usually parallel to the mucosal (medial) perichondrium of the thyroid or cricoid cartilage, and sometimes in a similar position in relation to the external (lateral) perichondrial layer of those cartilages (Fig. 35.16). Affected cartilages in descending order of frequency are the thyroid, the arytenoid and the cricoid cartilages. In some cases sinuses extended from gaps in the continuity of the cartilage medially to the laryngeal ventricle, where they became continuous with the airway of the larynx. A comparison of the sites of laryngeal damage found at pathology with the clinically observed position of the neoplasm has indicated that in many cases the radiation damage was

on the other side of the larynx to the clinically observed position of the tumour.

Microscopic Appearances

The pale-yellow infiltrate of the cartilage and of the surrounding connective tissue represents a large acute abscess in each case. Neutrophils of the abscess encroach on and erode the cartilage in an irregular fashion (Fig. 35.17). There are large empty spaces within or adjacent to the abscesses, presumably related to enzymatic lysis of the abscess material. This would correspond to the observation of gas bubbles adjacent to the thyroid cartilage in three of nine cases in a study of irradiation damage to the larynx by computerised tomography scan.[17]

In the vicinity of each abscess the cartilage shows an extensive area of tinctorial change, usually staining in an eosinophilic fashion. In some areas there is degeneration of chondrocytes, but in many areas these cells show only slight alterations, even close up to the edge of the abscess (Fig. 35.17). Small fragments of cartilage are sometimes seen loose within the abscess, but even here the chondrocytes, although often somewhat retracted from the wall of their lacunae in the cartilage, still show normally staining nucleus and cytoplasm (Fig. 35.18).

In the connective tissue around the abscess in each case there is an irregular deposition of fibrin. Collagen replacement of fibrin is frequent, and within the collagen, fibroblasts are seen, which are

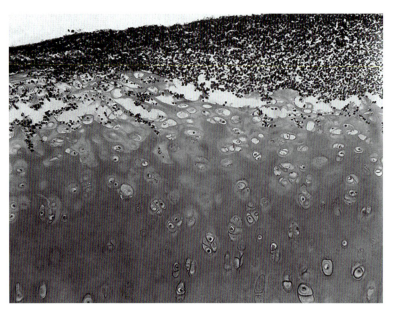

Figure 35.17 Edge of thyroid cartilage showing erosion by pus cells in a case of radiation damage. Note surviving cartilage cells up to region of pus

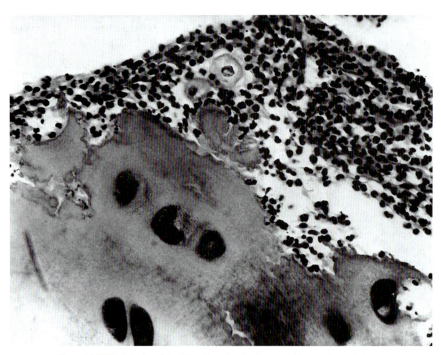

Figure 35.18 Eroded edge of thyroid cartilage showing loose, surviving cartilage cells in pus

often the "atypical" type frequently apparent after radiation damage. In some areas, fibrous replacement of areas of damaged cartilage has taken place. Granulation tissue and histiocytic cell infiltration are sometimes also present in the submucosal tissues adjacent to abscesses. Fibrosis, atrophy and regenerative changes of skeletal muscle, with numerous atypical giant cells of sarcolemmal origin, are frequently present in both the intrinsic laryngeal muscles adjacent to the necrotic cartilages and the extrinsic laryngeal muscles removed with the specimen. Myointimal proliferation of small arteries and arterioles is present in these areas. Venous blood vessels in the area are frequently telangiectatic, sometimes to such a degree as to be visible grossly as blood-filled cavities. The sinuses that communicate with the laryngeal ventricle are lined by squamous cell epithelium and in cases with such sinuses, colonies of Gram-positive cocci are present extensively in each abscess amid the neutrophils.

Pathogenesis

The foregoing observations would suggest that cartilage necrosis is secondary to the submucosal stromal changes. In many areas the perichondrial abscess encroaches on the cartilage, often with little degeneration of the chondrocytes adjacent to the abscess. Although the possibility of primary damage by the X-rays to the cartilage tissues cannot be completely excluded, the appearances are more in keeping with secondary damage to cartilage, possibly by lysosomal enzymes derived from the neutrophil leucocytes of the submucosal abscess. Thus the appearances described here indicate that radiation damage is an "erosion" of cartilage rather than "necrosis" of cartilage.

There is no pathological evidence that infection has a role in the induction of radiation damage, although it certainly plays a part in the later stages. In some cases the inflammatory changes of the submucosa are covered by a normal intact epithelium and it is difficult to see how organisms could have entered unless they came from the bloodstream. Colonies of bacteria are present amid the inflammatory exudate in each of the cases in which there is a sinus leading from the mucosal airway surface to the abscess cavity, suggesting that infection is produced by airway bacteria only. This is particularly prone to occur in the region of the lateral wall of the laryngeal ventricle, where the submucosa of the larynx is very thin. Following the rupture, a sinus may be formed along which cartilaginous debris may be shed, and the sinus may become partially lined by squamous epithelium, which grows from the airway mucosa.

It has been suggested by Keene et al.[16] that the presence of advanced supraglottic tumour is a necessary feature for radiation necrosis of cartilage to take place, yet seven out of 17 laryngectomised larynges with no tumour at all had necrosis in his study. There was no residual tumour at all in our cases in or near radiation-damaged areas.

The characteristic manifestation of a severe radiation reaction in the larynx is thus a perichondrial abscess. This process is a specific reaction of the perichondrium to ischaemia of the laryngeal mucosa and submucosa. A similar but less severe change takes place as a complication of laryngeal intubation (see Chapter 31) in which cartilage damage also may be found.

References

1. Larynx. In: American Joint Committee on Cancer: AJCC Cancer Staging Manual, 5th edn. Lippincott-Raven Publishers, Philadelphia, 1997, pp 41–46
2. Edmundson WF. Microscopic grading of cancer and its practical implication. Arch Dermat Syphil 1948;57: 141–150
3. Jakobsson PA, Eneroth CM, Killander D et al. Histologic classification and grading of malignancy in carcinoma of the larynx. Acta Radiol 1973;12:1–7
4. Bryne M, Koppang HS, Lilleng R et al. Malignancy grading of the deep invasive margins of oral squamous cell carcinomas has high prognostic value. J Pathol 1992; 166:375–381
5. Wiernik G, Millard PR, Haybittle JL. The predictive value of histological classification into degrees of differentiation of squamous cell carcinoma of the larynx and hypopharynx compared with the survival of patients. Histopathol 1991;19:411–417
6. Meyer-Breitung E, Burkhardt A. Tumours of the larynx. Histopathology and clinical inferences. Springer-Verlag, Berlin, 1988
7. Thaler ER, Montone K, Tucker J et al. Delphian lymph node in laryngeal carcinoma: a whole organ study. Laryngoscope 1997;107:332–334
8. Michaels L. Pathology of the larynx. Springer, Heidelberg, Berlin, New York, 1984
9. Lloyd GAS, Michaels L, Phelps PD. The demonstration of cartilaginous involvement in laryngeal carcinoma by computerized tomography. Clin Otolaryngol 1981;6: 171–177
10. Zbaren P, Greiner R, Kengelbacher M. Stoma recurrence after laryngectomy: an analysis of risk factors. Otolaryngol Head Neck Surg 1996;114:569–575
11. Harrer WV, Lewis PL. Carcinoma of the larynx with cardiac metastases. Arch Otolaryngol 1970;91:382–384
12. O'Brien PH, Carlson R, Stuebner EA et al. Distant metastases in epidermoid cell carcinoma of the head and neck. Cancer 1971;27:304–307
13. Lederman M. Radiotherapy of cancer of the larynx. J Laryngol Otol 1970;84:867–896
14. Stell PM, Morrison MD. Radiation necrosis of the larynx. Etiology and management. Arch Otolaryngol 1973;98: 111–113
15. Henk JM, Kunkler PB, Smith CW. Radiotherapy and hyperbaric oxygen in head and neck cancer. Final report of first controlled clinical trial. Lancet 1977;II:101–103
16. Keene M, Harwood AR, Bryce DP et al. Histopathological study of radionecrosis in laryngeal carcinoma. Laryngoscope 1981;92:173–180
17. Hermans R, Pameijer FA, Mancuso AA et al. CT findings in chondroradionecrosis of the larynx. AJNR Am J Neuroradiol 1998;19:711–718

36 Unusual Forms of Squamous Cell Carcinoma

The majority of squamous carcinomas of the larynx are composed of epidermoid elements with definite cytological changes of malignancy. In a few cases a major portion of the neoplasm shows a mesenchymal appearance without squamous cell differentiation – the spindle cell carcinoma. At the other extreme of the spectrum of malignancy is a highly differentiated epidermoid tumour, which, although behaving in an invasive fashion, is so well differentiated that a diagnosis of malignancy cannot be made on currently accepted cytological criteria. These tumours have a warty structure, which gives rise to the term verrucous squamous carcinoma. In this chapter we describe also some other less common variants of squamous cell carcinoma arising from the laryngeal mucosa, tumours that also can be encountered in other parts of the upper air and food passages. Lastly there will be a description of a well-differentiated squamous cell carcinoma that arises from the epithelium of the ventriculosaccular tract of the larynx.

Spindle Cell Carcinoma

Terminology

This variant of squamous cell carcinoma is histologically characterised by a squamous cell carcinoma and another underlying or adjacent spindle cell or pleomorphic component. Tumours with histology compatible with spindle cell carcinoma are not homogeneous but comprise: (1) *spindle cell carcinoma* in which a squamous cell carcinoma is associated with malignant spindle cells that are demonstrably epithelial; (2) *squamous cell carcinoma with pseudosarcomatous stroma* in which a squamous cell carcinoma is associated with atypical but non-neoplastic fibroblastic or fibrohistiocytic proliferation (Lane's pseudosarcoma); (3) the rare condition of *carcinosarcoma* in which a squamous cell carcinoma is associated with malignant spindle cells that are demonstrably mesenchymal.

Before describing the common form of squamous carcinoma with malignant spindle cells, a short account of the other two variants, which are much less common, will follow.

Squamous Cell Carcinoma with Pseudosarcomatous Stroma (Lane's Pseudosarcoma)

The squamous cell carcinoma with pseudosarcomatous stromal form of spindle cell carcinoma is a bulky lesion, which is almost invariably polypoid. It is rarely found outside the larynx. Histologically it consists of cells of atypical appearance that are shown to be fibroblastic or fibrohistiocytic in origin, and not epithelial, by immunohistochemistry and/or electron microscopy. Moreover, application of antibodies against proliferation-associated antigens (e.g. MIB-1) demonstrates a low proliferation index, not compatible with a malignant neoplasm. The overlying squamous epithelium may show an invasive squamous cell carcinoma; it often displays carcinoma in situ only, however. Thus, this variety of spindle cell carcinoma consists of a malignant surface epithelial neoplasm, and a benign, non-neoplastic, reactive fibroblastic proliferation.

True Carcinosarcoma

The true carcinosarcoma constitutes an even more rare type of spindle cell carcinoma.[1] An invasive squamous cell carcinoma is present and the bizarre cells in the bulky lesion are truly malignant mesenchymal cells (fibroblasts, chondrocytes, etc.). The morphology is thus similar to carcinosarcomas elsewhere in the body.

Squamous Carcinoma with Malignant Spindle Cells

The "real" spindle cell carcinoma (synonym sarcomatoid carcinoma) is a bimorphic carcinoma consisting of a malignant squamous cell epithelium overlying a polypoid tumour, the bulk of which consists of bizarre, neoplastic spindle cells that are epithelial.

Incidence

In Hyams' series of 39 laryngeal cases, 36 were in males and three in females[2] – a sex incidence similar to that for glottic carcinoma. A similar sex incidence was found in the series of 36 laryngeal spindle cell carcinomas reported by Lewis at al.[3] In a series of 2052 malignant laryngeal tumours, 12 (<1%) were spindle cell carcinomas.[4] Likewise, among 6255 laryngeal squamous cell carcinomas in the Armed Forces Institute of Pathology files, 81 cases (1.2%) were diagnosed as spindle cell carcinomas.[5]

Site

Although spindle cell carcinoma is most frequently encountered in the larynx, and particularly the glottis, it also occurs in the maxillary antrum, hypopharynx, the nasal and oral cavities, oesophagus, trachea, skin and breast.

Gross Appearances

The majority of laryngeal spindle cell carcinomas are polypoid, with a base ranging from a thin string-like stalk to a wide area of attachment. An infiltrative form is also occasionally seen.[6] Most of the lesions of spindle cell carcinoma are present on the vocal cord. Supraglottic and subglottic origins of spindle cell carcinoma are also sometimes seen. The surfaces of the tumour seen clinically are not ulcerated, but smooth, glistening pink to grey. The tumours are firm, with cut sections revealing a fibrous greyish-pink uniform parenchyma.

Microscopic Appearances

The diagnosis of spindle cell carcinoma requires identification of squamous cell carcinoma in some part of the tumour. In many cases, however, a diligent search with multiple sections is required, since malignant epithelium is frequently scarce and may be absent from the surface in many areas. Sometimes only carcinoma in situ without an invasive component is present, and a diagnosis of spindle cell carcinoma can only be suspected. Squamous cell carcinoma may be found only at the base stalk of the polypoid tumours.

In the conventional squamous carcinomatous areas, a "streaming" of malignant squamous cells from mucosal squamous carcinoma into adjacent malignant stroma may be seen (Fig. 36.1). The spindle cell component occupies the greater portion of the neoplastic mass, often extending over the entire tumour surface, making identification of the biphasic process difficult. The histological pattern of the spindle cell elements is extremely variable. At one end of the scale is a very cellular structure composed of abundant parallel bipolar cells, containing a large round or oval nucleus with prominent single or multiple nucleoli and bipolar cytoplasmic processes. Areas where the cells are more rounded are also present (Fig. 36.2). At the other end of the cellular spectrum are parts with a predominantly collagenous component and sparse spindle-shaped cells. The nuclear atypia in the latter serve to differentiate them from a benign or desmoplastic reaction. Giant cells may be found in variable numbers in addition to the spindle cell element. In the spindle cell component a prominent collagen and reticulin fibre network is revealed by special stains. Storiform or pericytoma-like patterns may be present. Intracytoplasmic hyaline globules are sometimes found in the sarcomatoid areas.[6] Abundant collagen is a frequent finding, whereas osteoid or cartilaginous tissue (Fig. 36.3) is not. The giant cells in spindle cell carcinoma are rarely multinucleated, in contrast to those seen in squamous cell carcinoma with pseudosarcomatous stroma (Lane's pseudosarcoma). The blood vessels show no tendency to radial arrangement and mitoses are infrequent. Occasionally the tumours can be myxoid, with a mucoid Alcian-blue-positive stroma between the cells. In most cases the

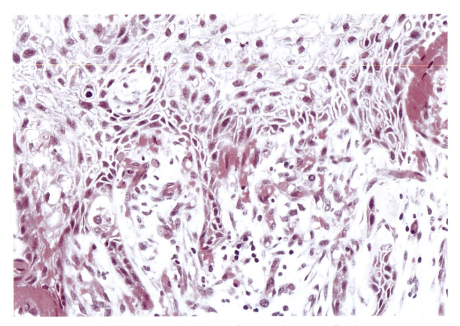

Figure 36.1 Spindle cell carcinoma. Origin from mucosal squamous cell carcinoma

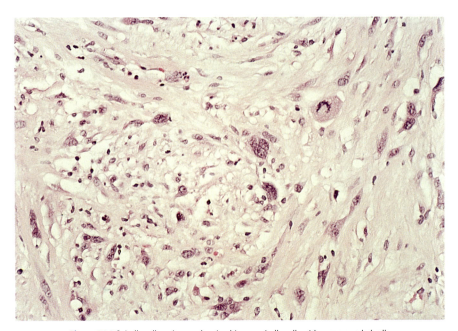

Figure 36.2 Spindle cell carcinoma showing bizarre spindle cells with some rounded cells

spindle cells stain positively for cytokeratins, and may also have a dual positivity for vimentin. The vimentin-positivity reflects that these bizarre fibroblast-like cells are carcinoma cells with true mesenchymal metaplasia. Electron microscopy also has demonstrated these cells to have epithelial characteristics with a relative abundance of desmosomes and tonofilaments.[7] The spindle cells have only a marginally lower Ki-67 index than the more readily

recognised squamous cell carcinoma cells from the overlying epithelium. The majority of the spindle cells are non-diploid, which again indicates that they are neoplastic and not reactive.[3]

In lymph node metastases from spindle cell carcinoma there may be a squamous carcinomatous element only, both the squamous and the spindle cell element, or the spindle cell component alone. Similar variations of malignant cell types may be

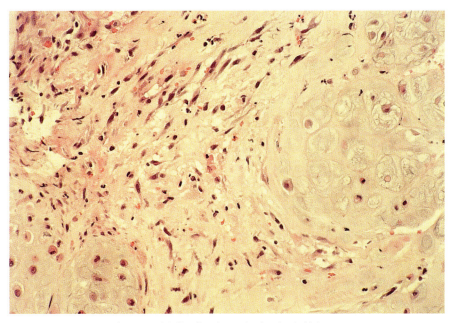

Figure 36.3 Spindle cell carcinoma showing chondroid change

seen in more distant metastases. Such histological findings tend to confirm the concept that this lesion is a variant of squamous cell carcinoma.

Natural History

Most but not all spindle cell carcinomas are relatively rapidly growing, polypoid and bulky. Irradiation therapy will not induce an anaplastic carcinoma with a more aggressive behaviour. It has been suggested that the prognosis of spindle cell carcinoma is better than that of squamous cell carcinoma, but other studies present a somewhat less optimistic future,[2] indicating that survival and reaction to treatment of spindle cell carcinoma are similar to those of conventional squamous cell carcinoma of the larynx, with particularly poor response to irradiation therapy alone. There is evidence that survival is inversely related to depth of invasion: in those patients whose tumours invade deeply, survival rate is low, whereas in those whose tumours are superficial, survival prospects are excellent.[6]

Verrucous Squamous Carcinoma

Definition and Site

Verrucous squamous cell carcinoma (Ackerman's tumour) is a highly differentiated variant of squamous cell carcinoma. It occurs most frequently in the oral cavity, where it constitutes 4% of all carcinomas.[8] It may develop in any mucosal surface of the ear, nose or throat, but particularly in the glottic area of the larynx, where it constitutes up to about 2% of all carcinomas.

Gross Appearances

The gross appearance is usually that of a warty, grey-white lesion with filiform projections. Clefts are seen on the cut surface, which extend from the surface into the substance of the growth.[8] Verrucous squamous carcinoma may arise from one, two or all three regions of the larynx (Figs 36.4–36.6).

Microscopic Appearances

The highly keratinising surface of the neoplasm, the frequent presence of papillary areas, and the apparent absence of dysplastic change in the squamous epithelium make this lesion difficult to recognise when it first presents. A diagnosis of squamous papilloma is frequently rendered by the pathologist at this time, and even after biopsy of one or more recurrences (see Chapter 33). Verrucous squamous carcinoma does, however, show a number of features in its histological picture that may suggest the correct diagnosis even at first presentation.

Rete ridges are often large, blunt ended and irregular; smaller offshoots of growth are also seen,

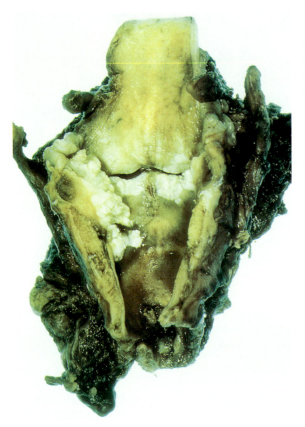

Figure 36.4 Verrucous squamous carcinoma of suproglottis, glottis and sub-glottis. Note whitish (keratinous) warty outgrowths

but narrow lines of cells invading into connective tissue in a "saw-tooth" fashion are characteristic of conventional squamous carcinomas, but not verrucous squamous carcinoma. Proliferating squamous masses often bulge outwards towards the surface in a papillary fashion, but the symmetrical form of a benign squamous papilloma, with several degrees of branching and the appearance of koilocytosis, a change present in almost all laryngeal papillomas and associated in them with human papillomavirus, demonstrable by immunohistochemistry and in situ hybridisation (see Chapter 33), is not shown by verrucous carcinomas. Under the higher powers of the microscope, features of verrucous squamous carcinoma may be detected in each layer of the squamous epithelium. The basal cells show vesicular nuclei usually containing a single eosinophilic nucleolus. These cells lie on a thin basement membrane, which, unlike squamous papilloma, does not appear hyalinised even in the papillary areas of the tumour, and in some areas is not present at all. The basal cells appear to be crowded and even to be bulging the basement membrane outwards. More superficially, between the basal layers and the surface keratinising cells, there are usually wide fields of squamous epithelium composed of cells that frequently have nuclei of 30–40 μm in diameter and abundant pale cytoplasm. The large size of these cells is the most diagnostic feature of the histological appearances (see below). This feature is also mirrored by the presence of prominent eosinophilic nucleoli in nuclei of cells at all levels. Superficially, keratin is produced, often in great abundance. This

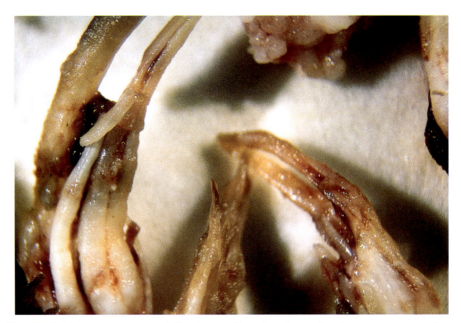

Figure 36.5 Claw-like excrescences composed of keratinous papillary outgrowths on surface of verrucous squamous carcinoma

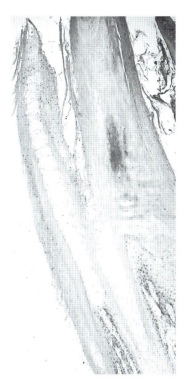

exudate beneath the tumour processes; lymphocytes and plasma cells (the latter often in great abundance) are the component cells.

When verrucous squamous carcinoma is studied in its location in a laryngectomy specimen, it is seen that the tumour grows in continuity with the normal epithelial lining by the development of a sudden acanthosis with the features described above. The degree of invasion is not great, the tumour being present often as a superficial spreading lesion. Invasion of cartilage is not seen (Figs 36.7–36.10).

Enlarged Malpighian Cells

Although apparently very well differentiated, observation of the component squamous epithelial cells of verrucous squamous carcinoma repeatedly confirms the greater size, particularly of the cells of the intermediate zone, as compared with the cells of squamous papilloma or other benign squamous cells. We have attempted to quantitate this observation by comparing sizes of various parameters of the cells of this zone in verrucous squamous carcinoma with the same parameters of cells of benign squamous papilloma in the same zone.[9] The most significant difference was found in the mean cell areas. This measurement was made on a number of cells in photographs of cases of verrucous carcinoma and in cases of benign squamous papilloma of the larynx. There was an obvious and significant difference

Figure 36.6 Section of verrucous carcinoma shown in Fig. 36.5. Note long thin keratinous outgrowths on surfaces of papillae

is present in some fields with an externally pointed appearance – the "church spire" effect. Parakeratosis is frequent. There is always a dense mononuclear cell

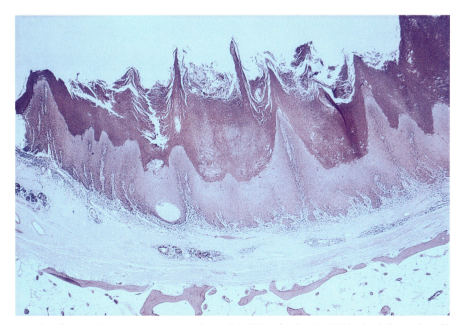

Figure 36.7 Low-power view of supraglottic verrucous squamous carcinoma. Note thick surface keratin with "church-spire" protrusions of keratin, blunt downgrowths with no deep tongues of invasion and brisk deep inflammatory response. The underlying thyroid cartilage is separated from the neoplasm by normal submucous glandular and pericartilaginous fibrous tissue

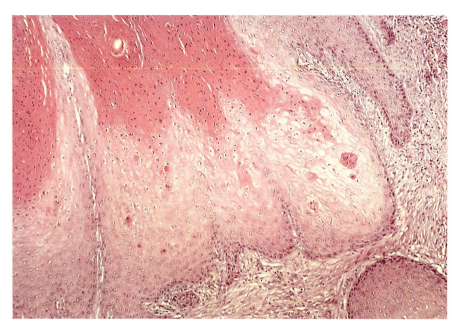

Figure 36.8 Verrucous squamous carcinoma showing blunt downgrowths

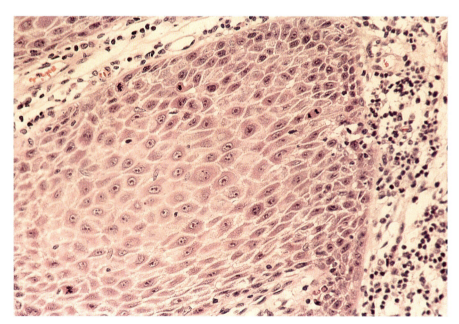

Figure 36.9 Verrucous squamous carcinoma showing enlarged cells of malpighian layer

between the mean cell areas of most verrucous squamous carcinomas and those of squamous papillomas, the verrucous carcinoma cells being much larger. The majority of the former also showed a wider range between –1 and +1 standard deviations than in the squamous papillomas. This observation is probably also significant in verrucous squamous carcinoma, indicating a greater range of cell sizes in this malignant lesion.

The measurement of cell areas may thus be a useful one in the diagnosis of any case in which the possibility of verrucous squamous carcinoma exists. Care should, however, be exerted in this regard in that raised keratotic plaques on the vocal cords, which have been referred to as verrucous hyperplasia,[10] may also show a similar degree of cellular enlargement to that of verrucous carcinoma and, indeed, it has been suggested that these plaques may

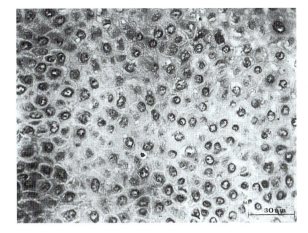

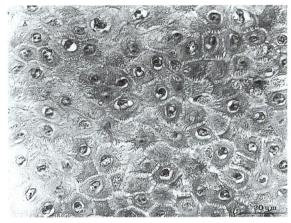

Figure 36.10 Cells from malpighian layer of squamous papilloma of larynx (*above*) are smaller than those of verrucous squamous carcinoma (*below*)

be precursors of that carcinoma[10,11] (see Chapter 33).

Natural History

Verrucous squamous carcinoma is said not to metastasise either to lymph nodes or by the bloodstream. Two matters of practical importance arise in connection with the natural history of this tumour. Firstly, on account of its exaggerated differentiation, the tumour may be mistaken by the histopathologist for a benign lesion, particularly squamous papilloma, and particularly if only a superficial biopsy specimen is examined. Recurrence and local invasion after several inadequate attempts at local resection may take place before the true nature is realised. Secondly, it has been suggested that treatment of verrucous squamous carcinomas by radiotherapy may convert this neoplasm into a rapidly growing anaplastic metastasising entity. The evidence for this has always been scanty, and as more and more patients with verrucous carcinoma have

been successfully treated, with long follow-up, by radiotherapy, claims for the existence of this complication have now disappeared.

Treatment

Irradiation is thus a useful mode of therapy for verrucous carcinoma and the trend is to treat the lesion as if it were a squamous carcinoma of the usual variety – by radiation therapy if it is a limited growth, usually on the glottis, or by surgical excision (often total laryngectomy) if it is more extensive. In view of its superficial quality, with little tendency to deep invasion, it is likely that more localised surgical excision might prove rewarding and recent reports support a conservative surgical resection for verrucous carcinoma whenever possible.[12]

Significance

The above description of verrucous squamous carcinoma has been given as if it represented a specific entity. Yet conventional squamous carcinomas are seen with areas showing microscopic appearances identical with verrucous squamous carcinoma. More worrying are those cases showing verrucous squamous carcinoma alone on laryngoscopic biopsy, but which, on examination of a larger specimen, show areas of conventional squamous carcinoma. It has been indicated above that, although verrucous squamous carcinoma is seemingly composed of completely mature epidermoid cells, these cells are, in fact, larger than benign epithelial cells and may have other subtle features of dedifferentiation such as enlarged nucleoli.

Verrucous squamous carcinoma of the larynx is an unusual form of laryngeal carcinoma, and more study of this lesion is required before a definite statement can be made as to its exact relationship to conventional squamous carcinoma. For the present, however, we would suggest that verrucous squamous carcinoma is a highly differentiated neoplasm within the broad spectrum of squamous cell carcinoma, which, in keeping with its apparent excellent differentiation, has a less aggressive activity.

Basaloid Squamous Cell Carcinoma

This high-grade variant of squamous cell carcinoma was first recognised in the 1980s as a separate entity occurring in the upper respiratory tract.[13] Basaloid squamous cell carcinoma is defined as a carcinoma consisting of a mixture of basaloid and squamous cell components.

Site and Incidence

Although basaloid squamous cell carcinoma has a strong predilection for the hypopharynx, base of tongue and supraglottic larynx, it is now evident that it may occur anywhere in the upper respiratory tract. There is a male predominance. The number of cases reported in the literature has long since exceeded 100, and includes lesions in the nasal cavity, oesophagus, tonsils and buccal cavity, many of which commenced in the floor of the mouth.[14-16]

Pathological Appearances

Laryngeal basaloid squamous cell carcinoma often appears as an exophytic, polypoid and centrally ulcerated mass. Microscopically the basaloid component is usually the more prominent, and consists of small cells with hyperchromatic nuclei and scanty cytoplasm. The cells are arranged in lobular masses or cords, often with small cystic spaces containing mucoid material, which stains with periodic acid–Schiff and/or Alcian blue. There is peripheral palisading, focal squamous differentiation, often numerous mitoses, and areas of necrosis (Figs 36.11–36.13). In simple terms, basaloid squamous cell carcinoma has the features of a mixture of basal cell carcinoma and squamous cell carcinoma of the skin. Stromal hyalini-

sation is a common finding. The squamous component, which may be invasive or in situ, can be defined by two or more of the following: (1) keratin pearl formation, (2) individual cell keratinisation, (3) intracellular bridging and (4) cells arranged in a pavement or mosaic pattern.[13]

Basaloid squamous cell carcinoma is positive for cytokeratins, often for epithelial membrane antigen and carcinoembryonic antigen, and occasionally there is focal positivity for S-100.[17] The differential diagnosis is primarily with adenoid cystic carcinoma, adenosquamous carcinoma (see below), poorly differentiated squamous cell carcinoma and small cell neuroendocrine carcinoma. High molecular weight cytokeratin reactivity is reported to differentiate basaloid squamous cell carcinoma more consistently from small cell undifferentiated carcinoma than the reactivity of the latter with neuroendocrine markers.[18] When located in the sinonasal tract, basal cell ameloblastoma may be confused with basaloid squamous cell carcinoma.

Natural History

Basaloid squamous cell carcinoma is an aggressive variant of squamous cell carcinoma and carries a worse prognosis than does regular squamous cell carcinoma. In a series of 15 basaloid squamous cell carcinomas of the larynx and hypopharynx, local recurrence was seen in three patients, and five of the nine patients with cervical lymph node metastases also developed distant metastases. The determined

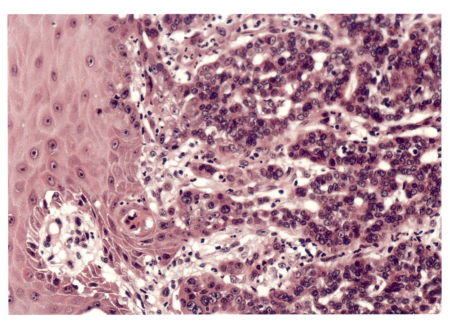

Figure 36.11 Basaloid squamous carcinoma. Origin from hyperplastic squamous epithelium

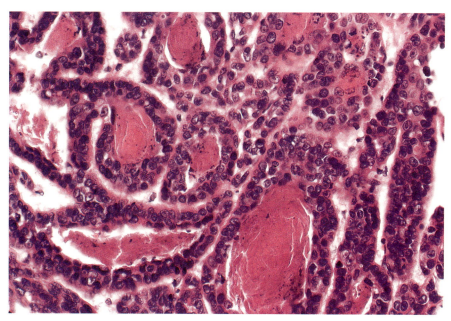

Figure 36.12 Basaloid squamous carcinoma. Cystic spaces with luminal secretion

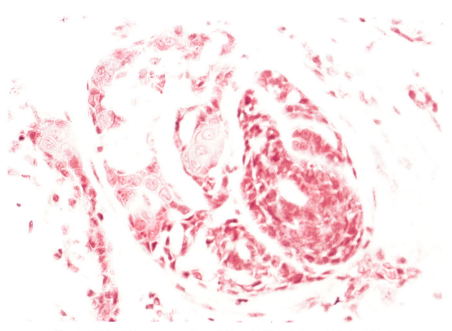

Figure 36.13 Basaloid squamous carcinoma. Epidermoid differentiation amid the basaloid cells

5-year survival was estimated at only 17.5% (Kaplan-Meier method).[19] A recent study demonstrated bcl-2 protein expression together with c-myc amplification to be present in 43.5% of basaloid squamous cell carcinomas but in none of the typical squamous cell carcinomas ($p<0.001$). This partly explains its high proliferative activity but also frequent spontaneous apoptosis.[20] The local recurrence rate is said to be similar in basaloid squamous cell carcinoma to that of conventional squamous cell carcinoma. However, even "early" basaloid squamous cell carcinoma recurs distantly rather than locally or regionally. The higher distant metastatic rate and poorer overall survival rate call for an extensive metastatic survey of these patients before surgery is recommended.[21]

Adenoid Squamous Cell Carcinoma

Adenoid squamous cell carcinoma is a low-grade variant of squamous cell carcinoma with pseudo-glandular lumina or spaces resulting from acantholysis of the tumour cells. There is thus no true glandular differentiation but there may be focal positive periodic acid–Schiff staining. Mucicarmine and Alcian blue stains, however, are negative. This tumour is usually located in the skin of the head and neck, and only very rarely in the larynx.[22,23] Adenoid squamous cell carcinoma has in the past been termed acantholytic squamous cell carcinoma, adenoacanthoma or pseudoglandular squamous cell carcinoma. The treatment for laryngeal adenoid squamous cell carcinoma is that of conventional squamous cell carcinoma.

Adenosquamous Carcinoma

Adenosquamous carcinoma is a highly malignant tumour with histological features of both adeno-carcinoma and squamous cell carcinoma. Adeno-squamous carcinoma has an aggressive growth and frequent metastases. Although adenosquamous carcinoma is not differentiated from mucoepider-moid carcinoma in the Armed Forces Institute of Pathology fascicle,[5] a clear distinction between the two entities is made in the World Health Organization classification.[24] However, the authors of the Armed Forces Institute of Pathology fascicle does state in regard to this lesion that such "… neoplasms might be better termed adenosquamous carcinoma", and also refers to a publication on this entity.[25] Many cases of adenosquamous carcinoma are reported from the pancreas, prostate, lung, rectum, gallbladder and small intestine. These sites of origin are organs rich in glandular structures, which might imply that this tumour entity arises in ductal and/or glandular structures, and then develops squamous metaplasia.[26] Adenosquamous carcinoma is not, however, very rare in the upper respiratory tract and about 12 cases have been reported from the oral cavity.[27] Hence the tumour may also represent a carcinomatous change in the surface squamous epithelium, in association with adenocarcinoma arising from the ducts or acini or the minor salivary glands, i.e. a kind of hybrid tumour. The largest series of laryngeal adenosquamous carcinoma consists of 21 patients, showing a strong male predominance (6:1) and it is most common in elderly patients (median 57 years).[25]

Microscopic Appearances

The distinct histological feature of this neoplasm is that, unlike mucoepidermoid carcinoma, glandular and squamous components are separate from each other. In adenosquamous carcinoma there is overt squamous cell carcinoma, or sometimes carcinoma in situ, and also adenocarcinoma. The adenocarci-nomatous component comprises the characteristic mucin-secreting cells, and the glandular elements are often lined by basal or columnar cells. The tumour should thus be distinguished from the low-grade adenoid squamous cell carcinoma (see above) and mucoepidermoid carcinoma (see Chapter 42).

Natural History

Adenosquamous carcinoma is an aggressive neo-plasm. Although the neoplasm is termed mucoepi-dermoid carcinoma in many reports, a distinction has often been made between low-grade and high-grade "mucoepidermoid carcinoma", the latter pre-sumably representing adenosquamous carcinoma. As is the case when adenosquamous carcinoma is located in other organs, surgery combined with radiotherapy and/or chemotherapy is advocated.[28,29]

Giant Cell Carcinoma

Primary giant cell carcinomas of the larynx are extremely rare and only an occasional case report is to be found in the literature.[30] Most malignant laryngeal giant cell tumours are malignant fibrous histiocytomas or other mesenchymal neoplasms (see Chapter 43). Histologically giant cell carcinoma has certain resemblances to giant cell carcinoma of the lung. The giant cells are often both bizarre and multinucleated. This latter feature may help in dis-tinguishing giant cell carcinoma from spindle cell carcinoma. The cells tend to have abundant eosino-philic cytoplasm, sometimes containing debris and leucocytes. Immunohistochemistry is most often necessary to discriminate giant cell carcinoma from rhabdomyosarcoma, malignant fibrous histiocytoma or other mesenchymal neoplasms.

Clear Cell Carcinoma

Laryngeal clear cell carcinoma is not a variant of squamous cell carcinoma, but a tumour of laryngeal minor salivary gland origin, or a metastatic neoplasm (see Chapter 43). However, there may be focal areas with clear cells in laryngeal squamous cell carcinoma, probably representing a metaplastic or degenerative process.

Ventriculosaccular Carcinoma

There exists in the larynx a second epithelial layer in addition to that of the airway – the lining of the tract of the ventricle and saccule.

The ventricle and saccule have a common embryological origin and are conspicuous in the early human larynx and in phylogenically related species. It would seem quite feasible that the action of carcinogenic factors should lead to a tumour process that is confined to this distinct anatomical tract. Yet, although carcinoma of the saccule or ventricle is sometimes referred to in the literature, it receives little detailed attention. Olofsson and van Nostrand, in their study of 139 serially sectioned larynges, stated that this entity "must be extremely rare".[31] Micheau et al. mentioned cancer of the ventricle in their report on 120 cases of laryngectomised carcinoma, and also "cancer developing on a laryngocele" as a separate entity, but it is difficult to perceive a connection between these two conditions in their study, and their meaning for the term "laryngocele" would not seem to be that in common usage.[32] There has been very little study of possible specific clinical features or natural history of this entity, and of its gross and microscopic pathology. The pathological and clinical features of a series of cases of ventriculosaccular carcinoma have been recorded and data given on the survival of these patients.[33]

Gross Appearances

After opening the larynx from behind in a case of ventriculosaccular carcinoma, tumour is usually present in the ventricle, often filling it and covered by the stretched lips of the false cord and true cord, above and below respectively. The saccular component of the tumour is displayed in the posterior view of the larynx before transverse slicing as a vertical bulge in the anterior supraglottic mucosa above the false cord, covered by normal mucosa (Fig. 36.14). Transverse slices of the larynx show a band of pale-grey tumour of mainly uniform thickness, which surrounds the lumen of the ventricle and saccule. Parts of mucosa may appear free of tumour. These areas correspond microscopically to zones of normal respiratory epithelium lining the saccule, and are usually on its medial surface. In one case a

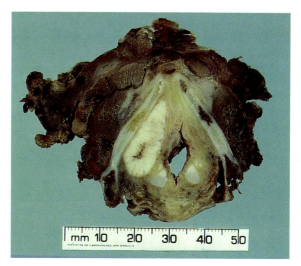

Figure 36.14 Saccular component of ventriculosaccular carcinoma of the larynx in transverse slice. The lateral edge of the carcinoma lies against the thyroid cartilage, but does not invade it

laryngocele has been observed with carcinoma arising multifocally from its epithelium.[33]

Microscopic Appearances

Microscopic observation of ventriculosaccular carcinoma confirms the gross impression of origin of the carcinoma from the ventricular mucosa in all cases, and from the saccular mucosa in most (Figs 36.15, 36.16). The level of the carcinoma may extend upwards to terminate either below or above the level of the notch of the thyroid cartilage. In a few cases the carcinoma may extend, with the saccule, to a level even above that of the hyoid bone.

The microscopic appearances of the tumour show certain similarities within the group, suggesting, perhaps, a distinct form of squamous cell carcinoma. There is a malignant epidermoid neoplasm arising from the epithelial lining of the ventricle and, in most cases, the saccule (Fig. 36.15). There are intervals in the surface lining of the ventriculosaccular tract with no neoplasm. These areas are lined by normal respiratory epithelium. At their edges these normal zones suddenly give way to a malignant squamous epithelial lining. Tumour tissue is aligned to the contour of the saccule or ventricle.

The carcinoma is characterised by deep clefts communicating with the surface and often filled with large amounts of keratin material representing the accumulated debris of desquamated surface squamous epithelial cells. The clefts are quite frequent and present regularly along the extent of the tumour, giving it a folded appearance in the low-

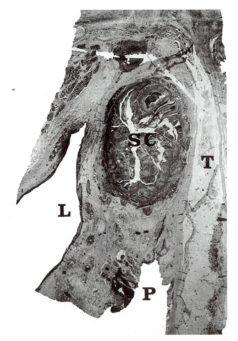

Figure 36.15 Saccular component of ventriculosaccular carcinoma in transverse slice. Note deep clefts of squamous neoplasm. *L*, lumen of larynx; *P*, piriform fossa; *T*, thyroid cartilage; *SC*, saccular carcinoma[33]

cases it is little thicker than a somewhat hyperplastic stratified squamous epithelium, so that the neoplasm resembles a florid form of squamous carcinoma in situ. The basal cell layer of the carcinoma is, in some cases, smooth; in others it forms corrugations; in still others there are numerous short, thin strands of tumour at its growing edge. In all cases, however, the general line of the deep boundary of the neoplasms runs approximately parallel to that of the lumen, without any deep tongues of extension into the tissues away from the main tumour mass. The cells of the carcinomas in all cases show atypia characteristic of malignancy, but mitotic figures are unusual. Individual cell keratinisation is present in the majority of these cancers.

Clinical Features

The age incidence of ventriculosaccular carcinoma seems to be similar to that of carcinoma of the laryngeal airway; Michaels and Hassmann's ten cases[33] had a median and average age of 58 years. Two of the patients were non-smokers and a third smoked ten cigarettes a day. The smoking history of the others was not available.

All the ten patients with known history had the major symptom of hoarseness. At direct laryngoscopy the most noteworthy feature is that in eight of the ten patients the neoplasm was thought to be

power view of the microscope. The thickness of the tumour from the surface of the saccule to the basal layer varies considerably from case to case, but is uniform in a particular transverse section. In some

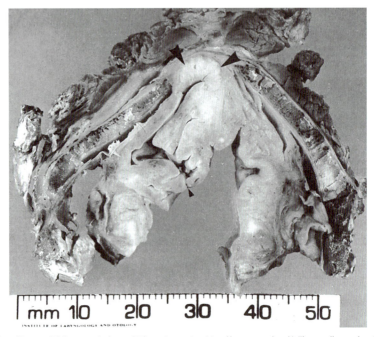

Figure 36.16 Transverse slice of larynx with laryngocele from which carcinoma is arising (*large arrowheads*). The *small arrowhead* points to a communicating channel between the laryngocele lumen and the laryngeal airway[33]

arising from the vocal cord. In only three cases was the tumour reported to be in the ventricle at laryngoscopy. The vestibular fold, epiglottis and subglottis were thought to be involved by tumour in four, three and three cases respectively.

Movement of the vocal cord at indirect laryngoscopy was decreased in three cases and absent in four. In two cases the vocal cords were thought to be mobile.

It would seem that ventriculosaccular carcinoma appears as a supraglottic mass on standard tomography. Only some of the most recent cases have been examined by computed tomography. Demonstration by this method of thickening in the paraglottis on one side together with a smooth laryngeal lining over the thickening would seem to be suggestive of the presence of a saccular neoplasm.

In none of the ten cases of Michaels and Hassmann[33] who were followed up after treatment for varying periods up to 27 years was there any recurrence of tumour locally or at a distance after laryngectomy; there were no cervical lymph node metastases at any stage of the disease, and there were no bloodstream metastases. In one case symptoms were present for at least 6 years before the laryngectomy, but a positive biopsy could not be obtained during this time.

Treatment by radiotherapy seemed to produce no beneficial effect and the treatment carried out in all the patients reported by Michaels and Hassmann was that of total laryngectomy.

Thus, we are dealing with a neoplasm arising in the ventriculosaccular tract of the larynx that is characterised by clinical and pathological features indicating slow growth and feeble invasiveness. How may it be diagnosed before definitive treatment is carried out? It would seem that the presence of some of the following features in a patient with a laryngeal neoplasm with or without vocal cord paresis may indicate a diagnosis of ventriculosaccular carcinoma of the larynx: (1) a tumour in the ventricle; (2) the presence of an anterior vertically elongated supraglottic bulge, covered by normal mucosa; (3) a paraglottic swelling covered by a smooth laryngeal lining on imaging; and (4) biopsy appearances of a low-grade squamous carcinoma of "folded" type.

It is possible that if a definite diagnosis of ventriculosaccular carcinoma could be made before laryngectomy, a more limited form of surgical therapy could be carried out in such a way as to retain some voice production. It seems likely, however, that total laryngectomy will continue to be used until the limited invasiveness that is suggested as a characteristic of ventriculosaccular carcinoma has been confirmed in further cases.

References

1. Klijanienko J, Viehl P, Duvillard P et al. True carcinosarcoma of the larynx. J Laryngol Otol 1992;106:58–60
2. Hyams VJ. Spindle cell carcinoma of the larynx. Can J Otolaryngol 1975;4:307–313
3. Lewis JE, Olsen KD, Sebo TJ. Spindle cell carcinoma of the larynx: review of 26 cases including DNA content and immunohistochemistry. Hum Pathol 1997;28:664–673
4. Ferlito A, Altavilla G, Rinaldo A et al. Basaloid squamous cell carcinoma of the larynx and hypopharynx. Ann Otol Rhinol Laryngol 1997;106:1024–1035
5. Hyams VJ, Batsakis JG, Michaels L. Tumors of the upper respiratory tract and ear. Atlas of tumor pathology, 2nd series, fascicle 25. Armed Forces Institute of Pathology, Washington, D.C., 1988
6. Leventon GS, Evans HL. Sarcomatoid squamous cell carcinoma of the mucous membranes of the head and neck: a clinicopathologic study of 20 cases. Cancer 1981;48:994–1003
7. Hellquist HB, Olofsson J. Spindle cell carcinoma of the larynx. APMIS 1989;97:1103–1113
8. Dockerty MB, Parkhill EM, Dahlin DC et al. Tumors of the oral cavity and pharynx. Atlas of tumor pathology, section IV, fascicle 10b. Armed Forces Institute of Pathology, Washington, D.C., 1968
9. Cooper JR, Hellquist HB, Michaels L. Image analysis in the discrimination of verrucous carcinoma and squamous papilloma. J Pathol 1992;166:383–387
10. Murrah VA, Batsakis JG. Proliferative verrucous leukoplakia and verrucous hyperplasia. Ann Otol Rhinol Laryngol 1994;103:660–663
11. Michaels L. The Kambic-Gale method of assessment of epithelial hyperplastic lesions of the larynx in comparison with the dysplasia grade method. Acta Otolaryngol (Stockh) 1997;527(suppl):17–20
12. Spiro RH. Verrucous carcinoma, then and now. Presidential Address. Am J Surg 1998;176:393–397
13. Wain SL, Kier R, Vollmer RT et al. Basaloid-squamous carcinoma of the tongue, hypopharynx, and larynx: report of 10 cases. Hum Pathol 1986;17:1158–1166
14. Hellquist HB, Dahl F, Karlsson MG et al. Basaloid squamous cell carcinoma of the palate. Histopathology 1994;25:178–180
15. Barnes L, Ferlito A, Altavilla G et al. Basaloid squamous cell carcinoma of the head and neck: clinicopathological features and differential diagnosis. Ann Otol Rhinol Laryngol 1996;105:75–82
16. Wieneke JA, Thompson LD, Wenig BM. Basaloid squamous cell carcinoma of the sinonasal tract. Cancer 1999;85:841–854
17. Banks ER, Frierson HF Jr, Mills SE et al. Basaloid squamous cell carcinoma of the head and neck. A clinicopathologic and immunohistochemical study of 40 cases. Am J Surg Pathol 1992;16:939–946
18. Morice WG, Ferreiro JA. Distinction of basaloid squamous cell carcinoma from adenoid cystic and small cell undifferentiated carcinoma by immunohistochemistry. Hum Pathol 1998;29:609–612
19. Ferlito A, Altavilla G, Rinaldo A et al. Basaloid squamous cell carcinoma of the larynx and hypopharynx. Ann Otol Rhinol Laryngol 1997;106:1024–1035
20. Sarbia M, Loberg C, Wolter M et al. Expression of Bcl-2 and amplification of c-myc are frequent in basaloid squamous cell carcinomas of the esophagus. Am J Pathol 1999;155:1027–1032
21. Winzenburg SM, Niehans GA, George E et al. Basaloid squamous carcinoma: a clinical comparison of two histologic types with poorly differentiated squamous cell carcinoma. Otolaryngol Head Neck Surg 1998;119:471–475

22. Hertenstein JC, Fechner RE. Acantholytic squamous cell carcinoma. Arch Otolaryngol Head Neck Surg 1986; 112:780–783

23. Batsakis JG, Huser J. Squamous carcinomas with glandlike (adenoid) features. Ann Otol Rhinol Laryngol 1990;99:87–88

24. Shanmugaratnam K, Sobin LH. Histological typing of tumours of the upper respiratory tract and ear. WHO international histological classification of tumours, 2nd edn. Springer-Verlag, Berlin, Heidelberg, New York, 1991

25. Damiani JM, Damiani KK, Hauck K et al. Mucoepidermoid-adenosquamous carcinoma of the larynx and hypopharynx. Head Neck Surg 1981;89:235–243

26. Aranha GV, Yong S, Olson M. Adenosquamous carcinoma of the pancreas. Int J Pancreatol 1999;26:85–91

27. Scully C, Porter SR, Speight PM et al. Adenosquamous carcinoma of the mouth: a rare variant of squamous cell carcinoma. Int J Oral Maxillofac Surg 1999;28:125–128

28. Snow RT, Fox AR. Mucoepidermoid carcinoma of the larynx. J Am Osteopath Assoc 1991;91:182–184

29. Fujino K, Ito J, Kanaji M et al. Adenosquamous carcinoma of the larynx. Am J Otolaryngol 1995;16:115–118

30. Ferlito A, Friedmann J, Recher G. Primary giant cell carcinoma of the larynx. A clinico-pathologic study of four cases. ORL J Otorhinolaryngol Relat Spec 1985;47:105–112

31. Olofsson J, van Nostrand AWP. Growth and spread of laryngeal and hypopharyngeal carcinoma with reflections on the effect of preoperative irradiation. 139 cases studied by whole organ sectioning. Acta Otolaryngol (Stockh) 1973;308 (suppl):1–84

32. Micheau C, Luboinski B, Sancho H et al. Modes of invasion of cancer of the larynx. A statistical, histological and radioclinical analysis of 120 cases. Cancer 1976;38:346–360

33. Michaels L, Hassmann E. Ventriculosaccular carcinoma of the larynx. Clin Otolaryngol 1982;7:165–173

37 Non-epidermoid Epithelial and Neuroectodermal Neoplasms

Non-epidermoid Epithelial Neoplasms

Most of the benign and malignant epithelial neoplasms of the larynx are epidermoid, but a small proportion are not. The latter may arise from the respiratory epithelium, which covers most of the larynx, or from the cells lining the subepithelial glands, which are abundant in the larynx, particularly in the false cord and adjacent to the saccule.

Benign Forms

Surface Epithelial Origin

Cylindric Cell Papilloma

Cylindric cell papilloma, which is seen in the nose and paranasal sinuses, is composed of proliferated papillary formations of respiratory epithelium (see Chapter 15). Such a lesion does not arise in the larynx in a pure state. However, similar neoplastic papillae of cylindric cells develop in conjunction with squamous cell papilloma of the larynx (see Chapter 33). These changes are found only in cases of squamous papillomatosis of widespread development in the larynx, with frequent recurrences. The neoplasm in these cases can, therefore, better be described as "mixed cylindric cell and squamous cell papillomatosis".

Subepithelial Gland Origin

Both intraepithelial and subepithelial glands are present in the larynx in large numbers, particularly in the supraglottis. The intraepithelial glands are mounds of goblet cells with a central lumen. It is not known whether they can give rise to neoplasms. The subepithelial (seromucous) glands are simple or branched tubes with ducts opening onto the surface. Secretory terminal pieces composed of mucous and serous elements, similar to salivary glands, are present on the branched glands. Benign neoplasms arising from subepithelial glands of the larynx do occur, but are rare. As these glands are homologous with salivary glands, it would be expected that they would give rise to both monomorphic and pleomorphic adenomas. Monomorphic adenomas of the larynx would seem to be very rare. The so-called "oncocytic cystadenoma"[1] is almost certainly a retention cyst of columnar epithelium, with associated oncocytic change of the cyst lining and the adjacent subepithelial glands, together with chronic inflammatory change (see Chapter 29).

Pleomorphic Adenoma

Pleomorphic adenomas are rare. They grow in most cases on the epiglottis, although they have been seen in other parts of the larynx.[2] Their microscopic appearance is similar to that of pleomorphic adenoma of major and minor salivary glands (see Chapter 41). They are benign and can be safely treated by local resection.

Malignant Forms

Surface Epithelial Origin

Malignant tumours almost certainly derived from respiratory epithelium are of two types – cylindric

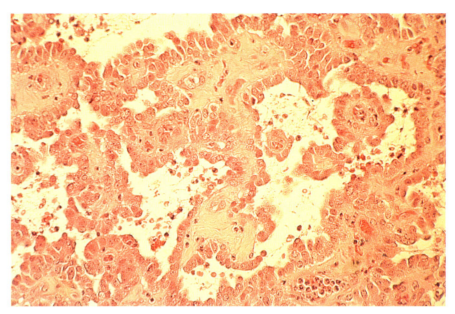

Figure 37.1 Papillary adenocarcinoma of thyroid presenting as a laryngeal tumour

(or cylindrical) cell carcinoma[3] and adenocarcinoma with papillary appearances. Both are essentially tumours of the nose (see Chapter 17) and are not seen in the larynx. Adenocarcinomas of surface origin are difficult to distinguish from adenocarcinomas of glandular origin. A papillary pattern in an adenocarcinoma might be considered an indication of surface epithelial origin, but such patterns are hardly ever present in primary laryngeal tumours. A papillary adenocarcinoma presenting in the larynx is most likely to be derived from a thyroid primary that has invaded into the laryngeal lumen (Fig. 37.1).

Subepithelial Gland Origin

Malignant tumours originating from subepithelial glands are in the form of adenocarcinomas and of adenoid cystic carcinomas. A third group of non-epidermoid carcinomas possibly also originating from subepithelial glands and now thought to be the most frequently occurring group – the neuroendocrine carcinomas – is considered separately below.

Frequency

These are rare neoplasms and are usually thought to constitute less than 1% of all laryngeal neoplasms.

Sites of Origin

Since the tumours arise from the epithelium of laryngeal subepithelial (seromucous) glands, they never arise on the true vocal cords, where such glands are not present. Adenocarcinomas and adenoid cystic carcinomas usually arise in the subglottis. A minority arise in the supraglottis.[4]

Clinical Features

The clinical features are similar to those of squamous carcinoma, affecting the same regions of the larynx. Subglottic tumours are usually advanced at diagnosis and produce obstruction of the airway. Supraglottic carcinomas produce sore throat, dysphagia and hoarseness. Pain is often prominent in adenoid cystic carcinoma, probably due to involvement of nerves by the tumour.

Gross Appearances

The tumours usually produce large non-ulcerated masses with either a smooth or a granular surface. There may be a polypoid configuration. On slicing, the tumours are seen always to invade the underlying intrinsic muscles, and invasion of the thyroid and cricoid cartilages, and epiglottic cartilage in the case of supraglottic tumours, is frequent. One or other lobes of the thyroid gland may be ultimately involved by deeply invading tumours.

Microscopic Appearances

Most non-epidermoid carcinomas are adenocarcinomas. A large proportion of carcinomas with an adenocarcinomatous pattern will be found to be neuroendocrine (see below). Of the rest muco-epidermoid carcinoma and adenocarcinoma not otherwise specified comprise the majority. The remaining glandular malignant tumours will show an adenoid cystic histological appearance.

Mucoepidermoid carcinomas may be of low grade or high grade and their appearances are identical to those described in salivary glands (see Chapter 42) (Fig. 37.2). Adenocarcinomas not otherwise specified may be very difficult to distinguish from neuro-endocrine carcinoma (see below) and reliance must be placed on immunohistochemical markers. Other salivary gland type adenocarcinomas such as acinic cell carcinoma and epimyoepithelial carcinoma are very rare in the larynx.[5] Adenoid cystic carcinomas are usually considered as a myoepithelial cell-derived variant of adenocarcinoma, with a very specific histological pattern (see Chapters 17 and 42). As in major and minor salivary glands, invasion of tumour along perineural spaces is frequently seen in histological sections of larynges bearing adenoid cystic carcinoma.

Natural History

Adenocarcinoma of the larynx has a bad prognosis. Lymph node and bloodstream metastases are common, and most patients die with metastases within 2 years of the onset in spite of radiotherapy and surgical treatment. Lymph node metastases are rare in adenoid cystic carcinoma. Recurrence usually follows local excision within 2 years, but in some cases a delay in recurrence for 5 years or more is seen (as in adenoid cystic carcinoma of minor salivary glands), and a similar delay may occur in the development of bloodstream metastases.

Metastatic Adenocarcinoma

Adenocarcinoma presenting in the larynx may be the result of bloodstream metastasis from a distant organ. Hypernephroma (carcinoma of the kidney) represents the commonest site of origin, and deposits from that source will usually be readily recognisable by the clear cytoplasm of the tumour cells, which contain both glycogen and lipid in abundance (see Chapter 22). Malignant melanoma sometimes metastasises to the larynx. Metastasis to laryngeal cartilage alone is quite common and may be without clinical symptoms. Such metastases are always to ossified cartilage, since unossified cartilage does not have a direct blood supply.

Neuroectodermal Tumours

Granular Cell Tumour ("Myoblastoma")

Granular cell tumour, which is commonly seen in surgical histology practice in such sites as the sub-cutaneous tissue and the tongue and other mucosal surfaces, also presents quite frequently in the larynx. As its name implies, it is composed of granular cells,

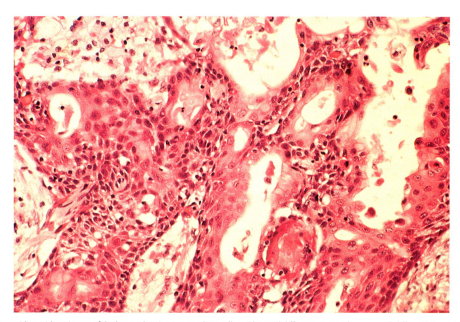

Figure 37.2 Mucoepidermoid carcinoma of the larynx showing intermediate cells, epidermoid differentiation and mucous cell differentiation with mucous glands and cysts

but its origin from primitive muscle cells has by no means been proven, and indeed even its neoplastic nature is not certain. A neuroectodermal, more specifically Schwann cell, origin has been suggested. On the basis of this possible origin, the granular cell tumour will be considered in this section, with tumours of probable neuroectodermal origin.

Incidence

Most cases present in the fourth decade, but some cases have been described in children.[6] The sex distribution is perhaps equal, but one large series has described a male bias.[7]

Site

The most common site is on the vocal cord. In many cases in the literature the lesion is stated to be in the posterior third. In some cases it has arisen from the arytenoid, supraglottic or subglottic regions.

Clinical Features and Treatment

Hoarseness is the usual symptom, but stridor has occurred in several cases, necessitating emergency tracheostomy. Local resection is usually all that is necessary to treat this. In ten cases, major surgical procedures have been required; two children required laryngectomy, and in eight patients a laryngo-fissure was carried out to remove the lesion. Radiotherapy has been used, but has no effect.

Pathological Appearances

The tumour was stated to vary in size from a small pea to a chestnut (in old-fashioned culinary pathology parlance). In the large Armed Forces Institute of Pathology series it was always less than 1 cm in diameter.[7] The dominant impression from gross descriptions of the lesion in the literature is that it is a sessile, raised swelling with a smooth mucosal surface arising from the vocal cord.

The histological characteristic of the lesion is the presence of rows of cells with granular eosinophilic cytoplasm. The nuclei are small, central and inconspicuous (Fig. 37.3). Interstitial fibrous tissue is commonly found, and the base of the lesion may thus give an impression of deep invasion, which belies the benign course of the disease. The cytoplasmic granules are eosinophilic by ordinary staining and positive by the periodic acid–Schiff method.

The appearance of the granules by electron microscopy is quite specific. They show great irregularity, being up to 1 μm diameter, with an internal structure of a complex nature showing powdery, vesicular, tubular and amorphous components (Fig. 37.4).

In the larynx, as in other mucosal surfaces, pseudo-epitheliomatous hyperplasia of the overlying squamous epithelium commonly, but not

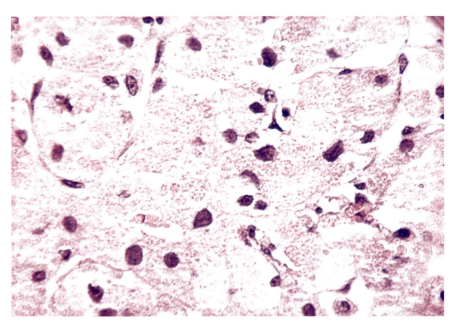

Figure 37.3 Granular cell tumour of the vocal cord showing large cells with eosinophilic granular cytoplasm and small, inconspicuous nuclei

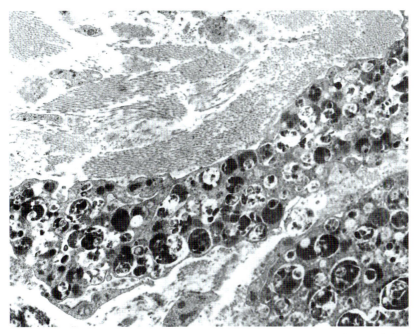

Figure 37.4 Electron micrograph of cytoplasmic processes of cell from granular cell tumour of the vocal cord. The cytoplasm is packed with irregular, dark-staining granules showing vesicles and fragmentation

always, takes place. The squamous cells do not have significant atypical features (Figs 37.5, 37.6).

Immunohistochemistry

All tumours have been found to be positive for S-100 protein and CD68 (a macrophage marker), and negative for keratin, desmin and actin.[8]

Differential Diagnosis

Granular cell tumour is a distinct lesion, but some of its features could give rise to difficulties in histological diagnosis. The differential diagnosis is usually from a histiocytic inflammatory lesion and an endocrine carcinoma. A few other lesions sometimes cause the histologist diagnostic problems. In an inflammatory formation, pleocytosis would be

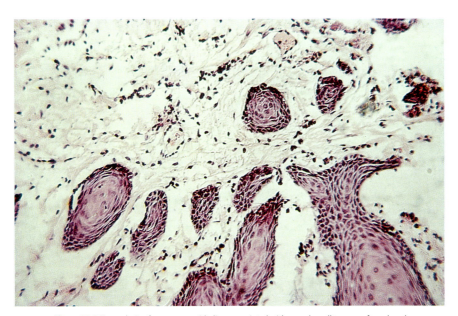

Figure 37.5 Hyperplasia of squamous epithelium associated with granular cell tumour of vocal cord

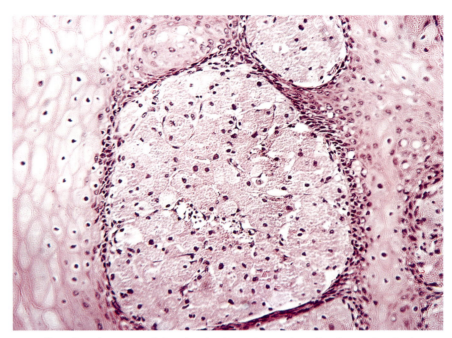

Figure 37.6 Higher power of hyperplasia of squamous epithelium of vocal cord in association with granular cell tumour. Note that there is no atypical change of the epithelium

present, while in granular cell tumour, the cells are uniform. In a neuroendocrine carcinoma, the nuclear size of the tumour cells is greater, the granularity of the cells is less obvious, and there is considerable vascularity. Periodic acid–Schiff staining does not show red cytoplasmic granularity in neuroendocrine carcinoma. Electron microscopy reveals small membrane-bound uniform granules in the latter. Malakoplakia – a lesion that has been identified on a few occasions in the upper respiratory tract and ear (see Chapter 2) but not in the larynx – might be confused with a granular cell myoblastoma. The diagnosis would be made by the presence of Michaelis-Gutmann bodies; but sometimes these structures are inconspicuous, the lesion consisting largely of histiocytic cells rather similar to those of granular cell tumour.

Squamous carcinoma may be erroneously diagnosed if a superficial biopsy shows the acanthotic squamous epithelium and the granular cells are not seen.

Neurogenic Tumours

Neurilemmomas (schwannomas) are tumours with a characteristic histological appearance. Neurofibromas are fibrous tumours with less specific features. They often show nerve fibres intermixed with the cellular elements. It may be difficult to designate particular tumours histologically into one or other of these categories. Intermediate and mixed forms

are found. The characteristic cell of each of these lesions is, moreover, the Schwann cell. For this reason, and the fact that many neurogenic tumours have been reported in the literature without designation of the particular category, the subject will be considered as "neurogenic" tumours of the larynx, including both types of neoplasm.

Incidence

Neurogenic tumours have been seen in all age groups from 3 months to 75 years.

Site

In the majority of cases, the lesion is situated in the aryepiglottic fold, bulging into the supraglottic space; it seems likely that a branch of the superior laryngeal nerve is involved in these cases. A few cases have involved the vocal cords.[9] Some neurofibromas, but not neurilemmomas, have been multinodular in the larynx.[10] Association with multiple neurofibromatosis (von Recklinghausen's disease) is encountered only rarely.[11]

Symptoms

The supraglottic position of most of the lesions will occasion initial symptoms of fullness or lump in the throat. Hoarseness and cough develop later, and when the airway is obstructed by the projecting supraglottic mass, stridor and respiratory distress become troublesome.

Treatment

Lateral thyrotomy has been recommended to approach and remove the mass after diagnosis has been made by biopsy.[9] Tracheostomy is usually necessary as a preliminary. A laryngectomy may be required if the tumour is very large.

Pathological Appearances

Neurogenic tumours appear in most cases as a supraglottic bulge covered by mucosa. The neurilemmomas are invariably firm spherical swellings with well-defined outlines. Neurofibromas may be more diffuse and less well defined. A major nerve trunk is sometimes identified in relation to the neoplasm in laryngeal neurogenic tumours (Fig. 37.7). Both types of tumour show a fibrous cut surface.

The histological appearances of a typical neurilemmoma are those of prominent Antoni A areas of palisaded Schwann cells, often whorled into Verocay bodies. Antoni B areas are almost invariably present in the same tumours and represent looser, reticular, often myxoid areas between the Antoni A regions (see Chapter 11). Neurofibromas are typically fibrous lesions with frequent nerve fibres traversing the tumour (Fig. 37.8). Sometimes a fibrous tumour will be seen with areas of nuclear palisading, representing the only indication of its neurogenic origin. Designation of such a case as neurofibroma or neurilemmoma may be very difficult. It has been stated that laryngeal neurogenic tumours are mostly of the neurofibromatous variety, but more proximally, in the mouth and pharynx, neurilemmomas will predominate.[12]

Neurofibromas may sometimes become malignant; neurilemmomas much more rarely so. In the larynx this eventuality is especially rare.

Neuroendocrine Carcinoma

Carcinoid tumours constitute a well-defined group of tumours that characteristically grow in the small intestine and vermiform appendix. On light microscopy they show a regular solid or trabecular arrangement of epithelial cells, and on ultrastructural examination there are neuroendocrine granules in the cytoplasm. A direct reducing effect on silver nitrate solution – the argentaffin effect – is produced by the tumour cells to give black cytoplasmic granules. Soluble substances, notably serotonin (5-hydroxytryptamine) are characteristically produced by the tumour cells and often cause symptoms when released into the bloodstream.

A morphologically similar neoplasm, which also has a tendency to produce polypeptide substances, grows in the bronchi, where it is usually regarded as one of the "adenomas" in spite of a slight propensity for metastases to develop. These bronchial tumours do not usually show the argentaffin reaction, but

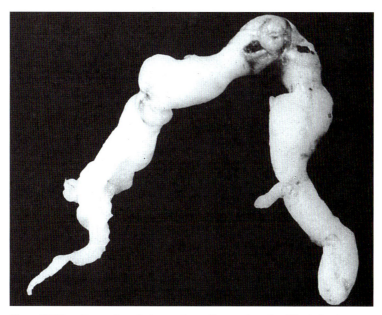

Figure 37.7 Neurofibroma of superior laryngeal nerve. The nerve is swollen diffusely along its course

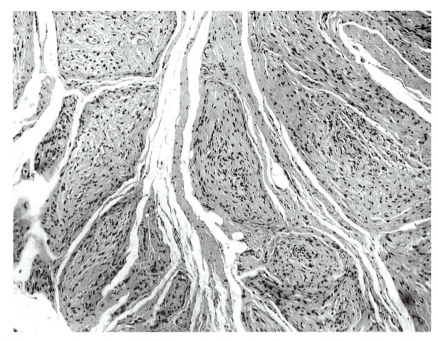

Figure 37.8 Histological appearance of tumour shown in Fig. 37.6. Groups of proliferated nerve fibres are set in a fibrous background. The appearances are those of a plexiform neurofibroma

frequently they are argyrophil, i.e. they will reduce silver solutions with the help of a reducing agent. Cells containing neuroendocrine granules normally may be found among both the surface epithelial cells (Kultschitsky cells) and the deep mucous glands of the bronchi, and it is possible that the carcinoid tumour may arise from these cells.

Small round and oat cell carcinoma is a frequent, poorly differentiated malignant tumour of the bronchus in which the tendency to tubule formation, the presence of neurosecretory cytoplasmic granules on electron microscopy and the positive reaction by immunohistochemistry to markers for neuroendocrine substances indicates an origin similar to carcinoid tumour of the bronchus. Intermediate forms between carcinoid tumour and oat cell carcinoma are well known in the bronchial neoplasms.

In the larynx similar forms of "neuroendocrine" neoplasms are now also recognised. Although uncommon, their incidence is second only to squamous carcinoma. These neoplasms may be considered to be of epithelial origin. An additional source of neuroendocrine tumours in the larynx is the paraganglia, which are known to be present normally (see Chapter 28). Paraganglia are of "neural", i.e. neuroectodermal, origin and may give rise to paraganglioma, as in other sites where paraganglia occur (see Chapter 5). Thus neuroendocrine neoplasms of the larynx may be classified as follows:[3]

1. Epithelial origin: typical carcinoid, atypical carcinoid, small cell carcinoma.

2. Neural origin: paraganglioma.

Typical Carcinoid

Typical carcinoid is very rare.[13] Most of the small number of described neoplasms of this type have arisen in the supraglottis. Microscopically the neoplasm is composed of nests of cells of bland appearance separated by a fibrovascular stroma. The Grimelius stain is positive (argyrophilia). On immunohistochemical study, neurone-specific enolase, chromogranin and synaptophysin give positive reactions.

This neoplasm usually grows slowly, but a very rare case with metastases has been described.[13]

Atypical Carcinoid

This neoplasm has also been referred to as large cell neuroendocrine carcinoma.[14] This tumour is less differentiated histologically and more aggressive in its behaviour than the typical carcinoid.

The majority of the cases are men. Almost all of these patients have been found to smoke cigarettes. The age range is 33–83 and mean age is 61 years.[14]

The usual symptoms are hoarseness and dysphagia. Sometimes referred pain to the ear is a prominent feature (glossopharyngeal neuralgia).

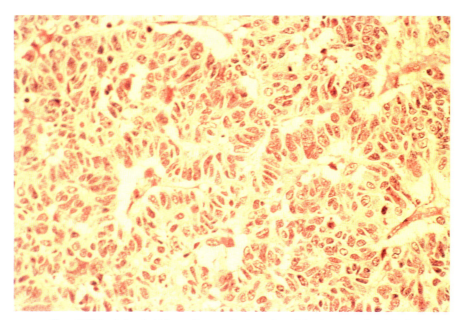

Figure 37.9 Atypical carcinoid (large cell neuroendocrine carcinoma) showing nests and acini of cells

Most of the tumours arise in the supraglottis. They are usually very small, most being less than 1 cm in diameter.[15] They may be polypoid, pedunculated, nodular or ulcerated. Microscopically the neoplasm is composed of epithelial cells forming nests, cords and acini (Fig. 37.9). The appearance of the cell nests may mimic the Zellballen pattern of paraganglioma and so lead to misdiagnosis. However, the component cells of atypical carcinoids are of malignant appearance and mitotic figures may be frequent.

Most of these neoplasms are argyrophilic and on electron microscopy all contain dense-core neurosecretory granules, which range from 90 to 250 nm in diameter. Neurone-specific enolase, chromogranin and Protein Gene Product 9.5 are usually positive on immunostaining and 50% are positive on staining for synaptophysin[15] (Fig. 37.10). Calcitonin is present in

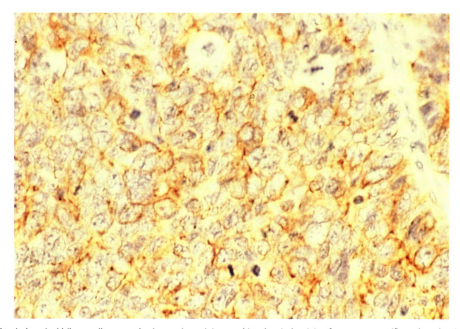

Figure 37.10 Atypical carcinoid (large cell neuroendocrine carcinoma). Immunohistochemical staining for neurone-specific enolase showing positive (red-staining) reaction of the cells

the majority.[14,15] The presence of calcitonin is a valuable adjunct in the differential diagnosis of these tumours from laryngeal paraganglioma.[14] Low molecular weight cytokeratin markers are usually positive, but high molecular weight markers are negative.

Metastasis to cervical lymph nodes is very common. Bloodstream metastases are also frequent, the main sites being liver, lungs, bone and brain. In some of the reported cases, multiple painful metastases to the skin have presented. In one case that we have seen the only relief that the patient could obtain was by the surgical excision of a large number of these skin metastases.

The mainstay of treatment is surgical excision, but the reaction to this is usually indifferent. Radiation therapy and chemotherapy have not proved to be effective.[16] Elective neck lymph node dissection is also necessary because of the high incidence of cervical metastases.

Survival at 5 and 10 years is 48% and 30% respectively.

Small Cell Neuroendocrine Carcinoma

Small cell neuroendocrine carcinoma is a well-described, but uncommon, neoplasm in the larynx;[17] the majority of patients are men over 50 years. The origins of these neoplasms are in all three regions of the larynx, but with a particular preference for the supraglottic region. Histologically the tumour resembles oat cell carcinoma of the bronchus, with small tumour cells showing little cytoplasm and containing darkly staining nuclei. Tubule formation may be present (Figs 37.11, 37.12). Argyrophilia is not present in the majority of these tumours. Ultrastructural examination shows neurosecretory granules between 100 and 380 nm in diameter. Positive staining for neurone-specific enolase is usually present, less frequently for the other neuroendocrine markers.

Small cell neuroendocrine carcinomas are very aggressive neoplasms, with a 2-year survival of 16% and a 5-year survival of only 5%.[18]

Paraganglioma

This neoplasm, probably arising from the paraganglia that are normally present in the larynx, has caused problems in the past by its confusion with atypical carcinoid. A study in 1991 clearly separated the two entities.[15] Paragangliomas may arise between the ages of 18 to 83 years, with a female to male incidence of approximately 3:1.[19] The great majority of these neoplasms arise in the supraglottis; a few have been described in the subglottis.

Grossly these tumours are red or blue submucosal masses around 2–3 cm in diameter.

The microscopic appearances are similar to those of paragangliomas of the carotid body, vagus nerve and jugular and tympanic paraganglioma in the presence of bland, uniform "Zellballen" and blood vessels (see Chapter 5). Paragangliomas are positive for neurone-specific enolase. Around the edge of the Zellballen, a row of slender elongated cells sug-

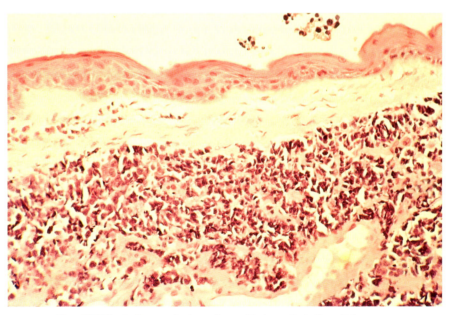

Figure 37.11 Small cell neuroendocrine carcinoma of the larynx situated beneath the mucosa

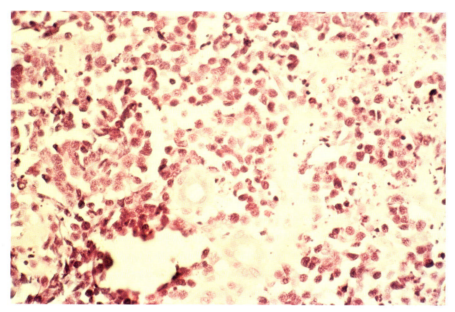

Figure 37.12 Small cell neuroendocrine carcinoma of the larynx showing some attempts at tubule formation

gestive of sustentacular cell origin can usually be discerned (Figs 37.13, 37.14).

Paragangliomas express all the usual neuroendocrine markers, including neurone-specific enolase, chromogranin, Protein Gene Product 9.5 and synaptophysin. These antibodies mark the chief cells. The peripheral sustentacular-like cells, in contrast, strongly express S-100 protein.

The most important ultrastructural feature of laryngeal paragangliomas is the presence of dense-core secretory granules up to about 290 nm in diameter. Occasional desmosomes may be present between the cell processes.

In marked contrast to atypical carcinoids, paragangliomas of the larynx are generally benign. In a very few cases metastasis has occurred. Bleeding

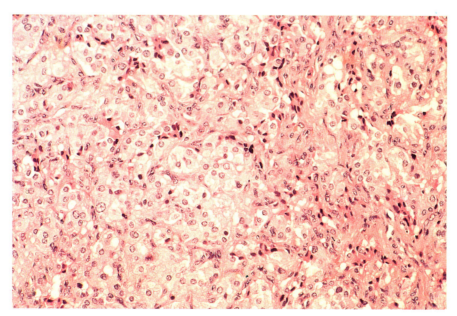

Figure 37.13 Paraganglioma of larynx. Note arrangement of cells into small packets – "Zellballen"

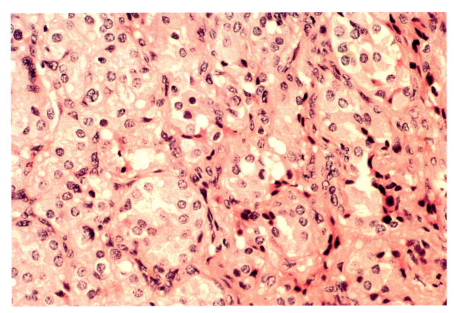

Figure 37.14 Higher power of paraganglioma of larynx shown in Fig. 37.13. Note regular cells and peripheral flattened sustentacular cells

may be a problem at biopsy, however, as at other sites of this highly vascular neoplasm (see Chapter 5).

Malignant Melanoma

Malignant melanomas are tumours arising from melanin-producing cells. The skin is the commonest site of origin for malignant melanomas, which are usually found in the epidermis. This neoplasm occasionally arises in the respiratory tract mucosa, particularly in the nose (see Chapter 18).

Melanocytes in Epithelium

Melanocytes (cells of dendritic appearance) have been observed in the epithelium of the larynx as melanin-containing dendritic cells in squamous epithelium of the supraglottic larynx after irradiation for carcinoma of the larynx, where it was felt that the irradiation had been a factor in their production.[20] Masson-Fontana silver stain for melanin in this study also revealed "appreciable numbers" of melanocytes in larynges from both Caucasian and African–American patients at autopsy. Melanocytes have also been observed in a biopsy specimen from the larynx of a single case of a patient with chronic laryngitis, but at post-mortem from 15 cases examination by the Swiss roll technique did not reveal a single larynx with dendritic silver-staining cells.[21]

Primary Malignant Melanoma

Primary malignant melanomas of the larynx are rare. It is likely that a large proportion of malignant melanomas that have been recorded in the larynx are metastatic to that organ from a primary site in the skin (see above). A compound nevus, i.e. a benign proliferation of melanocytes, has been reported in the larynx.[22]

Four cases of primary laryngeal mucosal malignant melanoma have been reported from the Armed Forces Institute of Pathology.[23] The patients were all males and ranged in age from 35 to 84 years. They had complained of hoarseness, haemoptysis, dysphagia or airway obstruction. The sites of involvement included the supraglottic larynx and the right true vocal cord. A history of cutaneous melanoma or of a melanoma at another site was not reported for any of the patients.

Histologically, the tumours were invasive and composed of pleomorphic malignant epithelioid cells with some spindle cells. Melanin was identified without staining in two patients and confirmed by Fontana stains in the other two. The immunohistochemical findings showed diffuse immunoreactivity with S-100 protein and HMB-45, but none for cytokeratin. Electron microscopy showed premelanosomes or melanosomes.

The patients were treated by laryngectomy supplemented with radiotherapy.

Follow-up information was available for three patients and all three died of metastatic disease within 36 months of diagnosis. Metastasis occurred to the brain, lungs, spine and regional lymph nodes.

Laryngeal mucosal malignant melanoma is thus a highly aggressive neoplasm.

References

1. Pinkerton PH, Beck JS. Eosinophilic granular cell (oncocytic) cysts of the larynx. J Pathol Bacteriol 1961; 81:532–534

2. Baptista PM, Garcia-Tapia R, Vazquez JJ. Pleomorphic adenoma of the epiglottis. J Otolaryngol 1992;21:355–357

3. Shanmugaratnam K, Sobin LH. Histological typing of tumours of the upper respiratory tract and ear. WHO international histological classification of tumours, 2nd edn. Springer-Verlag, Berlin, Heidelberg, New York, 1991

4. Cohen J, Guillamondegui OM, Batsakis JG et al. Cancer of the minor salivary glands of the larynx. Am J Surg 1985;150:513–518

5. Luna MA. Chapter 15. Salivary gland neoplasms. In: Ferlito A (ed) Surgical pathology of laryngeal neoplasms. Chapman & Hall Medical, London, 1996, pp 257–294

6. Conley SF, Milbrath MM, Beste DJ. Pediatric laryngeal granular cell tumour. J Otolaryngol 1992;21:450–453

7. Compagno J, Hyams VJ, Ste-Marie P. Benign granular cell tumours of the larynx: a review of 36 cases with clinicopathologic data. Ann Otol Rhinol Laryngol 1975;84:308–314

8. Lassaletta L, Alonso S, Ballestin C et al. Immunoreactivity in granular cell tumours of the larynx. Auris Nasus Larynx 1999;26:305–310

9. Cummings CW, Montgomery WW, Balogh KJ. Neurogenic tumours of the larynx. Ann Otol Rhinol Laryngol 1969;78: 76–95

10. Koc C, Luxenberger W, Humer U et al. Bilateral ventricular neurofibroma of the larynx. J Laryngol Otol 1996;110: 385–386

11. Chang-Lo M. Laryngeal involvement in Von Recklinghausen's disease: a case report and review of the literature. Laryngoscope 1977;87:435–442

12. Ash JE, Beck MR, Wilkes JD. Tumors of the upper respiratory tract and ear. Atlas of tumor pathology, section 4, fascicles 12 and 13. Armed Forces Institute of Pathology, Washington, D.C., 1964

13. El-Naggar AK, Batsakis JG. Carcinoid tumour of the larynx. A critical review of the literature. ORL J Otorhinolaryngol Related Spec 1991;53:188–193

14. Woodruff JM, Huvos AG, Erlandson RA et al. Neuroendocrine carcinomas of the larynx. A study of two types, one of which mimics thyroid medullary carcinoma. Am J Surg Pathol 1985;9:771–790

15. Milroy CM, Rode J, Moss E. Laryngeal paraganglioma and neuroendocrine carcinoma. Histopathology 1991;18:201–209

16. Woodruff JM, Senie RT. Atypical carcinoid tumour of the larynx. A critical review of the literature. ORL J Otorhinolaryngol Related Spec 1991;53:194–209

17. Pardo Mindan FJ, Algarra SM, Lozano BR et al. Oat cell carcinoma of the larynx. A study of six new cases. Histopathology 1989;14:75–80

18. Gnepp DR. Small cell neuroendocrine carcinoma of the larynx. A critical review of the literature. ORL J Otorhinolaryngol Related Spec 1991;53:210–219

19. Ferlito A, Milroy CM, Wenig BM et al. Laryngeal paraganglioma versus atypical carcinoid tumour. Ann Otol Rhinol Laryngol 1995;104:78–83

20. Goldman JL, Lawson W, Zak FG et al. The presence of melanocytes in the human larynx. Laryngoscope 1972;82: 824–835

21. Busuttil A. Dendritic pigmented cells within human laryngeal mucosa. Arch Otolaryngol 1976;102:43–44

22. Schimpf A, Musebeck K, Mootz W. Naevus zellnaevus (compound Naevus) im Larynxbereich (Plica ventricularis). [In German] Z Haut Geschlechtskrankheiten 1969;44:137–144

23. Wenig BM. Laryngeal mucosal malignant melanoma. A clinicopathologic, immunohistochemical, and ultrastructural study of four patients and a review of the literature. Cancer 1995;75:1568–1577

38 Neoplasms of Vascular, Connective and Muscular Tissue, Cartilage and Bone

Vascular Neoplasms

Vascular neoplasms arise from either lymphatic or blood vessels. Lymphangiomas are rare and usually arise from extension of cystic hygroma of the neck into the larynx (see Chapter 45). In a series of 160 cystic hygromas, ten (6%) extended into the larynx.[1] Lymphangioma confined to the larynx is very rare. Reported cases have presented in young children as respiratory obstruction, necessitating laser removal of the swelling from the laryngeal lumen.[2]

Neoplasms of blood vessels may be either benign (i.e. haemangioma) or malignant (i.e. haemangiosarcoma). Two types of tumour in which blood vessels make up part of the neoplastic element – haemangiopericytoma and Kaposi's sarcoma – will also be considered in this chapter.

Haemangioma

Haemangiomas in the adult larynx are unusual and clinically not distinctive lesions. In infants, on the other hand, laryngeal haemangiomas represent a distinctive and dangerous entity. It is, therefore, useful to subdivide laryngeal haemangiomas into adult and infantile types. The adult form includes lesions found in older children and adolescents.

Adult Form

There are two non-neoplastic lesions of the vocal cords that show a predominant content of blood vessels: (1) pyogenic granuloma of the posterior one-third of the vocal cord over the vocal process (a lesion that may be related to previous intubation or contact ulcer) and (2) a vascular vocal cord polyp (see Chapter 31). In both of these conditions gross appearances are those of a vascular, protuberant lesion on the cord, and biopsy will show an abundance of capillary blood vessels. These lesions may, therefore, be confused with haemangioma of the vocal cord and it is likely that in some of the reports of vocal cord haemangioma in adults, this has given rise to misinterpretation. Supraglottic haemangiomas do grow occasionally in adults, and in that situation are less likely to present diagnostic difficulties. Because of problems of haemorrhage they should be treated with care and, in fact, complete removal is not usually necessary if symptoms are slight.

A rare form of benign haemangioma – cavernous haemangioma – of the larynx with aggressive behaviour, involving the hypopharynx as well as the larynx, was described in children.[3]

Infantile Form

Angiomas are common lesions in the skin of infants. Other organ systems may be involved by the haemangiomas, including the central nervous system, abdominal organs, skeletal system and ocular system. The cutaneous lesions are usually noted soon after birth. They enlarge for the first 8 months or so of life and then, if left alone, will slowly involute.

The larynx may be the site of a similar lesion in infancy. Males and females are affected equally, and the lesion is almost always subglottic. The growth of infantile haemangioma in this position is dangerous because, since the subglottis is very narrow in the infant, airway obstruction soon takes place. Frequently the tumour is not visible, even on direct

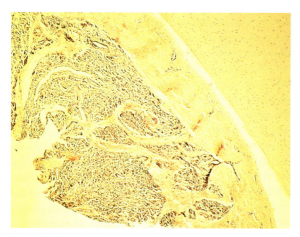

Figure 38.1 Subglottic haemangioma from an infant aged 18 months. The lesion is composed of closely packed capillaries and extends to the cricoid cartilage perichondrium on the *right edge*

laryngoscopy and the infant may die of respiratory obstruction without the diagnosis having been suspected.[4] Even at necropsy the haemangioma may not be seen grossly or may appear too small to be a cause of respiratory obstruction, as the blood drains from the vessels after death and the lesion shrinks.[5] Microscopically the angioma appears as small sinusoidal or capillary blood channels. Usually arranged in lobules, it is situated in the submucosa or on the luminal side of the cricoid cartilage perichondrium, in contact with the latter (Figs 38.1, 38.2). If, as is usually the case, the lesion is composed of capillaries, the endothelial cells may be swollen and the lumina difficult to identify. The adjacent mucosa may be ulcerated due to the pressure effects of an endotracheal tube used in treatment (see Chapter 31).

Treatment of the condition requires tracheostomy if there is significant airway obstruction. Resection of the haemangioma and adjacent subglottis, including cricoid cartilage, may be performed at a later date. Ablation may not be necessary; tracheostomy and waiting for the angioma to involute may be sufficient.[6]

Haemangiosarcoma

The terminology of malignant vascular tumours has been irregular, and the following terms have been used as synonyms for this condition: haemangiosarcoma, haemangioendothelioma, angiosarcoma, haemangioendotheliosarcoma, lymphangiosarcoma.

Pathological Appearances

The lesion is very rare in the larynx. Haemangiosarcoma usually has a haemorrhagic and cystic gross appearance. In the larynx in one of the few reported cases,[7] the tumour was widely invasive in the supraglottic larynx. In another reported case, the tumour widely infiltrated the soft tissues of and around the larynx, proceeding anteriorly into the pre-epiglottic space and posteriorly into the piriform fossae, although laryngeal cartilage was not invaded.[8]

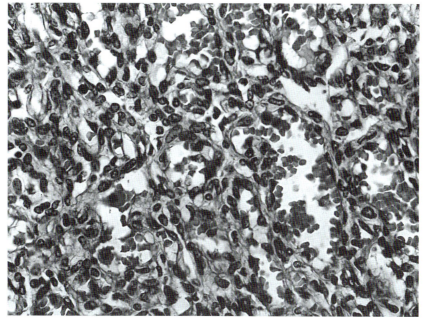

Figure 38.2 Higher power of Fig. 38.1. Some capillaries contain blood while others are closed and empty

Microscopically a spectrum of appearances can be recognised in haemangiosarcomas, from a well-differentiated angiomatous pattern to a poorly differentiated solid pattern (Fig. 38.3). It is important to identify that the actual endothelial cells lining blood vessels have malignant features. Immunohistochemistry with factor VIII, Ulex europaeus I and CD31 antibodies shows strong expression of the malignant endothelial cell and the cells of the solid areas, while the tumour cells are negative for cyto-keratins. Both of the cases of laryngeal haemangiosarcoma of the larynx cited above had metastasised early and the patients died as a result of the neoplasm within 1 year.

Haemangiopericytoma

Haemangiopericytoma is a neoplasm composed of normal blood vessels surrounded by spindle-shaped

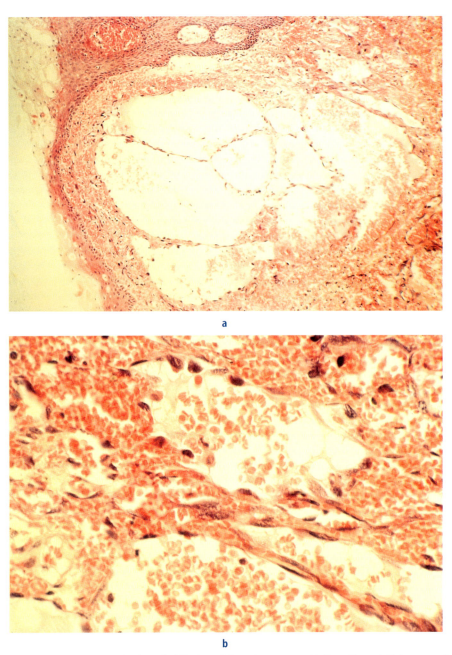

Figure 38.3 a Angiosarcoma showing large, irregular, thin-walled blood vessels beneath squamous epithelium of larynx. **b** Higher power of **a** showing highly atypical endotheial cells lining blood vessels

or round tumour cells, which are thought to be derived from the pericytes of Zimmermann. Since the very existence of the latter cells is in doubt, it is not surprising that the existence of the tumour entity itself is often doubted. Be that as it may, the neoplasm to which this term has been applied has only very rarely been identified in the larynx.[9] The latter author describes one case in which the larynx was widely involved from the aryepiglottic fold to the subglottis. Histologically the blood vessels are abundant, but lined by normal endothelial cells. The position of the latter cells may be confirmed by reticulin stains. The tumour cells lie between the normal blood vessels. Clearly there is ample scope for a variety of sarcomatous neoplasms and even undifferentiated carcinomas to be misinterpreted as haemangiopericytomas.

Kaposi's Sarcoma

Kaposi's sarcoma is a neoplasm with histological features comprising a mixture of spindle cells, vascular slits and branching vascular channels. This neoplasm was first described in the skin of the feet of Jewish and Mediterranean men, but has since become commonly observed in African males. In most cases it remains local, but visceral and lymph node involvement occurs in some, and approximately 15% of the patients have fatal visceral lesions in which the larynx may be one of the involved organs.

The lesion usually involved the epiglottis as a reddish, protuberant mass. Histologically the neoplasm shows moderately atypical spindle-shaped cells surrounding slit-like spaces containing red cells (Fig. 38.4). The tumour cells frequently stain positively for factor VIII, indicating an origin of this tumour from vascular endothelium.

Kaposi's sarcoma is now much more frequently seen as a manifestation of AIDS in homosexual men. It has recently been discovered to be caused by infection with a herpes virus – HHV8 – which actually infects the endothelial and spindle cells of Kaposi's sarcoma in AIDS patients.[10]

The neoplasm in AIDS is characterised by a greater tendency to involve the skin of the head and neck, and lymphadenopathy and other visceral involvement are more common than in the non-HIV-infected cases. Although involvement of the larynx is regarded as rare in HIV-infected patients,[11] the lesion may be seen quite frequently at fibreoptic examination or at autopsy of AIDS sufferers. It appears as purple or haemorrhagic, raised areas in the epiglottis, supraglottis or vocal cords and affects also the oropharynx and posterior tongue.[12]

Fibroblastic Lesions

Fibroblastic lesions, non-neoplastic and neoplastic, are uncommon in the larynx. In fact the numbers of reported cases are so small that any assessment of their behaviour in relation to gross and histological appearance is difficult. A similar range of lesions is encountered to that of the nose and paranasal sinuses (see Chapter 26).

Non-neoplastic Fibroblastic Lesions

The great majority of collections of fibrocytic cells with collagen are reactive in nature or fibromatoses.

Inflammatory Myofibroblastic Tumour

Synonyms for this condition are pseudotumours, inflammatory pseudotumours and nodular fasciitis.[13] These lesions may appear in any part of the larynx as a firm polypoid mass. Histologically they show oval to spindle cells set in a collagenous and/or myxoid stroma. There is always an accompanying inflammatory exudate of lymphocytes, plasma cells and macrophages (Fig. 38.5). There is usually no recurrence after surgical excision. The aetiology is unknown.

Fibromatosis

The most important lesion of fibroblasts in the non-neoplastic category is represented by the fibromatoses. These infiltrating masses of collagenous fibrous tissue are characterised by the absence of inflammatory cells, and the benign, non-neoplastic appearance of the component fibrocytes. This is a rare lesion of the larynx, growing usually in young children.[14] The fibromatoses may be locally infiltrative in the larynx and recur after removal. Microscopically the component tissue is composed of mature fibrocytes and abundant collagen.

Neoplastic Collagenous Lesions

Solitary Fibrous Tumour

A very rare neoplasm in the larynx is the "solitary fibrous tumour"[15] (see Chapter 20). Patternless spindle cells with focal vascular areas comprise the histological basis of this neoplasm. There is a notable immunoreactivity with antibodies to CD34 antigen.

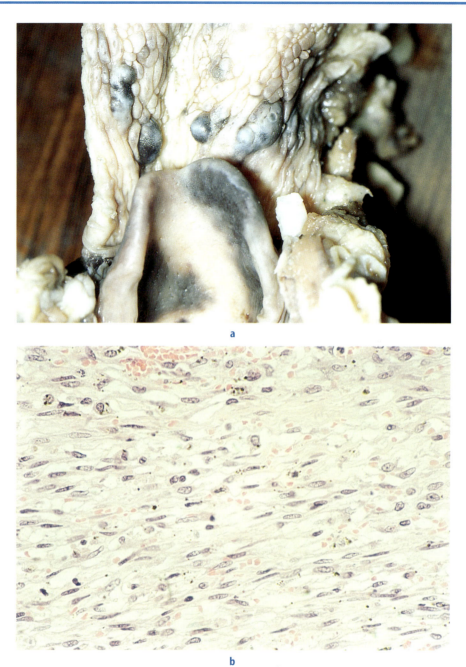

Figure 38.4 Kaposi's sarcoma. **a** Post-mortem specimen from a patient with AIDS showing multiple bluish swellings over base of tongue, pharynx and posterior surface of epiglottis. **b** The neoplasm is composed of moderately atypical spindle cells between vascular spaces

Fibrous Histiocytomas

The classification and histology of fibrous histiocytomas is discussed in Chapter 20. Cases of laryngeal fibrous histiocytoma that have been reported have arisen from both the glottis and subglottis. The tumour is made up of fibroblastic cells frequently arranged in a cartwheel (storiform) fashion and histiocytic cells containing lipid or haemosiderin or

with multiple nuclei as Touton giant cells. Electron microscopy shows fibroblast-like cells with abundant rough endoplasmic reticulum, histiocyte-like cells with numerous lysosomes and transitional cells with characteristics of both the fibroblast-like and histiocyte-like cells.[16]

Fibrous histiocytomas, including fibroxanthomas, occurring in the larynx should be regarded as potentially locally invasive, especially when they

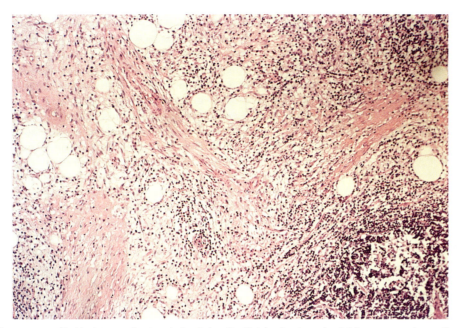

Figure 38.5 Inflammatory myofibroblastic tumour showing spindle cells (myofibroblasts) set in a dense chronic inflammatory exudate, and bundles of collagen

grow rapidly, recur locally and show a cellular histological pattern, but metastasis does not occur.

Fibrosarcoma

Malignant fibroblastic tumours are described as "fibrosarcoma". Small numbers of high-grade fibrosarcomas have been described in the larynx.[17] Previous radiotherapy to glottic carcinoma has sometimes been a factor.[18] Fibrosarcomas have grown in patients mainly over the age of 50 years. Most of these tumours arose from the anterior part of the true vocal cord or anterior commissure or both. They were usually nodular or pedunculated. Few were ulcerated. Microscopically they are composed of elongated malignant cells in bundles, often with interlacing fascicles – the "herring-bone" pattern. The rate of growth is related to the degree of differentiation. Those lesions composed of poorly differentiated fibrosarcomas grow by spread of the tumour along fascial planes and eventually penetrate muscle outside the larynx. Bloodstream metastasis is very unusual, but nearly all patients with such poorly differentiated tumours die from local recurrence within 3 years of presentation.

It must be pointed out that the term fibrosarcoma has formerly embraced several entities, some of which have now been recognised as distinct from that condition. In the larynx a pedunculated lesion with a malignant fibroblastic histological appearance growing in the region of the anterior vocal cord is most likely to be a spindle cell carcinoma. This lesion is recognised by the presence of a squamous carcinomatous component in some parts of the neoplasm, or at least by a surface malignant (i.e. intraepithelial carcinomatous) appearance with the impression of the malignant spindle cells emanating from the surface component (see Chapter 36). It must be admitted that cases are seen in which the surface epithelium is of doubtful malignancy, and a definite classification of the malignant neoplasm as either spindle cell carcinoma or fibrosarcoma cannot be made. Since there is a strong likelihood that the lesion is a spindle cell carcinoma, such malignancies should be treated on the same lines as a squamous cell carcinoma of similar size and position, i.e. by irradiation or surgery.

Synovial Sarcoma

In the development of a joint lining, the primitive mesenchymal cells in the vicinity of the joint cavity differentiate into an inner synovial layer and an outer connective tissue layer. The biphasic property of these mesenchymal cells – the development of both epithelial-like and connective tissue-like components – is a particular mark of the synovial cell, which is manifested in neoplasms derived from synovium, the synovial sarcomas. It is noteworthy that most synovial sarcomas do not arise from adult synovial membranes, and actual involvement of a joint cavity by the neoplasm is infrequent. It seems likely that undifferentiated mesenchymal cells may differentiate in the direction of synovioblastic cells and so give rise to synovial sarcoma, even in regions where adult synovium is not normally present.

Most of the synovial sarcomas presenting to oto-laryngologists are in the neck (see Chapter 45). In the larynx, synovial sarcoma is an extremely rare neoplasm. Microscopically the neoplasm consists of fusiform cells and also epithelioid cells arranged in nests or pseudo-acini containing mucin. Dystrophic calcification and calcospherites are characteristic findings in synovial sarcoma. The laryngeal synovial sarcomas, like the same tumour at other sites, shows on cytogenic analysis a reciprocal translocation between chromosomes X and 18, the detection of which can be of diagnostic value. A malignant outcome is to be expected in this tumour unless it is completely removed surgically at an early stage.

Neoplasms of Adipose Tissue

Although adipose tissue is a normal feature of the larynx, particularly in the false cord, neoplasms derived from this tissue are distinctly rare. Most of the lipomas affecting the larynx have extended from the hypopharynx. In a few patients the origin of the lipoma is from the aryepiglottic fold.

Grossly lipomas are light-coloured, encapsulated, smooth, lobulated swellings situated in the submucosa of the larynx. Broad fibrous trabeculae project inward from the capsule between the fat lobules. Microscopically the tumours are composed of fat cells, which vary greatly in size, and other connective tissue elements.

Liposarcomas are unusual in the head and neck and extremely rare in the larynx. Those described in the larynx were sited only in the supraglottis.[19] Histologically they were all well-differentiated, being composed of neoplastic lobules of adipocytes of varying size and shape traversed by fibrous bands. Atypical cells and lipoblasts were present in some areas. The neoplasms did not metastasize, but multiple recurrences were a feature.

Myogenic Neoplasms

Neoplasms made up of muscle cells conform to the two types of muscle tissue found in the body – smooth and striated muscle. In each group, benign and malignant forms are found. The head and neck is the usual site for muscle tumours of the striated variety. In the larynx all neoplasms of muscle are rare. Myogenic neoplasms of the nose are described in Chapter 19.

Neoplasms of Smooth Muscle

Benign Leiomyoma

Smooth muscle neoplasms fall into three possible patterns:

1. Those composed of smooth muscle cells only.
2. Vascular leiomyomas.
3. Epithelioid leimyomas (leiomyoblastomas).

Leiomyoma

Leiomyomas are well-demarcated, spherical tumours with a firm consistency. Microscopically they are composed of interlacing bundles of smooth muscle with fibrous tissue in varying amounts between the bundles. Smooth muscle cells are recognised as slender spindle cells with elongated nuclei showing rounded ("cigar-shaped") ends and fine cytoplasmic fibrils.

These lesions present usually in adults in the false cords. In some cases they are pedunculated. Larger tumours distend the aryepiglottic folds and expand the piriform fossa or protrude from the ventricle. Most tumours can be removed endoscopically. No recurrence of these benign neoplasms need be expected.[20]

Vascular Leiomyoma

Vascular leiomyomas are not uncommon in the forearms and legs, but are very rare indeed in the larynx. They differ from the more usual leiomyoma in the presence of a number of blood vessels with thick coats composed of smooth muscle cells, which merge with the smooth muscle cells in the main tumour substance. The tumours may bleed profusely before and especially during removal.[20]

Epithelioid Leiomyoma (Leiomyoblastoma)

In these tumours, usually found in the stomach, the smooth muscle cells display a vacuolated cytoplasm, the groups of cells together forming an epithelioid pattern (see Chapter 19). This neoplasm is extremely rare in the larynx, the few cases reported being on the vocal cord.[21]

Leiomyosarcoma

The malignant form of smooth muscle tumour, leiomyosarcoma is also rare in the larynx. In one case, the tumour extended from the false cord into the subglottis, and in another it was confined to the false cord.[20] In most of the cases, rapid recurrence, invasion and metastasis to cervical lymph nodes and by the bloodstream took place.

The rate of growth is related to the degree of differentiation. The better-differentiated cases may be cured by radical surgery, but even in these the outcome is unpredictable, since metastases may appear several years after surgery. Radiotherapy does not appear to be of value. The histological appearance of leiomyosarcomas is similar to that of leiomyomas. Nuclear atypicism and mitotic figures are the hallmarks of malignancy, and the severity of the former and the number of the latter give an indication of the degree of malignancy of the neoplasm.

Leiomyosarcomas are difficult to distinguish from other mesenchymal malignant tumours, particularly fibrosarcoma. Immunohistochemical investigation is required. The tumour cells are positive with antibodies against vimentin, desmin and smooth muscle actin antigens. Electron microscopy may be of help in the recognition of leiomyosarcoma. In the cells of that neoplasm (as indeed in all smooth muscle cells) on ultrastructural examination the cytoplasm characteristically shows parallel actin filaments, fusiform dense bodies among the filaments, and attachment plaques along the plasmalemma membrane.[22]

Neoplasms of Striated Muscle

Benign Rhabdomyoma

Patients with tuberose sclerosis often develop nodules of striated muscle in their myocardium. These nodules are distinct from true rhabdomyomas, which are rare, presenting mainly in the head and neck region. The larynx is an occasional site of presentation for benign rhabdomyoma. Two forms of rhabdomyoma are recognised: adult and fetal. In both, cross-striations are infrequent in the tumour cells, but the presence of muscle-specific actin, myoglobin and desmin antigens by immunohistochemistry helps in the recognition of the tumour cells as being of skeletal muscle origin. The site of origin of rhabdomyomas may be anywhere in the larynx.

Adult Rhabdomyoma

Adult rhabdomyoma occurs predominantly in males with a median age of 60 years.[23] This lesion is well circumscribed or encapsulated. Histologically adult rhabdomyomas are composed of large, uniform, round to polygonal cells with abundant acidophil, fibrillary cytoplasm and large vesicles, often peri-pheral nuclei and prominent acidophil nucleoli. Cross-striations are difficult to find in these neoplasms. Glycogen is plentiful in the cytoplasm of the cells and may be demonstrated by the periodic acid–Schiff stain with and without diastase. A feature of this tumour is the so-called "spider cells" in which there is a large peripheral cytoplasmic clear zone transversed by thin cytoplasmic strands extending from the central acidophilic cytoplasm to the periphery. These areas have probably come about by the loss of glycogen in the periphery of the cells by solution during fixation and processing (Fig. 38.6).

The differential diagnosis of this tumour is usually from granular cell tumour. In the latter the tumour cells are smaller and have inconspicuous nucleoli (see Chapter 37).

Adult rhabdomyoma is a benign tumour of the larynx and may be treated by simple surgical removal with excellent prospect of cure.

Fetal Rhabdomyoma

Fetal rhabdomyoma tends to occur in a younger age group than adult rhabdomyoma and with relatively fewer male cases.[24] In the few cases described in the larynx, fetal rhabdomyoma has appeared as a vocal cord polyp. Fetal rhabdomyomas have been divided into myxoid and cellular varieties.[25] The myxoid type is largely composed of immature cells containing little or no visible cytoplasm with small round to oval and occasionally spindle-shaped nuclei. Strap and ribbon cells showing cross-striations are also present in moderate numbers (Fig. 38.7). The other type of fetal rhabdomyoma – the cellular variety – is composed of closely packed interlacing bundles of spindle cells. It has not been described in the larynx. Fetal rhabdomyoma is a benign, unaggressive lesion.

Rhabdomyosarcoma

In its embryonal form, rhabdomyosarcoma is a relatively common tumour of the orbit, nasopharynx and middle ear of children (see Chapter 25). The larynx, however, is a rare site for this malignant neoplasm.[26]

These tumours tend to be bulky, sessile or pedunculated lesions with smooth surfaces, particularly occurring in the glottic region. Histologically the embryonal type may appear as a tumour composed of small oval undifferentiated mesenchymal cells; there may be some spindle-shaped or strap-shaped cells showing cross-striations. Glycogen is usually abundant in the cytoplasm of many of the tumour cells.

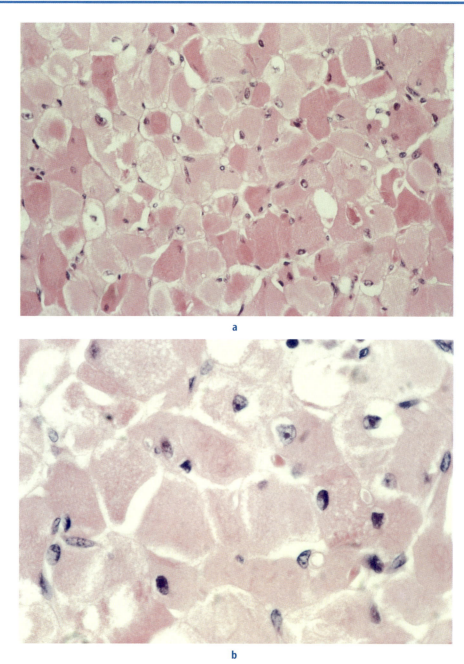

Figure 38.6 Adult rhabdomyoma of supraglottic larynx. **a** The constituent cells show abundant acidophil cytoplasm. Some of them are "spider cells", with thin cytoplasmic strands around the periphery. **b** Higher power of **a**. Cross striations are not visible. c Immunochemical staining for desmin is strongly positive and brings out the numerous cross-striations

(Figure 38.6 c, see opposite)

The more differentiated rhabdomyosarcoma – the pleomorphic rhabdomyosarcoma – is likewise rare in the larynx. It shows a higher proportion of strap-shaped or racquet-shaped differentiated striated muscle cells. Nuclei in both forms show markedly malignant features with mitotic figures, often atypical.

These highly malignant neoplasms exhibit a strong tendency to local recurrence and lymph node and distant metastases, in spite of vigorous local surgical therapy. It seems that, unlike rhabdomyosarcoma of the ear and nasopharynx, there is a fair chance of curing laryngeal rhabdomyosarcoma if a radical operation can be carried out sufficiently early.[20]

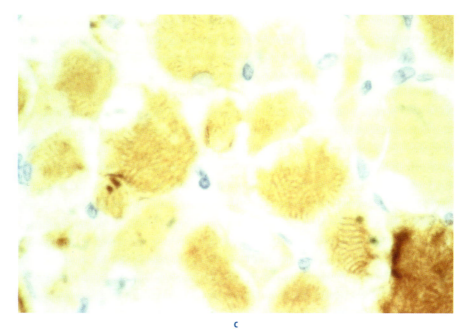

c

Figure 38.6 c

Alveolar Soft Part Sarcoma

Also known as malignant granular cell myoblastoma, alveolar soft part sarcoma is a malignant tumour that usually occurs in the muscles of the extremities, but which occasionally presents in the head and neck. While the tissue of origin is unknown, the tumour will be considered here with muscular neoplasms.

The tumour is characterised by the arrangement of the cells in compact groups composed of 5–50 cells. The component cells are large, polyhedral and eosinophilic, with finely granular cytoplasm. The nuclei are eccentrically situated, vesicular and contain one or more distinct nucleoli (Fig. 38.8). Large crystals are present by light and electron microscopy in the cytoplasm of the majority of cases.[27] Metastasis often occurs; in some cases local lymph node metastasis is reported, but more frequently this stage is bypassed and bloodstream metastases are the first sign of spread.

In the few cases in which alveolar soft part sarcoma has been reported in the larynx, the tumour has been sited in the supraglottis.[28]

Cartilaginous Neoplasms and Bone-Producing Lesions

Neoplasms of the laryngeal cartilage are surprisingly rare in spite of the considerable bulk of that tissue. Almost all the tumours are derived from and composed of hyaline cartilage. Metaplastic formations of elastic cartilage in the soft tissues of the larynx are considered separately in this chapter (see below).

Neoplasms of Hyaline Cartilage

Benign and malignant neoplasms of hyaline cartilage are found in the larynx. Although extreme degrees of malignancy are easy to recognise, the distinction between benign chondromas and low-grade chondrosarcomas is often not easy, and the two types of tumour will be considered as one entity.

Frequency

All publications on this subject are agreed that laryngeal chondroma and chondrosarcoma are rare. The experience of the present authors is that a single case presents at their institutions but once every 2 or 3 years. It should be pointed out that any type of such assessment must be weighted towards an artificially high incidence of the cartilaginous tumours, since cases of such an unusual entity tend to gravitate to specialist laryngological centres at the expense of some cases of the frequently occurring squamous carcinoma, which would usually be treated at local centres. A more balanced figure is that laryngeal chondrosarcoma represents 0.5% of

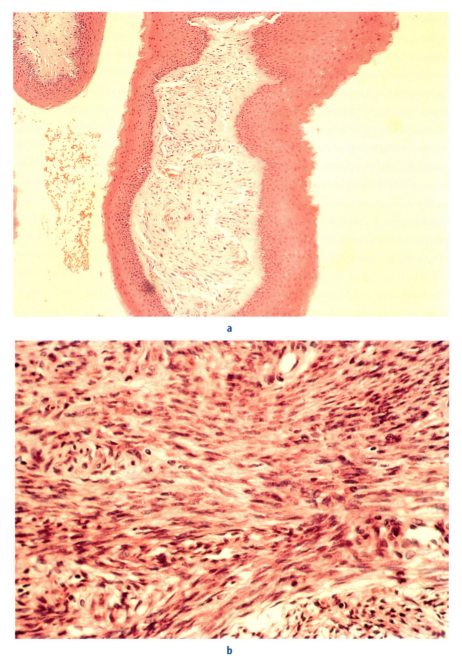

Figure 38.7 Fetal rhabdomyoma.**a** Myxoid variety, which presented as a polyp of the vocal cord.**b** Cellular variety showing abundant closely packed spindle cells. This was found in the nasopharynx.**c** End-to-end arrangement of nuclei in spindle cells.**d** Area of differentiated striated muscle in vocal cord fetal rhabdomyoma
(Figure 38.7 c and d, see opposite)

all laryngeal tumours.[29] Thus chondromatous neoplasms of the larynx must be very rare indeed.

in a large series of chondrosarcomas was 63 years, with a range of 44–91 years.[30]

Incidence

All series of cartilaginous tumours of the larynx show an increased incidence in males. The mean age

Site

By far the most usual site of origin of cartilaginous neoplasms in the larynx is the posterior lamina of

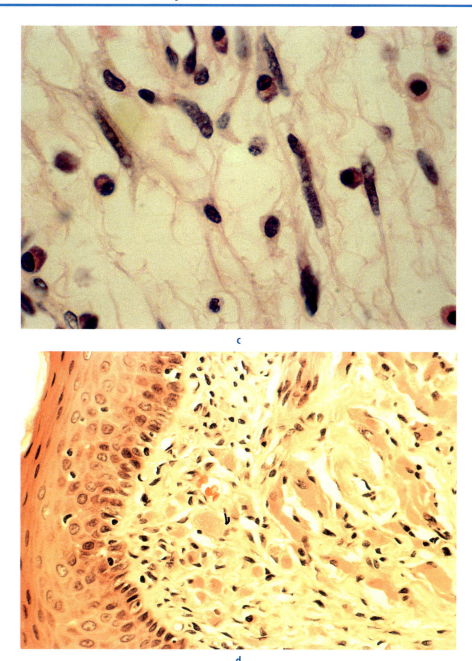

c

d

the cricoid cartilage; a smaller number arise from the thyroid cartilage. The arytenoid cartilage is rarely a site of cartilaginous tumour origin, although there are described cases[31,32] and a further one is shown below. Epiglottic cartilage origin is excessively rare[33] and the development of metastases in such a case is unique.[34]

Clinical Features

Hoarseness is likely to be a feature when vocal cord movement or vibration is affected by the tumour mass. Symptoms of airway obstruction are present in all cricoid lamina tumours, since the tumours tend to grow forward from the cricoid lamina and

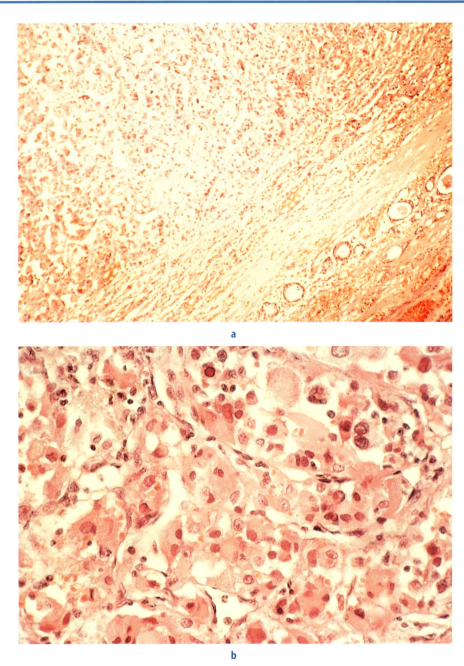

Figure 38.8 Alveolar soft part sarcoma of larynx. **a** Groups of large eosinophilic cells near laryngeal glands. **b** Large eosinophilic cells with finely granular cytoplasm

obstruct the subglottic lumen of the larynx. Thyroid cartilage neoplasms may grow inwards towards the lumen to produce airway obstruction, or outwards, where they may be detected as a mass related to the laryngeal framework on palpation of the neck.

The lesions are usually recognised on computerised tomography imaging study of the larynx as a smooth-surfaced, homogeneously dense tumour, which is occasionally ulcerated. There is frequently a significant degree of mottled calcification.

Biopsy Findings

Biopsy of a mass protruding into the laryngeal airway is frequently carried out at direct laryngoscopy. In some cases the presence of highly atypical cartilage cells in the biopsy fragment may enable a diagnosis of chondrosarcoma to be made easily. In other cases cartilage showing only slightly atypical changes may be obtained in the biopsy material, and the pathologist may be under the impression that this is normal cartilage removed at a rather deep bite by the biopsy forceps. In the process of bronchial biopsy, normal cartilage is frequently removed and its presence is of no significance in the pathological assessment. In the larynx, however, cartilage is rarely removed at endoscopic biopsy unless it is pathological, usually as a result of either perichondritis (see Chapter 35) or a cartilaginous neoplasm.

Gross Appearances

The majority of neoplasms of hyaline cartilage in the larynx will be seen as smooth protrusions of the cricoid lamina projecting from the posterior subglottic wall into the lumen. On opening the larynx, the tumour is seen to be arising from the central portion of the cartilage, usually on one side, but sometimes involving both sides of the cricoid lamina. The lesion has a faint bluish or grey hyaline appearance with a gently lobulated surface. Thyroid and arytenoid cartilage neoplasms present focal bulges from these cartilages with similar cut-surface appearances (Fig. 38.9).

Microscopic Appearances

Normal cartilage is composed of cells with small nuclei and basophilic cytoplasm. The cells may be situated in small clusters, but are always surrounded by large amounts of metachromatic hyaline ground substance containing fine collagen fibres. The cells in normal cartilage may be swollen, but this affects the cytoplasm only, and the nuclei remain small.

Cartilage cells are often more abundant at the growing edge near the perichondrium.

The growth pattern of normal cartilage is imitated in the cartilaginous tumours. These usually grow in lobules surrounded by loose connective tissue and vascular septa. There is often a thin rim of bone around the edges of the tumour lobules and little evidence of infiltration of adjacent cartilage.

In a chondroma the pathologist is satisfied by the resemblance of all cartilage cells to normal cells. In chondrosarcoma the differences from normal may be quite subtle. These differences were summarised by Lichtenstein and Jaffe,[35] and their severity provides an indication of the propensity for aggressive growth of laryngeal cartilage neoplasms. These criteria are as follows:

1. There are too many cells.
2. The cells and nuclei are too irregular, i.e. pleomorphism is present.
3. Nuclei stain too darkly.
4. Large or giant cells with single, double or multiple nuclei are present.

Attempts have been made to grade these tumours as an indication of the approach to treatment that should be adopted,[31] but with the exception of the "dedifferentiated" chondrosarcoma (see below), this is probably unnecessary because of generally good response to conservative surgical therapy. Areas of amorphous calcification are frequently found in chondrosarcoma of the larynx (Fig. 38.10). Osteoid or woven bone may also be seen in any chondroid lesion, but by themselves are of no significance in the assessment of possibly increased malignant tendency in these lesions.

Dedifferentiated Chondrosarcoma

The presence of substantial areas of an additional malignant mesenchymal component,[36] as well as the biopsy changes of a malignant cartilaginous tumour, have been shown to indicate a more serious outlook for the patient with the development of cervical lymph node and bloodstream – even bone – metastases. This dedifferentiated histological change in the neoplasm can develop months or years after the initial presentation of a chondrosarcoma of standard histological type.[34,37]

Treatment and Natural History

The benign tumours do not recur after adequate excision. Chondrosarcomas may recur after limited treatment, but conservative surgery would seem to

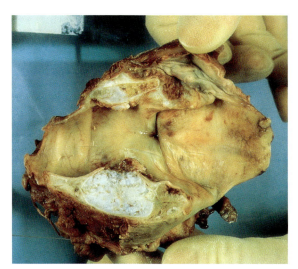

Figure 38.9 Chondrosarcoma of cricoid lamina. Larynx opened through the cricoid lamina, which is expanded by a pale grey tumour of hyaline appearance.

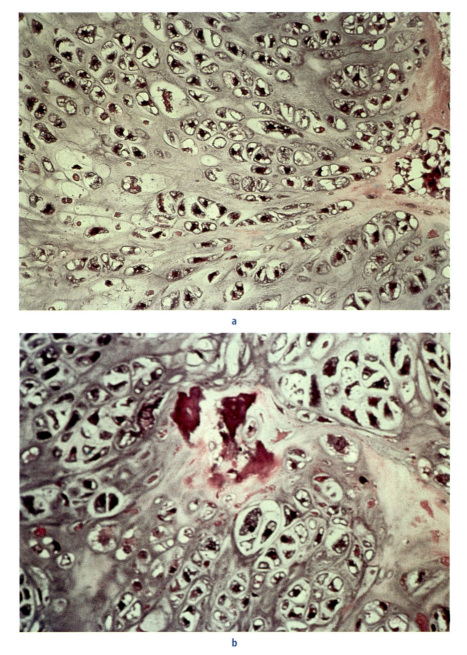

Figure 38.10 Microscopic appearance of chondrosarcoma of the larynx. **a** The cells are larger, more darkly staining, more numerous and more variable than those of normal cartilage. **b** There is an area of calcification among the cells

be adequate and laryngectomy can be safely deferred until one or even two recurrences have been experienced, since in low-grade chondrosarcoma recurrence is a slow process. In a large series of 44 cases the overall 5-year survival was 90.1%, which did not differ significantly from the expected natural survival of the patients.[30] Laryngectomy was performed as primary treatment for chondrosarcoma in six patients and only 15 of the patients (34%) required total laryngectomy. Of the patients

with chondrosarcoma, 40% had tumour recurrence or symptomatic tumour progression at an average of 4.5 years after diagnosis. There were no metastases.

Neoplasms of Elastic Cartilage

It is not certain that neoplasms of elastic cartilage even exist. Most elastic cartilaginous new forma-

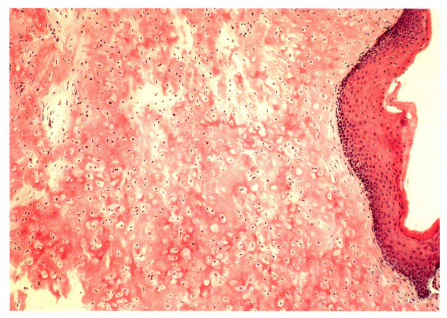

Figure 38.11 Elastic cartilage metaplasia in connective tissue of false cord, which normally consists of glands and adipose and connective tissue

tions of the larynx grow from the soft tissues, not from cartilage.

Elastic Cartilage Metaplasia

Nodules of elastic cartilage are quite commonly found in the false cord or true cord. In the true cord their presence rarely causes a clinical problem. In the false cord such nodules may produce symptoms and may be detected radiologically or observed as smooth bulges protruding into the laryngeal lumen at direct laryngoscopy.

Histologically these lesions are seen as adult elastic cartilage (Fig. 38.11). Fibroblasts at the periphery of the lesions show a transition to chondrocytes in the main part of the lesion.[38] It has been suggested, since almost 80% of patients with symptomatic chondrometaplasia had previously had endotracheal intubation,[39] that the lesion is the result of trauma.

Osteosarcoma

Osteosarcoma is an extremely rare neoplasm in the larynx. It is likely that some of the cases described as such do not, in fact, represent osteosarcoma, but some other bone-producing condition. Any bone-producing malignant mesenchymal neoplasm should at first be suspected as spindle cell carcinoma, and careful observation made of the covering epithelium for areas of squamous carcinoma or carcinoma in

situ. Not only bone but also cartilage may be produced in spindle cell carcinoma, and the conjunction of these hard tissues with the sarcoma-like tissue of the carcinoma may closely imitate osteosarcoma (see Chapter 36).

A well-authenticated case of osteosarcoma of the larynx has been described in a 62-year-old man with respiratory obstruction due to a large tumour filling the glottis and subglottis.[40] Histologically the tumour was composed of spindle cells showing numerous mitoses, osteoid, a little bone and chondroid tissue. In spite of subtotal laryngectomy, the patient died after 3 months with local recurrence and cervical lymph node, but not bloodstream, metastases. Spindle cell carcinoma was carefully excluded as there was nowhere any relationship of hyperplastic squamous epithelium to the neoplasm. A case of laryngeal osteosarcoma has been described, which grew after irradiation of nasopharyngeal carcinoma.[41]

References

1. Cohen SR, Thompson JW. Lymphangiomas of the larynx in infants and children. A survey of pediatric lymphangioma. Ann Otol Rhinol Laryngol Suppl 1986;127:1–20
2. Papsin BC, Evans JN. Isolated laryngeal lymphangioma: a rare cause of airway obstruction in infants. J Laryngol Otol 1996;110:969–972
3. Bridger GP, Nassar VH, Skinner HG. Hemangioma in the adult larynx. Arch Otolaryngol 1970;92:493–498
4. Ferguson CF, Flake CG. Subglottic hemangioma as a cause of respiratory obstruction in infants. Trans Am Bronchoesoph Ass 1961;41:27–47

5. Cameron AH, Cant WHP, MacGregor ME, et al. Angioma of the larynx in laryngeal stridor of infancy. J Laryngol Otol 1960;74:846–857

6. Sherrington CA, Sim DK, Freezer NJ et al. Subglottic haemangioma. Arch Dis Child 1997;76;458–459

7. Pratt LW, Goodof II. Hemangioendotheliosarcoma of the larynx. Arch Otolaryngol 1968;87:484–489

8. Sciot R, Delaere P, Van Damme B et al. Angiosarcoma of the larynx. Histopathology 1995;26:177–180

9. Schwartz MR, Donovan DT. Hemangiopericytoma of the larynx: a case report and review of the literature. Head Neck Surg 1987;369–372

10. Porter SR, Di Alberti L, Kumar N. Human herpes virus 8 (Kaposi's sarcoma herpesvirus). Oral Oncol 1998;34:5–14

11. Schiff NF, Annino DJ, Woo P et al. Kaposi's sarcoma of the larynx. Ann Otol Rhinol Laryngol 1997;106:563–567

12. Mochloulis G, Irving RM, Grant HR et al. Laryngeal Kaposi's sarcoma in patients with AIDS. J Laryngol Otol 1996;110:1034–1037

13. Sclafini AP, Kimmelman CP, McCormick SA. Inflammatory pseudotumour of the larynx: comparison with orbital inflammatory pseudotumour with clinical implications. Otolaryngol Head Neck Surg 1993;109:548–551

14. Rosenberg HS, Vogler C, Close LG et al. Laryngeal fibromatosis in the neonate. Arch Otolaryngol 1981;107:513–517

15. Safneck JR, Alguacil-Garcia A, Dort JC et al. Solitary fibrous tumour: report of 2 new locations in the upper respiratory tract. J Laryngol Otol 1993;107:252–256

16. Kuwabara H, Saito K, Shibanushi T et al. Malignant fibrous histiocytoma of the larynx. Eur Arch Otorhinolaryngol 1994;251:178–182

17. Batsakis JG, Fox JE. Supporting tissue neoplasms of the larynx. Surg Gynecol Obstet 1970;131:989–997

18. Nageris B, Elidan J, Sherman Y. Fibrosarcoma of the vocal fold: a late complication of radiotherapy. J Laryngol Otol 1994;108:993–994

19. Wenig BM, Weiss SW, Gnepp DR. Laryngeal and hypopharyngeal liposarcoma. A clinicopathologic study of 10 cases with a comparison to soft-tissue counterparts. Am J Surg Pathol 1990;14:134–141

20. Kleinsasser O, Glanz H. Myogenic tumours of the larynx. Arch Otorhinolaryngol 1979;225:107–119

21. Hellquist HB, Hellqvist H, Vejlens L et al. Epithelioid leiomyoma of the larynx. Histopathology 1994;24:155–159

22. Paczona R, Jori J, Tiszlavicz L et al. Leiomyosarcoma of the larynx. Review of the literature and report of two cases. Ann Otol Rhinol Laryngol 1999;108:677–682

23. Kapadia SB, Meis JM, Frisman DM et al. Adult rhabdomyoma of the head and neck: a clinicopathologic and immunophenotypic study. Hum Pathol 1993;24:608–617

24. Kapadia SB, Meis JM, Frisman DM et al. Fetal rhabdomyoma of the head and neck: a clinicopathologic and immunophenotypic study of 24 cases. Hum Pathol 1993;24:754–765

25. Di Sant'Agnese PA, Knowles DM. Extracardiac rhabdomyoma: a clinicopathologic study and review of the literature. Cancer 1980;46:780–789

26. Ruske DR, Glassford N, Costello S et al. Laryngeal rhabdomyosarcoma in adults. J Laryngol Otol 1998;112:670–672

27. Shipkey FH, Lieberman PH, Foote FW et al. Ultrastructure of alveolar soft part sarcoma. Cancer 1964;17:821–830

28. De Sautel M, Gandour-Edwards R, Donald P et al. Alveolar soft part sarcoma: report of a case occurring in the larynx. Otolaryngol Head Neck Surg 1997;117:S95–97

29. Hoffer ME, Pribitkin E, Keane WM et al. Laryngeal chondrosarcoma: diagnosis and management. Ear Nose Throat J 1992;71:659–662

30. Lewis JE, Olsen KD, Inwards CY. Cartilaginous tumours of the larynx: clinicopathologic review of 47 cases. Ann Otol Rhinol Laryngol 1997;106:94–100

31. Huizenga C, Balogh K. Cartilaginous tumours of the larynx. A clinicopathologic study of 10 new cases and a review of the literature. Cancer 1970;26:201–210

32. Hyams VJ, Rabuzzi DD. Cartilaginous tumours of the larynx. Laryngoscope 1970;80:755–767

33. Kasanzew M, John DG, Newman P et al. Chondrosarcoma of the epiglottis. J Laryngol Otol 1988;102:374–377

34. Jacobs RD, Stayboldt C, Harris JP. Chondrosarcoma of the epiglottis with regional and distant metastasis. Laryngoscope 1989;99:861–864

35. Lichtenstein L, Jaffe HL. Chondrosarcoma of bone. Am J Pathol 1943;19:553–589

36. Bleiweiss IJ, Kaneko M. Chondrosarcoma of the larynx with additional malignant mesenchymal component (dedifferentiated chondrosarcoma). Am J Surg Pathol 1988;12:314–320

37. Brandwein M, Moore S, Som P et al. Laryngeal chondrosarcomas: a clinicopathologic study of 11 cases, including two "dedifferentiated" chondrosarcomas. Laryngoscope 1992;102:858–867

38. Hill BJ, Taylor CL, Scott GBD. Chondromatous metaplasia in the human larynx. Histopathology 1980;4:205–212

39. Burtner D, Goodman M, Montgomery W. Elastic cartilaginous metaplasia of vocal cord nodules. Ann Otol Rhinol Laryngol 1972;81:844–847

40. Morley AR, Cameron DS, Watson AJ. Osteosarcoma of the larynx. J Laryngol Otol 1973;87:997–1003

41. Sheen TS, Wu CT, Hsieh T et al. Postirradiation laryngeal osteosarcoma: case report and literature review. Head Neck 1997;19:57–62

39 Hypopharynx: Anatomy, Histology and Pathology

Anatomy

The hypopharynx extends from the level of the hyoid bone above to that of the lower border of the cricoid cartilage below. For purposes of classification of the position and extent of carcinoma, the hypopharynx is divided into three areas:

1. Pharyngo-oesophageal junction (postcricoid area).
2. Piriform sinus.
3. Posterior pharyngeal wall.[1]

The anatomical extent of each of these areas is given in Table 39.1.

The hypopharynx is a mucosal lined tube related to muscle laterally and posteriorly and to laryngeal cartilages anteriorly. The muscle is the inferior constrictor. It arises anteriorly from the oblique line on the lateral side of the thyroid cartilage and the tendinous arch between the inferior tubercle of the oblique line and the cricoid cartilage. The lower part of the inferior constrictor is known as the cricopharyngeus muscle and is particularly important in the causation of pharyngeal diverticulum (see below). The posterior attachment of the inferior constrictor on each side is to the pharyngeal raphe, a thin midline vertical tendon.

Histology

The epithelium covering the hypopharynx is stratified squamous with a high content of glycogen, giving the cells a clear appearance. Lymphocytes are often numerous immediately beneath the epithelium of the piriform fossa, and occasionally form lymphoid follicles (Fig. 39.1). The submucosa contains glands that open on the surface by occasional ducts. The glands are composed of both mucous and

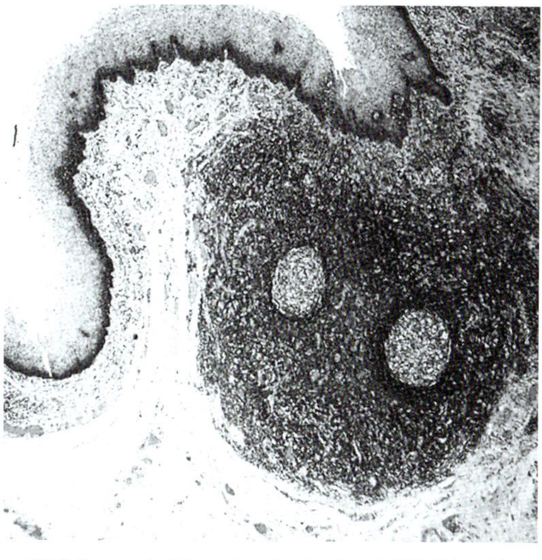

Figure 39.1 Mucosa of piriform sinus showing lymphoid follicles with germinal centres

---

Table 39.1. Anatomical sites of hypopharynx[1]

1. *Pharyngo-oesophageal junction (post-cricoid area)*
Extends from the level of the arytenoid cartilages and connecting folds to the inferior border of the cricoid cartilage

2. *Piriform sinus*
Extends from the aryepiglottic fold to the upper end of the oesophagus. It is bounded laterally by the thyroid cartilage and medially by the surface of the aryepiglottic fold and the arytenoid and cricoid cartilages

3. *Posterior pharyngeal wall*
Extends from the level of the vallecula to the level of the cricoarytenoid joints

---

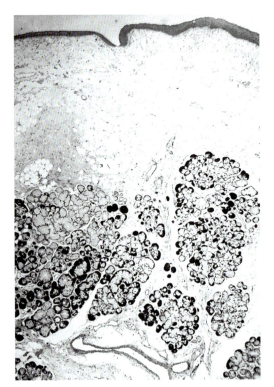

Figure 39.2 Submucosal glands of piriform fossa, composed of serous and mucous acini

serous acini (Fig. 39.2). There is a very rich plexus of lymphatic vessels in this region, which accounts for the ease with which hypopharyngeal cancer spreads by the lymph stream. The inferior constrictor muscle is striated.

Pharyngeal Diverticulum

These are diverticulae of the mucosa of the hypopharynx, which herniate through the muscle to produce a pouch. Rarely they occur in infants and are probably congenital; however, the great majority present late in adult life. They are, therefore, examples of "false" or "pulsion" diverticulae, representing herniations of the mucous membrane through a weakened area or defect of the muscularis.

The diverticulum is always present at the posterior wall of the hypopharynx immediately above the cricopharyngeus. In this region, known as Killian's dehiscence, the muscle is normally deficient (Fig. 39.3) and it is likely that a rise in pressure within the lumen of the hypopharynx gives rise to the bulge of the mucosa. The disturbance may be related to contractions of the cricopharyngeus muscle below the site of the pouch. Grossly the diverticulum is an oval smooth structure with a smooth inner and outer surface. The orifice in the

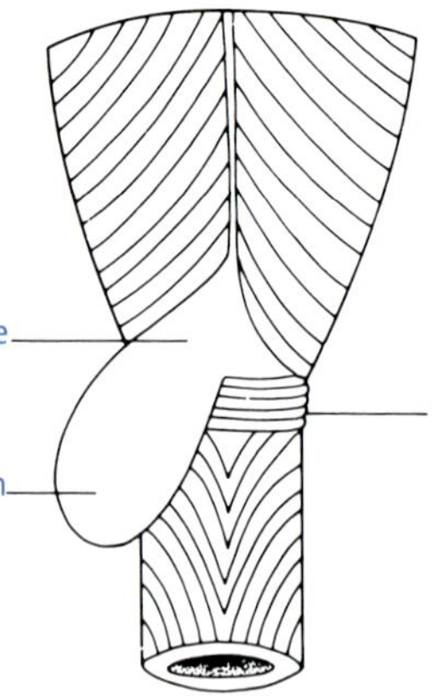

Figure 39.3 Diagram of posterior wall of hypopharynx and oesophagus to show the position of the pharyngeal pouch at Killian's dehiscence, which is in the region of the junction of the cricopharyngeus with the rest of the inferior constrictor

hypopharynx is wide. The lumen contains altered food contents. Microscopically the mucosal lining is of normal squamous epithelium and the wall is fibrous. Chronic inflammatory infiltration is frequently found beneath the squamous epithelial covering (Fig. 39.4).

The main complaint of patients suffering from a hypopharyngeal diverticulum is dysphagia due to compression of the pharynx against the cricoid cartilage by the swollen pouch. Aspiration of food into the lungs leading to infection is a serious complication.

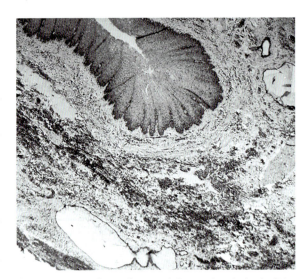

Figure 39.4 Section of surgically removed pharyngeal pouch, showing lining by squamous epithelium and markedly dilated submucosal glands with fibrosis and chronic inflammation beneath the epithelium. There is extensive haemorrhage due to operative trauma

Complicated by Carcinoma

Carcinoma, usually stratified squamous, but sometimes glandular, is occasionally found in a hypopharyngeal diverticulum, but the basis for the association of the two conditions is not known.

Cricopharyngeal Dysphagia

Cricopharyngeal dysphagia is a condition affecting patients of all ages and is characterised by difficulty in swallowing. Diagnosis is made by the presence of an indentation of the hypopharynx seen at barium swallow examination, which is caused by the failure of the muscle to relax. The condition is not associated with a pharyngeal diverticulum. Treatment is by a surgical incision into the cricopharyngeus (myotomy).

The histological changes in the cricopharyngeus muscle in cases of cricopharyngeal dysphagia were said to be those of degeneration and regeneration of muscle fibres, being associated with an interstitial fibrosis, which is sometimes severe[2] (Fig. 39.5). However, in another study, evidence of a generalised myositis, a variety of mild pathological changes in the cricopharyngeus muscle, or no abnormality at all, were found in patients with symptoms of cricopharyngeal dysphagia.[3] The basis for cricopharyngeal dysphagia is thus still unclear.

Piriform Sinus Fistula

Piriform sinus fistula is a congenital tract arising from the apex of the left piriform sinus and ending in or near the thyroid lobe of the same side. The fistula provides a pathway for infection to enter the thyroid gland and can lead to acute suppurative thyroiditis. This may be assuaged by antibiotics, but recurrence is frequent and a permanent cure can be effected only by surgical removal of the piriform sinus fistula.

Histologically the fistula is a hollow tube lined by stratified squamous, columnar or ciliated epithelium. It frequently contains mucous glands, thyroid follicular structures and thymic tissue. It terminates, often with branching, into the thyroid lobe on the same side.[4] C cells (neuroendocrine cells demonstrated immunohistochemically to contain calcitonin) are found in the thyroid tissue mainly near the termination of the fistula and sometimes these cells are found under the lining epithelium of the fistula.[4,5]

An explanation of the finding of solely left-sided congenital piriform sinus fistula with the thyroid changes is obtained by consideration of the development of the C cell system in the thyroid gland. The fourth pharyngeal pouch, which communicates with the primordial hypopharynx, forms dorsal and ventral diverticulae on each side. The dorsal part loses connection with the pharynx to become parathyroid glands. The ventral part forms the

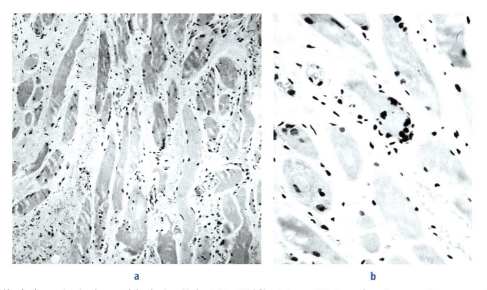

Figure 39.5 Muscle changes in cricopharyngeal dysphagia. **a** Moderate interstitial fibrosis is seen. **b** Features of muscle regeneration are present in this field, including numerous sarcolemmal and central nuclei

ultimobranchial bodies. In man and lower vertebrates the right ultimobranchial body is poorly developed. Neuroectodermal cells enter the left ultimobranchial body, which makes connection with the thyroid gland and produces the C cell system in the thyroid gland. It would thus seem likely that piriform sinus fistula is derived from the ultimobranchial body.

Sideropenic Dysphagia (Plummer-Vinson or Paterson-Brown Kelly Syndrome)

The features of this syndrome are dysphagia and iron deficiency anemia; hence "sideropenic dysphagia" is more descriptive than the more frequently used eponyms.

Clinical Features

Most patients are middle-aged females; children and adolescents between the ages of 14 and 19 with this condition have recently been reported.[6] Swallowing difficulty is mainly for solids. Clinical features of anaemia including koilonychia, chelosis and a smooth, red oral mucosa are present. Most patients show a microcytic hypochromic anaemia with a low serum iron. Achlorhydria is present in the majority. In three-quarters of patients there is a web – a smooth fold of mucosa – seen on barium swallow in the postcricoid mucosa.

On direct pharyngoscopy the mucosa of the hypopharynx appears atrophic. A web, when present, is seen as a thin crescentic membrane usually arising from the anterior or lateral walls of the hypopharynx. It narrows the lumen of the hypopharynx to a variable degree. Alternatively the hypopharynx may be constricted for several centimetres of its vertical extent.[7] Other medical conditions are often present, particularly Sjögren's syndrome and rheumatoid arthritis.

Pathological Appearances

The epithelium of the hypopharynx shows areas of atrophy and thinning, with other areas of keratosis. There is chronic inflammation of the subepithelial tissue. The web has been examined on only a few occasions and found to be composed of fibrous tissue covered by mucosa.[8]

Natural History

It is still not clear whether the iron deficiency causes the pharyngeal changes, including the web[7] or whether they are the primary lesion in this condition.[9] The most worrying aspect of this disease for the clinician is the tendency for the development of postcricoid carcinoma. However, in a long-term follow-up of 76 patients with sideropenic dysphagia, who were carefully treated with iron therapy and control of blood loss, McNab Jones[7] found that only one developed postcricoid carcinoma. On the other hand, in a survey of more than 300 cases of postcricoid carcinoma, he found evidence of one- to two-thirds having preceding sideropenic dysphagia. Gastric cancer may also be a sequel of sideropenic dysphagia.

Squamous Cell Carcinoma of the Hypopharynx

The only neoplasm encountered in the hypopharynx with any frequency is squamous cell carcinoma. All other tumours, benign and malignant, are rare.

Age and Sex Incidence

Most of the patients with hypopharyngeal carcinoma are men. Because of its relationship to sideropenic dysphagia, a disease almost entirely of females, carcinoma with a postcricoid location is found mainly in women. The age incidence of hypopharyngeal carcinoma in general is from 55 to 65 years.[10]

Clinical Features

The main feature is difficulty in swallowing, sometimes with a sensation of a foreign body in the throat. Pain may be present in the throat or even in the ear.

Aetiology

Sideropenic dysphagia has a relationship to postcricoid carcinoma. Between one-third and two-thirds of postcricoid carcinomas display evidence of that syndrome. The risk of cancer to sufferers of sideropenic dysphagia is, however, very small (see above).

A recent report suggests that the Epstein-Barr virus (EBV) may play a role in the development of hypopharyngeal carcinoma in a similar fashion to that of nasopharyngeal carcinoma[11] (see Chapter 24). Messenger RNA in situ hybridisation showed that five of 12 cases of hypopharyngeal carcinoma expressed EBV mRNA. Moreover, both tumour cell lines from two cases of hypopharyngeal carcinoma and five tumours formed by these cultured cells in nude mice expressed EBV transcripts and immuno-fluorescence staining showed expression of EBV-related nuclear antigen-2 and latent membrane protein-1 in the original tumours and the cell lines, as well as in the nude mouse tumours. Study by reverse transcription polymerase chain reaction also showed EBER1 and LMP1 expression. The tumour type studied was identified only as "squamous", not the lymphoepithelial type of undifferentiated carcinoma resembling nasopharyngeal carcinoma (see below).

Origin

It is commonly stated that hypopharyngeal carcinoma has three main sites of origin: piriform sinus, postcricoid area and posterior pharyngeal wall. An anatomical description of these sites is given above. In 85 resected specimens of hypopharyngeal carcinoma at the Royal National Throat, Nose and Ear Hospital, London, however, we found that in the majority (60%) the tumours involved more than one of these sites and usually all three. The piriform fossa was involved alone in 32%. Postcricoid and posterior hypopharyngeal wall alone were the sites of origin in only a small numbers of cases. These figures are in contrast with the findings of Olofsson and van Nostrand[12] and of Harrison.[13] In the Olofsson and van Nostrand series, piriform sinus tumours are in the majority, while in the series of Harrison it is the postcricoid carcinomas that are the most numerous. The two reported studies were based on microscopic serial sections of the larynx and hypopharynx specimens embedded in paraffin wax or celloidin respectively, while our results were derived from gross and microscopic examination of horizontal slices of specimens prepared by the method given in Chapter 28. The technical differences between the three studies are not sufficient to account for the marked differences in the location of the neoplasms within the hypopharynx.

The lower end of the hypopharyngeal neoplasm is often continuous with tumour arising from oesophageal squamous epithelium. The upper end is frequently continuous with tumour arising from the aryepiglottic folds, from the epiglottis and even, in an occasional case, from the vallecula and base of tongue.

Gross Appearances

At all sites, hypopharyngeal carcinoma is usually seen as a flat plaque with a well-defined somewhat raised edge (Figs 39.6, 39.7). The cut surface reveals a pale grey band of variable thickness. There may be superficial ulcerations or papillary surface formations of tumour.

Local Invasion

Invasion of the hypopharyngeal wall and adjacent structures by locally arising carcinoma takes place in a direction at right angles to the surface of origin of the tumour. The muscular wall of the hypopharynx provides no resistance to the neoplasm and is breached in almost every case. The thyroid, and even more so, the cricoid and arytenoid cartilages in

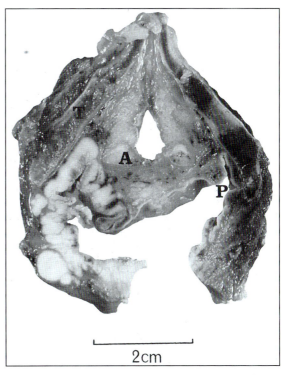

Figure 39.6 Transverse slice of laryngopharyngectomy specimen showing squamous carcinoma of hypopharynx arising from the left piriform sinus and the posterior wall. The hypopharynx has been opened from behind. Note that the tumour takes the form of a continuous, thick, surface field with two zones of submucous spread. Part of the field extends into the larynx between the left ala of the thyroid cartilage (*T*) and the left arytenoid cartilage (*A*). *P*, piriform sinus

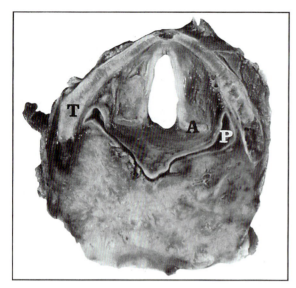

Figure 39.7 Transverse slice of laryngopharyngectomy specimen showing squamous carcinoma arising from the whole width of the posterior wall of the hypopharynx. *A*, right arytenoid cartilage at level of true vocal cords; *P*, right piriform sinus; *T*, left ala of thyroid cartilage

its origin, enter the submucosa of the trachea, pass upward to the vocal cord and produce death by constriction of the glottis (Fig. 39.8).

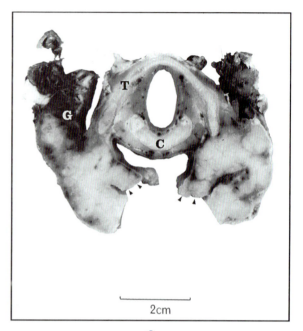

2cm

a

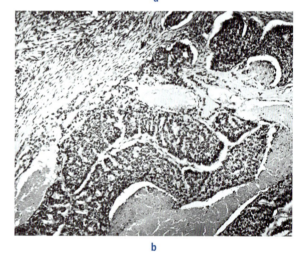

b

Figure 39.8 Carcinoma arising in pharyngeal diverticulum in pharyngolarygectomy specimen. **a** Transverse slice in cricoid region. Tumour arises from the diverticulum, which is shown by *arrowheads*. The posterior pharyngeal wall epithelium is seen as a fine, discrete line and does not give origin to the neoplasm. The left lobe of the thyroid gland (*G*) is invaded by tumour. The hypopharynx has been opened from behind by cutting through tumour posterior to the diverticulum. *C*, cricoid cartilage; *T*, left ala of thyroid cartilage. **b** The neoplasm shows a glandular pattern with an appearance similar to large cell neuroendocrine carcinoma of the larynx (see Chapter 37). Immunochemical staining and electron microscopy gave no further information, however, because the specimen had been stored in formaldehyde for 20 years before investigation

the adjacent larynx are resistant to invasion by hypopharyngeal carcinoma, but when this does take place the survival rate is markedly reduced. Such prognostic information is valid only when the patient's symptoms have been mild; in the presence of severe illnesss, regardless of invasion of laryngeal cartilage, the prognosis is very poor.[14]

The main pathway for invasion in piriform sinus carcinoma is anteriorly through the soft tissue and into the larynx. This is a natural pathway since the sinus is a normal invagination into the larynx between the thyroid alae and the arytenoid cartilages. Thus invasion forward, into the supraglottic and glottic regions, occurs in many cases of piriform sinus carcinoma. The thyroarytenoid and lateral cricoarytenoid muscles are often infiltrated and in some cases tumour may grow into the region of the saccule, where a natural pathway exists for its further invasion in an upward or downward direction (see Chapter 35).

Carcinoma originating in the postcricoid region (including the cases where this is one of two or more sites of origin) has a tendency to grow forward and invade the posterior cricoarytenoid muscle. Rarely the cricoid cartilage is invaded by this neoplasm.

The thyroid gland is frequently invaded by hypopharyngeal carcinoma growing in multiple sites. This is because of the close proximity of the gland to the lateral wall of the hypopharynx.

We have observed an abscess derived from the neoplasm to track for a considerable distance from

Microscopic Appearances

Squamous carcinoma of the hypopharynx arises, like that at other sites, from a field of surface squamous epithelium. Although no studies are available of the early preinvasive stages, comparable to those of the larynx (see Chapter 34), it is likely that a precursor of this neoplasm is carcinoma in situ of the hypopharyngeal epithelium. Invasive squamous carcinoma at this location is often bordered by a wide zone of carcinoma in situ. Such areas are similar in appearance to those of invasive carcinoma but they show a thinner, less hyperplastic malignant epithelium. In fact the point of change from intraepithelial to invasive carcinoma is difficult to identify.

Hypopharyngeal squamous carcinoma may vary from being well to poorly differentiated. Undifferentiated carcinoma resembling undifferentiated carcinoma of the nasopharynx (lymphoepithelioma) is rare in the hypopharynx, but when it occurs it is sited in the piriform sinus. Evidence for EBV in this particular type of carcinoma is, so far, equivocal,[15,16] unlike the unspecified squamous type in which five of 12 hypopharyngeal carcinomas were found to show evidence of the virus[11] (see above). It should be noted that lymphoid tissue may be found beneath squamous epithelium in the normal piriform sinus, giving that structure some resemblance to the nasopharynx (see above).

Submucous spread has been stressed as an important form of extension in carcinoma of the hypopharynx. It is a form of invasive carcinoma in which tumour is present beneath the mucosa, but does not arise from the overlying epithelium. In some cases with this appearance the neoplasm has indeed arisen from the overlying epithelium, but continuity with the epithelium has been destroyed by previous irradiation.

Invasion of the thyroid gland may be observed microscopically as a broad mass of tumour tissue, which seems to compress the thyroid, or as narrow tongues of tumour, which infiltrate between the thyroid follicles.

Spindle Cell Carcinoma

Spindle cell carcinoma occurs occasionally in the hypopharynx. The gross and histological features are similar to those of the laryngeal variety (see Chapter 36). Spindle cell carcinomatous areas are sometimes found adjacent to those of regular squamous carcinoma.

Basaloid Squamous Cell Carcinoma

Basaloid squamous cell carcinoma is an aggressive variant of squamous cell carcinoma showing both basaloid areas with small cystic spaces and areas of typical squamous cell carcinoma. The hypopharynx as well as the larynx is a favoured region for this growth[17] (see Chapter 36).

Adenosquamous Carcinoma

This aggressive neoplasm is described in the larynx (see Chapter 36), but may also be found in the hypopharynx.[18]

Spread

In contrast to the laryngeal region, the piriform sinuses are rich in lymphatic vessels. Permeation of these vessels is frequently seen in histological sections of hypopharyngeal carcinoma. The majority of patients with this type of cancer have metastatic involvement of the cervical lymph nodes. Bloodstream metastases develop in some 20–40% of patients with hypopharyngeal carcinoma within 9 months of the diagnosis. Lungs, mediastinum, bones and liver are the most common sites of metastasis.[10]

Other Neoplasms

Other benign and malignant neoplasms are very rare in the hypopharynx.

References

1. Spiessl B, Beahrs OH, Hermanek P et al. UICC TNM Atlas. Illustrated guide to the TMN/pTNM classification of malignant tumours. Springer, Berlin, Heidelberg, New York, 1992
2. Cruse JP, Edwards DAW, Smith JF et al. The pathology of a cricopharyngeal dysphagia. Histopathology 1979;3: 223–232
3. Laurikainen E, Aitasalo K, Halonen P et al. Muscle pathology in idiopathic cricopharyngeal dysphagia. Enzyme histochemical and electron microscopic findings. Eur Arch Otorhinolaryngol 1992;249:216–223
4. Miyauchi A, Matsuzuka F, Kuma K et al. Piriform sinus fistula and the ultimobranchial body. Histopathology 1992;20:221–227
5. Himi T, Kataura A. Distribution of C cells in the thyroid gland with pyriform sinus fistula. Otolaryngol Head Neck Surg 1995;112:268–273

6. Mansell NJ, Jani P, Bailey CM. Plummer-Vinson syndrome – a rare presentation in a child. J Laryngol Otol 1999;113: 475–476

7. McNab Jones RF. The Paterson-Brown Kelly syndrome. Its relationship to iron deficiency and postcricoid carcinoma. J Laryngol Otol 1961;74:529–543, 544–561

8. Shamma'a MH, Benedict EB. Esophageal web. A report of 56 cases and an attempt at classification. N Engl J Med 1958;259:378–384

9. Stell PM. In: Maran AG, Stell PM (eds) Clinical otolaryngology. Blackwell Scientific, Oxford, 1979, pp 368–381

10. Barnes L, Gnepp DR. Chapter 5 XV. Diseases of the larynx, hypopharynx and oesophagus. In: Barnes L (ed) Surgical pathology of the head and neck. Marcel Dekker, New York, 1985, pp 193–197

11. Shimakage M, Sasagawa T, Yoshino K et al. Expression of Epstein-Barr virus in mesopharyngeal and hypopharyngeal carcinomas. Hum Pathol 1999;30:1071–1076

12. Olofsson J, van Nostrand AW. Growth and spread of laryngeal and hypopharyngeal carcinoma with reflections on the effect of preoperative irradiation. 139 cases studied by whole organ serial sectioning. Acta Otolaryngol (Stockh) 1973;308 (suppl):7–84

13. Harrison DFN. Pathology of hypopharyngeal cancer in relation to surgical management. J Laryngol Otol 1970;84: 349–367

14. Deleyiannis FW, Piccirillo JF, Kirchner JA. Relative prognostic importance of histologic invasion of the laryngeal framework by hypopharyngeal cancer. Ann Otol Rhinol Laryngol 1996;105:101–108

15. MacMillan C, Kapadia SB, Finkelstein SD et al. Lymphoepithelial carcinoma of the larynx and hypopharynx: study of eight cases with relationship to Epstein-Barr virus and p53 gene alterations, and review of the literature. Hum Pathol 1996;27:1172–1179

16. Frank DK, Cheron F, Cho H et al. Nonnasopharyngeal lymphoepitheliomas (undifferentiated carcinomas) of the upper aerodigestive tract. Ann Otol Rhinol Laryngol 1995;104:305–310

17. Ferlito A, Altavilla G, Rinaldo A et al. Basaloid squamous cell carcinoma of the larynx and hypopharynx. Ann Otol Rhinol Laryngol 1997;106:1024–1035

18. Sanderson RJ, Rivron RP, Wallace WA. Adenosquamous carcinoma of the hypopharynx. J Laryngol Otol 1991;105: 678–680

F

Major Salivary Glands

40 Development; Histology; Non-neoplastic Swellings

Development

The major salivary glands arise by budding from oral ectoderm, with the possible exception of the submandibular glands, which may be of endodermal derivation. The anlage for the parotid and submandibular glands appears in the sixth/seventh week; the sublingual gland appears in the ninth. The glands migrate and have reached their final position by about the end of the twelfth week. In this context it may be mentioned that the "organ of Chievitz" appears earlier than the parotid anlage, and develops from the buccal sulcus. It has often been mistaken for the parotid anlage but presents epithelial pearls that are formed and then usually degenerate soon after birth. The epithelial structures are associated with nerve fibres.

General Histology

The human salivary glands consist of the paired parotid, submandibular and sublingual glands, and numerous minor or accessory salivary glands. Depending on the histological type of the acinar unit, the glands are divided into serous, mucinous or seromucinous salivary glands. The parotid gland (in the adult) is purely serous in type. However, on rare occasions pure mucinous acini may be observed intermingled in the parotid parenchyma. The submandibular and sublingual glands are mixed, the former being predominantly serous and the latter predominantly mucinous. The minor salivary glands are nearly all of seromucinous type (Table 40.1).

The parotid and submandibular glands are well-encapsulated glands and contain numerous septa that divide each gland into lobes and lobules. The facial nerve divides the parotid gland into a deep portion and a larger, flattened superficial portion. The parotid gland, which is the largest of the salivary glands, weighs between 14 and 28 g. The submandibular gland weighs 7–8 g, the sublingual gland 3 g. The duct system is similar in the parotid and submandibular gland, while intercalated ducts are infrequent or absent in the sublingual gland. In the parotid gland the numerous excretory ducts form a main duct (Stensen's duct), which is approximately 7 cm long and follows a twisted course, crossing both the masseter and buccinator muscles before opening into the oral cavity. The main duct from the submandibular gland (Wharton's duct) is shorter (approximately 5 cm) and opens in a small papilla on each side of the frenulum linguae. The main duct of the sublingual gland is called Bartholin's duct. It opens into the mouth through both the submandibular duct and several separate small ducts (ducts of Rivinus), which may open separately into the mouth in the plica sublingualis. All major salivary glands have interlobular connective tissue containing blood vessels, nerves and a few parasympathetic ganglia. The minor salivary glands are all of the mixed type, with the exception of some glands in the vicinity of the circumvallate papillae (von Ebner's gland), which are serous, and some in the palate, in the paratonsillar tissue, and at base of the tongue, which are purely mucous. The minor salivary glands are widespread and found not only in the lips, buccal mucosa, palate or tongue, but also in the whole upper respiratory tract, including the nose.

The salivary glands are composed of four different elements – serous and mucous cells, differentiated ductal cells and myoepithelial cells. Between the acinar and ductal structures there is interstitial

Table 40.1. Anatomical site and histology of salivary glands

Gland	Site	Duct opening	Histology
Parotid	Styloid process-mandible-mastoid-process	Vestibule	Serous
Submandibular	Submandibular triangle	Floor of the mouth (side of frenulum)	Mixed, mainly serous
Sublingual			
large gland	Floor of mouth	Duct of submandibular	Mixed, mucous
small gland	Floor of mouth	Plica sublingualis	Mixed, mucous
Anterior lingual (Blandin or Nuhn)	Tongue	Tongue	Mixed
Posterior lingual	Tongue	Tongue	Mixed
Weber's gland	Base of tongue	Tongue	Mucous
Von Ebner's gland	Tongue, circumvallate papillae	Circumvallate groove	Serous
Palatal	Palate	Palate	Mucous
Buccal	Cheeks	Vestibule	Mixed
Labial	Upper and lower lips	Vestibule	Mixed

connective tissue carrying both vessels and nerves. There is also lymphoid tissue consisting mainly of diffusely distributed lymphocytes, mucosa-associated lymphoid tissue, and in the parotid glands some intraglandular lymph nodes.

Acinar Unit

The acinar units may be purely serous, purely mucous or mixed. The serous acini are composed of rather large, slightly triangular cells with their base directed outwards. These pear-shaped groups of epithelial cells are surrounded by a distinct basement membrane. The serous acinus is smaller than the mucinous acinus, its cells containing secretory granules that are periodic acid–Schiff-positive, correlating in numbers with the phase of the secretory cycle. These basophilic secretory granules contain zymogen, in contrast to those of the lacrimal gland, which contain eosinophilic lysozyme-producing granules. The zymogen granules are composed mainly of amylase (ptyalin), which splits starch into water-soluble carbohydrates. The secretion is a watery liquid containing mainly proteins, ptyalin and salts but no mucus. Besides amylase, a large number of different enzymes have been demonstrated in the serous cells, e.g. glucosidase, acid phosphatases, esterases, glucuronidase, lactoferrin, lysozyme. However, steroid C-21 hydroxylase seems to be exclusively present in the duct system and absent in the serous and mucinous acinar cells, as well as in the myoepithelial cells. Ultrastructurally the serous cell is rich in microvilli and the apical plasma membrane is folded, while the lateral plasma membrane interdigitates with the neighbouring cells. The acinar cell in a mucinous acinus is characterised by being a rather large cell with vacuoles, and does not so often have the typical triangular shape as the serous cell. The clear cytoplasm is rich in both acid and neutral sialomucins, which stain positively for Alcian blue and mucicarmine and for periodic acid–Schiff, respectively. The amount of the sialomucins varies. In a mixed acinus the mucinous cells have serous caps towards the periphery (serous demilunes or crescents of Gianuzzi). In contrast to that of the serous cell, the plasma membrane of the mucinous cell is ultrastructurally seen to be devoid of microvilli. The principal electron microscopic feature of the mucinous cell is the electron-translucent secretion droplet, consisting of a membrane-bound fluid mass.

Duct System

All salivary glands have a system of branching ducts, in which the saliva produced in the acini is mixed with water and electrolytes. The part nearest to the acinus is called the intercalated duct. Distal to the intercalated duct is the striated duct. The intercalated and striated ducts are intralobular. The most distal portion of this duct system is the excretory duct. The intercalated duct is short. Its cuboidal or flattened cells have rather prominent nuclei, which usually are centrally located in the cells. The duct is usually lined with a single layer of these cells, and surrounded by an irregular layer of myoepithelial cells. Ultrastructurally the cells contain elongated mitochondria and a scanty rough endoplasmic reticulum and proximally a prominent Golgi apparatus suggesting a secretory function. The striated duct is identified by a columnar single layer of epithelium, often with a second outer row of cuboidal cells. Basal filaments (striations) are prominent. Ultrastructurally the striated cells are characterised by infoldings of the basal membrane producing the light microscopic appearances of striations. The cells often possess protrusions at their apical end, the so-called blebs, but are not so well developed in purely mucinous salivary glands as in serous glands. The convoluted granular ducts are modified striated ducts showing granules in the outer part of the cell. The excretory ducts consist of pseudostratified cylindrical cells with occasional goblet cells. Ultrastructurally there is a very infolded basal membrane. As the duct approaches the mucous membrane, the epithelium becomes stratified squamous. The simplicity of the excretory duct system reflects its function, transport of saliva.

Myoepithelial Cells

Myoepithelial cells are slender and spindle-shaped. They lie between the glandular or intercalated duct cells and the basement lamina, always located on the epithelial side of the basal lamina. The myoepithelial cell is of ectodemal origin but may be regarded as cell modified by a mesenchymal potential with a fine structure similar to that of smooth muscle, and even an ability to contract. It has no known secretory activity but can store glycogen. This dual function is reflected by the fact that the mesenchymal mucin in tumours such as pleomorphic adenoma is produced by the myoepithelial cell.[1] The acinar myoepithelial cells play an important role in the formation of and propulsion of saliva. The contraction of the intercalated duct by associated myoepithelium reduces the ductal resistance by dilatation and shortening of the ductular portion of the secretory unit. The origin of and whether or not the myoepithelial cell is pluripotential are still not entirely clarified. Although it has been long realised that this cell is a major component of salivary "mixed" tumours, there is increasing evidence that it originates from the same ectodermal precursor cell as the intercalated duct cells.[2] The myoepithelial cells contain several enzymes such as alkaline phosphatase and phosphorylase, and also fibrils similar to myofibrils composed of microfilaments measuring up to 7 nm and consisting of actin, tropomyosin and myosin and an intermediate filament of 10–12 nm width, consisting of both prekeratin and vimentin. The presence of vimentin is not constant. Vimentin is usually absent in normal myoepithelium but appears early in several salivary gland neo-

plasms. Desmin is not present. Monoclonal antibodies against metallothionein (MT, a metal binding protein) have been reported to be fairly specific for myoepithelial cells. However, ordinary mucosal squamous cells (basal and parabasal layer) and squamous cell carcinomas also stain positively for MT. Myoepithelial cells may be attached to the neighbouring epithelial cell by desmosomes, at the same time merging with the connective tissue. The myoepithelial cell plays an important role in the histogenesis of many salivary gland tumours,[3] e.g. pleomorphic adenoma, myoepithelioma, adenoid cystic carcinoma and epithelial-myoepithelial carcinoma. In general, tumours with a prominent myoepithelial component are those with a low to intermediate grade of malignancy. High-grade carcinomas, such as ductal adenocarcinoma or primary squamous cell carcinoma, show few myoepithelial cells.[2] Four major types of modified myoepithelial cells can be recognised particularly in neoplasms, but also sometimes under non-neoplastic conditions (Fig. 40.1).

1. The stellate or myxoid cell (as in pleomorphic adenoma, see Chapter 41).

2. Spindle-shaped (as in myoepithelioma, see Chapter 41).

3. A clear cell variant type (as in epithelial-myoepithelial carcinoma, see Chapter 42).

4. The so-called hyaline or plasmacytoid cell (as in pleomorphic adenoma and minor salivary gland neoplasms, see Chapters 41 and 42).

The morphologically different types of myoepithelial cell may also have slightly different immunohistochemical profiles. Whether the so-called reserve cell, which has been described to be located below the epithelial cells and above the basement membranes of ducts and acini, really is a separate cell type, or merely represents a flattened myoepithelial cell, is still under debate.

Normal Immunocytochemistry

The acinar cells are usually positive with anti-cytokeratin antibodies, but negative or weakly positive for S-100 and epithelial membrane antigen (EMA). The mucinous cells of the acinar structures in seromucinous glands, but not the serous cells, are often positive for epidermal growth factor receptor as well. The ductal cells are positive for anti-cytokeratin antibodies and EMA, but negative for S-100. The myoepithelial cells share many characteristics in common with both an epithelial cell and the smooth muscle cell. They are positive for S-100, smooth muscle actin, several anti-keratin anti-

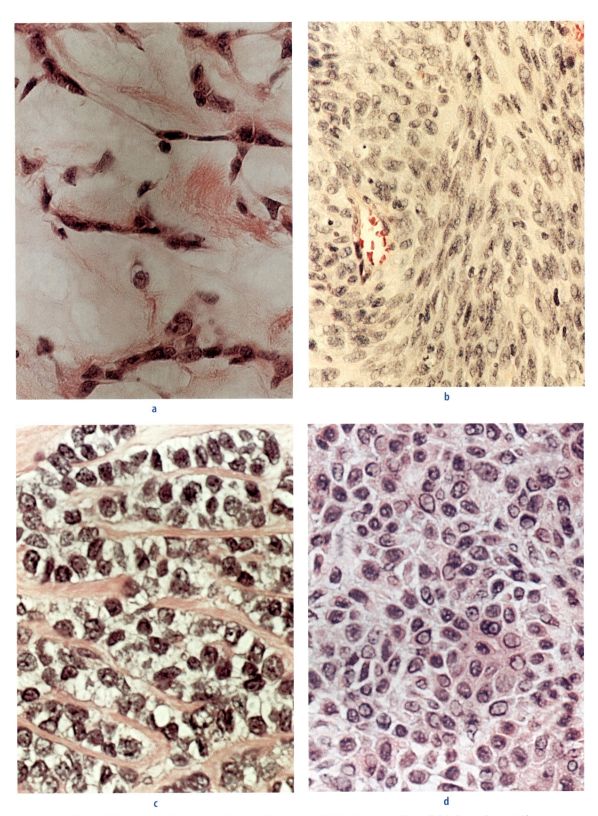

Figure 40.1 Types of modified myopepithelial cells. **a** Stellate or myxoid. **b** Spindle-shaped. **c** Clear cell. **d** Hyaline or plasmacytoid

bodies, e.g. 312C8-1, and particularly cytokeratin 14,[2,4,5,6] but are usually negative for desmin and vimentin. They are, however, as is the case with mucinous cells, positive for epidermal growth factor receptor. There is, however, not a single antibody that can specifically mark human myoepithelial cells. The localisation of antigens in normal salivary glands is not only of academic interest but provides a baseline for the study of neoplastic lesions.[7] The neu (c-erbB-2) oncoprotein has occasionally been demonstrated in normal salivary ductal and myoepithelial cells. However, membrane immunostaining for c-erbB-2 protein is negative in normal salivary tissue, and negative in most salivary gland neoplasms, except in certain high-grade adenocarcinomas (see Chapter 42).

Saliva

In basic terms the essence of the saliva is produced in the acini, and then mixed with water and electrolytes in the striated ducts. There is a continuous resting secretion of saliva into the mouth by all the salivary glands. However, most of the saliva is secreted from the major salivary glands. The three main roles of the saliva are to prepare the food for digestion by enzymatic action, to act as a protective agent for the oral mucosa and teeth, and to help the individual in tasting (assessment of the quality of) the food. The main digestive enzyme is alpha-amylase, but smaller amounts of many other enzymes are also present.

Non-neoplastic Swellings

Salivary Heterotopia

Salivary heterotopia can be classified as intranodal and extranodal. Intranodal heterotopia is much more common than extranodal heterotopia. The most common site is the lymph nodes near the parotid gland. The salivary gland tissue consists mainly of ductal elements, but acinar structures may be found, particularly those composed of serous cells. Intranodal heterotopia is one explanation for aberrant salivary gland tumours, and when malignant the lesion may present a difficult problem in distinguishing a primary salivary from a metastatic lesion.

Heterotopic salivary gland in the middle ear is one of the most common extranodal heterotopias and presents as a soft mass usually discovered during the evaluation of conductive hearing loss. The salivary gland tissue may extend into the Eustachian tube and the mastoid. Many cases have associated ossicular abnormalities. The morphology is that of normal salivary gland tissue covered by normal middle ear mucosa (see Chapter 5). Resection of the lesion cannot always be recommended, as in a large proportion of cases, the salivary gland tissue involves the facial nerve. Furthermore the ectopic salivary gland tissue enlarges very slowly so that radical resection is not usually necessary. Intraosseous heterotopic salivary glands are usually found in the posterior mandible and rarely in the anterior mandible. These lesions are more or less always incidental radiographic findings, are asymptomatic and do not require treatment. However, they may constitute a problem in differential diagnosis, thus necessitating fine needle aspiration or biopsy. Other extranodal salivary heterotopias are found along the medial border of the sternocleidomastoid muscle, in the pituitary and in the cerebellopontine angle.

Metaplastic Changes

Sebaceous

Sebaceous glands, either as glands with well-defined basement membranes or as isolated sebaceous cells, are normal findings in salivary tissue (Fig. 40.2). The

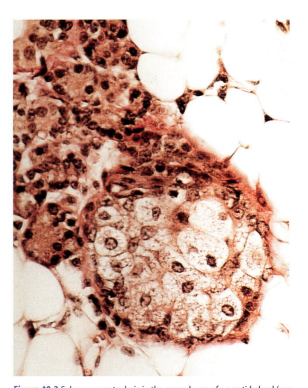

Figure 40.2 Sebaceous metaplasia in the parenchyma of a parotid gland (van Gieson)

sebaceous gland is linked to an interlobular duct. Sebaceous metaplasia may, however, occur not only as glandular formations in the vicinity of interlobular ducts, but as a metaplastic process of the salivary parenchyma.

Oncocytic

Oncocytic cells may be found among ducts and the epithelial cells of the acini. The transformation of epithelial cells into oncocytes was formerly regarded as a degenerative process, but is more likely to be a re-differentiation. The cells develop an intensively eosinophilic granular cytoplasm, which is due to increased numbers of mitochondria. Oncocytosis may be focal, usually in ducts, but occasionally also in acini, and is more common with advancing age. Oncocytic metaplasia may also occur as multifocal nodular oncocytic hyperplasia with several oncocytic nodules engulfing normal acinar tissue. Not infrequently there is a mixture of oncocytic and clear cell metaplasia, or even of clear cell metaplasia only.

Clear Cell

Clear cell metaplasia occurs in both normal salivary tissue and in salivary tumours (Fig. 40.3). In normal tissue, clear cells resulting from storage of glycogen may be found in the intercalated ducts. In the acini a similar occurrence may be produced by swelling and vacuolar change of the cytoplasm and this is also common in sialadenitis.

Myxoid

Myxoid or chondroid metaplasia may occur and should not be misinterpreted as pleomorphic adenoma. Usually the metaplastic areas are small and lack the capsule of adenomas.

Glandular

Glandular hyperplasia is a rare non-neoplastic event that may occur in mucous glands of the palate. The lesions do not recur after surgical excision and their aetiology remains obscure. The change may be seen in association with drug abuse or amalgam tattoo of the gingiva. In amalgam tattoo the gingiva shows as a dark region against the lighter background of the hyperplastic glands.

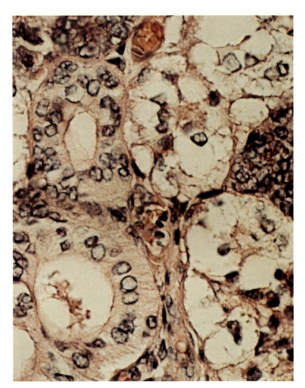

Figure 40.3 Clear cell metaplasia in which several large clear cells are seen. Note the proximity to the ducts

Secretory Immune System

The immune function of the salivary glands is complex and is related to the presence of mucosa-associated lymphoid tissue (MALT). This system is complex and not yet entirely elucidated. Brandtzaeg has systematically studied and clarified several aspects of the immune system of both the gut and the upper respiratory tract.[8] The extranodal MALT located in the salivary glands may be called SALT (salivary-associated lymphoid tissue, similar to GALT in the gut and BALT in the bronchi) and may have implications in certain salivary gland lymphoid neoplasms. The extranodal lymphoid tissue in salivary gland may also be part of a larger system in this region, NALT (nasal-associated lymphoid tissue). Brandtzaeg describes the lymphoid tissue, either distributed diffusely or in regional lymph nodes (Waldeyer's ring), as one part of this immune system. The specific secretory component (an epithelial receptor for polymeric Ig) produced by epithelial cells is the other.[8,9]

Mucosal Immune System

In the mucosa of the gut and also of the upper respiratory tract, epithelial cells (including epithelial salivary gland cells) have been shown to contain membrane-associated IgA and secretory component (SC). The SC can be regarded as an epithelial receptor for polymeric Ig. Free SC has been demonstrated intracellularly, whereas both free SC and IgA-complexed SC are found both on the membranes and in the apical portion of the cytoplasm. As early as 1974, Brandtzaeg proposed that SC would act as a specific surface receptor for dimeric IgA. This complex becomes partially stabilised in the cell membrane. The complex would then be capable of entering the gland lumen via the epithelial cell cytoplasm.[8]

The secretory immune system thus is a combined product of IgA produced by plasma cells and a secretory component produced by glandular epithelial cells.[9] The SC is a glycoprotein of approximately 83 kD and may be free or coupled to IgA. The free secretory component has been identified in the epithelium that lines duct-like structures, but not in myoepithelial cells, nor in mucinous acini. The transport of plasma cell-produced IgA through epithelial cells depends on the intracellular production of the SC. Thus secretory IgA (sIgA) is an external secretion and as such will be exposed to proteolytic enzymes. The secretory component will, however, increase the resistance to enzymatic degradation. Recent studies have shown that the expression of SC on human epithelial cells is regulated by certain cytokines, particularly IL-4 and IFN-gamma. This interaction between cytokines and epithelial cells may result in enhanced translocation of large amounts of locally produced (polymeric) IgA through epithelial cells into external secretions.

Histo- and Morphogenetic Aspects of Neoplastic Salivary Gland Diseases

The cell of origin, i.e. a stem cell or the morphohistogenetic cell of origin, that gives rise to particular salivary gland neoplasms, is still a subject of dispute. Central to the histogenetic concepts has been the determination of what type of cell in the normal salivary gland is involved in the induction of neoplasia. However, the exact population of cells in various salivary glands responsible for cell renewal and neoplastic transformation has not been determined specifically. The process of cellular differentiation may be more important in determining the histologic growth patterns (classification of tumours) than the exact cell originally responsible for the tumour arising in that organ.

Reserve Cell Concept

In 1977, Regezi and Batsakis postulated the theory of the so-called reserve cell.[10] This theory implies that salivary gland neoplasms arise from a population of pluripotential "reserve" cells ("stem" cells) present in the intercalated duct system. A severe drawback, however, in this otherwise attractive theory is the lack of convincing documentation of the existence of the "reserve" cell.

Cell of Origin Concept

Several classifications of salivary gland neoplasms, including the former World Health Organization classification, are based on the morphological appearance of the tumour cells compared with its "cell of origin". The bicellular theory would, for example, imply that an acinic cell carcinoma arises from the intercalated duct reserve cells, so would several other adenocarcinomas. The major drawback with this semipluripotential reserve cell theory is, as mentioned above, that there has been little or no direct evidence to support this hypothesis. Furthermore, autoradiographic studies have shown that as well as duct basal cells, luminal cells at all levels of the duct system and even acinar cells are capable of DNA synthesis and mitosis. Thus it is evident that dividing cells are not limited to basal cells of excretory ducts and luminal cells of intercalated ducts.

Morphogenetic Concept

The other major theory concerning the histogenesis of salivary gland neoplasms postulates that duct basal cells, luminal cells at all levels of the duct system and even acinar cells are capable of mitotic activity, thus being able to give rise to all kinds of salivary gland neoplasms. Thereby this concept denies the bicellular reserve (stem) cell hypothesis of Batsakis.[11] The entire concept of the morphogenetic aspect in regard to the development of salivary gland neoplasms lies in the ducto-acinar unit. The ducto-acinar unit comprises the normal acinus (i.e. luminal epithelial cells, ductal and/or acinar), the associated intercalated duct and the myoepithelial cells found both around the acinus and around the intercalated duct. It is emphasised that terminal portions of the secretory apparatus, i.e. both acini and intercalated ducts, are associated with myoepithelium, the ducto-acinar/myoepithelial complex. Dardick and van Nostrand stress that rather than investigating the origin of particular salivary gland tumours (i.e. histogenesis), valuable information can be obtained from studies of the differentiation of cells and structural evolution of these neoplasms (morphogenesis).[12] Accepting the theory of morphogenesis, it has to be pointed out that in such a differentiated organ as the salivary gland, it is possible that any type of normal cell may give rise to a distinct neoplasm, and that none of the normal cells are exempt from this process. On the other hand, it is also possible that one or more types of the dividing cells, through differentiation, may give rise to a variety of tumours differing in morphology.

Tumour-like Lesions

In several series of fine needle aspirates from salivary gland lesions it has been shown that 20–25% of cases are non-neoplastic. Most of the non-neoplastic salivary gland lesions are similar to their counterparts elsewhere in the body and are well described in books on general pathology. Therefore, only a brief account of these conditions is given in this chapter.

Obstruction

There is a large heterogeneous group of benign, non-neoplastic obstructive diseases of the salivary glands, which clinically may simulate neoplasms. The three main causes for obstruction and thereby a possible swelling of the gland are calculi, cysts and strictures.

Calculi

Ductal obstruction by lithiasis may result in glandular distention and swelling and furthermore a predisposition to retrograde spread by bacteria giving rise to sialoadenitis. Calculi are present in almost two-thirds of patients with chronic sialoadenitis.[3] The vast majority of calculi occur in the major salivary glands, of which 80–92% are found in the submandibular gland, less than 20% in the parotid gland and only approximately 2% in the sublingual gland and minor salivary glands (Fig. 40.4). There are a number of case reports describing very large calculi, predominantly in the major salivary glands, but also in the minor salivary glands. The large stones are most frequently encountered in the submandibular gland, and some even have been asymptomatic despite their size. A submandibular calculus was asymptomatic but measured 5 cm in length and weighed 23.5 g.

So-called dystrophic calcification of the submandibular gland may occur. In these cases large

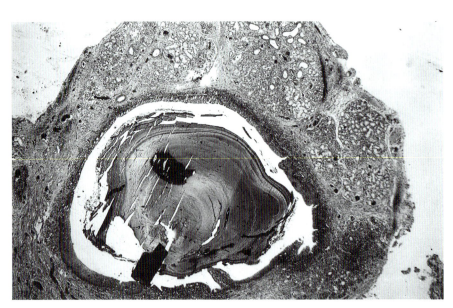

Figure 40.4 A calculus in duct of minor salivary glands of the upper lip. Note squamous metaplasia in bottom left of duct

areas of the gland may be replaced by calcium deposits. Whether this represents a progressive enlargement of a solitary sialolith or multicentric calcification remains unclear.

The most common site for calculi of the minor salivary glands is the anterior part of the mouth, especially close to the labial commissure (upper lip). They are usually asymptomatic and rather rare. However, well above 100 cases have been reported in the literature. Their size seldom exceeds 0.5 cm, and they appear as rather firm, movable submucosal nodules. The observation that microcalculi are present in normal human submandibular and parotid glands is of interest in regard to the aetiogenesis of calculi. They may form in autophagosomes in parenchymal cells and then pass into the lumina to be expelled in the saliva. Microcalculi can be found in serous acinar cells, striated duct cells, lumina and interstitium. Their size ranges up to 25 μm intracellularly, 70 μm luminally and 35 μm interstitially. They exhibit basophilia, are often laminated and stain positively by von Kossa's technique. A stone found on dissection of the glandular tissue is usually situated in a distended duct with metaplasia of the duct lining. Distended ducts are also often seen in the vicinity of a calculus. Squamous cell metaplasia is often seen in the larger ducts but rarely in the smaller ducts. The lumina of the acini become visible; first from distension and later from shrinkage and atrophy of the acinar cells, which lose their zymogen granules and resemble intercalated duct epithelium. There is often a pronounced periductal chronic inflammatory infiltrate. It has to be emphasised that the morphological picture of atrophy of acini, inflammation and fibrosis are findings observed in other conditions, notably Sjögren's syndrome.

The salivary gland stones are composed predominantly of calcium phosphate (hydroxyapatite) with small amounts of ammonium and magnesium. The most characteristic signs of sialolithiasis of the major salivary glands are recurrent episodes of swelling and pain, associated with eating and gradually disappearing after a couple of hours. However, symptoms caused by calculi of the parotid gland are less related to food intake than are those of the submandibular gland. The diagnosis is made through clinical history, palpation, and also sometimes by means of sialography and xeroradiography. Sometimes calcification of intravascular thrombi in vascular lesions of salivary glands may radiographically mimic sialolithiasis. In the parotid gland, in particular, mucous plugs are a common cause for gland obstruction, in fact more common than calculi. The mucous plugs are usually found within major ducts of the gland itself, whilst calculi more often are found in Stensen's duct. Treatment of calculi consists primarily of excisional biopsy for minor salivary gland stones, and in major salivary glands, where feasible, removal of the offending stone. However, after this latter procedure stones are often prone to recur. Particularly sialolithiasis of the submandibular gland lends itself better to surgical removal of the entire gland instead of excisional biopsy or removal of stone.

Cysts

In contrast to calculi, cysts are much more common in the minor salivary glands than in major salivary glands, and more than 75% of the cysts are found in the minor salivary glands.

Polycystic (Dysgenetic) Disease of the Parotid Gland. This is a rare developmental malformation of the parotid gland duct system in which the lobules are replaced by cystic spaces lined by flat, cuboidal or columnar epithelium.

Mucous Retention Cyst, Mucocele, Ranula. Mucous retention cyst, mucocele and ranula constitute a group of lesions whose nomenclature and pathogenesis have been somewhat controversial in the past. Obstruction of salivary ducts with consequent dilatation has previously been regarded as the cause of mucoceles and retention cysts. However, mucoceles (except those in the paranasal sinuses) lack an epithelial lining and an explanation of their pathogenesis of duct obstruction therefore seems inadequate in these cases.

Mucocele. Bhaskar et al. demonstrated that duct ligature in mouse salivary glands could not produce a lesion similar to the human mucous cyst.[13] On the other hand, by cutting a duct, and thereby causing an extravasation of mucus and saliva into the tissue, an extravasation cyst was formed. This cyst resembled most of the intraoral cysts and was lined not by epithelium, but by fibrous and granulation tissue. Occasionally, the granulation tissue may be very extensive, so creating a granuloma-like lesion, often referred to as Hamperl's granuloma. Like the experimentally induced cysts, mucoceles lined by granulation tissue are considered to be caused by trauma rather than by obstruction. The high incidence of this kind of cyst (cyst without epithelial lining) in the lower lip and the almost total absence of cysts with epithelial lining in this location also support the theory of Bhaskar and associates.[13] Furthermore, if calculi and obstruction leading to retention of mucus really were the major cause for these cysts, one would expect a much higher incidence in the major salivary glands, where calculi are so much

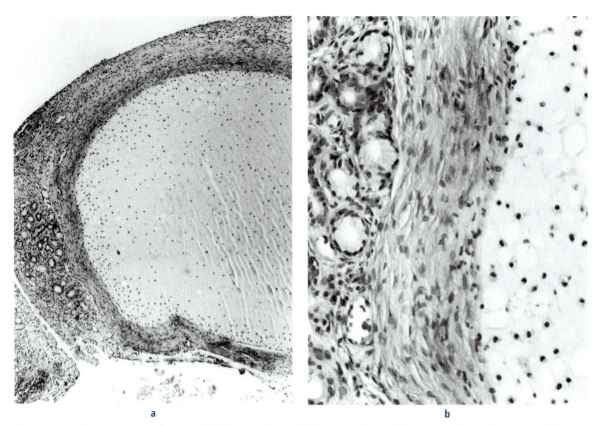

a   b

Figure 40.5 a Cyst from the lower lip without an epithelial lining, i.e. a "mucocele". **b** Higher magnification of the same cyst showing fibrous tissue and inflammatory cells constituting its lining

more common. Thus mucocele is the term preferably used for cysts without an epithelial lining and caused by trauma, and mucous retention cyst the term for the cysts with epithelial lining probably caused by obstruction (Fig. 40.5).

Mucous Retention Cyst. Salivary duct cysts occur mainly in the parotid gland and are lined by a duct epithelium, and also often filled with mucus.

Ranula. Ranula is a cyst of the floor of the mouth. There are two types, each of which has a different clinical behaviour and which requires a different regime of treatment. The simple ranula is usually a painless, superficial bluish nodule that may rupture spontaneously. This simple ranula is a true mucous retention cyst caused by obstruction of the duct of the sublingual gland and has an epithelial lining. The treatment is excision or marsupialisation of the wall. The other type of ranula, called plunging ranula, is caused by mucous extravasation and may penetrate into the fascial planes of the neck. It may have submandibular or cervical extensions and may even not be of salivary gland origin at all. Plunging ranulae are occasionally lined with a

cuboidal epithelium, but most often the wall consists of fibrous and granulation tissue as in the mucocele. The extent of a plunging ranula is dependent on time and since it is the result of mucous extravasation it may be considered to be a pseudocyst. The treatment of plunging ranula should include a meticulous dissection and excision in continuity with the sublingual gland.

Lymphoepithelial Cysts. Lymphoepithelial cysts are lined with a flattened multilayered epithelium surrounded by lymphoid tissue. The epithelium may occasionally be squamous with keratinisation. These cysts are filled with a serous fluid, lymphocytes and foam cells, and are found in the parotid gland or in the floor of the mouth.

Cystic Lymphoid Hyperplasia in HIV Infection. Bilateral confluent cystic cavities, usually in the parotid gland, occasionally in the submandibular salivary gland, lined by stratified squamous or columnar epithelium and filled with mucus are seen in the so-called cystic lymphoid hyperplasia of AIDS. A diffuse lymphoid infiltrate is invariably observed in the glandular tissue around the lymphoepithelial cysts and it is consistently associated with ectatic changes of the striated duct, suggesting that the lymphoid tissue proliferation – a characteristic feature of HIV infection – leads to obstruction of ducts.[14]

Neoplasia in Cysts. Development of tumours in salivary gland cysts is a rare event, although it has been suggested that certain distinct types of salivary gland cysts may be early manifestations of salivary gland neoplasia. There are few convincing cases of tumours arising in cysts, and examination of 1661 salivary gland cysts revealed only one case of development of a mucoepidermoid carcinoma of a parotid duct cyst.[15]

Branchial cyst and salivary gland fistula. Abnormalities in the development of the branchial apparatus may result in cysts. These are most often unilateral, although bilateral cysts may occur, particularly in children with fibrocystic disease of the pancreas. Cysts developing from the first branchial cleft appear in the preauricular region (see Chapter 2), while those originating from the second branchial cleft become manifest in the lower part of the parotid gland. These cysts are unilateral and are lined with a squamous, cuboidal or columnar epithelium, and accompanied by lymphoid tissue (see Chapter 45) (Fig. 40.6). The lumen is usually filled with fluid. Distinction has to be made between a branchial cyst (lymphoepithelial type) and benign lymphoepithelial lesion.

Salivary gland fistula manifests itself by unilateral swelling and discharge of saliva into the skin surface. Fistulae rarely open into the oral mucosa. The swelling is most often found in the area around the duct. Salivary gland fistulae most commonly affect the parotid gland and are nearly always caused by trauma.

Strictures

Strictures, other than congenital atresia of ducts, mainly occur in Stensen's and Wharton's ducts. Acute ulcerative papillary obstruction is caused by trauma; this may develop into chronic fibrotic stenosis by scarring. Another form of obstruction by stricture affects the duct rather than the papilla.

Inflammation

Although it can be difficult to decide whether inflammatory disorders are primarily infections with a secondary obstruction, or primarily obstruction with secondary infection, a number of specific non-specific inflammations are recognised in the salivary glands. The inflammatory process causes swelling of the salivary gland and may thereby mimic a neoplasm.

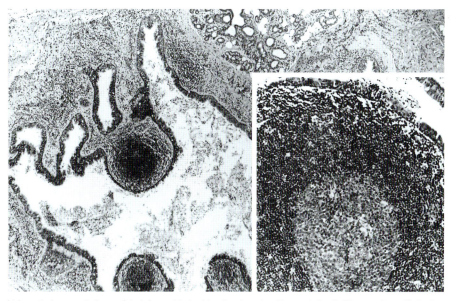

Figure 40.6 Branchial cyst in the preaurical part of the left parotid gland in a female patient. The cyst is lined with a pseudostratified columnar epithelium and lymphoid aggregates are frequent. Insert: higher magnification showing the lymphoid tissue with a germinal centre structure, and pseudostratified columnar epithelial lining

Virus Infection

Mumps is the most common viral infection and principally affects the parotid glands and to a certain degree also the submandibular glands. In spite of its name it is a systemic disease and biopsy specimens from a salivary gland with mumps are rare as the diagnosis usually is a clear-cut clinical one. The clinical diagnosis is reliable, particularly during epidemics, but the virus may be isolated from the urine a week after the salivary gland manifestations. Numerous other viruses, e.g. cytomegalovirus, influenza A, Cocksackie, and Echo virus, may cause a similar clinical picture of parotid swelling, but serologic tests for mumps are negative in these cases.

Bacterial Infection

Retrograde spread into the salivary ducts, particularly from the mouth, leads to a migration of bacteria to the glands. This is usually the case when there is an obstruction of the ducts. Acute bacterial infections, e.g. *Staphylococcus aureus* and *Streptococcus viridans* usually affect the entire oral cavity including the minor salivary glands. Chronic bacterial infections such as tuberculosis or syphilis may involve the entire oral mucosa but rarely the minor salivary glands and are most often confined to the parotid glands. Occasionally infection occurs during general anaesthesia, when it is known as "postoperative or nosocomial parotitis".

Immunological Disorders

Xerostomia

In patients with salivary gland hypofunction, the clinician must determine the cause for the hypofunction before treatment. Hypofunction usually falls into one of three conditions:

1. Intake of xerogenic drugs (e.g. certain antidepressive drugs).
2. Systemic disease (e.g. Sjögren's syndrome).
3. Irradiation to the salivary glands.

Drug-induced hypofunction is usually reversible and may be treated by alteration of the xerogenic drug medication, by use of gustatory stimuli, by increased mastication, or sialogenic drugs. Unfortunately, patients with salivary hypofunction caused by irradiation or sytemic disease often can be helped only by saliva substitutes.

Mikulicz Syndrome

Mikulicz syndrome, characterised by enlargements of salivary (and lacrimal) glands, is observed in a variety of disorders. It occurs in Sjögren's syndrome, sarcoidosis, malignant lymphoma, leukaemia and other disorders. Mikulicz syndrome is thus not a specific pathologic entity, but a hotchpotch of entities.

Sjögren's Syndrome

Although Sjögren's syndrome formally consists of conjunctivitis sicca, rhinitis sicca, pharyngolaryngitis sicca, polyarthritis, parotid enlargement and xerostomia, it implies in practice conjunctivitis sicca, xerostomia and (rheumatoid) arthritis. When rheumatoid arthritis is absent, it is known as primary Sjögren's syndrome. The morphological features of Sjögren's differ in the salivary glands with the progression of the disease. Early in the development of Sjögren's syndrome there is an accumulation of small lymphocytes around salivary ducts; soon they become accompanied by larger lymphocytes and plasma cells (Fig. 40.7). The mononuclear infiltrate eventually causes progressive swelling of the gland as acinar tissue is replaced. Proliferation starts from the ductal cells, and so-called epimyoepithelial islands appear in the lymphoid infiltrate. These cells are probably of ductal, not myoepithelial, origin. Fibrosis and acinar atrophy are not uncommon (Fig. 40.8).

This microscopic appearance is identical to that described in "benign lymphoepithelial lesion" and Mikulicz syndrome. The distinction between the different entities is thus based on clinical observa-

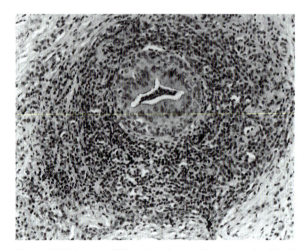

Figure 40.7 Early stage of Sjögren's syndrome with pronounced periductal inflammatory infiltrate composed predominantly of small lymphocytes

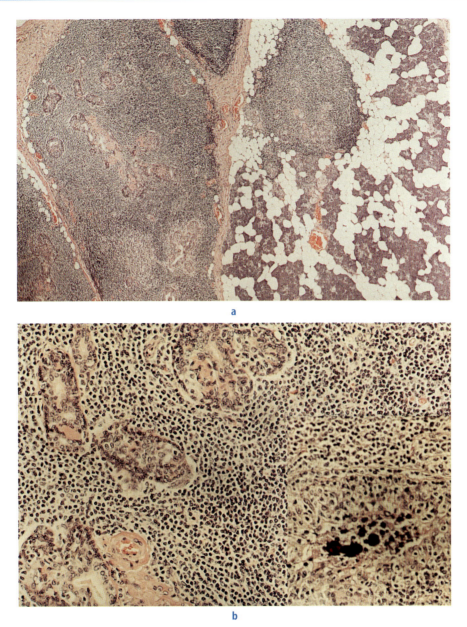

Figure 40.8 a Low-power view of parotid gland in Sjögren's syndrome showing part of a large focus of intense lymphocytic and plasma cell infiltration and a smaller one to the right of it. Note the epimyoepithelial islands. **b** Higher power view of epimyoepithelial islands in the inflammatory infiltrate. Insert: focus of calcification

tions. The European Community Study Group's recommendation on diagnostic criteria for Sjögren's syndrome is that salivary gland scintigraphy, parotid sialography and labial minor salivary gland biopsy are the most reliable tests in the diagnosis.[16]

Labial Salivary Gland Biopsy

Biopsy of the minor salivary glands (usually the lower lip) is a semiquantitative method for evaluat-ing foci of lymphocytes and plasma cells in the salivary gland in Sjögren's syndrome.[17] A single horizontal incision approximately 2 cm long is made between the midline and commissure. Following this, blunt dissection is carried out to free the sali-vary glands from the surrounding fascia. At least five small glands should be removed since, because of their small size, lymphocytic infiltration may not be present in all glands.

More than one focus of lymphocytes/4 mm^2 of minor salivary gland tissue accurately distinguishes

Sjögren's syndrome from normal controls. A focus of lymphocytes has been defined as an aggregate of 50 or more round cells. Focus score of 0 or 1 is normal. Scattered foci of lymphocytes may still yield a focus score of 0–1 if the number of lymphocytes in a given focus is small (<50 cells), or foci are widely spaced (>4 mm^2 of gland). Background glandular tissue must be normal as well.

Lymphoma in Sjögren's syndrome

Patients with Sjögren's syndrome have a higher incidence of malignant lymphomas, and the risk is more than 40 times higher than that of the normal population. In a series of 250 patients with Sjögren's syndrome, 41 had monoclonal gammopathy, four had pseudolymphoma, three had in situ monoclonal lymphoproliferation and 12 had malignant lymphoma.[18] Rearrangement of the rheumatoid factor-related germline gene Vg was found in 24 of 50 investigated genomic DNAs using peripheral leucocytes. The authors also suggest that the progression of Sjögren's syndrome from benign to malignant lymphoproliferation may be related to suppression of apoptotic death by bcl-2.

Benign Lymphoepithelial Lesion

In the early 1950s the term benign lymphoepithelial lesion was proposed to describe parotid gland lesions previously called Mikulicz syndrome. The microscopic appearance is as described above (Fig. 40.8). Despite the widely accepted term "epimyoepithelial islands", the cells in the islands are not myoepithelial cells but of several types, predominantly ductal cells. Benign lymphoepithelial lesion is sometimes associated with other lesions in the same specimen, e.g. sialolithiasis or adenomas. Malignant lymphoma may also be present.

In brief, patients with benign lymphoepithelial lesions may or may not have Sjögren's syndrome. On the other hand, patients with Sjögren's syndrome almost invariably have, or will develop, pathological features of benign lymphoepithelial lesion.

Necrotising Sialometaplasia

Necrotising sialometaplasia rarely affects the major salivary glands and manifests itself most often as an ulcer in the palate. The initial lesion may be ischaemia, surgery or trauma leading to necrosis. Microcopically, necrotising metaplasia is recognised by the presence of squamous metaplasia of ducts and acini of seromucinous glands accompanied by necrosis, sometimes with ulceration. Metaplastic squamous epithelium fills the ducts and acini, forming solid nests. These epidermoid nests can mimic invasive squamous cell carcinoma, or mucoepidermoid carcinoma (Fig. 40.9). There is often secondary inflammation and extravasation of mucus. Demonstration of intact glandular struc-

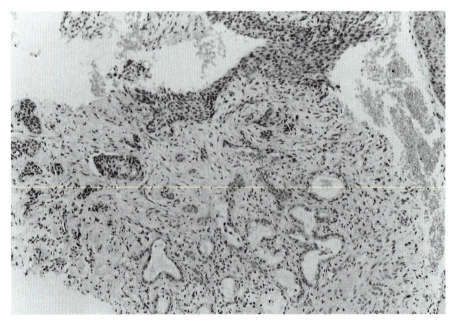

Figure 40.9 Necrotising sialometaplasia of the hard palate. Note necrosis (*upper right corner*) and several nests of metaplastic epithelium. There is a moderate chronic inflammation. The epithelial nests show benign cytological features and there are intact ducts and acini

tures with areas of necrosis and the absence of atypia in the metaplastic epithelium will give the correct diagnosis. The lesion may regress spontaneously, in 4–6 weeks, particularly if the initial trauma is removed.

Sialoadenitis and sialoadenosis

Sialoadenitis may be caused by bacteria, viruses, immune disorders, chronic sclerosis (Küttner tumour of submandibular gland) or irradiation. The microscopic appearance will depend upon which agents are causing the inflammation. Tuberculosis in some parts of the world is a common form of chronic sialoadenitis. The chronic bacterial and viral sialoadenitides are characterised by a heavy mononuclear inflammatory infiltrate. In chronic sclerosing sialoadenitis the most prominent microscopic feature is a periductal inflammation. Irradiation sialoadenitis, on the other hand, is characterised by an atrophy of acini and ducts, and a moderate inflammation only.

Sialoadenosis is, in contrast to sialoadenitis, a noninflammatory, non-neoplastic enlargement of the salivary gland. Sialoadenosis is usually bilateral and almost always associated with a system disease, e.g. malnutrition, drug abuse, hormonal disturbances, mucoviscidosis, etc. The microscopic appearance is dominated by a hypertrophy of acinar cells and the absence of inflammatory cells (Fig. 40.10).

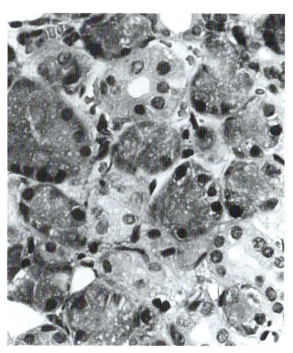

Figure 40.10 Sialoadenosis of the submandibular gland. Note the absence of inflammatory cells, the enlargement of the serous cells, which are tightly packed with granules

References

1. Azzopardi JG, Smith OD. Salivary gland tumors and their mucins. J Pathol Bacteriol 1959;77:131–140
2. Batsakis JG, Kraemer B, Sciubba JJ. The pathology of head and neck tumors: the myoepithelial cell and its participation in salivary gland neoplasia, part 17. Head Neck Surg 1983;5:222–233
3. Batsakis JG. Tumors of the head and neck. Clinical and pathological considerations, 2nd edn. Williams & Wilkins, Baltimore, London, 1979
4. Caselitz J, Osborn M, Wustrow J et al. Immunohistochemical investigations on the epimyoepithelial islands in lymphoepithelial lesions. Use of monoclonal keratin antibodies. Lab Invest 1986;55:427–432
5. Caselitz J, Walther B, Wustrow J et al. A monoclonal antibody that detects myoepithelial cells in exocrine glands, basal cells in other epithelia and basal and suprabasal cells in certain hyperplastic tissues. Virchows Arch (A) 1986;409: 725–738
6. Dardick I, Parks WR, Little J et al. Characterization of cytoskeletal proteins in basal cells of human parotid salivary gland ducts. Virchows Arch (A) 1988;412:525–532
7. Crocker J, Egan MJ. Immunohistochemistry of salivary gland tumors. Ear Nose Throat J 1989;68:130–136
8. Brandtzaeg P. Mucosal and glandular distribution of immunoglobulin components: differential localization of free and bound SC in secretory epithelial cells. J Immunol 1974;112:1553–1559
9. Brandtzaeg P. Human Secretory Component: II. Physiological characterization of free secretory component purified from colostrum. Scand J Immunol 1974;3:707–716
10. Regezi JA, Batsakis JG. Histogenesis of salivary gland neoplasms. Otolaryngol Clin North Am 1977;10:297–307
11. Dardick I, Burford-Mason AP. Current status of histogenesis and morphogenetic concepts of salivary gland tumorigenesis. Crit Rev Oral Biol Med 1993;4:639–677
12. Dardick I, van Nostrand APW. Morphogenesis of salivary gland tumors. A prerequisite to improving classification. Pathol Annu, part I. Appleton-Century-Crofts, Norfolk, Connecticut, 1987, pp 1–53
13. Bhaskar SM, Bolden TE, Weinmann JP. Experimental obstructive adenitis in the mouse. J Dent Res 1956;35: 852–862
14. Maiorano E, Favia G, Viale G. Lymphoepithelial cysts of salivary glands: an immunohistochemical study of HIV-related and HIV-unrelated lesions. Hum Pathol 1998;29:260–265
15. Seifert G. Mucoepidermoid carcinoma in a salivary duct cyst of the parotid gland. Contribution to the development of tumors in salivary gland cysts. Pathol Res Pract 1996;192: 1211–1217
16. Vitali C, Bombardieri S. The European Community Study Group on diagnostic criteria for Sjögren's syndrome. Sensitivity and specificity of tests for ocular and oral involvement in Sjögren's syndrome. Ann Rheum Dis 1994;53:637–647
17. Greenspan JS, Daniels TE, Talal N et al. The histopathology of Sjögren's syndrome in labial biopsies. Oral Surg Oral Med Oral Pathol 1974;37:217–230
18. Sugai S, Saito I, Masaki Y et al. Rearrangement of the rheumatoid factor-related germline gene Vg and bcl-2 expression in lymphoproliferative disorders in patients with Sjögren's syndrome. Clin Immunol Immunopathol 1994;72: 181–186

41 Benign Epithelial Neoplasms

Although many modern laboratory techniques such as cytopathology, immunohistochemistry, electron microscopy, frozen sections, chromosomal analysis and various molecular biological methods are available for the diagnosis of salivary gland neoplasms, routine haematoxylin and eosin-stained sections are still the most important and will in the majority of cases provide the diagnosis. The preliminary gross examination of specimens is important. As many sections as possible should be taken to ensure adequate sampling. Sections should be taken from the margins of macroscopically clear-cut neoplasms and especially from those that are indefinitely delineated. It is important to detect and study microscopically any lymph nodes in the specimen.

Pleomorphic Adenoma

Definition and Terminology

Since its first description by Billroth in 1859, terminology for this entity has veered to and fro between "mixed tumour" and pleomorphic adenoma. To label a neoplasm "tumour" may give rise to concern about its possible malignant potential. The term pleomorphic adenoma (complex adenoma) defines its benign, entirely epithelial origin, at the same time emphasising its variable histological picture. The so-called congenital pleomorphic adenoma (salivary gland anlage tumour), most often found in the midline of the nasopharynx of neonates and infants, is regarded by many as a hamartoma (see Chapters 23 and 43).

Site and Incidence

The majority of pleomorphic adenomas are situated in the parotid gland, particularly in its tail and inferior portions. A small number only arise in the submandibular gland, oral cavity and nasal cavity. A sublingual gland origin is very rare. The neoplasm shows a slight female predominance. It may be found at any age, even in the newborn; the peak age is about 40 years.

Pleomorphic adenoma is the most common salivary gland tumour in adults, irrespective of site. In children only haemangioma is more common than pleomorphic adenoma. In a compilation of some of the major series of salivary gland neoplasms in the literature, pleomorphic adenoma is found to comprise about 70% of all parotid tumours, about 50% of those in the submandibular gland and 40% in the oral cavity. Most series report pleomorphic adenoma to be mainly a parotid tumour (60–85%); approximately 10% only are situated in the submandibular gland, and only one case out of a thousand will be found in the sublingual gland. The remaining 5–30% are located in minor salivary glands, particularly in the cheek and upper lip. Occasionally pleomorphic adenomas may be found in lymph nodes in the neck, and in the nasal cavity (see Chapter 17). Even intra-osseous pleomorphic adenomas are described.

Histogenesis

This unique neoplasm is now generally accepted to be of purely epithelial origin, the plutipotent myoepithelial cell being the major neoplastic component. A salivary epithelial cell source is supported by immunohistochemical localisation of antigens from normal human saliva in the neoplastic cells, suggesting that pleomorphic adenomas are derived from distal gland cells and retain or develop a specific exocrine capability. Ultrastructural and immunohistochemical studies of pleomorphic adenomas have shown that they consist of a mixture of neoplastic ductular epithelial cells, rare acinar cells and myoepithelial cells.[1,2] A substantial population of stromal cells in pleomorphic adenomas have also been identified as dendritic cells of the interdigitating variety.

Clinical Features

Pleomorphic adenomas are slowly growing tumours often present for years before the patient seeks medical advice. They measure between 2 and 6 cm in diameter, but there are some huge ones on record, up to a massive 61 lb (27 kg) reported in the 1950s.

Pleomorphic adenoma is almost always a solitary lesion, although synchronous or metachromatous multiple involvement has been described. It may rarely be found in combination with other salivary gland neoplasms, usually Warthin tumour, but also with mucoepidermoid, acinic cell and adenoid cystic carcinoma. The most common clinical presentation is that of a painless, slowly growing, parotid mass, which is firm and mobile. The mobility may disappear. Recurrent pleomorphic adenomas are often fixed to the underlying tissue. Most are present in the superficial parotid lobe, but approximately 10% of parotid pleomorphic adenomas arise in the deep portion, when the tumour may present as a mass in the lateral part of the pharynx, in the soft palate, or in the tonsillar fossa.

Gross Appearances

Pleomorphic adenoma is a circumscribed, lobulated tumour with a capsule consisting of fibrous tissue of varying thickness, which gives the neoplasm a smooth surface. It is rarely multifocal. The multifocal appearance observed from time to time by the pathologist is usually artefactual and produced by cutting across finger-like protrusions of the nodular tumour. A recurrent pleomorphic adenoma following incomplete surgical removal, may indeed consist of multiple nodules. In contrast to pleomorphic adenoma, myoepithelial adenoma and myoepithe-lioma tend to have a more diffuse growth pattern, often lacking a capsule.

The appearance of the cut surface may reflect the cellular composition of the neoplasm. It may be solid and white in lesions with a predominant epithelial/myoepithelial component or bluish and semi-transparent corresponding to microscopic chondroid tissue. In areas with myxoid predominance the macroscopical appearance is soft and mucoid. Cysts are not infrequent. Pleomorphic adenomas are usually 2–6 cm in diameter in the major salivary glands, while in the minor salivary glands they usually are much smaller.

Microscopic Appearances

The histological appearances of pleomorphic adenoma vary not only from one tumour to another, but also in different parts of the same tumour. Such morphological diversity and complexity is one of the hallmarks of the neoplasm. By definition it consists of both epithelial structures and tissue of mesenchyme-like appearance (Fig. 41.1). The epithelial ducts are composed of inner duct-lining cuboidal cells and clear outer myoepithelial cells. This is also a feature not only of normal salivary gland tissue but also of epithelial-myoepithelial carcinomas and some adenoid cystic carcinomas. The ways in which epithelial and the myoepithelial cells are arranged determine the features of any particular neoplasm. The epithelial and myoepithelial structures are mixed with a variable amount of stromal tissue, which can be chondroid, myxoid, mucoid, fibroid, vascular, or a mixture of these. An equal amount of cellular and stromal tissue is found in about one-third of the neoplasms, one-fifth is predominantly cellular, and one-tenth is extremely cellular. There is no indication that a predominance of one or the other type of tissue has any bearing on the aggressiveness or otherwise of the tumour. Tumours of the minor salivary glands, including pleomorphic adenoma, especially those from the palate, often tend to be more cellular than their counterparts in the major salivary glands. We emphasise this fact in order to avoid a misdiagnosis of malignancy in a cellular adenoma of minor salivary gland origin.

The ductular component may not be evident when sections from only a single block are examined, which may give a cellular pleomorphic adenoma the features of a myoepithelioma. As with all salivary gland tumours, it is necessary to cut sections from several blocks to obtain an adequate histological diagnosis.

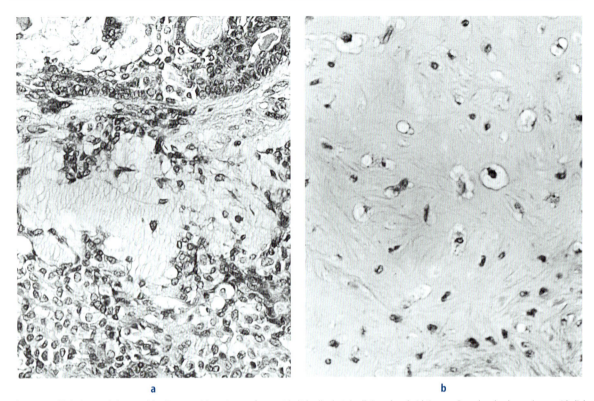

Figure 41.1 Typical case of pleomorphic adenoma with a mixture of myoepithelial cells, ductal cells in a chondroid tissue. **a** Round and polygonal myoepithelial cells and a bluish mucoid intercellular substance. A few ductal elements are seen in the right upper corner of the picture. **b** Higher magnification of the chondroid tissue. In the right lower corner the cartilaginous tissue is seen to merge from the myoepithelial "stromal" cells

Pleomorphic adenomas show at least three major microscopic patterns according to the arrangement of the epithelial cells; these cells may be mixed with tissue of mesenchymal appearance to any degree.

In some pleomorphic adenomas both the inner duct-lining cells and the outer myoepithelial cells are clearly visible. The lumina of the ducts usually contain clear fluid and sometimes eosinophilic periodic acid–Schiff-positive material. The myoepithelial cells are small, dark, flattened cells, sometimes spindle-shaped, and sometimes clear (Fig. 41.2).

In the second type, duct-lining cells, which are prominent columnar eosinophilic cells with rounded nuclei, are numerous, but myoepithelial cells are found in small numbers only around larger ducts (Fig. 41.3).

In the third (and most common) type of epithelial arrangement, myoepithelial cells are in the majority. In these cases the myoepithelial cells may be grouped in patches containing ductal structures or in large solid areas. They may be spindle-shaped as in myoepithelioma, or show clear cytoplasm as in epithelial myoepithelial carcinoma. In some cases the mucoid intercellular substance is replaced by hyaline material, which separates groups of myoepithelial cells and the appearances may then be similar to those of adenoid cystic carcinoma

(Fig. 41.4). When myoepithelial cells are very numerous and arranged in large solid masses they are fusiform, polygonal and stellate and sometimes difficult to distinguish from the interspersed ductal cells. This type of pleomorphic adenoma may cause diagnostic problems, particularly in small excisional biopsies, emphasising the importance of multiple blocks in the diagnosis of salivary gland neoplasms. When the myoepithelial cells are spindle-shaped cells there is a resemblance to leiomyoma even to the extent of their exhibiting an eosinophilic fibrillar cytoplasm. Sometimes a neoplasm consists of spindle-shaped myoepithelial cells only, with few ductal cells. In these instances it is better referred to as a myoepithelioma. When vacuolar degeneration of the myoepithelial cells into hydropic clear cells is present, the latter usually surround ducts, but may also appear as isolated small sheets or larger aggregates.

The amount of mesenchyme-like cartilage or myxoid tissue varies considerably from one tumour to another. A transitional zone between myoepithelial cells and this tissue is usually present, suggesting a metaplasia of the former. In some pleomorphic adenomas only a meticulous search will reveal mesenchymal tissue. In others the reverse is the case and scanty, stellate myoepithelial cells are found

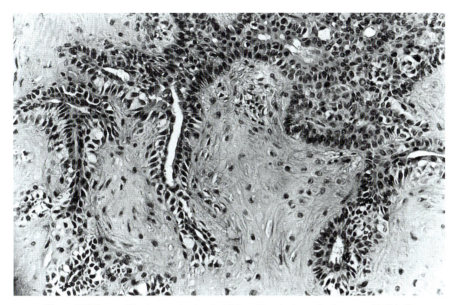

Figure 41.2 Pleomorphic adenoma showing duct-lining cells and outer, partly clear myoepithelial cells

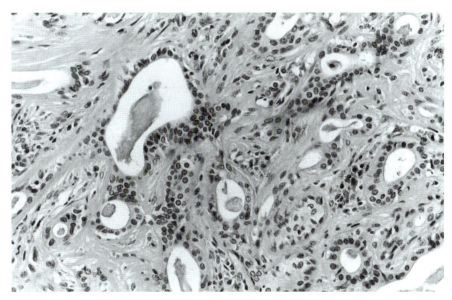

Figure 41.3 Pleomorphic adenoma with predominant ducts and some scattered myoepithelial cells

dispersed in a large amount of mucoid tissue (Fig. 41.5). The exact chemical nature of the mesenchymal component has been a source of debate ever since pleomorphic adenoma was first described in the last century.

Other metaplastic changes take place in pleomorphic adenomas apart from the transformation of myoepithelial cells to mesenchyme that is invariably present. Squamous metaplasia is found in approximately 25% of pleomorphic adenomas,[3] as in many other salivary gland neoplasms, and is usually seen in larger ducts, as free-lying patches of epidermoid tissue, sometimes with keratin pearl formation. Oncocytic metaplasia occurs either as a lining of duct-like structures or as solid groups of oncocytes. Calcification and even ossification, and adipose infiltration, may on rare occasions be present in pleomorphic adenoma (Fig. 41.6). Sebaceous glands, presumably the result of metaplasia of cells of intercalated and striated ducts, may be found in pleomorphic adenomas, as well as in normal salivary gland tissue.

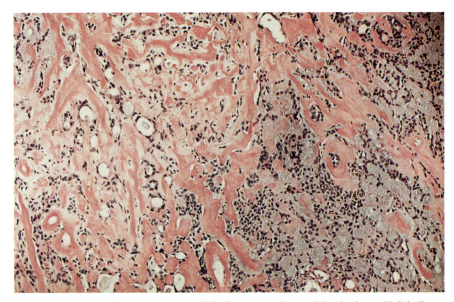

Figure 41.4 Pleomorphic adenoma dominated by hyaline stroma and scattered ductal and myoepithelial cells

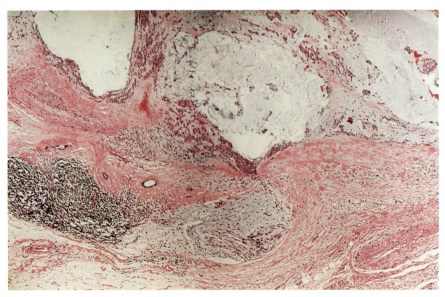

Figure 41.5 An example of a hypocellular pleomorphic adenoma with islands of mucoid substance and cystic changes (*top*). Inflammatory infiltrate (*left*) is not a common finding in pleomorphic adenoma

Crystals and Hyaline Cells

Crystalline structures may be found in pleomorphic adenomas. These may be tyrosine-rich crystalloids, collagen-rich crystalloids or oxalate crystals.

The so-called hyaline or plasmacytoid cell is an ovoid cell with eosinophilic hyaline cytoplasm resembling a plasma cell, which is found in some pleomorphic adenomas and is especially common in those neoplasms arising in minor salivary glands (Fig. 41.7). It represents a modified myoepithelial cell and seems to be unique to pleomorphic adenoma, apart from the closely related myoepithelioma. Its presence is diagnostically useful, especially in fine needle aspirates.

Immunohistochemistry

In the normal salivary gland, vimentin is positive in the stromal parts only, and not in the epithelial or myoepithelial cells. There is a coexpression of cyto-

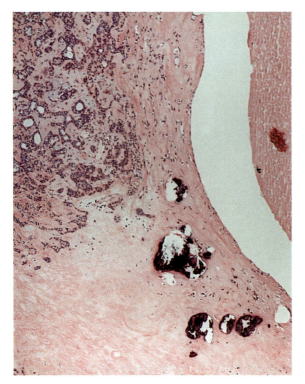

Figure 41.6 Cystic pleomorphic adenoma with deposits of calcium salts

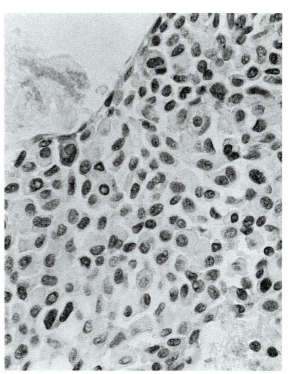

Figure 41.7 Hyaline cells in a palatal pleomorphic adenoma. The cells have eccentrically located nuclei giving them an appearance similar to that of plasma cells

keratin and vimentin in the epithelial and myo-epithelial cells of most pleomorphic adenomas, which is not restricted to the modified myoepithelial cells of the neoplasm, but is also present in the outer cells of the tubuloductal structures. Vimentin may thus be used as an early marker of modified myoepithelium in pleomorphic adenoma. Other antibodies have been shown to mark myoepithelial tumour cells in salivary gland neoplasms. These include S-100 protein, different cytokeratins, actin, myosin, lysozyme and lactoferrin, desmin, glial fibrillary acidic protein, a monoclonal antibody to liver metallothionein (L2E3), neurone-specific enolase, and Tumour-Associated Glycoprotein (TAG-72). Cytokeratin, S-100 protein and smooth muscle actin are at present the most reliable and a panel composed of these markers is thus recommended. However, in spite of this immunoprofile, the diagnosis of pleomorphic adenoma still rests on its histological appearance.

Mucopolysaccharide Content

Pleomorphic adenoma is rich in mucopolysaccharides which may be of biological significance. Two main types of mucin are present: duct-associated epithelial mucin containing a high content of neutral glycoprotein and mesenchymal mucin containing highly-sulphated glycosoaminoglycans. There is no relationship between the glycosoaminoglycan content and the state of differentiation of the pleomorphic adenoma.

Differential Diagnosis

The most important problem in relation to the histological diagnosis of pleomorphic adenoma is the possibility of the lesion being carcinoma in pleomorphic adenoma, or malignant myoepithelioma. A cellular tumour with atypia, even though sometimes discrete, together with a history of previous pleomorphic adenoma, is likely to be a recurrent pleomorphic adenoma. If an invasive growth pattern (to be distinguished from a multinodular one) is present, the process is best regarded as one of malignancy in pleomorphic adenoma. The presence of mitoses alone is not sufficient for the diagnosis of carcinoma ex pleomorphic adenoma or malignant myoepithelioma. Myoepithelioma may mimic the appearance of pleomorphic adenoma, but ductal structures are generally present only in pleomorphic adenoma. In cases of infarcted pleomorphic adenoma large areas may be necrotic and the tissue not readily identifiable (Fig. 41.8). With sufficient

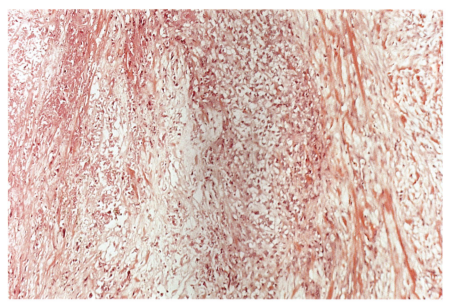

Figure 41.8 A case of infarcted pleomorphic adenoma. Note the necrotic nature of the tumour, but myoepithelial-like cells can still be appreciated in the centre of the photograph

numbers of blocks the true nature of the lesion usually becomes obvious.

Fine Needle Aspiration

A typical aspirate from a pleomorphic adenoma has a gelatinous, rather thick consistency, which is due to the acellular stromal substance. In Giemsa-stained smears the characteristic feature of pleomorphic adenoma, the fibrillary myxoid stromal substance, will appear as an intensively red to dark purple-staining amorphous material. Uniform crowded epithelial cells with well-defined cytoplasm are intermingled with this mucoid substance. There are single plasmacytoid cells, and clusters of hyperchromatic cells, which are lying free or merging with the fibrillary mucoid substance.

In cases of pleomorphic adenoma with predominance of myoepithelial cells, the cytopathology may be similar to myoepithelioma or basal cell adenoma (see below). A careful search in May Grünwald Giemsa-stained sections will, in most cases, reveal the fibrillary mucoid substance. Aspirates containing debris, squamous cells or other signs of cystic change are not unusual. Rarely the aspirate from a pleomorphic adenoma may contain mucous globules surrounded by monomorphous epithelial cells, making a distinction from adenoid cystic carcinoma difficult. Epidermoid cells or intracellular mucus may give rise to confusion with mucoepidermoid carcinoma.

Therapy and Prognosis

The treatment of pleomorphic adenoma is complete surgical excision. If it is not situated in the superficial parotid lobe, or in certain minor salivary glands, this procedure is not always readily performed. If completely removed it will not recur, but with unsatisfactory surgery there is a high risk of recurrences due to spillage at the operation or residual tumour left behind. In these latter cases radiotherapy immediately after the operation may be of benefit. An expected 5-year recurrence-free rate has been calculated at 96.6% and a 10-year recurrence-free rate at 93.2%.[4]

Malignant Transformation

The frequency of malignancy developing in pleomorphic adenoma has been assessed at between 2 and 10%.[5,6] The risk of malignant transformation increases the longer an untreated tumour has been present. Three different types of malignancy may originate in a pleomorphic adenoma. One is a pathological oddity in which a histologically benign neoplasm metastasises without any alteration in histological character. In the second both the epithelial and stromal elements are malignant and the lesion is a true malignant mixed tumour. The third type, the situation in the overwhelming majority of cases, is the carcinoma ex (in) pleomorphic adenoma, usually a poorly differentiated ductal adenocarcinoma and only rarely other types of carcinomas, e.g. mucoepidermoid carcinoma, malignant myoepithelioma, clear cell carcinoma, epidermoid carcinoma, adenoid cystic carcinoma (see Chapter 42).

Myoepithelioma

Until recently adenomas were divided only into pleomorphic and monomorphic types, with oncocytomas and Warthin tumour sometimes being separated from the monomorphic group. The clinical behaviour of adenomas other than pleomorphic was difficult to evaluate by this schema. The World Health Organization (WHO) classification,[3] including as it did, rare but clearly defined and noncontroversial entities, improved the clinicopathologic correlation of these tumours.

Definition and Terminology

Myoepithelioma is defined as a tumour composed of myoepithelial cells, alone or with the addition of small numbers of ductal structures, growing in a mucoid and/or myxoid-vascular stroma. Myoepithelial cells vary in appearance and can be spindle-shaped, hyaline, epithelioid or clear. Although at first thought to lack myxoid or chondral elements, such stromal changes have more recently been observed in these tumours. Thus myoepithelioma is similar to pleomorphic adenoma, apart from a scarcity of duct-like structures. Neoplasms otherwise compatible with myoepithelioma but comprising duct structures in considerable numbers are better classified as pleomorphic adenomas.[7]

Site and Incidence

Myoepithelioma is most commonly found in the parotid gland and palate. Occasionally it is seen in the submandibular and sublingual glands and in the minor salivary glands of the gingiva, the lip, nose, larynx and in the lacrimal gland.

Histogenesis

It seems likely that any of the various cells found in the normal salivary gland can serve as a precursor for neoplasia, the myoepithelial cell included. The myoepithelial cell can assume a variety of cytologic forms (see below), all of which may occur in myoepithelioma. The myoepithelial cell is also a common component in a variety of salivary gland tumours other than myoepithelioma.

Clinical Features

Myoepitheliomas have no distinctive clinical features and usually present as slowly growing, asymptomatic masses. The age and sex distribution is similar to that of pleomorphic adenoma.

Microscopic Appearances

Myoepitheliomas consist of one or several of the morphologically different types of the modified myoepithelial cell: spindle-shaped, epithelioid, plasmacytoid (hyaline) and clear cells (see Chapter 40). Different architectural patterns add a further degree of complexity to this tumour entity. Myoepitheliomas are of two basic types: myxoid and nonmyxoid. The non-myxoid (or solid) myoepithelioma, the most common type, consists of modified myoepithelial cells arranged in nests separated by fibrous or hyalinised stroma. Most often the myoepithelial cell is spindle-shaped with eosinophilic cytoplasm (Fig. 41.9). In myxoid myoepithelioma the tumour cells have a more mesh-like or sieve-like architecture, and the tumour cells are haphazardly arranged. Both these types of myoepithelioma resemble pleomorphic adenoma, although in myoepithelioma duct structures are absent or few in number.

When myoepithelioma occurs in minor salivary glands it is often very cellular (cellular myoepithelioma) and tends to grow both in solid nests and in narrow, anastomosing cords of cells, which may be separated by a myxoid and vascularised stroma (Fig. 41.10). When the latter growth pattern predominates it may mimic invasion, and the distinction between benign and malignant proliferation in such a myoepithelioma may be difficult, particularly when cellular pleomorphism is slight and mitotic activity low. However, the malignant counterpart usually has microcysts and the stroma usually displays a sarcomatous appearance with cellular atypia, numerous and occasionally abnormal mitotic figures and invasion of adjacent salivary gland tissue.

Immunocytochemistry

Myoepithelioma shows a co-expression of high- and low-molecular weight cytokeratin filaments, and

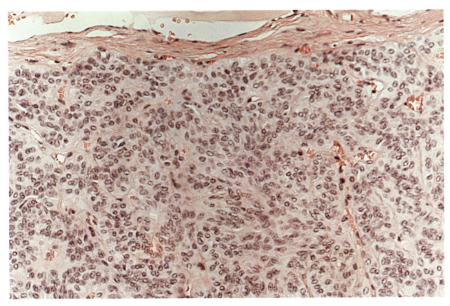

Figure 41.9 Parotid myoepithelioma consisting of solid masses of uniform myoepithelial cells. The cells are mainly spindle-shaped but some are also epithelioid and have a faintly eosinophilic cytoplasm. The cells are separated by a sparse amount of hypocellular stroma containing a few vessels. There are no duct-like structures in this part of the tumour

S-100 protein and smooth muscle actin are almost always present. Glial fibrillary acid protein and vimentin are also often expressed. Strong immunopositivity for type IV collagen and laminin is regularly seen in myoepithelioma, but they are also found in other salivary gland tumours and in basement membranes surrounding acini and the terminal duct system in normal salivary tissue.

Fine Needle Aspiration

The cytologic features of the neoplastic myoepithelial cell have been extensively studied in large series of pleomorphic adenomas, myoepitheliomas and a few malignant myoepitheliomas. Myoepithelioma in aspirates may be difficult to distinguish from pleomorphic adenoma with myoepithelial cell predominance. This has no bearing on the clinical management and outcome for the patient. The main objective of preoperative cytologic investigation is to distinguish benign from malignant tumours. An aspirate consisting of uniform myoepithelial cells isolated or arranged in clusters is likely to be derived from a myoepithelioma. The cells often have basophil cytoplasm and ill-defined cytoplasmic borders.

Therapy and Prognosis

Myoepitheliomas should wherever possible be classified separately from pleomorphic adenomas, but at

the same time it should be acknowledged that the former probably represent one end of the spectrum of pleomorphic adenoma. The natural behaviour of myoepithelioma is similar to pleomorphic adenoma: it is a benign neoplasm with a tendency to recur. Myoepithelioma is thought by some to have a more aggressive growth than pleomorphic adenoma, with a greater tendency to malignant transformation, but by others to be a more benign neoplasm.[3,8] Treatment is by surgical excision. A few progress to malignancy with metastases.

Warthin Tumour

Warthin tumour (adenolymphoma, cystadenolymphoma, papillary cystadenoma lymphomatosum) is a benign neoplasm composed of eosinophilic (often oncocytic) epithelial cells.

Site and Incidence

Warthin tumour is a commonly occurring neoplasm arising usually in the parotid gland. Other sites of origin are on record, although the interpretation of some of these lesions as Warthin tumours is open to doubt, including those in the submandibular gland, the palate, the buccal mucosa and lips and the nasopharynx. It could be argued that sialoadenoma papilliferum also, mainly found in the intraoral salivary glands, is a variant of Warthin tumour. Warthin tumour comprises more than 70% of non-

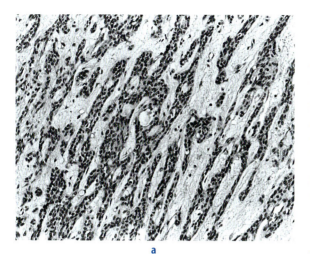

a

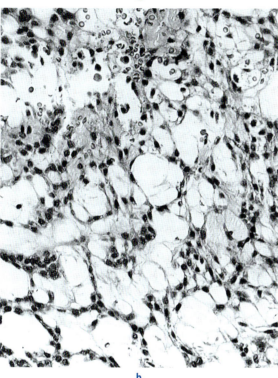

b

Figure 41.10 Non-solid myoepithelioma. **a** Palatal myoepithelioma with large amounts of myxoid stroma. The cells grow in strands and cords and there are very few duct structures. **b** Another non-solid myoepithelioma with micro- and pseudocysts. The cells are anastomosing, to some extent in a sieve-like pattern. The absence of cellular atypia and mitotic figures indicates the benign nature of this myoepithelioma

pleomorphic parotid adenomas, and 5–15% of all parotid neoplasms.

The majority of these tumours have been described in men, although some authors have recently indicated a substantial incidence in females. The peak age incidence is in the sixth and seventh decades, and they usually involve the lower part of the parotid gland. Bilateral or multiple Warthin tumours are observed in about 10% of cases. Although most bilateral Warthin tumours do not occur simultaneously but are metachronous, some simultaneously bilateral cases have been reported. Synchronous extra-parotid Warthin tumour has also been reported. Simultaneous occurrence of separate salivary gland tumours is rare and most of the cases cited in the literature have been Warthin tumour. A so-called combination tumour in the parotid gland was composed of a Warthin tumour and a sebaceous lymphadenoma, and likely represents a hybrid tumour (see Chapter 43).

Histogenesis

During late embryogenesis the parotid gland becomes encapsulated to include adjacent lymphatic tissue within the gland. Ducts (also acini in children) are therefore frequent findings in the normal intra-parotid lymph nodes. Such a process does not occur in any other major, or minor, salivary gland. Immunohistochemical as well as clinicopathological studies indicate that the epithelial structures of the Warthin tumour stem from both intercalated duct cells and ductal basal cells and the existence of these heterotopic ducts would also explain the high tendency for the neoplasm to be multifocal and bilateral. Mucoepidermoid and acinic cell carcinoma are other salivary gland neoplasms that on rare occasions may be encountered within a parotid lymph node, but these tumours are best considered as hamarblastomas.

It is still unclear whether the lymphoid tissue in Warthin tumour represents a normal lymph node, an immunological response to the proliferating epithelium, or a combination of both. Studies of the lymphoid stroma have shown features of an exaggerated secretory immune response, e.g. delayed hypersensitivity, perhaps similar to the lymphoid tissue in Hashimoto's thyroiditis. Contrary findings indicate that Warthin tumour can arise in a pre-existing lymph node. Immunocytochemical studies have shown strong immunoreactivity for Tenascin (an extracellular matrix glycoprotein) in the basement membrane zone of the epithelial component of Warthin tumour; this substance has not been observed in serous or mucinous salivary glands. Cytogenetic studies of Warthin's tumour have shown it to have three main stemline groups, one with a normal karyotype, a second with numerical changes only (loss of Y chromosome or trisomy or monosomy 5), and a third group involving structural changes with one or two reciprocal translocations.

Clinical Features

Warthin tumour presents as a painless parotid swelling, often egg-shaped, well-defined and mobile, and located in the posterior and inferior parts of the gland. Warthin tumour is usually less than 6 cm in diameter, but tumours larger than 10 cm in diameter have been described. The average period of awareness of the lump at diagnosis is 1–2 years.[9] In a minor proportion of cases pain is present, and many patients notice fluctuation in size of the tumour, especially when eating.

Gross Appearances

Warthin tumour is typically a round or oval mass covered by a thin capsule. The cut surface may show one or more large cystic spaces or may be composed a firm, solid and whitish tumour with a few small cysts. The cysts are filled with clear, serous or brownish fluid, or even sometimes cheesy material (Fig. 41.11).

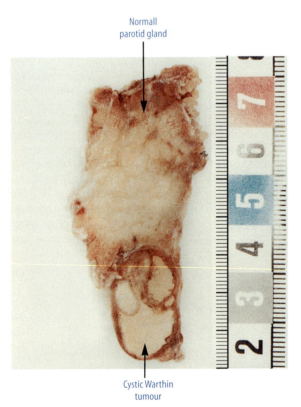

Normall
parotid gland

Cystic Warthin
tumour

Figure 41.11 Gross appearance of parotid gland with a Warthin tumour with cystic change at lower pole

Microscopic Appearances

The tumour is composed of strands of epithelial cells with frequent papillae (Fig. 41.12). The inner layer of the strands comprises finely granular, oncocytic columnar cells and an outer layer of more cuboidal cells. Large amounts of lymphoid tissue are present between the strands (Fig. 41.13). The luminal cells often form small blebs resembling apocrine secretion. Rarely cilia are present. Concentrically laminated bodies resembling corpora amylacea may be present. The tumour is usually surrounded by a thin capsule, which may be incomplete. Distended cysts may be associated with attenuation of the epithelium. The cysts are usually filled with an eosinophilic secretion or amorphous material; sometimes cholesterol clefts and accompanying inflammatory and multinucleated giant cells are present. A subclassification into typical Warthin with an equal ratio of epithelium and lymphoid stroma, stroma-poor tumours that have a lymphoid component of less than 30%, stroma-rich Warthin tumours that have a lymphoid component of more than 70% of the tumour mass and a fourth metaplastic type with large areas of squamous epithelium has been proposed. Germinal follicles are absent from the lymphoid follicles in 40% of cases. In infarcted Warthin tumours there are areas of necrosis and squamous and mucous metaplasia sometimes creating an appearance that can be mistaken for mucoepidermoid carcinoma; the appearances resemble also the metaplastic type of Warthin tumour. Granulomatous change is said to be present in 40% of cases.[9]

Adjacent to the main Warthin tumour one may see minute Warthin tumours arising from ductal elements within lymphoid tissue, which sometimes seems to be diffusely distributed and not encapsulated as in a lymph node. Such an observation throws doubt as to whether Warthin tumour indeed arises from inclusions of salivary gland tissue in lymph nodes.

A predominance of T lymphocytes, similar to the findings in normal and reactive lymph nodes, has been described by some, indicating an origin in pre-existing lymph nodes, but others have found a predominance of B lymphocytes. The latter, together with a concomitant reduction of T lymphocytes, has led to the suggestion that the lymphocytes in Warthin tumour may be a cellular infiltrate reactive to the neoplastic epithelium.

Differential Diagnosis

Ductal oncocytosis in an otherwise papillary tumour (e.g. papillary cystadenoma and metastatic

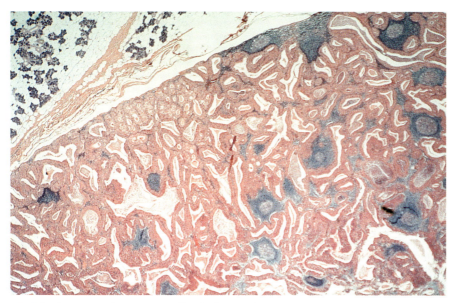

Figure 41.12 Warthin tumour with sparse amount of lymphoid tissue. A distinct capsule is not seen. Parotid gland at upper left corner

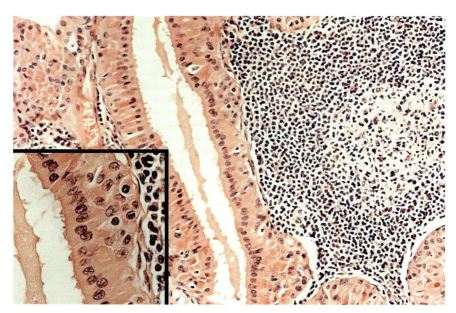

Figure 41.13 Photomicrograph of Warthin tumour showing the epithelium with two cell layers. The outer oncocytic columnar cells have a pseudociliated appearance and the inner layer is of cuboidal basal cells. A germinal follicle is evident in the lymphoid tissue. Insert: higher magnification of the epithelium

papillary carcinoma of the thyroid), and oncocytic change in epithelial hyperplasia associated with lymphoid aggregates, are alternative diagnostic possibilities in some Warthin tumours. The infarcted (metaplastic) type of Warthin tumour with squamous metaplasia may resemble a ruptured epidermoid or lymphoepithelial cyst.[9]

Fine Needle Aspiration

Fine needle aspirates of Warthin tumours typically consist of cystic fluid with lymphocytes, scattered fragments of lymphocytes, and epithelial cells, often granular and oncocytic. The oncocytic cells are often arranged in cohesive, irregular sheets with a tendency for peripheral palisading of the cells. The cells have abundant cytoplasm and rather small, round nuclei. Furthermore, there are amorphous and granular debris. Occasionally, malignant-appearing, stratified squamous-like cells may be present due to reparative foci or metaplastic changes, and care has to be taken not to misinterpret these cells as representing a squamous cell carcinoma.

Therapy and Prognosis

Warthin tumour is a benign neoplasm usually cured by surgical excision. Recurrence rate may be difficult to assess due to the frequently multifocal nature of Warthin tumour, but can be estimated at between 5.5% and 12%.[10] No malignant changes were reported in three large series of 357, 278 and 275 cases of Warthin tumour. A few convincing cases of malignancy arising in Warthin tumour were carcinomas. Coexistence with a malignant lymphoma, e.g. Hodgkin's disease, may occur. Confidence in the benign character of almost all Warthin tumours is such that at many institutions no surgical treatment is carried out after the fine needle aspiration diagnosis has been made.

Oncocytoma

Oncocytoma, or oncocytic adenoma, is a tumour consisting of polyhedral eosinophilic cells, the so-called oncocytes. In clear cell oncocytoma, a rare variant, the polyhedral cells have clear cytoplasm but still show granular positivity of mitochondria on phosphotungstic acid haematoxylin staining. Non-neoplastic oncocytic transformation of epithelial cells is commonly seen in the ageing parotid gland. It is not a degenerative process but rather a redifferentiation of the cells with proliferation of mitochondria in an attempt to increase their output of high-energy phosphate. A related process is hyperplasia of oncocytic buds from ductal epithelium, leaving normal acinar tissue at the periphery and going on to produce non-encapsulated oncocytic nodules (multifocal nodular oncocytic hyperplasia; see Chapters 29 and 40).

Site and Incidence

Oncocytoma is a rare neoplasm usually arising in the parotid gland of elderly patients. It represents less than 1% of epithelial tumours of all salivary glands. A few cases have been described in the sub-mandibular gland and even fewer in minor salivary glands (nasal - see Chapter 17 - palatal or oral). Oncocytic metaplasia of benign salivary gland tumours (pleomorphic and basal cell adenomas) is far more common than oncocytoma itself.[11]

Histogenesis

Oncocytic change should be considered as a meta-plastic rather than a degenerative process and a neoplasm could conceivably originate from a hyperplasia of oncocytes. The exact cell of origin still remains unclear, although the intercalated duct reserve cell has been proposed. The chromosomal abnormality found in benign oncocytomas of the parotid gland, a trisomy 7, must be interpreted as neoplasia-related and not as an expression of ageing or degeneration. The oncocyte is capable of proliferation and therefore, theoretically, has the capacity of becoming neoplastic. This seems more likely than the concept that the oncocytic changes constitute a secondary event in already malignant transformed cells.

Oncocytomas can be induced in kidneys of rats by the use of N-nitrosomorpholine, and the process seems to start with oncocytic hyperplasia, indicating that this process may become eventually transformed into oncocytoma.

Clinical Features

Oncocytomas are clinically indistinguishable from pleomorphic adenomas. They are usually well-demarcated and present as a smooth, firm swelling, usually less than 4 cm in the superficial parotid lobe. The tumour is freely movable and not attached to underlying structures.

Gross Appearances

Oncocytoma is a solid tumour and most often solitary, although bilateral in a small proportion of cases. It usually is brown-red in colour, and surrounded by a thin, wispy fibrous capsule, rarely by a distinct one.

Microscopic Appearances

The tumour is composed entirely of oncocytically transformed acini and ducts, which form a solid or trabecular growth in which residual normal salivary tissue occasionally may be seen. On rare occasions a

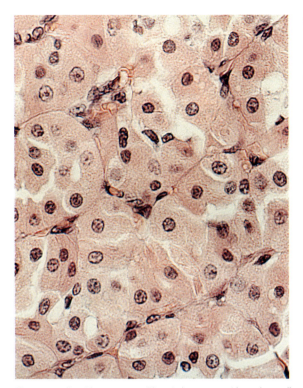

Figure 41.14 Parotid oncocytoma with typical oncocytes with regular, small nuclei and abundant, granular eosinophilic cytoplasm

papillary growth pattern is observed, giving a picture very similar to Warthin's tumour except for the absence of lymphoid tissue. The tumour cells are polyhedral with small, dark nuclei and eosinophilic cytoplasm (Fig. 41.14). Areas of clear cell differentiation are found in most oncocytomas, if many sections are examined. A rare variant, called clear cell oncocytoma,[12] has been described. This consists of a circumscribed tumour mass of polyhedral cells with clear cytoplasm. The clear cell oncocytoma often shows a positive reaction for glycogen if stained by periodic acid–Schiff, before and after diastase. The cytoplasmic granularity due to the mitochondria is best demonstrated with phosphotungstic acid haematoxylin. The importance of recognising clear cell oncocytoma is that it is probably the only benign clear cell neoplasm of salivary glands.

A diagnosis of oncocytoma can be confirmed by electron microscopy when the cells will be found to contain numerous mitochondria (up to 60% of the total cell volume) and by a positive immunoreactivity for anti-mitochondrial antibody.

Differential Diagnosis

Oncocytoma should be distinguished from nonneoplastic hyperplasia of oncocytic cells, a normal feature of salivary gland tissue in elderly subjects. These nodules are not encapsulated, normal acinar tissue is often found at their periphery and there is usually clear cell differentiation. Keeping the possibility of multifocal hyperplasia in mind, care has to be taken also not to misdiagnose an oncocytic satellite focus in the vicinity of an oncocytoma as a sign of invasive activity by the latter.

In respect to neoplasms the main differential diagnoses are acinic cell carcinoma, pleomorphic adenoma and mucoepidermoid carcinoma with oncocytic changes, and metastases from oncocytic carcinoma cells of the thyroid, kidney or liver. Unlike acinic cell carcinoma, oncocytoma does not have well-differentiated acinar cells and also contains glycogen. If chondroid or myxoid metaplasia, spindle or plasmacytoid myoepithelial cell differentiation, or keratin formation, are present, the tumour is best classified as an oncocytoid pleomorphic adenoma. The term oncocytoid should be used for cells resembling oncocytes but not fulfilling the histochemical requirements for the oncocyte. The diagnosis of mucoepidermoid carcinoma has to be considered should intracytoplasmic sialomucin be present, and should phosphotungstic acid haematoxylin staining for mitochondria be negative. Oncocytic carcinoma exists but is exceedingly rare (see Chapter 42).

Fine Needle Aspiration

The cytologic appearance of oncocytoma is characterised by the presence of cohesive clumps of benign oncocytic cells with small nuclei, similar to those found in Warthin tumour, but without associated lymphocytes.

Therapy and Prognosis

Being mainly a solitary lesion, surgical excision will cure in most instances.

Basal Cell Adenoma

Basal cell adenoma is defined as a tumour composed of basaloid cells with prominent basal cell layer resting on a distinct basement membrane-like structure.[3] During the last two decades many authors have used the terms basal cell adenoma, monomorphic adenoma, and canicular adenoma, synonymously. In an earlier classification the general term monomorphic adenoma was recommended to be used for any benign salivary gland tumour other than pleomorphic adenoma showing a distinct epithelial basement membrane. However, the new WHO classification clearly defines basal cell adenoma as a distinct entity with recognisable histological features.[3]

Site and Incidence

Basal cell adenomas represent 1.8–7.5% of all salivary gland tumours. They are most commonly found in the superficial portion of the parotid gland; in minor salivary glands most often in the lips, particularly the upper lip. Basal cell adenoma tends to occur in elderly patients with a peak incidence in the sixth, seventh and eighth decades, in a rather older age group than for pleomorphic adenoma. There is a slightly increased frequency in females.[5,10]

Histogenesis

These tumours may arise from secretory ductal cells or lining ductal epithelial cells, because of the resemblance to eccrine spiroadenoma of the skin. Other studies have suggested that basal cell adenoma arises from epithelial cells of the intercalated ducts, which also could explain certain resemblances to adenoid cystic carcinoma.[13]

Clinical Features

The tumours are small, usually less than 3 cm, and are clinically indistinguishable from pleomorphic adenoma.

Gross Appearances

Basal cell adenoma is well-circumscribed and the capsule smooth and glistening.

Microscopic Appearances

The histological hallmarks of a basal cell adenoma are basaloid cells with a prominent basal cell layer, and a distinct basement membrane structure. There are no myxoid, mucoid or chondroid stromal elements as found in pleomorphic adenomas. The growth pattern may vary, and at least four different types can be recognised (Fig. 41.15). The trabecular and the tubular variants are most common. In the trabecular type the basaloid cells are arranged in anastomosing thin and narrow, sometimes broader

nests of cells. In tubular adenomas small duct-like structures are present. Combinations of these two growth patterns often exist in the same tumour. A third type is a solid variant resembling a basal cell carcinoma of the skin with solid nests of crowded tumour cells surrounded by a palisaded outer layer. Squamous metaplasia is seen from time to time in this type. The solid variant of basal cell adenoma as well as the trabecular type may have areas with cribriform growth pattern. The membranous type (dermal analogue tumour) resembles the dermal cylindroma and not infrequently coexists with tumours of the skin, e.g. eccrine cylindroma, trichoepithelioma. The tumour shows islands or of epithelial cells with basophilic nuclei and scanty cytoplasm. There is peripheral palisading. Larger cells with paler-staining nuclei may be present near the centre of the epithelial islands. In most cases an extracellular, often hyalinised material is observed as droplets, as deposits around vessels, or as larger masses in which small pyknotic nuclei are found. In all types of basal cell adenomas, cysts may be present, as in adenoid cystic carcinoma.[14]

Differential Diagnosis

An important differential diagnosis of basal cell adenoma, particularly in minor salivary glands of the hard palate or in the sinonasal tract, is ameloblastoma. However, the cells of ameloblastoma usually show a resemblance to stellate reticulum and although peripheral palisading is a feature of that neoplasm, thickened basement membrane is not. Pleomorphic adenoma with little stromal component may give rise to diagnostic difficulty. The most important differential diagnosis is adenoid cystic carcinoma with its profoundly different biological behaviour. Two notable guidelines are the palisaded peripheral cells in the basal cell adenoma, and the frequent perineural invasion found in the adenoid cystic carcinoma.

Basal cell adenoma may on rare occasions become transformed into a low-grade malignant neoplasm, basal cell adenocarcinoma, which may resemble adenoid cystic carcinoma or malignant myoepitheliomas.

Fine Needle Aspiration

In fine needle aspiration material from basal cell adenoma, the appearances should be distinguished from adenoid cystic carcinoma, and sometimes a distinction from that of pleomorphic adenoma is necessary. The hyaline globules surrounded by neoplastic cells, typical for adenoid cystic carcinoma,

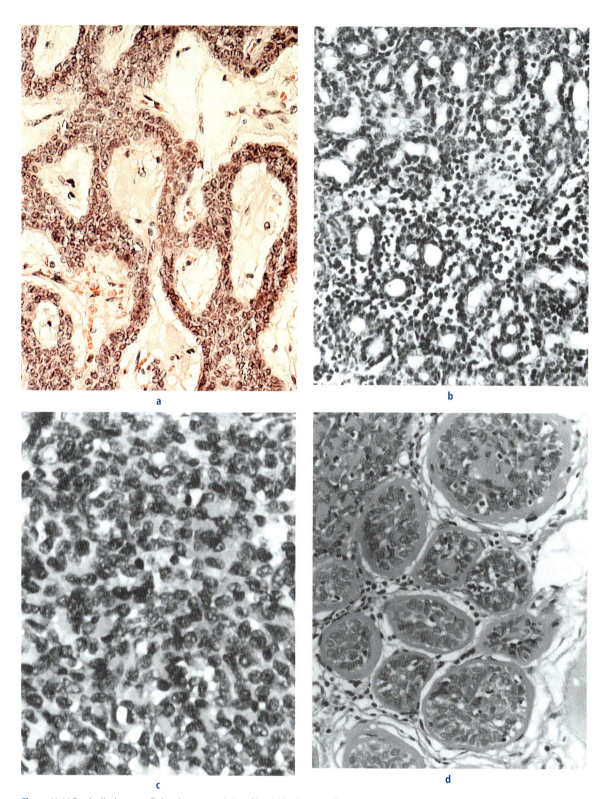

Figure 41.15 Basal cell adenoma. **a** Trabecular type consisting of basaloid cell tumours forming anastomosing cords, often with two cell layers only. There is no distinct basement membrane-like structure. **b** Tubular type has round tubules, and there may be an inflammatory infiltrate. **c** Solid variant of basal cell adenoma, devoid of typical tubules and anastomisng cords. **d** Membranous type of basal cell adenoma with a thick hyaline membrane surrounding each lobule of small cells

can also be found in basal cell adenoma. The main cytological difference lies in the much greater atypia seen in adenoid cystic carcinoma. Pleomorphic adenoma shows greater cytologic heterogeneity than that found in basal cell adenoma.

Therapy and Prognosis

The basal adenoma is a benign tumour, which responds well to local excision only. The membranous type may rarely become transformed to a locally aggressive tumour of low-grade malignancy and without regional or distant metastases.

Canalicular Adenoma

Canalicular adenoma is defined as a benign neoplasm composed of columnar epithelial cells arranged in anastomosing, often bilayered, strands with a loose and highly vascular stroma.

Site and Incidence

The majority of these tumours arise in the upper lip and some in the buccal mucosa, but this neoplasm is rare in the parotid gland, in contrast to basal cell adenomas. Almost all cases of canalicular adenoma occur in patients over 50 years of age, the mean age being 65 years.[3,10]

Clinical Features

Canalicular adenoma is quite often multifocal or multinodular and most often it presents as a small, slowly growing, painless nodule in the upper lip. The lesion may fluctuate in size and is therefore not seldom mistaken clinically for a mucocele. Unlike basal cell adenoma there is no known association with dermal cylindroma.

Gross Appearances

The circumscribed lump is usually encapsulated, but is occasionally unencapsulated, especially in the larger lesions.

Microscopic Appearances

The epithelial cells are columnar or cuboidal, containing cytoplasm that is weakly eosinophilic, with scattered granules that stain positively with periodic acid–Schiff. The nuclei are regular and round or oval, and rarely show vesicles. The cells are arranged in anastomosing, often bilayered strands, in a fashion similar to trabecular basal cell adenoma, but unlike the latter there are no tubular structures. The most distinctive feature is the oedematous, lightly basophilic, non-fibrous stroma with numerous vessels and sometimes a few scattered inflammatory cells (Fig. 41.16). The stroma stains positively with

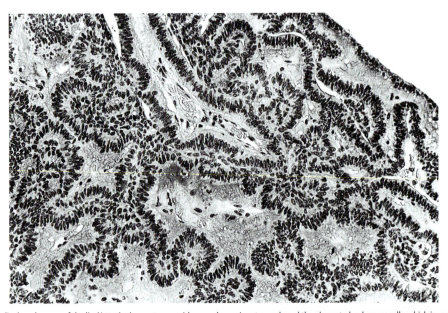

Figure 41.16 Canalicular adenoma of the lip. Note the loose stroma with several prominent vessels and the elongated, columnar cells, which in several areas show two layers. The nuclei tend to be located towards one end of the cells and the cytoplasm is pale eosinophilic

Alcian blue, periodic acid–Schiff and mucicarmine. On rare occasions psammona bodies may be present, particularly in papillary areas of the tumour.

Fine Needle Aspiration

Adenomas other than pleomorphic adenoma have cytologic features that can be unique and recognised in fine needle aspiration . An aspirate of canalicular adenoma, often clinically assessed as a mucocele of the lip, shows columnar, slightly eosinophilic cells without atypia, and a rich amount of ground substance but no fluid.

Therapy and Prognosis

The treatment of choice is complete surgical excision, and in spite of its tendency to be multifocal, canalicular adenoma rarely recurs. Malignant change does not occur in canalicular adenoma. We have encountered a case of canalicular adenoma in juxtaposition to adenoid cystic carcinoma, thus a "hybrid tumour" (see Chapter 43).

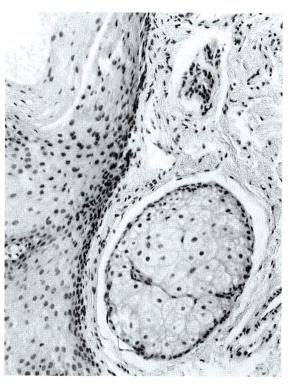

Figure 41.17 Fordyce's spot in the lip showing a sebaceous gland and the overlying mucosal epithelium

Sebaceous Adenoma

Sebaceous adenoma is a rare, benign neoplasm composed of regular sebaceous cells without atypia. In sebaceous lymphadenoma there are circumscribed nests of sebaceous cells in a lymphoid stroma showing a similarity to Warthin tumour. Cystic sebaceous lymphadenoma, on the other hand, is a cyst with sebaceous metaplasia of the duct-lining cells and an underlying lymphocytic infiltrate. Foci of sebaceous differentiation can be seen in other salivary gland neoplasms, most often in pleomorphic adenoma, mucoepidermoid carcinoma and Warthin tumour.[3,10]

Clinical Features

The tumours present as small, painless swellings.

Microscopic Appearances

Sebaceous gland formations (Fig. 41.17) (Fordyce's spots) are common in the mouth and particularly on the vermilion of the upper lip. These are choristomas. Sebaceous cells and glandular formations are present normally in the parotid and the submandibular glands in particular, but also occasionally in the sublingual gland.

Sebaceous adenoma is a well-circumscribed neoplasm composed of benign sebaceous cells. The glandular formations vary considerably in size, and the nests of sebaceous cells are usually surrounded by thin rims of connective tissue. There may be cysts or ectatic salivary ducts with foci of sebaceous cells. Sebaceous lymphadenoma is composed of multiple nests of sebaceous cells and ducts, embedded in a lymphoid tissue with an appearance somewhat similar to Warthin tumour.

Mucoepidermoid carcinoma may contain cystic spaces and clear cells, not only lining the cysts but forming small nests. Many of the clear cells, however, contain intracellular mucin that is not seen in sebaceous tumours.

Therapy and Prognosis

Adequate excision is sufficient therapy, and neither sebaceous adenoma nor sebaceous lymphadenoma have any tendency to recur if properly excised.

Ductal Papilloma

There are three different types of true papillary tumours of the salivary glands, namely inverted ductal papilloma, intraductal papilloma and sialadenoma papilliferum.[3]

Site and Incidence

Many salivary gland tumours, including papillary cystadenoma, Warthin tumour and low-grade polymorphous adenocarcinoma, may show a papillary growth pattern, but ductal papillomas are very rare. The majority of true salivary gland papillomas occur in the minor salivary glands, the lip and palate being the most common.[10] Rare cases have been described in the parotid gland.

Histogenesis

Inverted ductal papilloma is often seen as an extraglandular tumour and it hence seems very likely that it originates from the ductal epithelium of the excretory ducts. The intraductal papilloma also probably stems from ductal cells. As regards sialadenoma papilliferum, an origin from the excretory ductal cells has been proposed.[10] Other proposals include derivation from excretory duct reserve cells, myoepithelial cells or primitive precursor cells, capable of multidirectional differentiation. It has also been considered by some as a non-neoplastic lesion.

Clinical Features

Because of their rarity there is little information available on the clinical features of these benign neoplasms. Sialadenoma papilliferum, however, appears to be more common in men than in women, and usually occurs in elderly patients, although it has been reported in a 2-year-old child.

Microscopic Appearances

Inverted ductal papilloma resembles inverted papilloma of the sinonasal tract. They are small, firm nodules with an intact overlying mucosa. Inverted papilloma is a well-circumscribed tumour consisting of predominantly stratified squamous epithelium but also basaloid and goblet cells are arranged in papillary configurations into a luminal cavity. Microcysts may be present.

Intraductal papilloma is similar to intraductal papilloma of the breast. Intraductal papilloma is usually a cystic lesion with a lining typically of one or two layers of columnar or cuboidal cells with interspersed goblet cells. There are numerous intraluminal papillary fronds with thin fibrovascular cores (Fig. 41.18). Occasional areas of the cyst lining can also be of intermediate or squamous cell type.

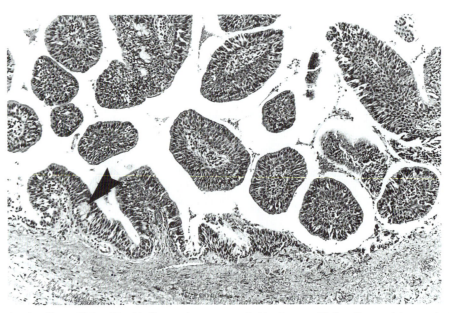

Figure 41.18 Intraductal papilloma with branching thin fibrovascular cores covered with columnar epithelium. There are interspersed goblet cells in the epithelium (*arrow*)

Sialadenoma papilliferum is a small, exophytic lesion, similar to a squamous papilloma. It shows double-layered papillary exophytic projections, microcysts, and often continuity with the surface epithelium and so resembles cutaneous syringocystadenoma papilliferum.[3] Sialadenoma papilliferum is characterised by proliferation of ductal epithelium, both in an exophytic and endophytic fashion. The papillary projections are covered with stratified squamous epithelium, often parakeratotic, and the epithelium merges with the ductal epithelium. The papillary projections are supported by fibrovascular cores, often with a pronounced inflammatory infiltrate. The ductal structures may be dilated and numerous. The proliferation of the ductal elements in the tissue beneath the cystic lining, and absence of a capsule, may give a false impression of invasion.

Therapy and Prognosis

The prognosis of all types of ductal papillomas is excellent with a very low recurrence rate. In spite of its morphologic similarity to sinonasal inverted papilloma, salivary inverted ductal papilloma is not similarly prone to recurrence. The cases of sialadenoma papilliferum reported in the literature have been benign and local recurrences are exceptional. Malignant transformation probably does not occur, although a possible malignant variant of sialadenoma papilliferum with metastasis to a cervical lymph node, and also a case of papillary adenocarcinoma that possibly could have arisen from an intraductal papilloma have been reported.

Cystadenoma

The new WHO classification defines two types of benign cystadenoma, papillary and mucinous.[3] Papillary cystadenoma closely resembles Warthin tumour but is devoid of the lymphoid element. Mucinous cystadenoma, like papillary cystadenoma, is a multicystic tumour, but is lined by goblet cells. There are no atypia, nor any invasion, in either of the two types of cystadenoma.

Site and Incidence

Cystadenomas are most common in the sixth through eighth decades. The parotid gland is the most common site for cystadenoma, but it is also found in the other major and in minor salivary glands.[10] Papillary cystadenomas, although rare in salivary glands outside the larynx, can only occa-

sionally be found in major salivary glands, the palate and the tonsillar region. Laryngeal "papillary cystadenomas" often show oncocytic metaplasia and are reactive cystic lesions with hyperplasia rather than true neoplasias (see Chapter 29).

Microscopic Appearances

Papillary cystadenoma shows similarities to Warthin tumour but lacks the lymphoid stroma and has a more variable appearance. Cyst linings are tall columnar to cuboidal and even flattened cells, and oncocytic cells are often seen. Goblet cells are interspersed between the columnar cells. Mucinous cystadenoma, like papillary cystadenoma, is a multicystic tumour but is lined with goblet cells. Mucinous cystadenoma usually lacks a capsule.

Differential Diagnosis

Papillary and mucinous cystadenocarcinoma are distinguished by their infiltrative growth, nuclear atypia and mitoses, which are not present in cystadenomas. Likewise, low-grade mucoepidermoid carcinomas show invasive growth, and also certain epidermoid differentiation (see Chapter 42).

Therapy and Prognosis

Conservative excision is recommended. Occasional recurrences have been described.

References

1. Erlandson RA, Cardon-Cardo C, Higgins PJ. Histogenesis of benign pleomorphic adenoma (mixed tumor) of the major salivary glands. An ultrastructural and immunohistochemical study. Am J Surg Pathol 1984;8:803–820
2. Dardick I, van Nostrand APW. Myoepithelial cells in the salivary gland tumors – revisited. Head Neck Surg 1985;7:395–408
3. Seifert G, Sobin LH. Histological typing of salivary gland tumors. WHO international histological classification of tumors, 2nd edn. Springer-Verlag, Berlin, Heidelberg, New York, 1991
4. Hickman RE, Cawson RA, Duffy SW. The prognosis of specific types of salivary gland tumors. Cancer 1984;54:1620–1624
5. Thackray AC, Lucas RB. Tumors of the major salivary glands. Atlas of tumor pathology, 2nd series, fascicle 10. US Armed Forces Institute of Pathology, Washington, D.C., 1974
6. Hellquist HB, Michaels L. Malignant mixed tumor. A salivary gland tumor showing both carcinomatous and sarcomatous features. Virchows Arch (A) 1986;409:93–103
7. Dardick I, Thomas MJ, van Nostrand AWP. Myoepithelioma – new concepts of histology and classification: a light and

electron microscopic study. Ultrastruct Pathol 1989;13: 187–224

8. Sciubba JJ, Brannon RB. Myoepithelioma of salivary glands: report of 23 cases. Cancer 1982;49:562–572

9. Eveson JW. Cawson RA. Warthin's tumor (cystadenolymphoma) of salivary glands. A clinicopathologic investigation of 278 cases. Oral Surg Oral Med Oral Pathol 1986;61: 256–262

10. Ellis GL, Auclair PL, Gnepp DR (eds) Surgical pathology of the salivary glands. Major problems in pathology, vol 25. WB Saunders Co, Philadelphia, London, Toronto, 1991

11. Palmer TJ, Gleeson MJ, Eveson JW et al. Oncocytic adenomas and oncocytic hyperplasia of salivary glands: a clinicopathological study of 26 cases. Histopathology 1990;16: 487–493

12. Ellis GL. "Clear cell" oncocytoma of salivary gland. Hum Pathol 1988;19:862–867

13. Luna MA, Mackay B. Basal cell adenoma of the parotid gland: case report with ultrastructural observations. Cancer 1976;37:1615–1621

14. Batsakis JG, Luna MA, El-Naggar A. Pathology consultation. Basaloid monomorphic adenomas. Ann Otol Rhinol Laryngol 1991;100:687–690

42 Malignant Epithelial Neoplasms

The vast majority of malignant epithelial neoplasms of salivary glands can be allocated to the categories of acinic cell carcinoma, mucoepidermoid carcinoma or adenoid cystic carcinoma. All of the other neoplasms described in this chapter are rare.

Acinic Cell Carcinoma

Definition and Terminology

Acinic cell carcinoma is defined as an epithelial tumour of low-grade malignancy composed of cells differentiated towards serous acinar cells. Originally considered benign, its malignant potential has been acknowledged since the early 1950s.[1] In keeping with terminology applied to other glandular neoplasms, this condition should strictly speaking be called acinic cell adenocarcinoma.

Site and Incidence

Acinic cell carcinomas, although not common, constitute 13–16% of all malignant salivary gland tumours. A slightly increased incidence in females has been observed. Acinic cell carcinoma is second only to Warthin tumour among salivary tumours in its tendency to bilateral involvement. Acinic cell carcinoma is also the second most common malignant salivary gland tumour to arise in children, mucoepidermoid carcinoma being the most common. Most acinic cell carcinomas occur in the parotid gland, but are also found in minor salivary glands, although rarely in the palate.[2–5]

Clinical Features

Acinic cell carcinomas are slowly growing neoplasms and are usually less than 3 cm at presentation but may be 10 cm or more. Swelling is the principal symptom, but pain is not uncommon. Facial nerve paralysis is rare.

Gross Appearances

The tumours are firm, rubbery or soft. Some are circumscribed or encapsulated but the majority have ill-defined borders. Cystic areas are frequently seen on the cut surface.

Microscopic Appearances

Four types of cells may be present in acinic cell carcinoma. The acinar cells of acinic cell carcinoma appear similar to those seen in normal salivary gland tissue, i.e. relatively large cells with basophilic to amphophilic cytoplasm showing numerous dark-staining granules, which are stained red by periodic acid–Schiff. Electron microscopy has demonstrated that the granules are stages in saliva production, corresponding to the pre-enzyme granules of the normal acinic cell. The nuclei are usually rather small and centrally placed.

Vacuolated cells are also frequently seen, which are unique to acinic cell carcinoma among salivary gland neoplasms, and are most frequent in those tumours with a microcystic and papillary cystic growth pattern. The vacuoles contain mucopolysaccharides, but are without lipids or glycogen. In some acinic cell carcinomas the granules may be absent or eosinophilic, resembling intercalated duct cells.[1,2] Clear cell differentiation is seen in less than 10% of cases; it never replaces the entire tumour. The clear cells also display the characteristic periodic acid–Schiff-positive cytoplasmic zymogen granules (see Chapter 43) (Fig. 42.1).

A fourth cell type encountered in acinic cell carcinoma is the non-specific glandular cell, which lacks features of any of the other three cell types. These

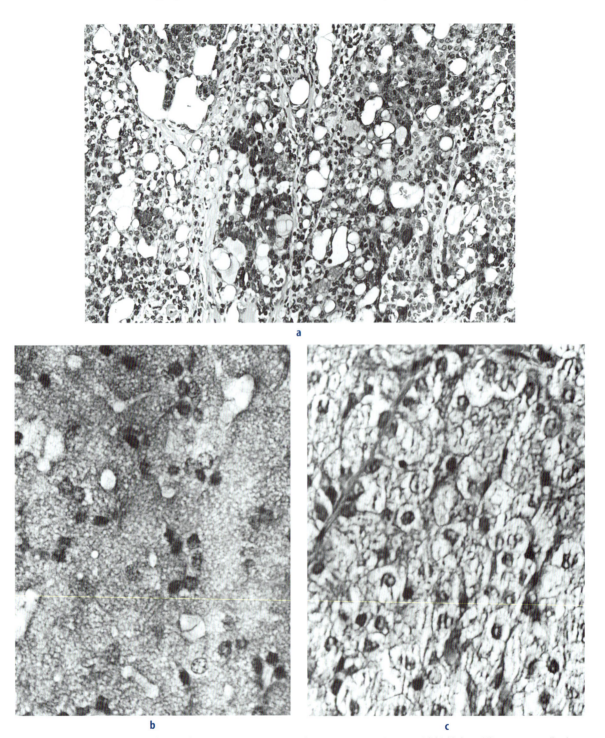

Figure 42.1 a Acinic cell carcinoma with a mixed solid and microcystic pattern. There are numerous microcysts with highly basophilic content as well as larger spaces and scattered darkly basophilic acinar cells. **b** Part of the solid areas of this tumour showing closely packed large, granular acinar cells. **c** From another area of the solid part of the same tumour where the cells are of clear cell appearance

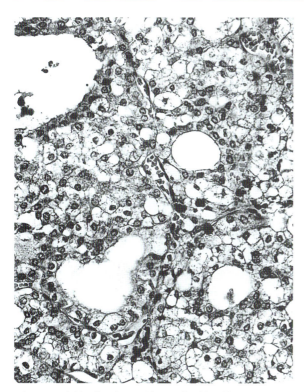

Figure 42.2 Acinic cell carcinoma with intercalated duct-like arrangements

(psammoma-like bodies) and diffuse dystrophic-type calcifications in a collageneous stroma, which can be abundant and hyalinised. Mitotic figures are unusual in acinic cell carcinoma, reflecting its low proliferative rate and low-grade malignancy.

Four main growth patterns: solid, microcystic, papillary cystic, follicular, and combinations thereof have been recognised, although little or no prognostic value can be obtained from such a subclassification.[1] Acinic cell carcinoma with a solid growth pattern, the most common variant, is composed of well-differentiated, usually uniform basophilic acinar cells, predominantly in a glandular or indefinite arrangement. Necrosis is a common finding, but is not necessarily a sign of rapid growth and more aggressive clinical behaviour and, contrary to what is found in most salivary gland tumours, is the presence of numerous lymphocytes with some plasma cells (Fig. 42.3). The solid type of acinic cell carcinoma may sometimes show a sparse microcystic pattern. The microcystic pattern shows a large number of small cystic spaces. These microcystic spaces probably result from the coalescence of intracellular vacuoles of ruptured cells. The microcysts may be filled with mucinous or proteinaceous material.

Acinic cell carcinomas with a papillary-cystic growth pattern are less frequent than the solid and microcystic variants. The cysts are large and papillary growths of epithelial cells supported by thin vascular stalks extend into the cystic spaces. Immunostaining with thyroglobulin can be of help in distinguishing a papillary-type acinic cell carcinoma from metastatic papillary thyroid carcinoma.

cells show the most pronounced atypia, with prominent nucleoli and mitotic activity. The cytoplasm is usually eosinophilic. They may form duct-like structures (Fig. 42.2). Occasionally differentiated myoepithelial cells are present. Calcium deposits are frequent. They present both as calcospherites

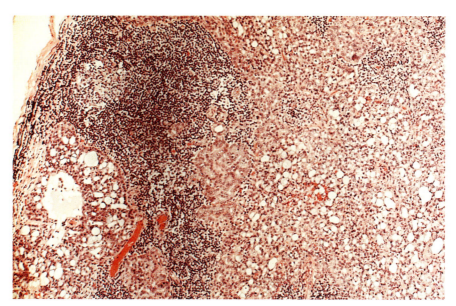

Figure 42.3 A microcystic acinic cell carcinoma. Note the numerous lymphocytes, which are even producing a lymphoid follicle with germinal centre in the left upper corner. Lymphocytes are often present in acinic cell carcinomas and their presence does not denote an intranodal origin

A follicular growth pattern is the least common in acinic cell carcinoma. The structure resembles thyroid follicles with septa of epithelial cells surrounding spaces containing a homogeneous eosinophilic material. The epithelial cells are cuboidal or slightly elongated, and the luminal cell surfaces are convex, imparting a scalloped border to the secreted material. This can be misdiagnosed as metastatic follicular thyroid carcinoma.

Recently an apparently distinct subgroup of acinic cell carcinoma has been described, called well-differentiated acinic cell carcinoma associated with lymphoid stroma. The tumours showed a dense lymphoid stroma with germinal centres, and a thin fibrous pseudocapsule, mimicking intraparotid lymph node containing a metastasis.[6] Real lymph node metastasis of acinic cell carcinoma may be poorly differentiated and difficult to diagnose unless there is information about the existence of a primary.

Immunohistochemistry

Immunocytochemistry may be of help as many acinic cell carcinomas stain positively for amylase. However, several other salivary gland tumours may occasionally be positive for amylase, including some monomorphic adenomas, salivary duct carcinoma and, very rarely, pleomorphic adenoma.

Molecular Biology

Attempts have been made to correlate the nuclear DNA pattern of acinic cell carcinoma in relation to prognosis but without success. Nucleolar organiser regions associated protein (Ag-NORs) has been used as a marker for the proliferation rate of acinic cell carcinoma and related to prognosis. In certain series correlation with prognosis was found, in others not. Several types of gene products, e.g. c-erbB-2 oncoprotein, have also been investigated in the search for prognostic factors with regard to acinic cell carcinomas, but so far with no great success. However, estimation of the proliferation rate by Ki-67 immunostaining has been shown to be an independent prognostic factor.[7,8]

Fine Needle Aspiration

In typical cases of acinic cell carcinoma the aspirate contains much material, consisting of cohesive clusters of cells with abundant cytoplasm, often granular or vacuolated. The cells are regular with medium-sized nuclei, which display moderate atypia. There are bare tumour cell nuclei, possibly myoepithelial cells, and single separate cells. The background is clean but often contains lymphocytes.

Therapy and Prognosis

The incidence of local recurrence of acinic cell carcinoma depends upon several factors including the type of surgery applied. Formerly salivary gland neoplasms were excised by limited resections, such as enucleation. Accordingly many tumours were incompletely resected, frequently recurred and were associated with a low 20-year survival rate. Parotidectomy, superficial or total, is the modern treatment of choice with a cumulative survival of 90–100% at 5 years, 85% at 10 years, and 65–80% at 15 years, thus having the best survival of all carcinomas of salivary gland origin.[4]

Mucoepidermoid Carcinoma

Definition and Terminology

Although usually described as a distinctive entity, mucoepidermoid carcinoma presents a wide variety of appearances. It is defined as a tumour comprising a mixture of mucus-secreting cells, squamous cells and cells of intermediate type, present in varying proportions. Different degrees of histological differentiation of mucus-secreting and epidermoid components are present, but it has been shown that even the highly differentiated forms of mucoepidermoid carcinoma are malignant neoplasms. Early attempts were made with some success to classify the neoplasm into different prognostic groups, but some denied the malignant nature of the lowest grade, which led to the whole entity being referred to as mucoepidermoid "tumour", a nomenclature that unfortunately was validated by the first World Health Organization (WHO) Classification in 1972. The term mucoepidermoid carcinoma has been restored and is now widely accepted.

Site and Incidence

Although one of the most common of malignant salivary gland neoplasms, mucoepidermoid carcinomas are unusual neoplasms comprising only approximately 10% of all salivary gland tumours. Most are located in the parotid gland, but some are found in minor salivary glands, mucoepidermoid carcinoma being the commonest malignant intra-oral salivary gland tumour. Very rarely, centrally occurring mucoepidermoid carcinoma of the jaws may be encountered and also within intraparotid lymph nodes.[9,10]

Histogenesis

It has been suggested that the epidermoid and mucous cells of mucoepidermoid carcinoma arise from an undifferentiated cell associated with salivary gland excretory ducts. However, experimentally many cells from different salivary gland epithelia, even acinar cells, are found to be capable of cellular proliferation.[11] The apparent absence of myoepithelial cells in mucoepidermoid carcinoma casts doubt on the concept of segregation of mucoepidermoid carcinoma from the many other entities said to originate from the intercalated duct reserve cell. The intermediate cells of mucoepidermoid carcinoma are almost certainly the counterpart of the modified myoepithelial cells of pleomorphic adenoma. Since all parts of the duct system have luminal and basal/myoepithelial cells, and myoepithelial cells are even present on intralobular striated ducts, mucoepidermoid carcinoma as well as other neoplasms could develop from a variety of cell types in any segment of the ducts and yet have similar histological appearances.[11] Mucoepidermoid carcinoma may also arise in a pre-existing benign salivary gland neoplasm, e.g. from Warthin tumour and pleomorphic adenoma. The karyotypic abnormality t(11;19) appears to be intimately associated with the mucoepidermoid phenotype, and has been reported in mucoepidermoid carcinomas regardless of site. The frequency of mucoepidermoid carcinoma has been reported as disproportionately high among atomic bomb survivors (at high radiation dose; 1950–1987), suggesting a causal role for ionising radiation for mucoepidermoid carcinoma in contrast to other salivary malignancies.

Clinical Features

Most are movable, painless swellings. Oral neoplasms may mimic mucoceles. Fixation to the surrounding tissues, pain and facial paralysis may be present in parotid tumours. The mean interval between initial swelling and histological verification of the neoplasm has been found to be 6.4 years, but more malignant variants manifest themselves on average only 1.5 years previously. More recent experience gives this interval for all mucoepidermoid carcinomas at less than 1 year.[10] Parotid tumours are

1–2 cm, sometimes as large as 4 cm, and occasional long-standing but high-grade tumours are larger than 5 cm.

Gross Appearances

Most mucoepidermoid carcinomas are poorly circumscribed and many are cystic, often with intracystic haemorrhage.

Microscopic Appearances

Mucoepidermoid carcinoma is composed of three distinctive cell types, namely mucous cells, intermediate cells and squamous cells. The proportion of the three cell types varies. In solid types of mucoepidermoid carcinoma, the epidermoid and intermediate cells predominate, while mucous cells are more frequent in tumours that are mainly cystic. Mucoepidermoid carcinoma shows both solid and glandular components with macro- and microcystic spaces, the contents of which stain positively with periodic acid–Schiff, with and without diastase, Alcian blue and mucicarmine. The glands and cystic spaces are lined with mucous cells and surrounded by sheets of squamous and intermediate cells.

The mucous cells are columnar or cuboidal goblet cells, which line the cysts or form solid masses. They often have pale, eosinophilic, foamy cytoplasm resembling normal acinar cells. When mucous cells are sparse, or not well differentiated, visualisation of mucin by special stains can be diagnostic. Mucous cells lining cysts can be a single layer or multilayered. Occasionally the mucous cells acquire a signet-ring cell appearance.

The intermediate cells, which may be the counterpart of the modified myoepithelial cells of pleomorphic adenoma[11] are smaller than mucous cells and are often situated below the mucous cells. The nuclei are usually dark staining with sharply demarcated cytoplasmic borders

The epidermoid cells are larger cells, often showing intercellular bridges and occasionally keratinisation and individual keratin pearls.

Oncocytic metaplasia is rare in mucoepidermoid carcinoma, but hydropic degeneration with the development of areas of clear cells is not unusual, and may even be a dominant feature of the neoplasm. The clear cells have small nuclei, often pyknotic and centrally placed. An abundant lymphoid stromal component is also relatively common, particularly as an inflammatory infiltrate adjacent to a macrocystic mucoepidermoid carcinoma.

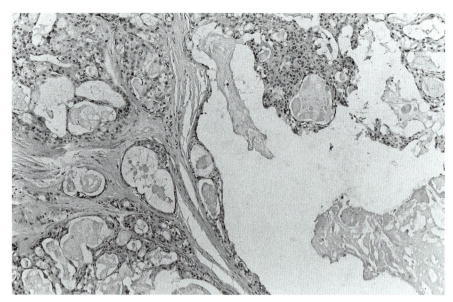

Figure 42.4 A low-grade (well-differentiated) mucoepidermoid carcinoma with a large cyst and smaller ones all containing mucus, mucous cells and intermediate cells

The tumours are classified into well-differentiated or low-grade tumour, and poorly differentiated or high-grade tumour. The well-differentiated type is usually less than 4 cm in diameter, circumscribed but non-encapsulated, and predominantly cystic. More than 50% of the tumour cells are well-differentiated epidermoid and mucus-producing cells. There are few mitoses and minimal nuclear polymorphism (Figs 42.4–42.7). The poorly differentiated type is usually larger than 4 cm, with ill-defined margins, being solid rather than cystic, with areas of haemorrhage and necrosis. These neoplasms show numerous mitoses, and pronounced nuclear polymorphism (Fig. 42.8). Less than 10% of the tumour cells consist of mucus-producing cells, which often are not readily identified without special stains. The high-grade neoplasms are said to show infiltrative permeation rather than infiltration by a broad pushing margin,[1] but in practice both types of infiltration, or either one, may be found in low- or high-grade neoplasms.

Mucoepidermoid carcinomas also have been separated into three grades of malignancy. The three-level grading defines mucoepidermoid carci-

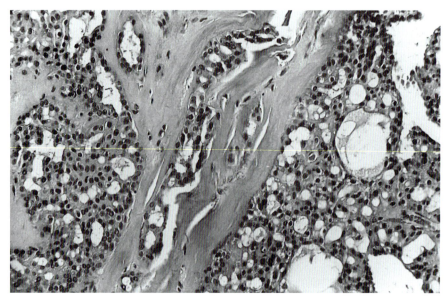

Figure 42.5 A low-grade mucoepidermoid carcinoma from the lip showing infiltrative growth, microcystic pattern and intermediate cells

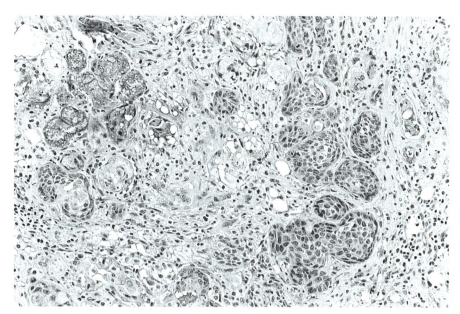

Figure 42.6 Low-grade mucoepidermoid carcinoma. There are nests of epidermoid cells but no keratin pearls, and few mucous cells. Mucoepidermoid carcinoma like this can mimic necrotising sialometaplasia, should the lesion be palatal and the biopsy specimen too small

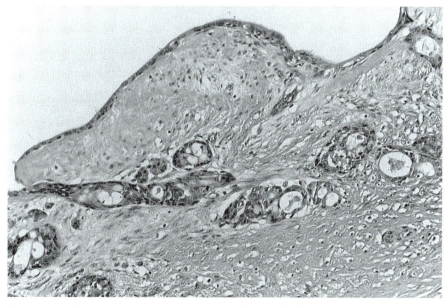

Figure 42.7 A large low-grade parotid cystic mucoepidermoid carcinoma lined by flattened cuboidal epithelium. Invasion by both mucinous and intermediate cells is present, which differentiates this low-grade carcinoma from a benign parotid cyst, which is lined by similar epithelium

nomas as low-grade (well-differentiated) tumours, intermediate-grade tumours (Fig. 42.9) and high-grade (anaplastic) tumours. The three-level system has a better bearing on prognosis[9,12,13] and incorporates histological features that are readily recognisable. It also emphasises the intermediate cell population as an integral histogenetic and histologic component, and it separates out the poorly differentiated type associated with a dismal prognosis.

The morphological criteria for the three-level grading system are outlined in Table 42.1. It should be pointed out that some gradings of mucoepidermoid carcinoma indicate that macrocysts are never associated with high-grade malignancy. Macrocysts are, in fact, present in some high-grade lesions. A macrocystic mucoepidermoid carcinoma in which the cells display moderate atypia should be graded as intermediate grade. An argument against a three-level grading system is that the intermediate-

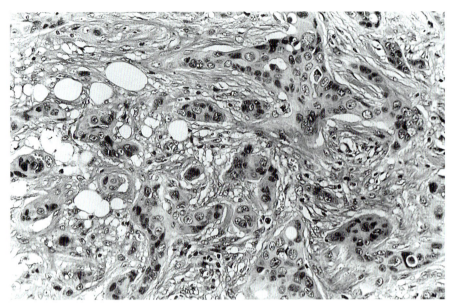

Figure 42.8 Parotid high-grade (poorly differentiated) mucoepidermoid carcinoma with pronounced atypia. These tumours tend to be solid, but microcysts are present

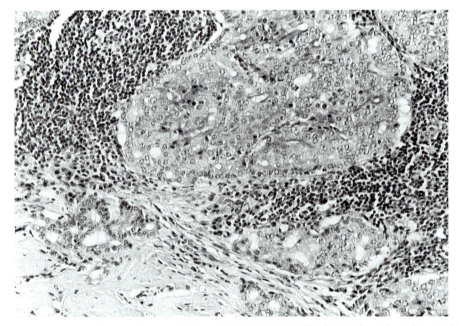

Figure 42.9 Mucoepidermoid carcinoma of intermediate-grade malignancy. The tumour consists mainly of intermediate cells mostly arranged in solid nests. The cells display moderate atypia and there are few mitoses. Note the inflammatory infiltrate, which can be pronounced even in a non-cystic mucoepidermoid carcinoma

grade tumours still have to be treated as high grade, thus diminishing the clinical value of a three-level histological grading. We therefore adhere to the two-level grading recommended by WHO.[1]

A study relating to the assessment of intraoral mucoepidermoid carcinomas was based on the presence or absence of the following five features: (1) cellular anaplasia, (2) four or more mitotic figures per ten high-power fields, (3) neural invasion, (4) necrosis and (5) an intracystic component of less than 20%. Use of these criteria gave a good estimate of prognosis. A similar study of parotid mucoepidermoid carcinomas also revealed correlation with clinical outcome.[14,15]

Table 42.1. Histological grading of mucoepidermoid carcinomas (modified from Batsakis and Luna[13])

Low-grade	Intermediate-grade	High-grade
Cells		
Differentiated mucous and epidermoid cells Minimal with intermediate cells	Intermediate cells dominate, with or without epidermoid differentiation	Few differentiated cells, <10% of cells are mucous cells
Little or no pleomorphism Rare (extremely) mitoses	Little to moderate pleomorphism Few mitoses	Pronounced pleomorphism Numerous mitoses
Structure		
Macro- and microcysts	No macrocysts, fewer microcysts, solid nests of cells	No macrocysts Predominantly solid, microcysts present
Invasion		
Broad-fronted, often circumscribed invasion	Usually well defined and uncircumscribed	Diffuse, soft tissue, perineural, intravascular

Immunohistochemistry

As a rule, mucoepidermoid carcinomas stain uniformly for keratins (both low- and high-molecular weight) and occasionally, focally, for vimentin. A co-expression of other intermediate filaments, desmin and glial fibrillary acidic protein (GFAP) is generally not a feature of mucoepidermoid carcinoma, although occasionally present. Involucrin, a marker for epithelial cell differentiation and usually absent in normal salivary gland tissue, has been demonstrated in the intermediate and epidermoid cells, but not the mucous cells, of mucoepidermoid carcinoma. The myoepithelial differentiation is minimal, as evidenced by the limited expression of S-100, GFAP, myosin and smooth muscle actin. Thus immunohistochemistry has limited value in the histological diagnosis of mucoepidermoid carcinomas, and at present it is useful neither in its recognition, nor in its subclassification.

Differential Diagnosis

If the sections taken from the surgical specimen show very few, or no, glandular elements, or show large squamous areas, the tumour may be mistaken for squamous cell carcinoma. Positive immunostaining with involucrin will not distinguish the tumour from other salivary gland neoplasms, nor would positivity for vitamin B12 R-binder, nor tenascin. Stains for mucin are probably the best support in the diagnosis of mucoepidermoid carcinoma in these cases. A cribriform pattern with basement membrane-like hyaline material surrounding sheets of tumour cells, which is found in adenoid cystic carcinoma, is lacking in mucoepidermoid carcinoma. Moreover, in the solid type of adenoid cystic carcinoma the cells are more atypical than are those of mucoepidermoid carcinomas with predominantly solid areas (intermediate cells). Adenosquamous carcinoma, a highly malignant tumour arising from mucous membrane or ducts of minor salivary glands, has histological features of both adenocarcinoma and squamous cell carcinoma, and it may constitute a difficult differential diagnosis to high-grade mucoepidermoid carcinoma. However, the glandular and squamous components of an adenosquamous carcinoma, although in close proximity, are still distinct, contrary to those of mucoepidermoid carcinoma, in which these structures are intimately admixed within individual glandular or cystic structures. Furthermore, intermediate cells are not a feature of adenosquamous carcinoma. Acinic cell carcinoma may have certain histological similarities to mucoepidermoid carcinoma. Acinic cell carcinoma usually has microcysts, clear cells and mucin-secreting cells, but no epidermoid cells, unlike mucoepidermoid carcinoma. Furthermore, the cells of an acinic cell carcinoma usually contain amylase, which is not the case with mucoepidermoid carcinoma. Rarely pleomorphic adenoma may mimic mucoepidermoid carcinoma. However, a careful search for the mesenchymal component and the myoepithelial proliferation of the former will allow separation of the two entities. Necrotising metaplasia constitutes another source of confusion. This may be distinguished by the preservation of normal lobular architecture of glandular tissue amongst the nests of hyperplastic epidermoid epithelium and an inflammatory reaction (see Chapter 40). Certain cystic lesions, e.g. intraoral mucoceles, ruptured retention cysts, mucinous cystadenoma and parotid cysts may cause diagnostic difficulty in regard to low-grade mucoepidermoid carcinoma. If the latter is present, invasion beneath the flattened cuboidal epithelium of the cyst will be discovered on examination of sections from multiple blocks. To distinguish mucoepidermoid carcinoma from a mucinous cystadenoma, the presence of layers of intermediate cells beneath the mucinous cells that are lining the cystic lesion are diagnostic of the former.

Macrocystic low-grade mucoepidermoid carcinoma is rarely present in minor salivary glands.

Fine Needle Aspiration

Mucoepidermoid carcinoma is difficult to diagnose by fine needle aspiration biopsy, but there are certain features that can be indicative of that neoplasm. Using three of these criteria together, e.g. intermediate cells, squamous cells and overlapping epithelial groups, the sensitivity and specificity of accurately diagnosing mucoepidermoid carcinoma were 97% and 100%, respectively.[16] It may thus be stated that mucoepidermoid carcinoma shows variation in cell type (many cells with abundant cytoplasm), regular nuclei with occasional nucleoli, and a dirty background of mucus and debris. It must be said, nevertheless, that mucoepidermoid carcinoma is one of the most difficult salivary gland lesions to diagnose correctly by fine needle aspiration.[17]

Therapy and Prognosis

Mucoepidermoid carcinoma is of low radiosensitivity, and therefore primary radical surgical removal is advocated. In high-grade cases, adjuvant therapy is required, and whether this should consist of radiotherapy and/or chemotherapy is not yet fully established. In cases of the intermediate- and high-grade types, local recurrences are likely and metastases to cervical lymph nodes and lungs may develop. Mucoepidermoid carcinomas of lower malignancy grade follow a clinical course not unlike that of a pleomorphic adenoma, i.e. slow growth, fairly frequent recurrences and a rare ability to metastasise.

Investigation of the DNA patterns (DNA ploidy, S-phase, etc.) as well as Ag-NOR count have been performed in order to improve the possibility of predicting the biological behaviour and prognosis. Certain results are promising but not yet definite enough to be put into routine use. Observations made from multivariate analyses indicate that the clinical stage at the time of diagnosis is the most important prognostic variable, however. The histological features have been shown also to be independent factors that bear on the patient outcome.[4] Tumour recurrences usually appear during the first postoperative year. Recurrence rates of 6, 20 and 78% for grades 1, 2 and 3, respectively, have been found. A high incidence of cervical lymph node, pulmonary and cerebral metastases has been shown in the higher grades.

Contrary to several other salivary gland neoplasms the survival rate of this neoplasm can be judged with good accuracy after only 5 years' observation and has been assessed at 70%[1] and 92%.[9,18] The 5-year determinate cure rates were 92, 83 and 27% for low-, intermediate- and high-grade tumours, respectively, and in another study, 5-year cumulative survival rates for the three grades were 92, 47.7 and 0%, respectively.[18] In the latter study cumulative survival rates for 5, 10 and 15 years were all 0% for high-grade mucoepidermoid carcinoma. It may be concluded that distant metastases and death are unlikely to occur in patients with grade 1 and 2 carcinomas, but in grade 3 neoplasms less than 50% 5-year survival can be expected.

Adenoid Cystic Carcinoma

Definition and Terminology

Adenoid cystic carcinoma is a distinctive type of adenocarcinoma showing a sieve-like pattern of small malignant cells. Billroth in the mid 19th century termed it cylindroma ("Zylindrome") and the modern name, adenoid cystic carcinoma, was adopted much later, although several synonyms are still in use, such as cribriform adenocarcinoma, cylindromatous carcinoma, adenocarcinoma of cylindromatous type, adenocystic carcinoma and cylindroma.

Site and Incidence

Most adenoid cystic carcinomas are found in the major salivary glands and upper respiratory tract minor salivary glands. They occasionally occur in many other sites, e.g. lacrimal gland, mandible, breast, oesophagus, vulva and cervix, external auditory meatus, Cowper's gland, skin, prostate and lung. Adenoid cystic carcinoma is recorded as comprising from 7 to 18% of parotid malignancies, and from 33 to 58% of minor salivary gland malignancies. It is the most common malignant tumour of the submandibular gland, constituting 12% of all submandibular gland tumours, and also the most common malignant minor salivary gland tumour of the entire upper respiratory tract. In the oral cavity the palate is the most common site. In the sublingual gland, an uncommon site for neoplasms, adenoid cystic carcinoma is third in frequency after mucoepidermoid carcinoma and pleomorphic adenoma.[10]

There is a slight preponderance in females, and the majority of adenoid cystic carcinomas occur between 40 and 70 years of age. Occurrence in children and teenagers is very uncommon, although palatal adenoid cystic carcinoma has been reported in a 9-year-old boy, and a sublingual gland adenoid cystic carcinoma in a 16-year-old female.

Histogenesis

The tumour is thought to be composed of modified myoepithelial and ductal cells These may arise by a change of intercalated duct reserve cells into ductal luminal and myoepithelial cells.[19] A number of adenoid cystic carcinomas have been characterised cytogenetically. It appears that t(6;9) is a non-random aberration in adenoid cystic carcinomas and may constitute the primary cytogenetic abnormality.[20] Adenoid cystic carcinoma may also occasionally arise in a pleomorphic adenoma. In cases of the exceedingly rare hybrid tumours of salivary glands, adenoid cystic carcinoma is often one of the two tumours (see Chapter 43).

Clinical Features

In about one-third of patients with parotid gland neoplasms, pain and "spontaneous" paralysis of the facial nerve occur. A palpable mass in the parotid region is the most common clinical presentation. The patient has usually been aware of the tumour for months or even years before seeking medical advice. It is generally a slowly growing cancer, and fixation to skin occurs late.

Microscopic Appearances

Adenoid cystic carcinoma is composed of two rather distinct cell types: flat, spindle-shape cells with scanty cytoplasm lining the pseudocysts and ductal or luminal cells with broader, eosinophilic cytoplasm. A prominent stroma is present consisting of mucopolysaccharides, collagen-like fibres and basal lamina components such as fibronectin, laminin, type IV collagen and glycosaminoglycans. The two cell types are arranged in three possible patterns.

1. Most common is the cribriform (glandular) type, created by many cysts and pseudocysts scattered in cell islands. The pseudocysts (pseudolumens) often dominate; they have the appearance of having been "punched out" of the cell islands (Fig. 42.10) and contain proteoglycans and basal lamina components, a material that is hyaluronidase sensitive, Alcian blue positive and weakly periodic acid–Schiff positive after diastase digestion. The true cysts, on the other hand, contain secretory material that is diastase resistant, periodic acid–Schiff positive and mucicarmine positive and are lined by duct-like cuboidal or occasionally columnar cells.

2. The second arrangement is the tubular type of adenoid cystic carcinoma in which duct-like cells are arranged in tubular structures surrounded by a hyaline stroma. Outside the duct-like cells there are one or several layers of the

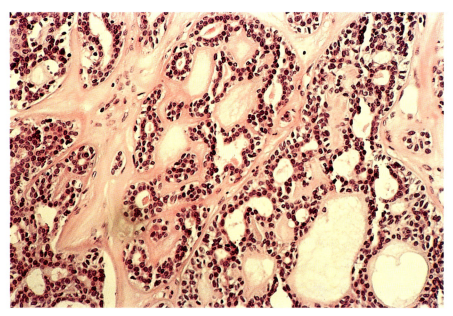

Figure 42.10 Typical cribriform pattern of a palatal adenoid cystic carcinoma

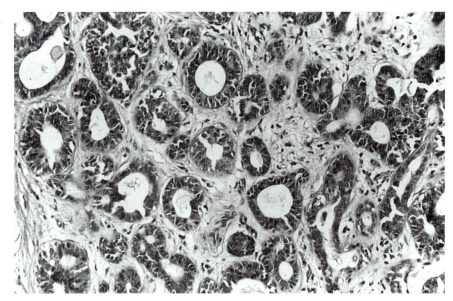

Figure 42.11 Adenoid cystic carcinoma with a predominantly tubular growth pattern. Many of the tubules have columnar cells forming ductal structures. Fewer myoepithelial type cells are present as compared with the cribriform pattern seen in Fig. 42.10

flat, spindle-shaped cells. The ductal structures often contain an eosinophilic material. Occasionally, not only the myoepithelial component, but also the ductal cells, tend to be hydropic and of clear cell appearance (Fig. 42.11). The tubules can occasionally be arranged longitudinally; the cells are sometimes arranged in a palisading pattern.

3. In the solid type there are few glandular structures or pseudocysts, and the cells are arranged in solid epithelial or epithelial/myoeithelial

nests of variable size. Between the islands of these often rather small cells there are strands of stroma. In cases showing solid growth only it is imperative to find areas with a cribriform or tubular pattern, otherwise the tumour might be classified differently, e.g. as malignant myoepithelioma. Most adenoid cystic carcinomas show a mixture of all three growth patterns. There may be areas of necrosis, sometimes of considerable size (Fig. 42.12). In all three types of adenoid cystic carcinoma, mitoses are scarce.

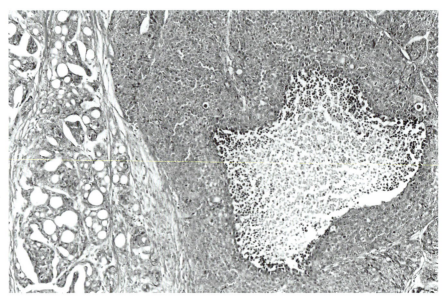

Figure 42.12 An adenoid cystic carcinoma showing predominantly solid pattern on the right with necrosis. On the left a mixed cribriform and tubular pattern is seen

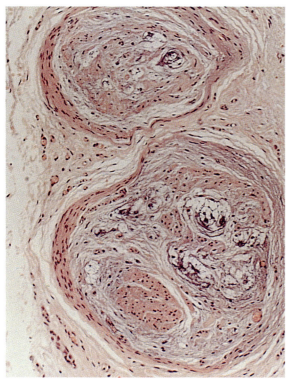

Figure 42.13 Intraneural growth of adenoid cystic carcinoma in two nerves

Neural invasion (both peri- and intraneural) is frequently observed (Fig. 42.13) and vascular invasion may also be present.

Immunohistochemistry

The two cell types present in adenoid cystic carcinoma may each show characteristic immunohistochemical profiles. The myoepithelial cells, but not the ductal cells, have been shown to be positive for certain proteoglycans such as chondroitin 6 sulphate and heparin sulphate, and positive for cytokeratins, S-100 and smooth muscle actin. The ductal cells also express several cytokeratins, including low molecular weight cytokeratins, and a variable degree of positive staining for epithelial membrane antigen (EMA), carcinoembryonic antigen and S-100 protein. Laminin, a glycoprotein that is the main constituent of basement membrane and a marker for this structure, and EMA, a marker of luminal surfaces of ducts and of glandular differentiation,[19,21] have confirmed the dual cellular patterns of adenoid cystic carcinoma. These features can occasionally be useful to differentiate the neoplasm from other adenocarcinomas. Adenoid cystic carcinoma may express c-erbB-2 and c-erbB-3 gene products, but not epidermal growth factor-R (EGF-R), a feature not shared by many salivary malignancies.

Differential Diagnosis

Many tumours may produce a cribriform growth pattern or may be composed of rather small, myo-epithelial-like cells. The differential diagnosis of adenoid cystic carcinoma may thus include adenoid and basaloid types of squamous cell carcinoma, pleomorphic adenoma, mucoepidermoid carcinoma, malignant myoepithelioma, salivary duct carcinoma and small cell neuroendocrine carcinoma. However, the most important differential diagnosis is that of polymorphous low-grade adenocarcinoma (PLGA, see below). Adenoid cystic carcinoma has a higher Ki-67 index than has PLGA,[22] and also usually a strong positivity for bcl-2. The solid type of adenoid cystic carcinoma should, moreover, be distinguished from basal cell adenocarcinoma, which is of low-grade malignancy.

Fine Needle Aspiration

The most typical features of a fine needle aspirate from adenoid cystic carcinoma are those of uniform, tightly cohesive cells with little pleomorphism, but which may show slightly hyperchromatic nuclei and prominent nucleoli, surrounding amorphous, hyaline globular structures. The cells tend to be round to ovoid with a basophilic cytoplasm. The aspirates are usually quite cellular, and a cribriform arrangement of the cells is often a striking feature.[17]

Treatment and Prognosis

Several morphological parameters have been studied in estimating the prognosis of adenoid cystic carcinoma, including grade of differentiation, histological subtype, presence of tumour in the resection margin, and percentage of area occupied by matrix-containing pseudolumens. A correlation between the extent of the solid component and patient outcome has been reported in a large number of studies. New prognostic criteria include flow cytometric DNA investigations and Ag-NOR counts. The potential role of DNA ploidy in the prediction of prognosis in patients with adenoid cystic carcinoma has been studied by several investigators, but there is considerable disparity of results with aneuploid rates ranging from 0 to 45%, and in some series an inability to correlate the presence of aneuploidy with adverse pathological factors or outcome.

With regard to the Ag-NOR method, normal salivary tissue gives low counts, benign salivary gland tumours have slightly higher counts, and adenoid cystic carcinoma considerably higher counts. It must be stressed, however, that there is a lack of reproducibility of the Ag-NOR method when performed in different laboratories in this as in other areas of tumour pathology. Apoptosis has a major influence on tumour growth and is in part regulated by the bcl-2 proto-oncogene. The expression of bcl-2 protein varies among salivary gland tumours but several adenoid cystic carcinomas show a strong immunopositivity for the bcl-2 protein. Recent studies have shown that reduced expression of E-cadherin in adenoid cystic carcinomas correlates with unfavourable prognosis,[23] whilst expression of oncoprotein p53 appears to be unrelated to prognosis. Single type of p53 point mutation (exons 5 and 6) has been demonstrated in recurrent adenoid cystic carcinomas, and adenoid cystic carcinomas show a relatively high incidence of loss of heterozygosity at the p53 gene, and also at the retinoblastoma gene, but no K-ras mutations at sites suspected of harbouring recessive oncogenes (see Chapter 43).

Adenoid cystic carcinoma is relatively slow-growing, has a high recurrence rate, is markedly infiltrative and has a pronounced tendency to grow along nerves. The prognosis is poor and in the early 1970s the probability of death from adenoid cystic carcinoma of the major salivary glands was considered to be 24% at 5 years and 43% after 15 years. The histological grading does not seem to play as important a prognostic role as the clinical staging, anatomical site and surgical management. The clinical stage probably has greater prognostic significance than grade in adenoid cystic carcinoma. Since adenoid cystic carcinomas have such a dismal long-term prognosis, the 15-year, and even the 20-year survival rate should be taken into account. Radiotherapy for adenoid cystic carcinoma of the head and neck gives little or no prognostic improvement but a combination of postoperative radiotherapy and hyperthermia has had promising results.

Epithelial-Myoepithelial Carcinoma

Definition and Terminology

The tumour consists of two cell types, ductal cells and clear myoepithelial cells. The tumour has been described under a variety of names including glycogen-rich adenocarcinoma and clear cell carcinoma. The term epithelial-myoepithelial carcinoma was first used in 1972.[24]

Site and Incidence

Epithelial-myoepithelial carcinoma arises predominantly in the parotid gland and has a slight female predominance. The submandibular gland is the second commonest site. Epithelial-myoepithelial carcinomas may, however, be encountered anywhere in the upper respiratory tract, and cases have been reported from the oral cavity as well as in the trachea, nose and paranasal sinuses. Epithelial-myoepithelial carcinoma constitutes approximately 0.5% of all salivary gland tumours, and has a peak incidence in later life, during the 6th, 7th and 8th decades.[1,5,10,24,25]

Histogenesis

Ultrastructural studies have substantiated the conclusion that the intercalated duct cell is the precursor of both cellular elements of epithelial-myoepithelial carcinoma.[23] Primitive myoepithelial cells contain large amounts of glycogen and basally orientated filamentous processes, and transformation of clear cells to myoepithelial cells with several transitional cell types has been observed.

Clinical Features

The commonest symptom is a painless mass in the parotid region, which has been present over a period of several months or years. Although neural invasion is common, facial paralysis and/or pain occur only occasionally.[25]

Gross Appearances

Most epithelial-myoepithelial carcinomas are solitary and multilobulated. They tend to be firm and show a whitish cut surface. The are usually well circumscribed but the capsule is frequently incomplete and small tumour nodules can be seen to extend through it.

Microscopic Appearances

Epithelial-myoepithelial carcinoma is composed of well-defined tubules of varying size, separated by various amounts of fibrous tissue. Two layers of cells line the tubules. The inner cell layer is composed of columnar cells, with a central or basal nucleus and eosinophilic cytoplasm. The outer layer, which may be of multiple rows, consists of polyhedral cells with clear cytoplasm overlying an external basement membrane (Fig. 42.14). The outer, myoepithelial clear cells stain positively with S-100, whilst the inner duct cells stain positively with several cyto-keratin antibodies. Collagenous tissue is often scarce in epithelial-myoepithelial carcinoma, consisting usually of the basement membrane only. Necrosis is often present. In some cases tubules are not well pre-served and are replaced by hyalinised stroma; the

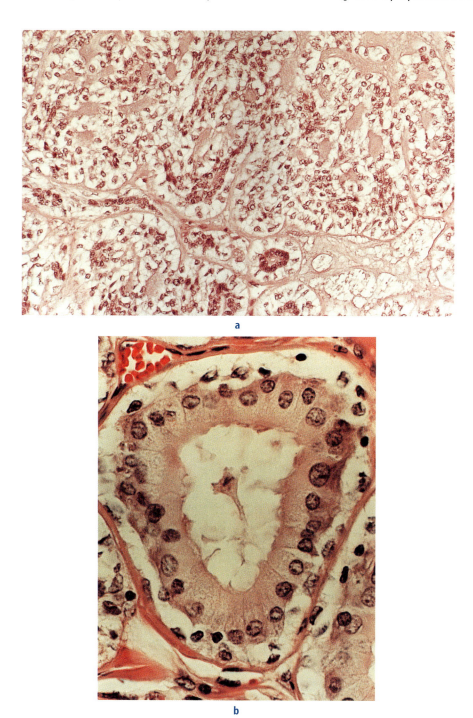

a

b

Figure 42.14 a Typical epithelial-myoepithelial carcinoma. In some areas the tubules are well separated, in others they form more solid masses. b Higher magnifi-cation of a well-developed and preserved tubule. Columnar cells with finely granular eosinophilic cytoplasm and round nuclei constitute the inner layer, and cells with clear cytoplasm the outer. The whole tubule is surrounded by a basement membrane

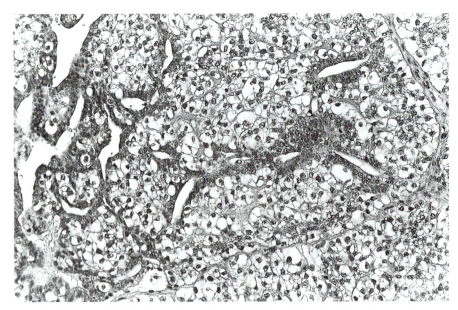

Figure 42.15 Epithelial-myoepithelial carcinoma mainly consisting of solid sheets of clear cells with some ducts, and almost no stroma

tumour showing in these cases proliferation of clear cells predominantly in solid sheets or trabeculae. In a few lesions there is an abundance of non-hyalinised stroma, and the proliferating clear cells are arranged in nodules, with few tubules (Fig. 42.15). In rare cases there are areas with pronounced hypertrophy of the ductal component with very little clear cell proliferation. Nuclear atypia are seen in the clear cells. The infiltration into adjacent tissue is usually that of nodular ingrowth but a diffuse infiltration may also occur.

Differential Diagnosis

In its classic form epithelial-myoepithelial carcinoma should not be confused with any other tumour. When the tumour is less well differentiated and typical tubules are difficult to find, it may mimic several other salivary gland tumours, including acinic cell carcinoma and other malignant neoplasms with clear cell components, especially carcinoma in pleomorphic adenoma and malignant myoepithelioma. Clear cell adenomas do not have a biphasic pattern and do not show infiltration. The clear cells of an acinic cell carcinoma are usually periodic acid–Schiff positive after appropriate digestion with diastase, and most acinic cell carcinomas are immunopositive to antibodies against amylase. In carcinoma arising from pleomorphic adenoma and malignant myoepithelioma, the stromal and epithelial complexity of these latter tumours is evident. Epithelial-myoep-

ithelial carcinoma differs from adenoid cystic carcinoma in not possessing hyaline material within oval or round spaces. Epithelial-myoepithelial carcinoma may occur as one of the two tumour entities in salivary hybrid tumours, but is exceedingly rare (see Chapter 43).

Therapy and Prognosis

Epithelial-myoepithelial carcinoma has hitherto been considered to be of low-grade malignancy. Mitoses are rare and cytological features are often bland. Perineural and vascular invasion may be present and recurrence and metastasis are not uncommon. In fact, recurrence rate is relatively high, being approximately 40% and a high metastatic rate has been reported.[25] Epithelial-myoepithelial carcinoma should be regarded as a neoplasm of intermediate-grade malignancy. The treatment should, therefore, consist not only of radical surgery, but also adjuvant therapy.

Salivary Duct Carcinoma

Definition and Terminology

This tumour of high-grade malignancy has a close morphological similarity to ductal breast carcinoma. It was described in 1968[26] and gained wider recognition first in the 1980s.

Site and Incidence

Salivary duct carcinoma is mainly a parotid tumour, but has also been described in the submandibular gland and in minor salivary glands. It is primarily a tumour of elderly men (male to female ratio 4–5:1), many cases occurring in the sixth and seventh decades. It has been regarded as being extremely rare but several recent reports indicate that it may not be so uncommon as previously thought. Salivary duct carcinoma may also arise in pleomorphic adenoma, and as part of hybrid salivary carcinoma. The latter is very rare but a palatal hybrid tumour consisting of adenoid cystic carcinoma and salivary duct carcinoma has been described (see Chapter 43).

Histogenesis

Salivary duct carcinoma is believed to arise from excretory ducts. In general, carcinomas arising from the intercalated duct portion of the salivary duct unit are biologically of low-grade malignancy (e.g. acinic cell carcinoma and polymorphous low-grade adenocarcinoma) while those originating from the excretory ducts are of high-grade malignancy.

Clinical Features

Pain is often associated with the presence of a parotid mass and also facial paresis. The patients most often only give a short history of a growing mass in the parotid region. Involvement of neck nodes already at the first presentation is not rare. Furthermore, histological examination of the parotidectomy specimen may reveal spread to intra- and periglandular lymph nodes. Salivary duct carcinoma thus is characterised by a rapid onset and rapid progression of disease.

Gross Appearances

Parotid tumours present as a white, firm mass, often larger than 3 cm, which may be partly circumscribed, or multifocal (Fig. 42.16).

Microscopic Appearances

Salivary duct carcinoma has a close morphological similarity to invasive ductal breast carcinoma. It is characterised by pleomorphic cells that form aggregates resembling distended ducts and solid nests and displaying combinations of solid, cribriform, papillary and comedo patterns, embedded in a desmoplastic, often hyaline, stroma (Fig. 42.17). Comedonecrosis is invariably present (Fig. 42.18). The cribriform and in situ-like formations are similar to those seen in some breast lesions. Ductal carcinoma in situ extending within the lobules of the parotid gland (cancerisation of lobules) is often present. A papillary growth pattern may predomi-

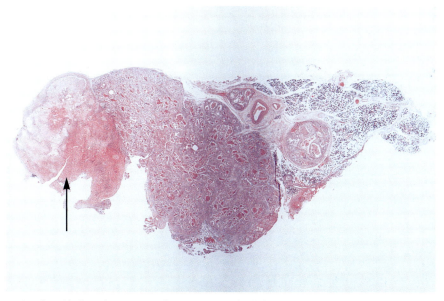

Figure 42.16 Macrosection of parotid salivary duct carcinoma. The tumour measured well above 3 cm, and a remnant of parotid gland tissue is seen to the right. Note that the bulk of the tumour is composed of ducts with eosinophilic comedonecrosis. There is an area of necrosis to the left (*arrow*). The tumour is multifocal with two smaller nodules, which are seen to the right of the main mass

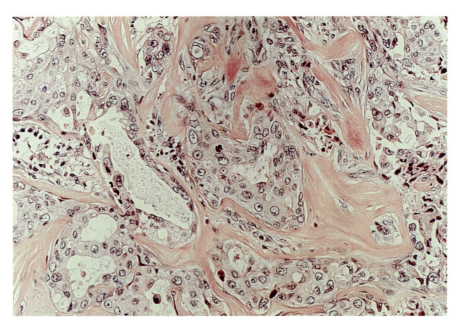

Figure 42.17 Salivary duct carcinoma with highly atypical cells showing numerous mitotic figures, comprising the ducts. Note the markedly hyalinised stroma

nate in some areas. The tumour cells are usually relatively large, polygonal and with an eosinophilic cytoplasm. The cell borders are well defined and the nuclei tend to be vesicular, some with prominent nucleoli. Mitotic activity is usually moderate to high,

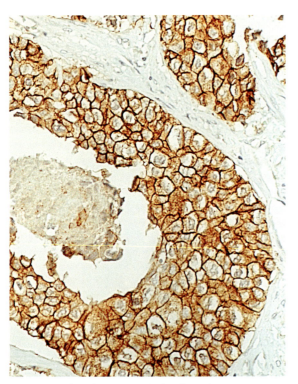

Figure 42.18 Salivary duct carcinoma displayed by C-erbB-2 immunostaining showing the positive membrane accentuation. Also note comedonecrosis

more than one mitotic figure per high-power field being present in some areas. In other areas the nuclei are more dark-staining with condensed chromatin. The invasive component is usually solid or microglandular and characteristically surrounded by desmoplastic stroma, as found with invasive mammary ductal carcinoma. Dense hyalinisation of the stroma is seen in most cases. Perineural invasion is common. On rare occasions one may see clear-cut evidence of previous or coexistent pleomorphic adenoma, most often as a separate sclerotic nodule.

Immunohistochemistry

Salivary duct carcinoma often shows overexpression of c-erbB-2 oncoprotein, as detected by membrane accentuation in immunocytochemical staining. Overexpression of c-erbB-2 is found rarely in other salivary gland carcinomas.[27,28] Salivary duct carcinoma also often expresses androgen receptor, gross cystic disease fluid protein (GCDFP-15) and CD44. Nevertheless, this immunophenotype does not completely exclude metastasis from breast carcinoma.[29] It is usually, but not always, negative for oestrogen and progesterone receptors.

Differential Diagnosis

Great care should be taken not to misdiagnose a metastatic breast carcinoma as salivary duct carcinoma. Other salivary carcinomas that may have necrosis, e.g. acinic cell carcinoma, epithelial-myoepithelial carcinoma, and a high-grade muco-epidermoid carcinoma may cause diagnostic problems. However, the presence in the same tumour of combinations of the different growth patterns described above, the comedonecrosis, and the desmoplastic stroma, are unique for salivary duct carcinoma, and not found in any other salivary gland neoplasm.

Therapy and Prognosis

Total parotidectomy followed by radiotherapy appears to be the treatment of choice, but few successes are reported in the literature. Ipsilateral neck dissection, adjuvant chemotherapy, and/or endocrine therapy similar to the treatment regime for ductal breast carcinomas could possibly benefit these patients. Local recurrence lymph node and distant metastasis are frequent. Many of the patients unfortunately die within the first 3–4 years after surgical treatment, giving this tumour the most dismal short-term prognosis of all salivary gland neoplasms.[30] There are, however, indications that salivary duct carcinoma may exist in a low-grade variant with a distinctive histology with predominant intraductal growth pattern. This tumour thus exhibits differentiation towards an intercalated duct-like cell phenotype, but its relationship to high-grade salivary duct carcinoma needs to be explored further.[31]

Polymorphous Low-Grade Adenocarcinoma

Definition and Terminology

Polymorphous low-grade adenocarcinoma (PLGA) is a tumour of low-grade malignancy characterised by bland cytological features and great diversity (polymorphous) of growth patterns. The morphology of PLGA was first described under that name in 1984,[32] but it had earlier been reported as lobular carcinoma and terminal duct carcinoma.

Site and Incidence

Although reported more frequently in recent years, there are relatively few cases of PLGA reported in the literature. A large study of intraoral minor salivary gland tumours revealed that PLGA accounts for one-quarter of all malignant salivary oral tumours, and that it is the second most common malignant salivary gland tumour of the oral cavity (mucoepidermoid carcinoma being the most common).[5] Polymorphous low-grade adenocarcinoma is essentially a neoplasm of minor salivary glands, but occurs sometimes in major salivary glands, de novo, or in association with carcinoma arising in pleomorphic adenoma. PLGA primarily develops in patients in their sixth and seventh decade and displays a female predilection (female/male ratio is approximately 2:1). The commonest site of origin is the palate, particularly the hard palate, and the buccal region is the second most common site, followed by the lips.[5,10] Outside the oral cavity PLGA has been reported in the sinonasal tract, nasopharynx and the lacrimal gland.

Histogenesis

Polymorphous low-grade adenocarcinoma is believed to arise from the intercalated duct portion of the salivary duct unit. Ultrastructural as well as immunocytochemical studies have shown evidence of derivation from both myoepithelial and ductal cells, thus supporting a multicellular concept of histogenesis. A recent study of 30 cases of PLGA indicates that it may originate from cells located at the acinar-intercalated duct junction.[33]

Clinical Features

Polymorphous low-grade adenocarcinoma is described as an indolent tumour, which is locally invasive and persistent, but rarely metastasises. It usually presents as a painless, rather small swelling, which may be associated with bleeding.

Gross Appearances

Polymorphous low-grade adenocarcinoma is usually well circumscribed, often 1–2 cm in size, but sometimes as large as 5–6 cm. The overlying mucosa is in most cases intact and not ulcerated.

Microscopic Appearances

The tumour is usually unencapsulated and shows invasion, which most often presents a single-file pattern. The most striking histological feature of PLGA is the variety of morphologic configurations within any one tumour and its bland cytological features. There are several distinct microscopic patterns, which may be found if sufficient blocks are taken from the tumour. These patterns include cribriform growth pattern, which may have duct-like structures either as tubules or forming trabeculae, mimicking adenoid cystic carcinoma. A lobular arrangement and with a tendency to palisading of cells can be present. The tumour cells can be arranged in solid nests resembling the solid type of adenoid cystic carcinoma. Papillary and cystic areas are usually prominent and often display oncocytic metaplasia, and sometimes mucinous or clear cell metaplasia. Intratubular calcification may occasionally be present. In yet other cases the papillary pattern is very scarce or absent, and these cases have been described as the non-papillary subtype of PLGA.[34] Necrosis is rare in all variants of PLGA. The stroma may be hyalinised in certain areas whilst mucinous change and haemorrhage can be seen in other parts of the tumour. The tumour cells are characteristically pale round to oval, and regular. The nuclei are often vesicular, and mitoses as well as prominent nucleoli are rare. The cytological features resemble those of a benign tumour rather than a malignant neoplasm (Figs 42.19–42.21).

Differential Diagnosis

The main difficulty in differential diagnosis arises in the palatal tumours. The histological features can be very similar to those of adenoid cystic carcinoma, and several blocks are often needed to identify the architectural polymorphism of PLGA. As in adenoid cystic carcinoma, perineural invasion is commonly seen. Perineural invasion thus does not distinguish adenoid cystic carcinoma from PLGA. If a small excisional biopsy or frozen section only is available, the differentiation may become impossible. Immunostaining with Ki-67 may help in differentiating these difficult cases, as PLGA tends to have a considerably lower proliferation index than adenoid cystic carcinoma.[22] Immunopositivity for bcl-2 is usually much more pronounced in adenoid cystic carcinoma than it is in PLGA. Papillary cystadenoma may constitute another differential diagnosis; this tumour, however, does not have the diversity of growth patterns that PLGA has. Metastatic papillary thyroid carcinoma may be confused with PLGA, because of cellular similarities of the two, both showing vesicular nuclei and a papillary growth pattern. Immunostaining for thyroglobulin, the location of the lesion, and careful examination of the thyroid gland will all be of substantial help in these cases. Occasionally PLGA may be confused histologically with cellular pleomorphic adenoma. Immunostaining for GFAP, often positive in pleomorphic adenoma, but not in PLGA, may help in the differential diagnosis. Also carcinoma in pleomorphic adenoma may show a great variation in growth patterns, mimicking PLGA. However, the cellular atypia and mitoses exclude it as a realistic alternative.

Therapy and Prognosis

Treatment of choice is essentially by radical surgery. The value of adjuvant radiotherapy has yet to be

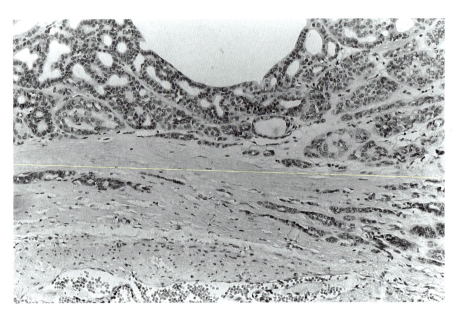

Figure 42.19 Polymorphous low-grade adenocarcinoma. Tubules and duct-like formations, as well as a cyst, are seen. The typical pattern of invasion with files a single or a few cells wide is seen below the main mass

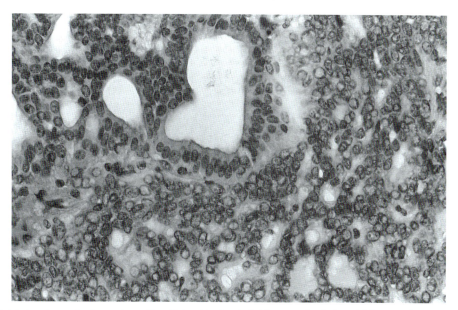

Figure 42.20 Polymorphous low-grade adenocarcinoma. The cells show bland cytological features and vesicular nuclei. No, or very few, mitotic figures are present

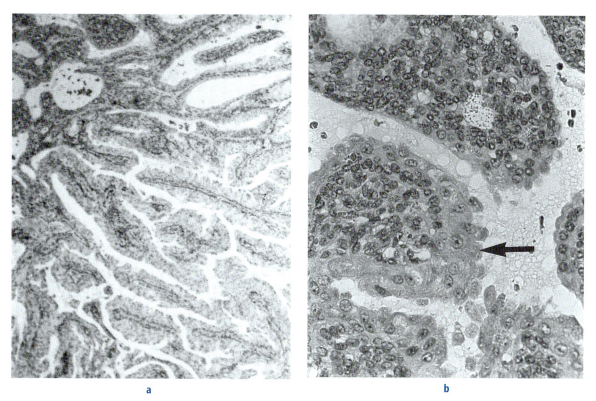

| a | b |

Figure 42.21 Polymorphous low-grade adenocarcinoma. **a** Pronounced papillary structure and **b** focal oncocytic metaplasia on the surface of the papillary structure, staining in an eosinophilic fashion in the original (arrow)

demonstrated. The local recurrence rate is approximately 25%. Spread to regional lymph nodes is unusual. Distant metastasis is rare, but has been reported.[10] Long-term studies are needed to ascertain that PLGA does not mimic the slow but relentless course of adenoid cystic carcinoma. Some indeed regard this tumour as a low-grade malignant variant of adenoid cystic carcinoma.

Basal Cell Adenocarcinoma

Definition and Terminology

Basal cell adenocarcinoma is defined as a neoplasm with similar cytological features to those seen in basal cell adenoma but with definite signs of a malignant growth pattern. Four morphological subtypes, comparable with those of basal cell adenoma, can be recognised: solid, tubular, trabecular and membraneous (see Chapter 41). The term basal cell adenocarcinoma seems to have been established as recently as 1990[35] and is now widely accepted, both as regards being a separate tumour entity and as regards its terminology.[1]

Site and Incidence

Basal cell adenocarcinoma is predominantly a parotid tumour, and is rare. It is found to occur predominantly in the sixth and seventh decades, without any sex preference. The Armed Forces Institute of Pathology (AFIP) Registry of 13,749 salivary tumours comprised only 43 basal cell adenocarcinomas. Thirty-nine of those were in the parotid; the remaining four were located in the submandibular gland.[10] Basal cell adenocarcinoma was previously almost exclusively reported from the major salivary glands. A few tumours located in the oral mucosa have been described, and the first series of basal cell adenocarcinoma of minor salivary glands and seromucinous glands of the head and neck region has now been published.[25] The latter study reported 12 cases of basal cell adenocarcinoma from a Portugese series of 1108 salivary gland neoplasms. Another important review of this topic in the same year has concluded that 16% of the 85 cases found in the literature up to that date were of minor salivary gland origin.[36] Since then, some further case reports and series have been published. Basal cell adenocarcinoma is thus not as exceptionally rare as first believed, comprising as it does 2–3% of all salivary gland malignancies, and it has a significant incidence in the minor salivary glands.

Histogenesis

It is generally assumed that the vast majority of basal cell adenocarcinomas arise de novo. Occasionally basal cell adenocarcinoma may arise from pre-existing basal cell adenoma, particularly the membranous type, or the dermal analogue tumour. Basal cell adenocarcinoma of the major salivary glands is also known to occur synchronously with cutaneous tumours (eccrine cylindroma, trichoepithelioma or eccrine spiradenoma).

Clinical Features

Basal cell adenocarcinoma usually presents as a slowly enlarging, asymptomatic parotid mass of several months' duration. Facial nerve involvement is not common.

Gross Appearances

The tumours are often cystic, usually 2–3 cm large, and often contain fluid. The fluid tends to be brownish, not infrequently haemorrhagic, and occasionally mucoid in consistency.

Microscopic Appearances

The predominating overall architectural pattern is mainly lobular, most often with a palisaded appearance at the periphery of the tumour nests. The tumour aggregates can be solid, or showing a tubular pattern (Figs 42.22, 42.23). In the solid tumour nests there may be small glandular lumina with secretory content. The tubular pattern with irregular double-layered structures may mimic epithelial myoepithelial carcinoma. A mixture of trabecular arrangement and membranous organisation is usually found in smaller areas of the tumours. In all types of basal cell adenocarcinoma there are two distinctive cell populations. The most common cell is small and basaloid with sparse cytoplasm, and with nuclei having a dense chromatin pattern. The other cell is larger, has a clear, slightly eosinophilic cytoplasm but a similar nucleus to that of the basaloid cell. Comedo-like necrosis is frequent (Fig. 42.23) and focal squamous metaplasia can be seen in as many as 25% of cases.[25]

Differential Diagnosis

The palisading pattern of basal cell adenocarcinoma distinguishes it from a solid adenoid cystic carcinoma. Basal cell adenoma shows no invasive features as does basal cell adenocarcinoma. Small cell carcinomas of salivary glands also constitute a differential diagnosis. There are two types of small cell carcinoma, one being neuroendocrine in derivation and one not (see below). The latter type exhibits bicellular composition of dark cells and clear, larger cells, and thus has several features in common with

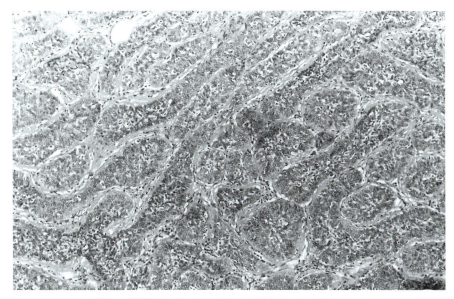

Figure 42.22 Basal cell adenocarcinoma with lobular and tubular pattern

basal cell adenocarcinoma. Basal cell adenocarcinomas are negative for neuroendocrine markers but show immunoreactivity cytokeratins, smooth muscle actin and S-100, i.e. an immunoprofile compatible with myoepithelial phenotype. Basaloid

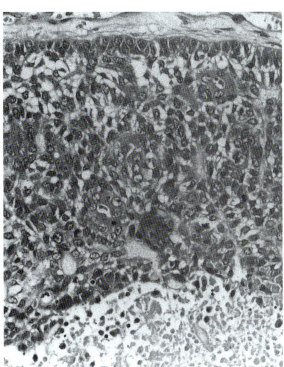

Figure 42.23 Higher magnification of basal cell adenocarcinoma showing peripheral palisading and necrosis

squamous cell carcinoma is yet another differential diagnosis; however, this tumour shows attachment to the overlying epithelium.

Therapy and Prognosis

Basal cell adenocarcinoma is a tumour of low-grade malignancy, although having a relatively high recurrence rate. Regional lymph node and distant metastasis are rare, and therefore local excision with free margins is the treatment of choice.

Papillary and Mucinous Cystadenocarcinoma

Definition and Terminology

These tumours of low-grade malignancy are morphologically characterised by their cystic nature. The papillary cystadenocarcinoma shows endocystic projections, whilst the mucinous cystadenocarcinoma have abundant mucus production. The mucinous type tends to have less pronounced cysts, and are often only called mucinous adenocarcinoma. Although papillary and mucinous cystadenocarcinoma were not recognised as separate entities before the 2nd edition of the WHO Classification,[1] tumours displaying those features were described and reported earlier.

Site and Incidence

Because it has been recognised only recently as a separate tumour entity, it is difficult to assess its incidence and predominant site of location. Papillary cystadenocarcinoma is thought to occur more frequently in the minor salivary glands. However, of the 23 cases of cystadenocarcinoma (both papillary and mucinous) diagnosed at the AFIP between 1978 and 1988, 12 were parotid tumours, four submandibular, one sublingual; the remaining six were found in minor salivary glands of the palate, gums and lips.[10] In a more recent and larger series of 57 salivary gland cystadenocarcinomas, 65% occurred in the major salivary glands and 35% in minor salivary glands.[37] Papillary cystadenocarcinoma is more common than mucinous cystadenocarcinoma.

Clinical Features

Cystadenocarcinomas are slowly growing unencapsulated tumours that present as painless swellings. Men and women are affected equally.

Microscopic Appearances

The papillary cystadenocarcinoma is defined by cysts and endocystic papillary projections. Papillary cystadenocarcinoma shows these two features only, unlike papillary salivary gland neoplasms, which have additional features (e.g. PLGA and mucoepidermoid carcinoma). Papillary cystadenocarcinoma is composed of cystic spaces into which papillae project. The papillae are lined with cuboidal or columnar epithelium (Fig. 42.24). Mucinous cystadenocarcinoma is defined as a tumour with abundant mucus production, and cuboidal or columnar cells line the cysts, which are partly or completely filled with mucus (Fig. 42.25). In mucinous cystadenocarcinoma epidermoid or intermediate cells are not present (as in mucoepidermoid carcinoma), and the mucus should occupy over 50% of the tumour.[1] The lesions are thus characterised by one or several cysts, and infiltrative growth in the adjacent cyst wall. In papillary cystadenocarcinomas the cystic spaces are filled with papillae with rather narrow, fibrous cores, which are lined with cuboidal, or low columnar cells, displaying nuclear pleomorphism and some few mitoses. Occasionally interspersed mucus secreting cells can be found. The papillary growths in the cyst lumina may sometimes be extensive with a rather pronounced complexity. In other cases the cyst-lining epithelium shows cribriform areas or "Roman arc" formations. Psammona bodies, vascular and perineural invasion are occasionally present. The distinction from a papillary cystadenoma is made by the infiltrative growth, nuclear atypia and mitoses.

Therapy and Prognosis

Cystadenocarcinomas should be regarded as of low-grade malignancy, and it would therefore seem

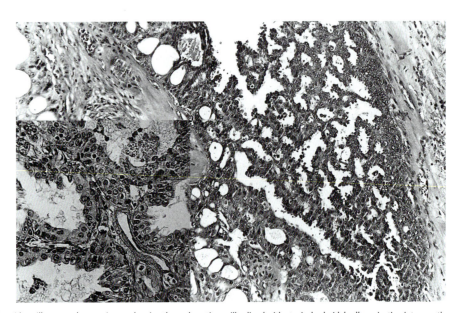

Figure 42.24 Parotid papillary cystadenocarcinoma showing the endocystic papillae lined with atypical cuboidal cells projecting into a cystic space. Insert: higher power showing the lining cells of the papillae

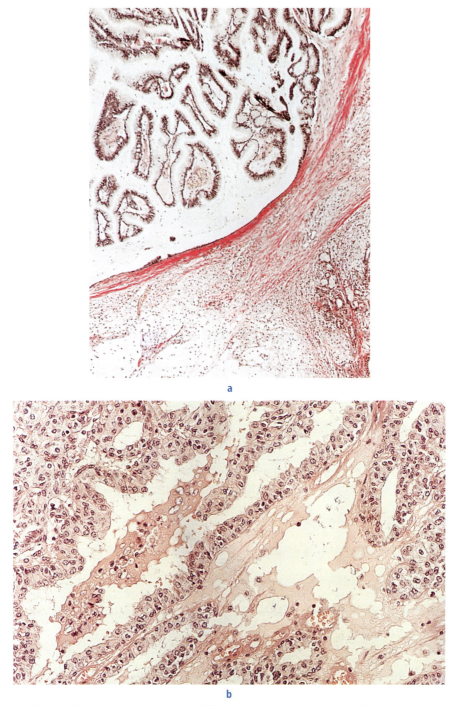

Figure 42.25 a Mucinous cystadenocarcinoma. **b** Higher power showing glandular spaces with excessive mucin

appropriate to apply similar treatment strategies to those of other low-grade salivary gland neoplasms. Recent reports, however, indicate that cystadenocarcinomas may have an indolent biological behaviour and exhibit a wider morphological spectrum than that described in the latest WHO classification.[37]

Carcinoma in Pleomorphic Adenoma

The concept of malignancy in pleomorphic adenoma is more complex than appears at first sight. Carcinoma in pleomorphic adenoma constitutes 3–4% of all salivary tumours and 10–12% of all salivary malignancies. The frequency of malignancy developing in pleomorphic adenoma has been assessed at between 2 and 10%.[38] The risk of malignant transformation increases the longer the tumour has been present. Pleomorphic adenoma, particularly those of minor salivary glands, can display hypercellularity, cellular atypia and necrosis. The diagnosis of malignancy in carcinoma in pleomorphic adenoma rests primarily on evidence of infiltration into surrounding tissue, and to a lesser extent on capsular invasion, increased number of, and atypical, mitoses, and vascular involvement. Evidence of remaining pleomorphic adenoma should be present.

There are three different types of malignancies that may arise. The overwhelming majority of cases are carcinomas. Most of these are rather poorly differentiated ductal carcinomas (Fig. 42.26), but several other types of carcinomas may arise (e.g. mucoepidermoid carcinoma, salivary duct carcinoma, adenoid cystic carcinoma and squamous cell carcinoma). It is likely that several of the tumours previously reported as carcinomas in pleomorphic adenomas are in fact myoepithelial carcinomas (see below). True carcinosarcoma is the second commonest malignancy arising in pleomorphic adenomas, and displays a morphology similar to that found in carcinosarcomas elsewhere in the body. The third type, the so-called metastasising pleomorphic adenoma, is a pathological oddity. It remains histologically "benign" at the primary site, as well as in local recurrences and distant metastases. It tends to metastasise rather widely to distant sites, and has typically a very long time interval (several decades) between primary tumour and metastases. In spite of its histology it may kill the patient.

Malignant Myoepithelioma

Definition and Terminology

Malignant myoepithelioma, or myoepithelial carcinoma, is defined as a malignant epithelial tumour composed of atypical myoepithelial cells. Malignant myoepitheliomas are distinguished from myoepitheliomas by their infiltrative, destructive and aggressive growth. The cells display increased mitotic activity and cytological pleomorphism.[1]

Site and Incidence

Malignant myoepithelioma is now considered to be very rare, most tumours occurring in the parotid gland in elderly patients.

Clinical Features

Malignant myoepitheliomas are characterised by an aggressive local growth rather than distant metastases. They appear to arise in two different clinical settings: either de novo or in a recurrent pleomorphic adenoma.[39]

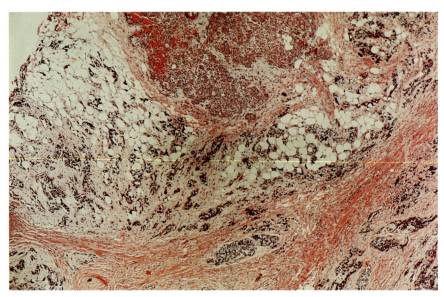

Figure 42.26 Poorly differentiated adenocarcinoma ex pleomorphic adenoma. Remnant of the pleomorphic adenoma is seen in the upper central part. The carcinoma is infiltrating connective tissue

Microscopic Appearances

The neoplastic cells show a wide morphological variety. They are spindle-shaped admixed with round and stellate cells. Many cells show epithelioid features, often with a clear cytoplasm. Others are plasmacytoid cells with eccentric nuclei and abundant eosinophilic cytoplasm. Most tumours are myxoid to a variable extent, and necrosis is relatively common. Squamous metaplasia is occasionally present. The cellular atypia is variable, and so is the number of mitotic figures. Infiltrative growth is thus imperative for the diagnosis of malignant myoepithelioma, as some of these tumours have bland cytological appearance and few mitoses (Fig. 42.27).

Several cases of monomorphic clear cell carcinomas of the salivary glands have appeared to be clear cell variants of malignant myoepithelioma.[40] These

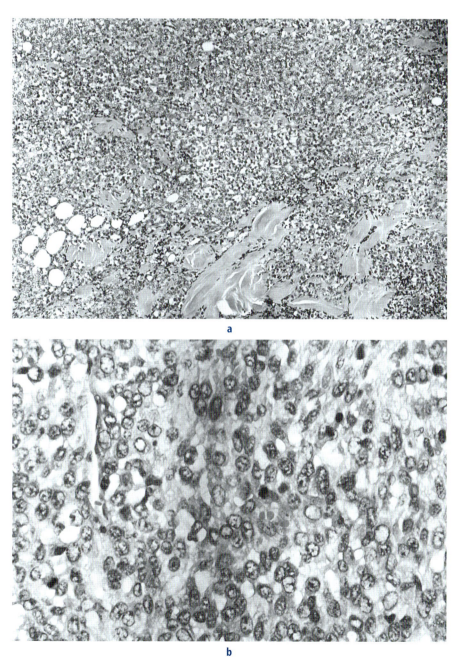

Figure 42.27 Malignant myoepithelioma **a** Low-power view of atypical myoepithelial cells and infiltration into connective tissue. **b** Higher power showing atypical myoepithelial cells, some epithelioid and some elongated, and some mitotic figures

clear cell carcinomas have an immunoprofile compatible with myoepithelial differentiation, e.g. positive immunoreactivity for cytokeratins, S-100 and smooth muscle actin. Vimentin may also be positive, and patchy positivity for GFAP, particularly in myxoid areas, can be seen.

Therapy and Prognosis

The study by Di Palma and Guzzi[39] indicates that malignant myoepithelioma is a low-grade malignancy when it arises from a pleomorphic adenoma, but more aggressive and having a higher metastatic potential when it arises de novo. Hence further studies including long-term follow-up are necessary to clarify the biological behaviour of this tumour. Taking the statement of Di Palma and Guzzi[39] into account, it is necessary to re-evaluate the prevailing opinion that all carcinomas arising in pleomorphic adenomas are highly aggressive.

Adenocarcinoma

The later WHO Classification[1] is orientated to the routine work of the surgical pathologist, and useful commentaries on this classification have also been published. It contains 18 clearly identifiable entities of primary malignant epithelial salivary gland tumours, but there are still cases of adenocarcinoma that do not readily fall into any of these categories. These adenocarcinomas have often been called adenocarcinoma NOS (not otherwise specified), but here we prefer to adhere to the nomenclature proposed by WHO and not use the extra explanatory qualifier of NOS.

Adenocarcinoma is defined as a carcinoma with glandular, ductal or secretory differentiation that does not fit into any of the other categories of salivary carcinoma. Its definition thereby seems clear and the diagnosis is thus reached by exclusion of any other possible diagnosis (Fig. 42.28). However, depending on the experience of the individual pathologist with regard to the morphological appearance of the other 17 salivary epithelial malignancies, the frequency by which salivary gland adenocarcinoma is diagnosed varies. It is obvious that many of the tumours reported as adenocarcinomas in the older literature, would today be classified as any one of the many subtypes given in the WHO Classification. Also, many pathologists have applied the new terminology for a limited number of years only, and therefore it is difficult to estimate the true incidence, biological behaviour and prognosis for this group of tumours. Adenocarcinoma thus constitutes a diminishing group of salivary carcinomas, but still has a significant incidence.

Oncocytic Carcinoma

Oncocytic carcinoma is exceedingly rare and only a few cases are reported in the literature, contrary to the far more common benign salivary oncocytoma (see Chapter 41). One might question whether this

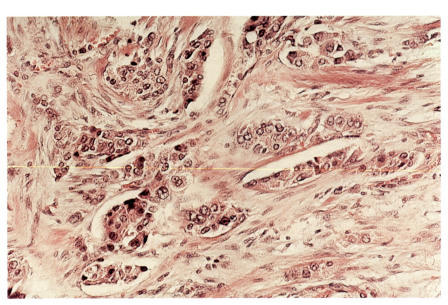

Figure 42.28 Parotid adenocarcinoma not otherwise specified showing malignant features of a glandular tumour, but not compatible with any readily classified subentity

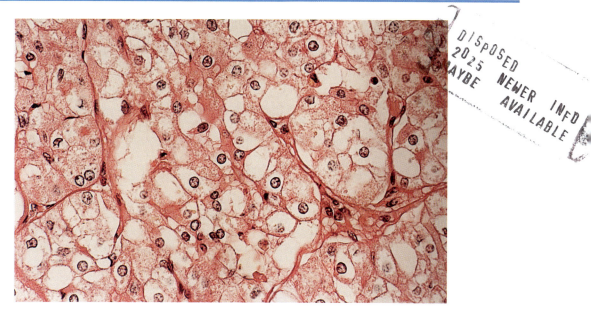

Figure 42.29 Parotid oncocytic carcinoma showing eosinophilic cells with nuclear aberrations and granular cytoplasm

lesion really represents a distinctive pathological entity, or, rather, is merely a phenotypic pattern that is shared with tumours with diverse lineages of differentiation.

The microscopic appearances are those of an invasive tumour consisting of rather large cells with variable shapes. The cells have an abundant eosinophilic, finely granular "oncocytic" cytoplasm. The nuclei are round to oval and variable in size, with coarsely clumped chromatin, and displaying atypia and evident nucleoli. Mitoses are not frequent and typical glandular formations are sparse (Fig. 42.29). The cells show a rather intense, finely granular immunoreactivity with anti-mitochondrial antibody, are cytokeratin and EMA positive, and may also stain positively for mucin. Neurone-specific enolase (NSE), GFAP and S-100 protein are reported to be negative.

Sebaceous Carcinoma

Sebaceous carcinoma of the salivary glands is composed of sebaceous cells of varying degrees of maturity. It is very rare, being almost exclusively found in the parotid gland, and regarded as having low-grade malignancy. The sebaceous cells display atypia and mitoses (Fig. 42.30). Sebaceous lymphadenocarcinoma is a recognised subentity of sebaceous carcinoma, and consists of a sebaceous lymphadenoma (see Chapter 41) with an adjacent carcinomatous component.[1] Sebaceous metaplasia, which occurs normally in salivary gland tissue, may also very occasionally be seen as small patches in some

tumours, and should hence be distinguished from sebaceous adenoma and sebaceous carcinoma (see Chapters 40 and 41).

Squamous Cell Carcinoma

The diagnosis of a primary salivary gland squamous cell carcinoma relies finally on clinical data. The morphology is that of a squamous cell carcinoma elsewhere in the body, and great care has to be taken to avoid confusion with metastasis from primary squamous cell carcinoma of the skin. Mucoepidermoid carcinoma with a predominant squamous component should readily be ruled out if sufficient numbers of blocks are taken from the tumour. Also several other salivary gland carcinomas may have foci of squamous metaplasia, e.g. carcinoma in pleomorphic adenoma, malignant myoepithelioma, etc.

Undifferentiated Carcinoma

Definition and Terminology

Salivary gland undifferentiated carcinoma is defined as a poorly differentiated malignant epithelial tumour, which is lacking any phenotypic expression by light microscopy by which it could be placed in any of the other carcinoma groups.[1] Undifferentiated carcinoma with lymphoid stroma is a special subtype, which is histologically indistinguishable from non-keratinising, undifferentiated nasopha-

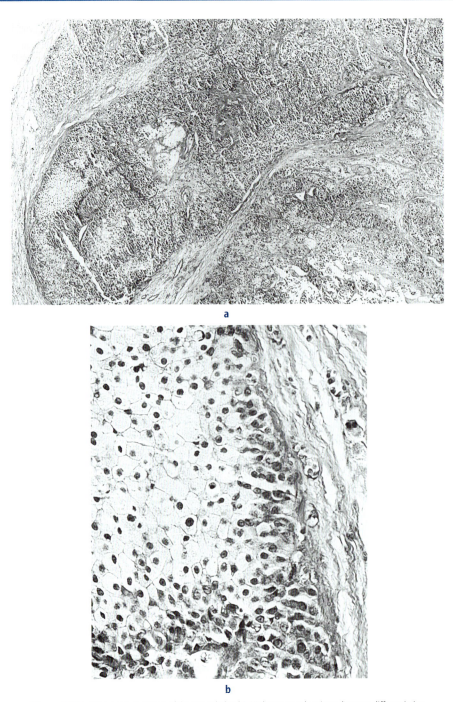

Figure 42.30 a Sebaceous carcinoma of the parotid gland. **b** Higher power showing sebaceous differentiation

ryngeal carcinoma with lymphoid stroma (lympho-epithelial carcinoma).

Site and Incidence

Undifferentiated carcinoma is rare, and since the first report in 1962, only 130–140 cases have been reported in the world literature. Some of these cases may in fact have been basal cell adenocarcinomas.[25] The incidence is highest among the Chinese, and the Inuit of Greenland and North America. The tumour is predominantly a parotid one, although on rare occasions occurring in the submandibular and minor salivary glands. The majority of tumours reported appear to be lymphoepithelial carcinoma.[41]

Histogenesis

The consistent association of Epstein-Barr virus with salivary gland lymphoepithelial carcinoma reported in the literature, suggests that the virus may play a causal role in this tumour. No such association is evident for undifferentiated carcinoma without lymphoid stroma, nor for any other salivary gland neoplasm.[41,42]

Microscopic Appearances

The tumour cells are relatively large, spheroid or spindle-shaped and are similar to those of undifferentiated carcinoma elsewhere in the body. The large spheroid cells have typical vesicular nuclei and prominent nucleoli, whilst the spindle-shaped cells may have dark, hyperchromatic cells. The tumour cells are arranged in irregularly or moderately well-defined masses, or as loosely connected cells. The tumour cells may or may not be accompanied by a lymphoid stroma.

Differential Diagnosis

The main differential diagnosis is malignant lymphoma (large cell, centroblastic, immunoblastic) but in most cases immunohistochemistry will solve the problem.

Therapy and Prognosis

The prognosis of salivary gland undifferentiated carcinoma is poor. The single most important clinicopathologic factor related to patient outcome is size of the primary tumour. In one series, all patients with carcinomas larger than 4 cm died.[43] Lymphoepithelial carcinoma is reported to have a much more favourable prognosis than undifferentiated carcinoma without lymphoid stroma.[41]

Small Cell Carcinoma

Definition and Terminology

Small cell carcinoma of salivary glands has been defined as a malignant tumour similar in histology, behaviour and histochemistry to the small cell carcinoma of the lung.[1] There are said to be two types of salivary small cell carcinoma distinguished by different immunophenotypes and different electron microsopic features. One type is immuno-reactive for neuroendocrine markers (NSE, chromogranin, synaptophysin, etc) and electron microscopy demonstrates neuroendocrine granules. The other type is a ductal variety without endocrine organelles and negative for neuroendocrine markers. However, further immunohistochemical studies have revised this concept, because most small cell carcinomas express at least one neuroendocrine marker. One may conclude that all small cell salivary gland carcinomas have neuroendocrine characteristics, even though dense core granules cannot be demonstrated in some of them ultrastructurally[44]. Hence, previous proposals that salivary gland small cell carcinomas comprise two categories, probably need to be re-evaluated.

Site and Incidence

Small cell carcinoma is very rare and only 50–60 cases have been reported. The vast majority of cases appear to be of "neuroendocrine type", and most are located in the parotid gland. Salivary small cell carcinoma has a peak incidence between 50 and 70 years of age, and a slight male predominance.

Histogenesis

The neuroendocrine-type small cell carcinoma has been thought to arise from neuroendocrine stem cells that have migrated from the neural crest to the salivary glands. Absent neuroendocrine differentiation by electron microscopy was felt to signify origin from ductal cells. Ultrastructural and light microscopic studies have shown glandular and squamous differentiation in cases with neuroendocrine differentiation. Demonstration of bidirectional neuroendocrine and squamous differentiation in salivary small cell carcinomas supports a hypothesis of a single multipotent stem cell rather than migrated neuroendocrine stem cells.

Microscopic Appearances

The histology is very similar to that of small cell carcinoma of the lung. The tumour thus consists of small, oval tumour cells with hyperchromatic nuclei and minimal cytoplasm. There may be areas with ductal structures, and also occasionally squamous differentiation. At least two neuroendocrine markers of the following list should be positive: NSE, synaptophysin, chromogranin, Phe 5, PGP 9.5 or Leu 7.

Regardless of site and morphological subtype of salivary small cell carcinoma, the possibility of metastasis from small cell of the lung has first to be excluded. Metastasis or involvement from a skin Merkel cell carcinoma has also to be considered. Merkel cell carcinoma displays consistently positivity for cytokeratin 20, and very often shows a punctate staining pattern. However, salivary gland small cell carcinoma may also occasionally express cytokeratin 20.[45] Other small round cell tumours, e.g. peripheral neuroectodermal tumours and extraskeletal Ewing's sarcoma, and malignant lymphoma, can usually be distinguished by their immunophenotype (positive MIC-2 and leucocyte markers, respectively), by electron microscopy or by genetic analysis. Basaloid squamous cell carcinoma and solid adenoid cystic carcinoma may sometimes constitute a differential diagnostic alternative.

Therapy and Prognosis

The prognosis is poor, currently with survival at 5 years of 30%, although this is better than the prognosis for other sites, with survival over 2 years being unusual. The cytokeratin 20 positivity observed in some salivary gland small cell carcinomas may suggest that they may be more closely related biologically to Merkel cell carcinoma than to pulmonary-type small cell carcinoma. This may explain why they are less aggressive than other small cell carcinomas.[45]

Familial Low-Grade Neuroendocrine Carcinoma

This tumour entity has only very recently been described, comprising a family living on the Isle of Man. Four sibs in a family, two brothers and two sisters, presented with low-grade malignant tumours of the submandibular gland in three cases, and in the minor salivary glands of the nasal cavities and maxillary sinuses in one.[46] Cervical neck node metastases have developed in all four cases; bloodstream metastases have developed in two. All four patients are still alive.

Microscopic Appearances

The tumours displayed medium-sized, rather regular cells. The cells were arranged in a loose manner, and dispersed among these cells, ductal structures were readily identifiable. Also, myoepithelial cells were found around the ductal elements (Fig. 42.31). Thus these tumours did not display the normal features of a salivary gland small cell neuroendocrine carcinoma, but rather those of a neuroendocrine carcinoma of the respiratory tract. All tumours contained numerous Grimelius-positive cells, and showed immunoreactivity for NSE and synaptophysin. In three of the cases electron microscopy was carried

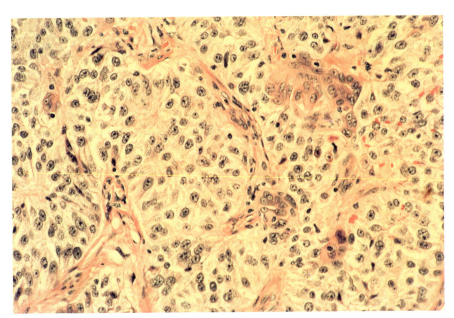

Figure 42.31 Familial low-grade neuroendocrine carcinoma showing loose collections of cells, having a neuroendocrine immunoprofile, and ducts with myoepithelial cells

out, and dense-cored, neurosecretory-like granules measuring 90–160 nm were detected. The distinction between low- and high-grade neuroendocrine carcinoma of the respiratory tract lies in the number of mitoses, extent of necrosis, and the MIB-1 index. In these reported four cases there were no areas of necrosis and very few mitoses.

There are several unusual features associated with this tumour. Three of the neoplasms were situated in the submandibular gland, a gland not very prone to malignancy as compared with the parotid gland. Secondly, the morphological picture of this neuro-endocrine tumour has not been described before in salivary glands, but resembles very much a low-grade, well-differentiated neuroendocrine carcinoma of the respiratory tract. Furthermore, three of the sibs and many of their children had enamel hypoplasia (amelogenesis imperfecta), and two of the four had inherited sensorineural hearing loss. Beyond any doubt these tumours represent a previously undescribed pleiotropic X-linked, or autosomal dominant syndrome of cancer. Genetic investigations are currently being carried out on blood and tissue material from this family.

References

1. Seifert G, Sobin LH. Histological typing of salivary gland tumours. WHO international histological classification of tumours, 2nd edn. Springer-Verlag, Berlin, Heidelberg, New York, 1991
2. Ellis GL, Corio RL. Acinic cell adenocarcinoma. A clinico-pathologic analysis of 294 cases. Cancer 1983;52:542–549
3. Eveson JW, Cawson RA. Salivary gland tumours. A review of 2410 cases with particular reference to histological types, site, age and sex distribution. J Pathol 1985;146:51–58
4. Spiro RH. Salivary neoplasms: overview of a 35-year experience with 2,807 patients. Head Neck Surg 1986;8:177–184
5. Waldron CA, El-Mofty SK, Gnepp DR. Tumours of the intra-oral minor salivary glands: a demographic and histologic study of 426 cases. Oral Surg Oral Med Oral Pathol 1988;66:323–333
6. Michal M, Skálová A, Simpson RH et al. Well-differentiated acinic cell carcinoma of salivary glands associated with lymphoid stroma. Hum Pathol 1997;28:595–600
7. Skálová A, Leivo I, von Boguslawsky K et al. Cell proliferation correlates with prognosis in acinic cell carcinomas of salivary gland origin. Immunohistochemical study of 30 cases using the MIB 1 antibody in formalin-fixed paraffin sections. J Pathol 1994;173:13–21
8. Hellquist HB, Sundelin K, Di Bacco A et al. Tumour growth fraction and apoptosis in salivary gland acinic cell carcinomas. Prognostic implications of Ki-67 and bcl-2 expression and of in situ end labelling (TUNEL). J Pathol 1997;181:323–329
9. Batsakis JG. Tumours of the head and neck. Clinical and pathological considerations, 2nd edn. Williams & Wilkins, Baltimore, London, 1979
10. Ellis GL, Auclair PL, Gnepp GR (eds) Surgical pathology of the salivary glands. Major problems in pathology, vol 25. W.B. Saunders Company, Philadelphia, London, Toronto, Montreal, Sidney, Tokyo, 1991
11. Dardick I, Byard RW, Carnegie JA. A review of the proliferative capacity of major salivary glands and the relationship to current concepts of neoplasia in salivary glands. Oral Surg Oral Med Oral Pathol 1990;69:53–67
12. Clode AL, Fonseca I, Santos JR et al. Mucoepidermoid carcinoma of the salivary glands: a reappraisal of the influence of tumour differentiation on prognosis. J Surg Oncol 1991;46:100–106
13. Batsakis JG, Luna MA. Histopathologic grading of salivary gland neoplasms: I . mucoepidermoid carcinoma. Ann Otol Rhinol Laryngol 1990;99:835–838
14. Auclair PL, Goode RK, Ellis GL. Mucoepidermoid carcinoma of intraoral salivary glands. Evaluation and application of grading criteria in 143 cases. Cancer 1992;69:2021–2030
15. Goode RK, Auclair PL, Ellis GL. Mucoepidermoid carcinoma of the major salivary glands: clinical and histopathologic analysis of 234 cases with evaluation of grading criteria. Cancer 1998;82:1217–1224
16. Cohen MB, Fisher PE, Holly EA et al. Fine needle aspiration diagnosis of mucoepidermoid carcinoma. Statistical analysis. Acta Cytol 1990;34:43–49
17. Warner Learmonth G. An atlas of cytopathology of the head and neck with clinical and histological correlations. Arnold, London, 1998
18. Jensen JO, Poulsen T, Schiødt T. Mucoepidermoid tumours of salivary glands. A long term follow-up study. APMIS 1988;96:421–426
19. Caselitz J, Schultze I, Seifert G. Adenoid cystic carcinoma of the salivary glands: an immunohistochemical study. J Oral Pathol 1986;15:308–318
20. Stenman G, Dahlenfors R, Mark J et al. Adenoid cystic carcinoma: a third type of human salivary gland neoplasm characterized cytogenetically by reciprocal translocations. Anticancer Res 1982;2:11–16
21. Chen J, Saku T, Okabe H et al. Basement membranes in adenoid cystic carcinoma. An immunohistochemical study. Cancer 1992;69:2631–2640
22. Skálová A, Simpson RH, Lehtonen H et al. Assessment of proliferative activity using the MIB1 antibody help to distinguish polymorphous low grade adenocarcinoma from adenoid cystic carcinoma of salivary glands. Pathol Res Pract 1997;193:695–703
23. Franchi A, Gallo O, Bocciolini C et al. Reduced E-cadherin expression correlates with unfavourable prognosis in adenoid cystic carcinoma of salivary glands of the oral cavity. Am J Clin Pathol 1999;111:43–50
24. Donath K, Seifert G, Schmitz R. Diagnosis and ultra-structure of the tubular carcinoma of salivary gland ducts. Epithelial-myoepithelial carcinoma of the intercalated ducts [In German]. Virchows Arch (A) 1972;356:16–31
25. Fonseca I, Soares J. Epithelial-myoepithelial carcinoma of the salivary glands. A study of 22 cases. Virchows Arch (A) 1993;422:389–396
26. Kleinsasser O, Klein HJ, Hubner G. Speichelgangcarcinome. Ein den Milchgangcarcinomen der Brustdrüse analoge Gruppe von Speicheldrüsentumore. Arch Klin Exp Ohren Nasen Kehlkopfheilk 1968;192:100–115
27. Hellquist HB, Karlsson MG, Nilsson C. Salivary duct carcinoma – a highly aggressive salivary gland tumour with overexpression of c-erbB-2. J Pathol 1994;172:35–44
28. Press MF, Pike MC, Hung G et al. Amplification and over-expression of HER-2/neu in carcinomas of the salivary gland: correlation with poor prognosis. Cancer Res 1994;54:5675–5682
29. Kapadia SB, Barnes L. Expression of androgen receptor, gross cystic disease fluid protein, and CD44 in salivary duct carcinoma. Mod Pathol 1998;11:1033–1038
30. Lewis JE, McKinney BC, Weiland LH et al. Salivary duct carcinoma. Clinicopathologic and immunohistochemical review of 26 cases. Cancer 1996;77:223–230

31. Delgado R, Klimstra D, Albores-Saavedra J. Low grade salivary duct carcinoma. A distinctive variant with a low grade histology and a predominant intraductal growth pattern. Cancer 1996;78:958–967

32. Evans HL, Batsakis JG. Polymorphous low-grade adenocarcinoma of minor salivary glands. A study of 14 cases of a distinctive neoplasm. Cancer 1984;53:935–942

33. Araújo V, Sousa S, Jaeger M et al. Characterization of the cellular component of polymorphous low-grade adenocarcinoma by immunohistochemistry and electron microscopy. Oral Oncol 1999;35:164–172

34. Frierson HF Jr, Mills SE, Garland TA. Terminal duct carcinoma of minor salivary glands. A nonpapillary subtype of polymorphous low-grade adenocarcinoma. Am J Clin Pathol 1985;84:8–14

35. Ellis GL, Wiscovitch JG. Basal cell adenocarcinomas of the major salivary glands. Oral Surg Oral Med Oral Pathol 1990;69:461–469

36. Muller S, Barnes L. Basal cell adenocarcinoma of the salivary glands. Report of seven cases and review of the literature. Cancer 1996;78:2471–2477

37. Foss RD, Ellis GL, Auclair PL. Salivary gland cystadenocarcinomas. A clinicopathologic study of 57 cases. Am J Surg Pathol 1996;20:1440–1447

38. Auclair PL, Ellis GL. Atypical features in salivary gland mixed tumours: their relationship to malignant transformation. Mod Pathol 1996;9:652–657

39. Di Palma S, Guzzo M. Malignant myoepithelioma of salivary glands: clinicopathological features of ten cases. Virchows Arch (A) 1993;423:389–396

40. Michal M, Skálová A, Simpson RHW et al. Clear cell malignant myoepithelioma of the salivary glands. Histopathology 1996;28:309–315

41. Sheen T-S, Tsai C-C, Ko J-Y et al. Undifferentiated carcinoma of the major salivary glands. Cancer 1997;80:357–363

42. Chan JK, Yip TT, Tsang WY et al. Specific association of Epstein-Barr virus with lymphoepithelial carcinoma among tumours and tumourlike lesions of the salivary gland. Arch Pathol Lab Med 1994;118:994–997

43. Hui KK, Luna MA, Batsakis JG et al. Undifferentiated carcinomas of the major salivary glands. Oral Surg Oral Med Oral Pathol 1990;69:76–83

44. Gnepp DR, Wick MR. Small cell carcinoma of the major salivary glands. An immunohistochemical study. Cancer 1990;66:185–192

45. Chan JK, Suster S, Wenig BM et al. Cytokeratin 20 immunoreactivity distinguishes Merkel cell (primary cutaneous neuroendocrine) carcinomas and salivary gland small cell carcinomas from small cell carcinomas of various sites. Am J Surg Pathol 1997;21:226–234

46. Michaels L, Lee K, Manuja SL et al. Family with low-grade neuroendocrine carcinoma of salivary glands, severe sensorineural loss, and enamel hypoplasia. Am J Med Genet 1999;83:183–186

43 Miscellaneous Neoplasms

Angiomas

Angioma, including haemangioma and lymph-angioma, is the most common benign mes-enchymal salivary gland tumour (45%), and represents about 50% of all salivary gland tumours in children, but less than 5% in adults. The age peak for angiomas is in the first and second decades of life. Only 10% of mesenchymal salivary gland tumours are sarcomas (see below). Angiosarcoma is very rare but has been described.[1]

Angiomas are most commonly found in the parotid gland region, the lesions being usually in the surrounding soft tissues rather than in the parotid glandular tissue itself. Angiomas produce a clinical swelling. Microscopy shows a vascular tumour in which the lining consists of benign endothelium without atypia, and stains positively with Factor VIII and CD31. Erythrocytes are seen in some of the vessels. The actual parotid tissue shows reactive changes of inflammation and slight fibrosis.

Hybrid Tumours

Salivary hybrid tumours are defined as being com-posed of two different tumour entities, each of which conforms to an exactly defined tumour cate-gory. These different neoplasms are not separated, but have an identical origin within the same topo-graphical area.[2] Hybrid tumours are very rare. Cases reported have shown the following combinations:

1. Basal cell adenoma and canalicular adenoma.
2. Basal cell adenoma and adenoid cystic carci-noma.
3. Salivary duct carcinoma and adenoid cystic carcinoma.
4. Adenoid cystic carcinoma and acinic cell carcinoma.
5. Adenoid cystic carcinoma and epithelial-myoepithelial carcinoma.

The prognosis is determined by the most high-grade malignant part of the hybrid tumour.

Giant Cell Tumours

Giant cell tumour is not a separate entity in the classification of salivary gland tumours, but several salivary neoplasms may have giant cells. Most giant cell reactions have been described in carcinoma ex pleomorphic adenoma, but also occur in pleo-morphic adenomas, acinic cell carcinoma and mucoepidermoid carcinoma. The giant cells have cytoplasmic vacuoles, irregularly dispersed nuclei and stain positively for CD68. Microscopy shows a foreign-body giant cell reaction or sarcomatoid osteoclast-like giant cell reaction, the latter with cells having a greater number of nuclei, often more than 20.[3]

Congenital Tumours

Congenital epithelial salivary gland tumours are exceptionally rare. The Salivary Gland Registry in Hamburg contains only three cases among a total of 6646 tumours. These cases were congenital basal cell adenomas with a morphology similar to the adult counterpart (see Chapter 41). The differential diagnosis primarily includes hamartoma, teratoma and sialoblastoma or embryoma.

Multiple Tumours

Multiple tumours of the salivary glands are not common. There are two categories. Multiple tumours with identical histology constitute the most common variety, particularly Warthin tumour and pleomorphic adenoma. Less frequently the tumours each display a different histology, and in this category Warthin tumours and pleomorphic adenomas most often are the tumour entities that show combinations with other adenomas or carcinomas of salivary gland type. In both categories the tumours can be uni- or bilateral, syn- or metachronous. The most common bilateral tumours are acinic cell carcinomas, basal cell adenomas and oncocytomas. Multiple salivary tumours should be distinguished from hybrid tumours (see above) and biphasically differentiated tumours (e.g. adenoid cystic carcinoma, epithelial-myoepithelial carcinoma, basaloid squamous cell carcinoma, etc.).

Clear Cell Tumours

Clear cell tumours of salivary gland origin are almost invariably malignant. There are, however, a few benign lesions that can have a significant proportion of clear cells, namely pleomorphic adenoma, myoepithelioma, oncocytoma, sebaceous adenoma and oncocytic hyperplasia. Metastatic carcinoma always has to be considered in the differential diagnosis, and in particular primary renal and thyroid carcinoma, but also malignant melanoma. In general, most salivary gland tumours can be diagnosed on routine haematoxylin and eosin stains, but clear cell tumours are an exception, and often require immunohistochemistry, special stains or electron microscopy.

Definition and Terminology

Clear cell tumour, or carcinoma, is not a diagnostic category, but a description of one or several salivary gland neoplasms or tumour-like lesions characterised by a significant population of cells possessing clear cytoplasm.[4] There are carcinomas that usually are not characterised by clear cells, but with rare clear cell variants, e.g. acinic cell carcinoma and mucoepidermoid carcinoma. On the other hand, there are salivary carcinomas that usually are characterised by clear cells, and these can be either monomorphic or dimorphic. Epithelial-myoepithelial carcinoma is an example of the dimorphic type (see Chapter 42). Monomorphic clear cell carcinomas are either epithelial (hyalinising clear cell carcinoma) or myoepithelial (clear cell malignant myoepithelioma). The term hyalinising clear cell carcinoma gained wider recognition first in 1996,[4] although it had been described earlier. Approximately 80 cases had been described in the literature before that date, most of them as case reports, but larger series have also been published.

Site and Incidence

Hyalinising clear cell carcinomas show low-grade malignancy and are most commonly situated in the minor salivary glands. Approximately one-third of tumours are found in the major salivary glands, particularly the parotid gland, but cases are also reported in the submandibular and sublingual glands. There is a female predominance. Intraosseous hyalinising clear cell carcinoma of the jaws has been described, and constitutes an important differential diagnosis to various odontogenic clear cell tumours.

Histogenesis

Ultrastructural studies indicate that the tumour cells are undifferentiated duct cells with few organelles and inclusion of glycogen granules.[4]

Microscopic Appearances

Hyalinising clear cell carcinoma is composed of polygonal, clear cells that are arranged in solid sheets and trabecular formations. The tumour cells are typically separated by a hyalinised stroma, which often form dense, desmoplastic collagen bands. The cells are rich in glycogen, and stain positively for cytokeratins and epithelial membrane antigen. The tumour cells are negative for S-100, alpha smooth muscle actin, and also mucin negative. Carcinoembryonic antigen is occasionally positive. The cells are relatively large, and have small to medium-sized, irregular nuclei. Mitoses are sparse.

A small number of similar clear cell tumours have been described, which are S-100 and alpha smooth muscle actin positive, contrary to the negativity found in typical hyalinising clear cell carcinoma. These tumours appear to arise primarily in the major salivary glands, and are considered to be in the category of clear cell malignant myoepithelioma.

Malignant Lymphoma

Lymphomas of the upper respiratory tract are most commonly found in Waldeyer's ring, and the general opinion is that lymphomas arising here should be considered as "nodal". Only some 5% of lymphomas of Waldeyer's ring are low-grade B-cell lymphoma of mucosa-associated lymphoid tissue type (see Chapter 22). Next to Waldeyer's ring, the salivary glands are the most common site for lymphomas, followed in incidence by the sinonasal tract. Approximately 40% of all malignant lymphomas of the head and neck occur in the salivary glands, and 5% of all extranodal lymphomas affect the salivary glands. Salivary gland lymphoma may be part of systemic spread of the disease, or the only manifestation of the disease. To accept a salivary gland lymphoma as primary the following criteria should be fulfilled:

1. No palpable superficial lymphadenopathy at presentation.
2. Normal white cell count.
3. No enlargement of mediastinal lymph nodes (by X-ray), or other lymph nodes, gut, liver or spleen.

The lymphoid tissue of salivary glands can be considered as part of the mucosa-associated lymphoid tissue (MALT). The salivary lymphoid tissue thus consists of diffusely distributed lymphocytes (and plasma cells) in the glandular parenchyma, intraepithelial lymphocytes and intra- and periglandular lymph nodes.

Salivary gland malignant lymphoma is very often associated with chronic immunosialadenitis, e.g. Sjögren's syndrome (see Chapter 40). Non-Hodgkin lymphomas constitute the vast majority of salivary gland lymphomas (85%), most of which are well differentiated (centrocytic-centroblastic lymphoma, immunocytoma, etc.). A substantial number of salivary gland lymphomas are low-grade B-cell lymphoma of MALT type,[5] and among the Hodgkin lymphomas, the nodular-sclerosing type is one of the most common. The salivary gland lymphomas should thus be classified as in lymphoid tissue elsewhere in the body, and a detailed description of their morphologies can be found elsewhere.

Secondary Carcinoma

The large majority of metastases to the salivary glands are from squamous cell carcinomas of the skin of the head and neck, but metastases from malignant melanoma are not infrequent. More rarely metastases occur from nasopharyngeal carcinomas and thyroid carcinomas. Most of the metastases are localised in the parotid gland, of which 60% are in the intra- and periglandular lymph nodes and the rest in the glandular parenchyma. Haematogenous spread to the salivary glands is uncommon but does occur, and then mainly as deposits from carcinomas in the breast, lung and kidney.

Non-Epithelial Tumours

Non-epithelial tumours of the salivary glands are classified according to the World Health Organization histological classification of soft tissue tumours.[1] The vast majority of non-epithelial tumours (90%) are benign; angiomas, lipomas and neural tumours being the most common. Malignant fibrous histiocytoma, malignant schwannoma and rhabdomyosarcoma are most frequent among the salivary gland sarcomas.[1]

References

1. Seifert G, Sobin LH. Histological typing of salivary gland tumours. WHO international histological classification of tumours, 2nd edn. Springer-Verlag, Berlin, Heidelberg, New York, 1991
2. Seifert G, Donath K. Hybrid tumours of salivary glands. Definition and classification of five rare cases. Eur J Cancer B Oral Oncol 1996;32B:251–259
3. Donath K, Seifert G, Roser K. The spectrum of giant cells in tumours of the salivary glands: an analysis of 11 cases. J Oral Pathol Med 1997;26:431–436
4. Seifert G, Donath K. Das hyalinisierende hellzellige Karzinom der Speicheldrüsen [In German]. Pathologie 1996;17:110–115
5. Isaacson PG. The MALT lymphoma concept. Updated Annals Oncol 1995;6:319–320

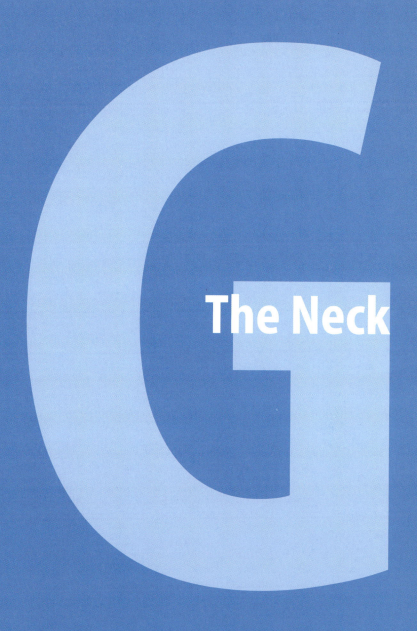

The Neck

44 Cervical Lymph Nodes

In this chapter an account of the histopathology of cervical lymph nodes is provided in respect of the role of the pathologist in the examination of neck dissection specimens from patients with cancer of the head and neck. The diagnostic pathology of other lymph node lesions such as malignant lymphoma is beyond the scope of this work.

Neck Dissection Specimens

Anatomy of Cervical Lymph Nodes

Carcinomas from many of the organs of the head and neck metastasise to the cervical lymph nodes. An important part of the surgical treatment of head and neck cancer is to remove en-bloc, affected and possibly affected cervical lymph nodes, a procedure referred to as radical neck dissection. Techniques aimed at reducing tissue loss by confining removal of cervical lymph to those at risk have been introduced over the past 30 years and are now common in head and neck surgical practice. It is important for the pathologist to have some knowledge of the modern terminology for cervical lymph node groups and of those that are removed in the standard operations, in order to carry out histopathological examination in the most useful fashion.

The lymph nodes removed by the radical neck dissection operation have been grouped into levels as follows.[1]

Level I

Submental

These comprise those lymph nodes that are within the triangular boundary of the anterior belly of digastric muscles on both sides and the hyoid bone, and this level is therefore central, not separate on left and right (Fig. 44.1).

Submandibular

This bilateral level is within the boundaries of the anterior and posterior bellies of the digastric muscle and the body of mandible. It includes the submandibular salivary gland specimen.

Level II

Upper Jugular Group: Upper Third of Internal Jugular Vein and Adjacent Accessory Nerve

This level extends from the carotid artery bifurcation or hyoid bone up to the skull base. Posteriorly it is bounded by the posterior border of the sternocleidomastoid and anteriorly by the lateral border of the sternohyoid muscle.

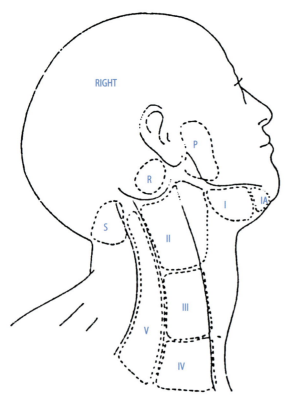

Figure 44.1 Levels of cervical lymph node groups on the right side of the neck except for level 1A, which is a midline structure. *P*, parotid preauricular group. *R*, retroauricular group. *S*, suboccipital group

Level III

Middle Jugular Group: Middle Third of Internal Jugular Vein

This level extends from the carotid bifurcation down to the omohyoid muscle or cricothyroid notch. Posteriorly it is bounded by the posterior border of the sternocleidomastoid and anteriorly by the lateral border of the sternohyoid muscle.

Level IV

Lower Jugular Group: Lower Third of Internal Jugular Vein

This level extends from the omohyoid muscle above to the clavicle below. Posteriorly it is bounded by the posterior border of the sternocleidomastoid muscle and anteriorly by the lateral border of the sternohyoid muscle.

Level V

Posterior Triangle Group: Along Lower Half Accessory Nerve and Transverse Cervical Artery – Also Includes Supraclavicular Nodes

This level extends posteriorly from the anterior border of the trapezius muscle to anteriorly the posterior border of sternocleidomastoid muscle.

The system of lymph node levels also separately identifies: P, parotid preauricular lymph nodes; R, the retroauricular lymph nodes; and S, the suboccipital lymph nodes (Fig. 44.1).

Classification of Neck Dissection Operations

Radical Neck Dissection

All lymph nodes from levels I through V are removed by the radical neck dissection operation. The following non-lymph node structures are also extirpated: accessory nerve, internal jugular vein and sternocleidomastoid muscle. Other lymph node groups in the neck are not removed.

Modified Radical Neck Dissection

This comprises the removal of all the lymph node groups routinely removed by radical neck dissection, but with preservation of one or more of the following structures normally removed at radical neck dissection: accessory nerve, internal jugular vein and sternocleidomastoid muscle.

Selective Neck Dissection

This operation entails the preservation of one or more lymph node groups that are normally removed at radical dissection:

1. Supraomohyoid neck dissection: removal of levels I, II and III only. The sternocleidomastoid muscle is removed with the specimen.
2. Posterolateral neck dissection: removal of levels II, III, IV and V and also the suboccipital and retroauricular lymph nodes.
3. Lateral neck dissection: removal of levels II, III and IV.
4. Anterior compartment neck dissection (used for thyroid gland cancer operations): removal of pretracheal, perithyroidal and precricoid (Delphian) lymph nodes.

Extended Radical Neck Dissection

Any of the above neck dissections can be extended to remove either further lymph node groups or vascular, neural or muscular structures that are not routinely removed in a neck dissection.

Gross Examination of Neck Dissection Specimens

It is good practice to pin out the neck dissection specimen on a cork board before fixation in order to preserve the anatomical relationships. If the specimen is one obtained at radical neck dissection, the submandibular salivary gland, sternomastoid muscle and internal jugular vein are present and these structures can be used as landmarks to identify the five lymph node levels. If some of these landmarks have not been excised, the lymph node levels may need identification by one of the surgical team. Boundaries of individual levels can be demarcated with India ink in the specimen before isolating individual nodes.

The lymph nodes are best identified by palpation in the adipose tissue followed by incision into each node that requires confirmation using a scalpel with a new blade. The mean numbers of lymph nodes that were found at each cervical lymph node level in 20 cadavers[2] are shown in Table 44.1. A mean total number of lymph nodes, amounting to 25 nodes, was found in these cadavers, who did not have head and neck neoplasms. It has been observed that the necks of patients who do have head and neck cancer may yield higher numbers than those, probably because of hypertrophy of minute, previously grossly undetectable, lymph nodes as a result of the immunological reaction to the cancer. Thus, in a study of radical neck dissections from 50 patients with advanced squamous carcinoma of the head and neck, up to 60 lymph nodes were identified per specimen, in spite of the fact that the carcinoma had been irradiated in each case.

Masses found in the dissection specimen to be larger than 3 cm are usually confluent lymph nodes.

Lymph nodes are sectioned wherever possible in their long axis to obtain the maximum area of the cut surface into the section. After embedding, ribbons are cut and mounted in step sections at three levels of the lymph node to obtain the maximum coverage in the search for carcinomatous metastases. The use of molecular techniques to detect p53 gene mutations has resulted in a yield of 21% more nodes positive for carcinoma in neck dissections that were previously negative for neoplasm,[3] but use of immunohistochemistry for detection of metastases has not yielded an increase of malignancy over the levels provided by routine histology.[4]

Sites of Origin of Metastatic Cervical Lymph Nodes

The primary sites of origin for metastases derived from head and neck cancers are listed in Table 44.2. It will be noticed that a frequent primary source is undifferentiated carcinoma of the nasopharynx. The origin of such metastases can frequently be suspected from the histological appearance of the neoplasm in the lymph node (see Chapter 24). On some occasions the metastatic tumour will have the appearance of a cyst filled with keratin and surrounded by lymphoid tissue. The lesion may be identified as a malignant transformation of a branchial cleft cyst. We believe that such a transformation does not occur and that the cystic change has occurred in a metastatic carcinoma in the lymph node (see Chapter 45). Such cystic stratified squamous carcinomatous metastases may not have a clinically obvious primary source. Under these circumstances the palatine tonsil is often the origin, a diagnosis that can be confirmed only by direct biopsy of the tonsil itself.

Table 44.1. Average lymph node numbers at the different levels, counted in 20 cadavers[2]

Level	Lymph nodes
I	2
II	7
III	5
IV	8
V	2
Total	24

Table 44.2. Malignant tumours metastatic to cervical lymph nodes

Frequent
Undifferentiated carcinoma of nasopharynx
Hypopharyngeal carcinoma
Laryngeal carcinoma
Oral carcinoma
Malignant melanoma
Papillary carcinoma of thyroid
Medullary carcinoma of thyroid

Occasional
Carcinoma of nose and paranasal sinuses
Carcinoma of external and middle ear
Adenoid cystic carcinoma of head and neck (only 15%)
Rhabdomyosarcoma of head and neck

Prognostic Factors in Cervical Lymph Node Metastases

Numerous studies have attested to the concept that progressive reduction in 5-year survival, increase of recurrence rate and numbers of distant metastases are enhanced by the following factors:

1. The presence of cervical lymph node metastases.
2. Multiple cervical lymph node metastases.
3. Increased size of cervical lymph node metastases.

Extracapsular Spread

Metastases first lodge in the subcapsular sinus of an affected lymph node and then spread to the body of the lymph node. When the node is filled with tumour, the latter may spread outside the capsule of the lymph node. Such extracapsular deposition of neoplasm may be detected in necks with advanced carcinoma as naked tumour masses unrelated to lymph node tissue or they may be found in relation to a lymph node from which they have been derived. The finding of extracapsular spread has often been thought to worsen the prognosis by making the neoplasm less amenable to surgical excision or by the tendency that extracapsular cancer has to involve vital structures, particularly blood vessels such as the internal jugular vein or the common carotid artery. The presence of extracapsular spread of neoplasm is thus important and should be recorded if found during the histological survey of neck dissection specimens.

In some lymph nodes invaded by cancer, extracapsular spread may occur with minimum or even no involvement of the body of the lymph node itself by growth of neoplasm from obstructed afferent lymphatic vessels.[5] This may be an explanation for the occasional finding of extranodal masses of tumour in the neck without nodal involvement. Some observers have found that the presence of extracapsular spread does not influence survival and neck recurrence of tumour[6] and may indeed be associated with improvement. Such findings may be the result of the use of combined treatment modalities that decrease the unexpected adverse local effects previously associated with extracapsular spread.

Reactive Adenopathy

The examination of large numbers of lymph nodes in neck dissection specimens will often lead to the finding of conditions other than metastasis of carcinoma within the lymph node. A list of such condi-

Table 44.3. Forms of reactive adenopathy (after Cousar et al.[8])

Reactive states in possible immunological response to malignant tumour[9]
Patterns 1–4

Reactive states with follicular hyperplasia
Rheumatoid arthritis
Sjögren's syndrome
Systemic lupus erythematosus
Histiocytic lupus erythematosus (Kikuchi–Fujimoto disease[10])
Kimura's disease
Cat-scratch disease
Toxoplasmosis
Syphilis
HIV infection
Angiofollicular hyperplasia (Castleman's disease)

Reactive states with interfollicular hyperplasia
Dermatopathic lymphadenopathy
Sinus histiocytosis with massive lymphadenopathy (Rosai-Dorfmann)
Drug reactions (especially to phenytoin)
Sarcoidosis
Lymph node infarction
Inflammatory pseudotumour
Mycobacterial spindle cell pseudotumour
Vascular transformation of lymph node sinuses
Bacillary angiomatosis (*Bartonella henselae* and *quintana*)

tions is provided in Table 44.3. Changes have been described that are regarded as reaction states in possible immunological response to the malignant tumour. Four reaction patterns have been described.[7] Pattern 1 is one of T cell predominance. The outer cortex shows follicles without germinal centres, there are increased numbers of lymphocytes throughout the cortical and medullary regions, reticular cells are prominent, as are endothelial cells in capillaries and postcapillary venules. Pattern 2 reflects activation of the humoral immune responses. There is marked hyperplasia of lymphatic follicles and germinal centres rich in large lymphoid cells. Medullary cords are enlarged and contain numerous plasma cells and plasmablasts. Pattern 3 is an unstimulated lymph node, sometimes partly replaced by adipose tissue, with no germinal centres, hypocellular cortex, unremarkable medullary cords and prominent medullary sinuses. Pattern 4 is one of lymphocytic depletion with decreased numbers of lymphocytes and absent germinal centres. There is some evidence that patients with cervical lymph nodes showing patterns 1 and 2 may have a better prognosis than patients with pattern 4, regardless of the presence or absence of metastases in the lymph nodes.

References

1. Robbins KT, Medina JE, Wolfe GT et al. Standardizing neck dissection terminology. Official report of the Academy's Committee for Head Neck Surgery and Oncology. Arch Otolaryngol Head Neck Surg 1991;117:601–605

2. Friedman M, Lim JW, Dickey W et al. Quantification of lymph nodes in selective neck dissection. Laryngoscope 1999;109:368–370

3. Brennan JA, Mao L, Hruban RH et al. Molecular assessment of histopathological staging in squamous-cell carcinoma of the head and neck. N Engl J Med 1995;332:429–435

4. Ambrosch P, Kron M, Fischer G et al. Micrometastases in carcinoma of the upper aerodigestive tract: detection, risk of metastasizing, and prognostic value of depth of invasion. Head Neck 1995;17:473–479

5. Toker C. Some observations on the deposition of metastatic carcinoma within cervical lymph nodes. Cancer 1963; 16:364–374

6. Pinsolle J, Pinsolle V, Majoufre C et al. Prognostic value of histologic findings in neck dissections for squamous cell carcinoma. Arch Otolaryngol Head Neck Surg 1997;123:145–148

7. Pohris E, Eichhorn T, Glanz H et al. Immunohistological reaction patterns of cervical lymph nodes in patients with laryngeal carcinomas. Arch Otorhinolaryngol 1987;244: 278–283

8. Cousar JB, Casey TT, Mason WR et al. Chapter 17. Lymph nodes. In: Diagnostic surgical pathology, 3rd edn. Lippincott Williams & Wilkins, Philadelphia, 1999, pp 709–777

9. Klimek T, Glanz H, Dreyer T. Histomorphologic characteristics of non-metastatic lymph nodes in patients with head and neck cancers according to their site in the neck. Acta Otolaryngol (Stockh) 1996;116:336–340

10. Kuo T-T. Kikuchi's disease (histiocytic necrotizing lymphadenitis): a clinicopathologic study of 79 cases with an analysis of histologic subtypes, immunohistology and DNA ploidy. Am J Surg Pathol 1995;19:798–809

45 Infections and Cysts

Actinomycosis

Actinomycosis is an infection caused by an anaerobic bacterium, *Actinomyces* sp., composed of thin branching fibres, akin to the hyphae of fungi, but much thinner in width. It is a commensal in the mouth and palatine tonsil. In the latter it may be seen normally as large Gram-positive masses of hyphae within the crypts, without any apparent pathological reaction apart from a few attached neutrophils. The commonest location for active infection by the organism is the immediate site of lymphatic drainage of the above, the anterior triangle of the neck, where the infection is manifested as an inflamed swelling with sinuses. Diagnosis is made by detection and microscopy of sulphur granules in the pus from the sinuses, biopsy of the lesion or prolonged anaerobic culture for the organism (see Chapter 30).

Cysts

Branchial Cleft Cyst

Incidence

Branchial cleft cysts occur equally in the sexes and may be found at any age between early infancy and 78 years.[1]

Clinical Features

Branchial cleft cyst masses are found in the upper lateral part of the neck as a fluctuant subcutaneous mass at the anterior border of the sternocleidomastoid muscle in its upper one third. When resected surgically the posterior segment of the cyst is deep to the anterior border of the sternocleidomastoid muscle. The tract derived from the cyst passes superolateral to the common carotid artery and the ninth and twelfth cranial nerves, ending near the middle constrictor muscle or at the tonsillar fossa, which it reaches by running between the internal and external carotid arteries. Occasionally branchial cleft cysts may be bilateral.

Gross Appearances

The branchial cleft cyst is unilocular with a thin capsule. The contents may be thick and mucoid or greasy yellow material.

Microscopic Appearances

Regauer et al.[1] made a study of 97 lateral neck cysts at different ages. The epithelial lined cyst is surrounded by lymphoid tissue and a thin fibrous pseudocapsule. The epithelium is of respiratory type in children under 4 years of age and the lymphoid tissue is scanty without secondary follicles. In adolescents the respiratory epithelial lining alternates with multilayered pseudostratified epithelium containing lymphocytes and Langerhans cells, and the lymphoid tissue has hyperplastic secondary follicles oriented towards the epithelial lining. In adults the epithelial lining is mostly stratified squamous with some areas of heaped-up pseudostratified epithelium and very scanty respiratory epithelium (Fig. 45.1). The respiratory epithelium is essentially

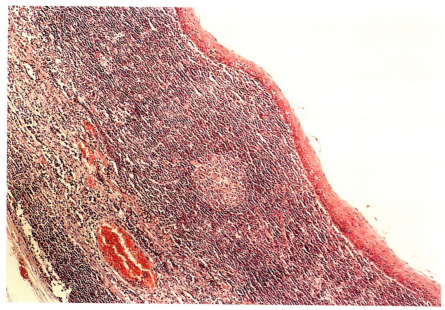

Figure 45.1 Branchial cleft cyst in an adult, showing a covering of stratified squamous epithelium and underlying lymphoid tissue with a secondary follicle

CK 18 positive, but CK 14 negative; with the development of multilayered and stratified squamous epithelium the latter becomes essentially CK 14 positive, but CK 18 negative. The submucosa becomes scarred and lymphoid tissue disappears altogether. Regauer et al. maintain that these changes occur in branchial cysts with developing age, the stratification and epidermoid change and lymphoid hyperplasia resulting from postnatal immunological stimulation.[1]

Development

Similar changes to those seen in branchial cleft cysts at different ages are observed in the palatine tonsil (see Chapter 26). Regauer et al. argue that, like the latter, the branchial cleft cyst develops from the second branchial pouch.[1]

An external sinus may be present rather than a deeper branchial cleft cyst. This presumably represents the opening of an non-obliterated branchial cleft and is usually seen in the lower one-third of the neck along the anterior border of the sternocleidomastoid muscle.

Carcinoma arising from Branchial Cleft Cyst

Cases are seen in which solitary cystic lesions with the histological appearance of squamous cell carcinoma are present in the neck with an accompanying strong lymphocytic infiltration. The absence of a primary source for the carcinoma in these patients has prompted the suggestion that these are branchial cleft cysts that have become malignant. Compagno and Hyams, from the Armed Forces Institute of Pathology, studied 22 of such cases and found that on detailed follow-up investigation, primary sources for the carcinoma were, in fact, discovered in 19.[2] Most of these were in the Waldeyer's ring region, but in some the primary was in the lung, larynx, thyroid and a major salivary gland. The suspicion that such solitary neck neoplasms are most likely to be metastases has, since that investigation, prompted a meticulous search for a primary in many of such cases, using modern methods of investigation including ultrasound, magnetic nuclear resonance and computerised tomography and even extensive biopsies of base of tongue, nasopharynx and tonsillectomy. In virtually every case a primary has been found.

A further study from the Armed Forces Institute of Pathology by Thompson and Heffner, involving 136 cases of predominantly cystic squamous carcinoma metastatic to jugulodigastric lymph nodes without an obvious primary site of origin at initial diagnosis, has cast more doubt on the branchiogenic origin of cystic cervical carcinoma.[3] It also provides useful information on the identification of the primary site of origin of the cystic lymph node metastases in relation to their histological appearance in the biopsy. Follow-up of the these cases revealed that in 87 (63%) the primary growth was at the base of tongue, the lingual or the faucial (palatine) tonsil. The other cases were derived from the nasopharynx, larynx, palate, palate or sinuses; in 27 cases the primary source of the neoplasm was not identified. Almost all the cases originating from the base of tongue, the lingual or the faucial (palatine) tonsil had a similar histopathological appearance of the cervical metastases with five characteristics:

1. The presence of large cysts as opposed to small or comedo-like cysts.

2. Largely cystic composition of the metastatic deposit, with only focal areas of solid growth.

3. Cysts lined by a single epithelial row of tumour cells with a uniform thickness throughout the cyst, except for occasional endophytic or irregular papillary exophytic proliferations.

4. Lining epithelium shows no surface maturation, and little or no keratinisation (Fig. 45.2).

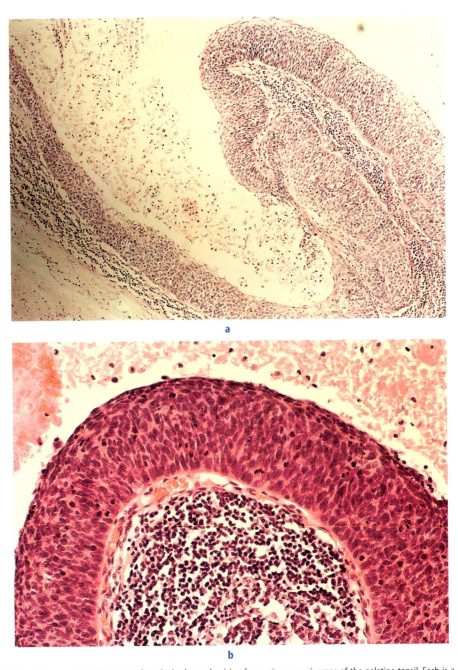

Figure 45.2 Cyst lining in two cystic carcinomatous deposits in the neck arising from primary carcinomas of the palatine tonsil. Each is a non-keratinising epithelium. Mitotic activity is present in **b**. Note underlying lymphoid tissue derived from lymph node in which this is a metastatic deposit

5. Degree of atypical change of the tumour epithelium mild and similar to that of the normal tonsillar crypt epithelium; mitotic activity is variable.

The authors indeed suggested that neoplasm arises from tonsillar crypt epithelium, which is closely associated with lymphocytes and dendritic reticulum cells (see Chapter 26). Those metastases that arose from areas outside Waldeyer's ring showed either much more keratinisation and many mitoses or a "lymphoepitheliomatous" appearance with syncytial sheets of tumour cells, large vesicular nuclei and prominent nucleoli characteristic of an origin from the nasopharynx (see Chapter 25). It seemed unlikely that there was such an entity as branchiogenic carcinoma.

Thymic Cysts

The thymus gland is derived from the third pharyngeal pouch at the sixth week of fetal life and descends into the thorax by the ninth week in relation to the pericardium. The persistence of a connection to the third pharyngeal pouch in the neck may account for cervical thymic cysts and remnants. These lesions may be found midline or anterior to the sternocleidomastoid muscle, where they may resemble a branchial cleft cyst. They may be connected to the thymus gland in the thorax or may communicate with the pharynx through an epithelial-lined tract.

Thymic cysts in the neck are usually unilocular with a thin fibrous wall and a lining of flattened squamous epithelium. Lymphoid tissue and Hassall's corpuscles are found in the wall of the cyst. Thymus remnants present as nodules in the lower neck at surgery. They are composed of fibrous tissue, lymphoid tissue and Hassall's corpuscles (Fig. 45.3).

Thyroglossal Duct Cyst

The most common congenital neck mass is the thyroglossal duct cyst. This presents in the midline along the path of embryological descent of the thyroid from the foramen cecum in the tongue usually through the hyoid bone to its final location. Thyroid tissue anywhere along the path has the potential for developing into a cyst (Fig. 45.4).

The presentation is that of a midline mass, usually in a child, but occasionally in an adult, measuring between 2 and 4 cm. It can be seen to elevate on tongue protrusion.

The lesion is treated by excision of the mass together with the midportion of the hyoid bone, after identifying the proportion of thyroid tissue within the lesion by a radioisotope technique.

The mass is composed of a collapsed cyst lined by columnar epithelium. In the fibrous tissue adjacent to the cyst small glands are usually evident. These frequently contain thyroid colloid. The fragment of hyoid bone should be decalcified and sectioned so as to seek thyroglossal duct tissue, which in some cases can be found within it (Fig. 45.5). This finding

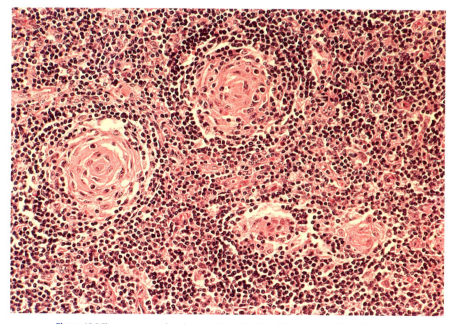

Figure 45.3 Thymus remnant from lower neck showing Hassall's corpuscles and lymphoid tissue

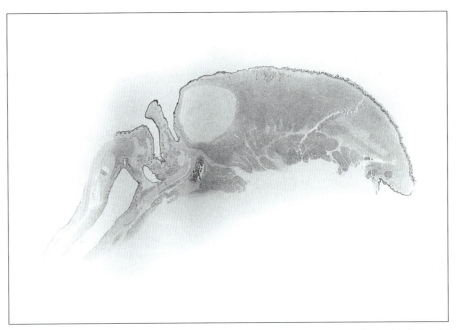

Figure 45.4 Autopsy specimen of coronal section through tongue and larynx showing a large thyroglossal duct cyst, filled with colloid, at the back of tongue. The patient was a 10-day-old baby who died suddenly of suffocation after having difficulty in swallowing and breathing since birth

explains the reduction in the numbers of cases in which recurrence of the cyst after surgery takes place when central hyoid bone is surgically removed with the mass.

Malignant change associated with a thyroglossal duct cyst is exceedingly rare.

Bronchogenic Cyst

Bronchogenic cyst is a benign congenital developmental abnormality of the embryonic foregut.[4] The most common extrapulmonary location of this lesion is the mediastinum but it is sometimes

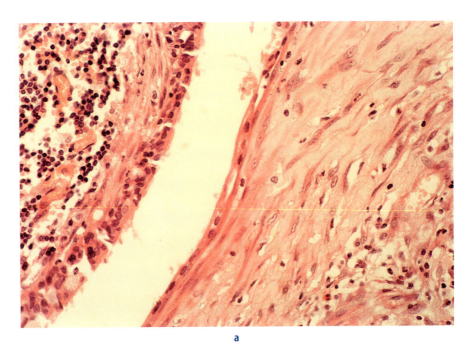

a

Figure 45.5 Thyroglossal duct cyst of neck. **a** Lining of cystic tumour composed both of stratified squamous epithelium and ciliated columnar. **b** Colloid follicles in the wall of the cyst. **c** Thyroglossal duct in midportion of the hyoid bone

(Figure 45.5 b and c, see opposite)

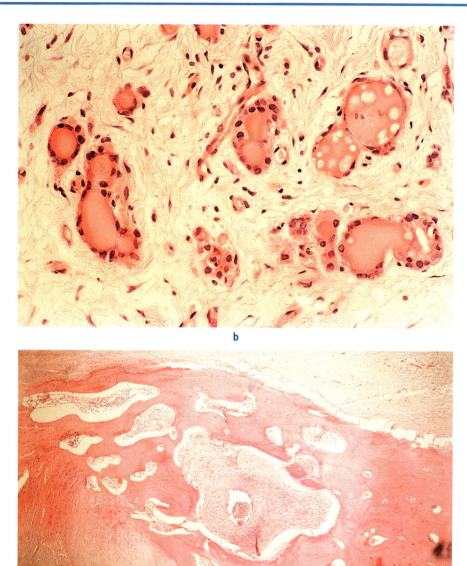

b

c

Figure 45.5 b, c

encountered in the neck, where it may be confused with a branchial cyst. The cyst is lined by ciliated pseudostratified epithelium, among which are goblet cells. In the wall of the cyst smooth muscle cells and, less frequently, cartilage may be found.

Cystic Neoplasm

Cystic hygroma

Cystic hygroma is the most common form of lymphangioma, most commonly found in the posterior cervical space. It is a congenital lesion, which typically extends into adjacent structures without respecting the fascial planes. It is usually multilocular and contains serous fluid. Microscopically it is composed of dilated lymphatic spaces surrounded by connective tissue that contains lymphocytes.

Complete excision is difficult and extirpation procedures are often followed by recurrence.

References

1. Regauer S, Gogg-Kamerer M, Braun H et al. Lateral neck cysts – the branchial theory revisited. A critical review and clinicopathological study of 97 cases with special emphasis on cytokeratin expression. APMIS 1997;105:623–630
2. Compagno J, Hyams VJ, Safavian M. Does branchiogenic carcinoma really exist? Arch Pathol Lab Med 1976;100: 311–314
3. Thompson LD, Heffner DK. The clinical importance of cystic squamous cell carcinomas in the neck: a study of 136 cases. Cancer 1998;82:944–956
4. Zvulunov A, Amichai B, Grunwald MH et al. Cutaneous bronchogenic cyst: delineation of a poorly defined lesion. Pediatr Dermatol 1998;15:277–281

Subject Index